Understanding Depression

A translational approach

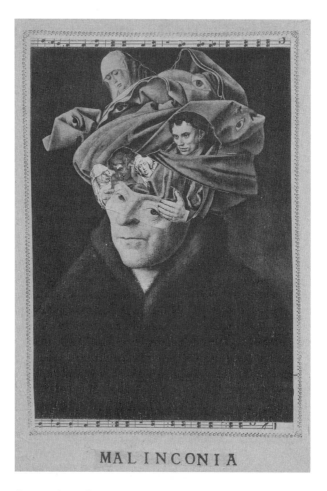

MALINCONIA

Javier Rodriguez (b. 1975). Malinconia. Commissioned for the Conference on 'Depression: Brain Causes, Body Consequences', in London, 2–3 April 2007, by Carmine M. Pariante. Text by Mathew Hurrell.

Malinconia, by Venezuelan artist Javier Rodriguez, deals with one of the most prominent mental health issues of recent times: depression. Malinconia is the Italian word for melancholy. Depression and melancholia can be viewed as one and the same thing.

The piece is a collage based on the Jan van Eyck painting Portrait of a Man with a Turban, a famous work of the Northern Renaissance. From the mouth down the picture is untouched retaining the classic Renaissance pose and stoic expression. But from the nose up the picture is a distortion: a confused jumble of images. This image of the Renaissance and all it entails – discovery, progress and a greater understanding of the universe – is juxtaposed with images of confusion and doubt, perfectly encapsulating the milieu that so often leads to melancholy: that greater knowledge leads not to greater understanding and certainty, but instead to more questions and uncertainty.

The most powerful part of the piece is the man's eyes. Slightly off-centre, they are where the face first becomes distorted. His eyes are the windows to his melancholia, their downward slant conveying his angst.

Peering from within the folds of the turban are four eyes, indicating a strong influence of the surrealist movement, who themselves were influenced by psychoanalysis.

Rodriguez's works are intricate compositions made from antique books. This mixture of old materials and modern technique perfectly encapsulates his sensibility of classic ideas in a contemporary context. Please visit http://www.javierrodriguez.co.uk to see his work.

Understanding Depression
A translational approach

Edited by

Carmine M. Pariante

Sections of Perinatal Psychiatry and Stress,
Psychiatry and Immunology (SPI-Lab),
Institute of Psychiatry,
King's College London,
London, UK

Randolph M. Nesse

Department of Psychology,
University of Michigan,
Ann Arbor,
MI, USA

David Nutt

Psychopharmacology Unit,
University of Bristol,
Bristol, UK

Lewis Wolpert

Department of Anatomy and Developmental Biology,
University College London,
London, UK

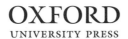
OXFORD
UNIVERSITY PRESS

OXFORD

UNIVERSITY PRESS

Great Clarendon Street, Oxford OX2 6DP

Oxford University Press is a department of the University of Oxford.
It furthers the University's objective of excellence in research, scholarship,
and education by publishing worldwide in

Oxford New York

Auckland Cape Town Dar es Salaam Hong Kong Karachi
Kuala Lumpur Madrid Melbourne Mexico City Nairobi
New Delhi Shanghai Taipei Toronto

With offices in

Argentina Austria Brazil Chile Czech Republic France Greece
Guatemala Hungary Italy Japan Poland Portugal Singapore
South Korea Switzerland Thailand Turkey Ukraine Vietnam

Oxford is a registered trade mark of Oxford University Press
in the UK and in certain other countries

Published in the United States
by Oxford University Press Inc., New York

British Library Cataloguing in Publication Data
Data available

Library of Congress Cataloging in Publication Data
Data available

Typeset in Minion
by Cepha Imaging Private Ltd., Bangalore, India
Printed in Great Britain
on acid-free paper by
The MPG Books Group

ISBN 978-0-19-953307-7 (Pbk.)

10 9 8 7 6 5 4 3 2

Oxford University Press makes no representation, express or implied, that the drug dosages in this
book are correct. Readers must therefore always check the product information and clinical procedures
with the most up-to-date published product information and data sheets provided by the manufacturers
and the most recent codes of conduct and safety regulations. The authors and the publishers do not
accept responsibility or legal liability for any errors in the text or for the misuse or misapplication of
material in this work. Except where otherwise stated, drug dosages and recommendations are for the
non-pregnant adult who is not breastfeeding.

Preface

Interdisciplinary efforts to integrate work from disparate fields is the way forward for depression research, but opportunities for experts from diverse areas to talk remain rare. In response, the editors decided to invite the world's authorities to address a few key questions that had, until now, never been addressed in the same scientific setting.

- *Why do all humans have a capacity for depression?*
- *Why has natural selection left mood regulation mechanisms so vulnerable to failure?*
- *Where is depression localised in the brain?*
- *Where is depression localised in the body?*
- *Does depression impact physical health, and, if so, what are the mechanisms?*
- *Are animal models helpful?*
- *Is bipolar depression different from unipolar depression?*
- *And, most important, how can we develop new antidepressants?*

On the 2nd and 3rd of April 2007, this conference became a reality. It not only brought together excellent speakers – and now authors of the chapters of this book – but also attracted wide attention from the scientific and the lay press. Thanks to Oxford University Press, we are delighted to be able to bring the questions – and the answers – to a much larger audience.

Carmine M. Pariante
Randolph M. Nesse
David Nutt
Lewis Wolpert

Contents

Contributors

Katherine J. Aitchison
MRC SGDP Centre, Institute of
Psychiatry at King's College London,
London, UK.

Jose Amat
Department of Psychology and
Center for Neuroscience,
University of Colorado, USA.

Michael V. Baratta
Department of Psychology and
Center for Neuroscience,
University of Colorado, USA.

Bettina Bewernick
Department of Psychiatry, University
Hospital, Bonn, Germany.

Elisabeth B. Binder
Department of Psychiatry
and Behavioral Sciences,
Emory University School of Medicine,
Atlanta, GA, USA; Department of
Human Genetics, Emory
University School of Medicine,
Atlanta, GA, USA; Max-Planck
Institute of Psychiatry,
Munich, Germany.

Sondra T. Bland
Department of Psychology and Center for
Neuroscience, University of Colorado, USA.

Nathalie Castanon
INRA, UMR 1286 PsyNuGen,
Université Victor Ségalen Bordeaux 2,
CNRS, Bordeaux, France.

Sabine Chourbaji
Central Institute of Mental Health (ZI),
Germany.

Stephan Claes
University Psychiatric Centre,
Catholic University Leuven,
Leuven, Belgium.

Antony J. Cleare
Reader in Affective Disorders,
Section of Neurobiology of Mood Disorders,
Department of Psychological Medicine,
Institute of Psychiatry at Kings College London,
London, UK.

Jason C. O'Connor
Laboratory of Integrative Immunology and
Behavior, Department of Animal
Sciences, College of Agricultural,
Environmental and Consumer Sciences,
and Department of Pathology,
College of Medicine, University of Illinois
at Urbana-Champaign, Urbana, USA.

Becky L. Conway-Campbell
Henry Wellcome Laboratories for
Integrative Neuroscience and Endocrinology,
University of Bristol,
Bristol, UK.

Philip J. Cowen
University Department of Psychiatry,
Neurosciences Building,
Warneford Hospital,
Oxford, UK.

Monica Kelly Cowles
Department of Psychiatry and
Behavioral Sciences,
Emory University School of Medicine,
Atlanta, USA.

Nick Craddock
Professor of Psychiatry,
Cardiff University, UK.

Bernard J. Crespi
Department of Biosciences, Simon Fraser
University, Burnaby, Canada.

John C. Christianson
Department of Psychology and
Center for Neuroscience,
University of Colorado, USA.

B. Czeh
Clinical Neurobiology Laboratory,
German Primate Center,
Leibniz Institute for Primate Research,
Göttingen, Germany.

A.M. van Dam
Free University Medical Center,
Department of Anatomy and
Neurosciences Amsterdam,
The Netherlands.

Robert Dantzer
Laboratory of Integrative Immunology
and Behavior, Department of Animal
Sciences, College of Agricultural,
Environmental and Consumer Sciences,
and Department of Pathology,
College of Medicine, University of Illinois
at Urbana-Champaign, Urbana, USA.

A.G. Dayer
Department of Neurosciences,
University Medical Center,
University of Geneva Medical School,
Geneva, Switzerland.

Timothy G. Dinan
Department of Psychiatry and
Alimentary Pharmabiotic Centre,
University College Cork, Ireland.

I.Nicol Ferrier
Institute of Neuroscience,
Newcastle University, Psychiatry,
Royal Victoria Infirmary,
Newcastle upon
Tyne, UK.

Peter Fitzgerald
Department of Psychiatry and Alimentary
Pharmabiotic Centre, University College
Cork, Ireland.

Sarah E. Gartside
Institute of Neuroscience, Newcastle
University, The Medical School,
Newcastle upon
Tyne, UK.

Peter Gass
Central Institute of Mental Health (ZI),
Germany.

Nicole Geschwind
Department of Psychiatry
and Neuropsychology,
South Limburg Mental Health Research
and Teaching Network, EURON,
Maastricht University, Maastricht,
The Netherlands.

Bhanu Gupta
MRC SGDP Centre, Institute of Psychiatry,
Kings College London,
London, UK.

Catherine J. Harmer
University Department of Psychiatry,
Neurosciences Building,
Warneford Hospital,
Oxford, UK.

Max Henderson
MRC Research Training Fellow,
Department of Psychological Medicine,
Institute of Psychiatry,
King's College London,
Weston Education Centre, London, UK.

Megan C. Holmes
Endocrinology Unit, University of
Edinburgh, Queen's Medical Research
Institute, Edinburgh, UK.

Matthew Hotopf
Professor of General Hospital Psychiatry,
Department of Psychological Medicine,
Institute of Psychiatry, King's College
London, Weston Education Centre,
London, UK.

Matthew T. Keener
Western Psychiatric Institute
and Clinic, School of Medicine,
University of Pittsburgh, Pittsburgh,
PA, USA.

Robert Keers
MRC SGDP Centre, Institute of Psychiatry,
Kings College London,
London, UK.

Keith W. Kelley
INRA, UMR 1286 PsyNuGen, Université
Victor Ségalen Bordeaux 2, CNRS,
Bordeaux, France.

Jacques Lestage
INRA, UMR 1286 PsyNuGen, Université
Victor Ségalen Bordeaux 2, CNRS,
Bordeaux, France.

Stafford L. Lightman
Henry Wellcome Laboratories for
Integrative Neuroscience and Endocrinology,
University of Bristol,
Bristol, UK.

Christopher A. Lowry
University of Bristol,
Psychopharmacology Unit, UK;
University of Colorado at Boulder,
Department of Integrative Physiology,
Boulder, Colorado, USA.

Paul J. Lucassen
Centre for Neuroscience,
Swammerdam Institute for Life Sciences,
University of Amsterdam,
Amsterdam, The Netherlands.

Steven F. Maier
Department of Psychology and
Center for Neuroscience,
University of Colorado, USA.

R. Hamish McAllister-Williams
Institute of Neuroscience,
Newcastle University, Psychiatry,
Leazes Wing, Royal Victoria Infirmary,
Newcastle upon Tyne, UK.

Peter McGuffin
MRC SGDP Centre, Institute of Psychiatry
at King's College London, London, UK.

P. Meerlo
Department of Molecular Neurobiology,
Center for Behavior and Neurosciences,
University of Groningen, Haren, The
Netherlands.

Andrew H. Miller
Department of Psychiatry and Behavioral
Sciences, Winship Cancer Institute, Emory
University School of Medicine, Atlanta, USA.

A.S. Naylor
Department of Physiology, Faculty of
Medicine and Health Sciences, The University
of Auckland, Auckland, New Zealand.

Charles B. Nemeroff
Department of Psychiatry and Behavioral
Sciences, Emory University School of
Medicine, Atlanta, USA.

Randolph M. Nesse
The University of Michigan, USA.

David Nutt
University of Bristol, Psychopharmacology
Unit, Bristol, UK.

Charlotte A. Oomen
Centre for Neuroscience, Swammerdam
Institute of Life Sciences, University of
Amsterdam, Amsterdam, The Netherlands.

Jim van Os
Department of Psychiatry and
Neuropsychology, South Limburg Mental
Health Research and Teaching Network,
EURON, Maastricht University, Maastricht,
The Netherlands; Division of Psychological
Medicine, Institute of Psychiatry, London, UK.

Michael J. Owen
Head of Department of Psychological
Medicine, Cardiff University, UK.

Thaddeus W.W. Pace
Department of Psychiatry and Behavioral
Sciences, Winship Cancer Institute, Emory
University School of Medicine, Atlanta, USA.

Carmine M. Pariante
Sections of Perinatal Psychiatry & Stress,
Psychiatry and Immunology (SPI-Lab),
Institute of Psychiatry, King's College
London, UK.

Frenk Peeters
Department of Psychiatry and
Neuropsychology, South Limburg Mental
Health Research and Teaching Network,
EURON, Maastricht University, Maastricht,
The Netherlands.

Mary L. Phillips
Western Psychiatric Institute and Clinic,
School of Medicine, University of Pittsburgh,
Pittsburgh, PA, USA; Department of
Psychological Medicine, Cardiff University
School of Medicine. Wales, UK.

Charles L. Raison
Department of Psychiatry and
Behavioral Sciences, Winship Cancer
Institute, Emory University School of
Medicine, Atlanta, USA.

Keith S. Reid
Institute of Neuroscience, Newcastle
University, Psychiatry, Royal Victoria
Infirmary, Newcastle upon Tyne, UK.

Robert R. Rozeske
Department of Psychology and Center for
Neuroscience, University of Colorado, USA.

Thomas E. Schlaepfer
Department of Psychiatry,
University Hospital, Bonn,
Germany.

Jonathan R. Seckl
Endocrinology Unit, University of Edinburgh,
Queen's Medical Research Institute,
Edinburgh, UK.

Daniel J. Smith
Clinical Senior Lecturer in Psychiatry,
Cardiff University, UK.

Andrew Steptoe
Department of Epidemiology and Public
Health, University College London, UK.

Brittany Thompson
Department of Psychology and
Center for Neuroscience,
University of Colorado, USA.

Rudolf Uher
MRC SGDP Centre, Institute of
Psychiatry at King's College London,
London, UK.

Linda R. Watkins
Department of Psychology and Center for
Neuroscience, University of Colorado, USA.

Marieke Wichers
Department of Psychiatry and
Neuropsychology, South Limburg Mental
Health Research and Teaching Network,
EURON, Maastricht University, Maastricht,
The Netherlands.

Crispin C. Wiles
Henry Wellcome Laboratories for
Integrative Neuroscience and Endocrinology,
University of Bristol,
Bristol, UK.

Grzegorz Wisniewski
Institute of Neuroscience, Newcastle
University, Psychiatry, Leazes Wing,
Royal Victoria Infirmary,
Newcastle upon Tyne, UK.

Lewis Wolpert
Cell and Developmental Biology, University
College, London, UK.

Caitlin S. Wyrwoll
Endocrinology Unit,
University of Edinburgh,
Queen's Medical Research Institute,
Edinburgh, UK.

Allan H. Young
LEEF Chair in Depression
Research and Director, Institute of
Mental Health, Department of
Psychiatry, University of British
Columbia, Vancouver, Canada.

Elizabeth A. Young
Molecular and Behavioral Neurosciences
Institute and Department of Psychiatry,
University of Michigan,
Ann Arbor, Michigan, USA.

Chapter 1

Experiencing depression

Lewis Wolpert

Depression varies from low mood to clinical depression. Severe depression is disabling and difficult to describe. Other symptoms such as local pain, feeling faint, and not being able to sleep are common. I describe my own experience.

If you can describe your severe depression you probably have not had one. It is indescribable and one enters a world with little relation to the real one. It was the worst experience in my life, even worse than the death of my wife from cancer. It is shameful to admit this but that was my experience (Wolpert, 2001). While she was dying I could do things to help her and I mourned afterwards. But with my depression there was nothing I felt I could do and I believed I would never get better. My mental state bore no resemblance to anything I had experienced before. I had had periods of feeling low but they were nothing like my depressed state. I was totally self-involved and negative and thought about suicide all the time. I just wanted to be left alone and remain curled up in my bed all day. I could not ride my bicycle and had panic attacks if left alone too long.

I also had numerous physical symptoms – my whole skin would seem to be on fire and I would on occasion twitch uncontrollably. Each new physical sign caused extreme anxiety. Sleep was very difficult and sleeping pills only seemed to work for a few hours. The future seemed hopeless and I was convinced that I would never recover and would probably end up completely mad.

Everyone has some story to tell as to why they get depressed. My own, I believe came from the difficulties I had in controlling my episodes of atrial fibrillation. The drug I had taken for several years no longer was as effective. My cardiologist changed my medication to flecainide and this gave me morning sickness and severe stomach cramps. I do believe it was this drug that precipitated my depression but the evidence is poor. I am a well-known hypochondriac and feared having a stroke. I also had a trip planned to South Africa, my country of origin, concerned with science and was terrified I would go into fibrillation far from medical help.

I persuaded a colleague at my medical school to give me an X-ray but all was in order. My doctor encouraged me to go and I cancelled the trip. I was distressed at letting my colleagues down and this increased my anxiety. I began to feel even more weird, and I was unable to sleep at all. I was clearly rather ill and called a psychiatrist friend from my medical school to visit me. He told me that I was severely depressed and put me on a tricyclic antidepressant. I read about its side effects and it became increasingly difficult for me to urinate. I ended up begging a urologist to hospitalize me. He did not but I came off the tricyclic antidepressant.

I spent most of my time at home thinking about death. It was weird that I should have been in this condition as I was generally very stable, happily married and with a fine job at the university. Then one night I had a dream about devils and woke up with a compulsion to kill myself. My wife and family got me into the Royal Free hospital by lunchtime and I was curiously relieved to be there. I was in the psychogeriatric ward and it was peaceful and I was well looked after. My psychiatrist put me on Seroxat® and assured me that I would recover – I did not believe her. I spent most of the time in bed for the first few days doing relaxation exercises, and then they let me go for little walks with a companion. They tried to give me cognitive therapy but it made no sense at that stage. I accepted that all my views were negative but this seemed perfectly natural considering the condition I was in. I thought of suicide all the time but did not know how to do it. As I was too scared of heights, jumping from my window which was high up was ruled out. I kept asking for electro-convulsive therapy which involves giving the brain electric shocks as I thought the drug would not work.

Nothing gave me pleasure and every decision, no matter how small, increased my anxiety. I had no emotions and was unable to cry but I did retain a macabre sense of humour. Sleep was very difficult but the staff gave me pills which left me dopey the next day. I got a bit better during the day and by evening could read and watch TV, but next morning I was back in the original bad state – a diurnal change classical for depression I was told. My hypochondria continued and I had Parkinson's disease as my hand trembled, and my foot flapped which they diagnosed as muscle weakness. My memory seemed to be failing and I was frightened that I was going insane. I also wondered what I was doing in a ward of old sick people, but at the same time was probably the sickest.

Over a period of three weeks I improved a bit and cognitive therapy began in the last week to make some sense. I returned home but remained indoors most of the time. My wife was angry that I was thinking of suicide and made a bargain with me. If I was no better in a year she would help me to die. I believed her and it reduced my suicidal thoughts.

I had cognitive therapy once a week and began to consider going back to work but was frightened I would not be able to cope. There was a meeting that I considered attending but was frightened I would panic and walk out. My therapist did a scenario with me about the meeting in which I walked out but the others did not mind. This enabled me to go and I survived and this was an important step in my recovery. I gradually got better and felt like Lazarus risen from the dead.

My wife was embarrassed about my depression. She had not told anyone about it as she thought it would be bad for my career – stigma is ever present. She just told them that I had a minor heart condition. For many the stigma of depression is a serious problem and I have been told by other depressives that they would not confide their condition to their bother or sister even though they had attempted suicide. Others were concerned that if their condition were known they would lose their job. One lady told me how she disguised her condition by appearing cheerful in public. I have to confess that prior to my illness I had a temporary technician in the department who had a severe depression that was so disruptive for those working with her, that I did not reappoint her. Carers of depressives all too often get depressed themselves.

But my recovery from my severe depression was not the end. I had read that only 10% of patients with a severe depression do not have a relapse and I believed that I would be in that group. Four years later, though I was working and travelling a lot, some of the symptoms of depression came back for no obvious reason. I tried St. Johns Wort but that did not help. I returned to my cognitive therapist who thought I was anxious about my impending retirement. I even visited her on the morning of my 70th birthday. Things got worse and my psychiatrist put me back on Seroxat® (paroxetine) and my decline continued. There were panic attacks and a cold tingling feeling would spread over my skin. I tried exercise which usually made me feel better but this made me exhausted and I entered a half-sleep state when I no longer had control of my thoughts. I felt I was going insane. I cancelled many of the meetings at which I was supposed to talk.

My new partner, my wife had died, found my condition very hard to deal with and she persuaded me against my will to consult a psychoanalyst. She had to drive me there and pick me up as I could not travel on my own. I refused to lie on the couch and found the interaction unfriendly, quite unlike my relationship with my cognitive therapist. Also I think psychoanalysis is without any scientific foundation. Fortunately after several weeks he took a long winter break and I got much better and did not go back. Since then there have been further episodes, but none really severe and I was prescribed Effexor® (venlafaxine) which I am still on. Exercise also works well for me.

Depression has a confusing number of different meanings and there is a lumpy continuum from feeling low to severe depression. Considering how many people have a severe depression it is surprising that there are virtually no good descriptions of depression in English novels. But writers have done well with their own depression. An outstanding example is William Styron's book *Darkness Visible*. He points out early on that 'the pain of severe depression is quite unimaginable to those who have suffered it, and it kills in many instances as it cannot be borne.'

Hamlet was clearly depressed:

> 'I have of late (but where fore I know not) lost all my mirth, foregone all custom of exercises ... the earth seems to me a sterile promontory ... it appears no other thing to me than a foul and pestilent congregation of vapours.'

John Stuart Mill (1962) wrote that Coleridge's poem, 'Dejection', was an accurate description of his state.

> A grief without a pang, void, dark and drear,
> A drowsy, stifled, unimpassioned grief,
> Which, finds no natural outlet or relief
> In word, or sigh, or tear.

Manley Hopkins poem is also excellent.

> No worst, there is none. Pitched past pitch of grief,
> More pangs will, schooled at forepangs, wilder wring.
> Comforter, where is your comforting?

Shelley described his suicidal feelings thus:

> Then would I stretch my languid frame
> Beneath the wild wood's gloomiest shade,
> And try to quench the ceaseless flame,
> That on my withered vitals preyed;

The poet John Clare was in an asylum for many years:

> I am! yet what I am none cares or knows,
> My friends forsake me like memory lost;
> I am the self-consumer of my woes,

And Tolstoy wrote that life had no meaning for him. Anne Sexton (1999) had manic depression and committed suicide:

> God went out of me
> as if the sea had dried up like sandpaper,
> as if the sun became a latrine.
> God went out of my fingers.
> They became stone.
> My body became a side of mutton
> and despair roamed the slaughterhouse.

All these descriptions are essentially based in terms of Western culture. To what extent is the experience of depression similar in other cultures? There are claims that in some cultures there is no word for depression. An important feature of depression is somatization which results in bodily symptoms similar to that of neurasthenia. In the 1980s, Arthur Kleinman (Kleinman, 1988) found that in China most cases of patients with neurasthenia were suffering from severe depression which was not an acceptable concept in China at that time. In India typical comments by depressed patients were that they could not tell anyone how they felt as it would lead to ill-treatment and people thinking lowly of the person (Raguram et al. 1996).

Since depression is common and disabling, particularly so as suicide is all too common, and since there is a strong genetic component involved, it is surprising that evolution has not reduced the incidence (Wolpert, 2008). It is hard for many to believe that so common a state does not have some advantage for the individual. I must confess that I can see no advantage to me that having a severe depression may have brought, other than having a better understanding of the condition. This debate is accurately described in Chapter 3 of this book.

There is no doubt that sadness is an adaptive emotion, but it is severe sadness, severe depression, that raises problems. Several hypotheses have been proposed to show that depression can have an advantage for the individual. One of the first was the social competition hypothesis (Price et al.1994). This sees depression as an adaptation whose function is to inhibit aggression by rivals and superiors when one's status is low. It is a means of yielding when there is social competition and thus reduces the efforts by the aggressor. It is hard to see how this could actually function in any current human society, and why depression should be so physically and psychologically debilitating. In terms of these ideas, just giving in would be sufficient. It also is completely at variance with women having twice the incidence of depression as men, depression in children, and the increased chance of a depression in adulthood if a child is abused or neglected – all these argue against depression being used to yield to social competition, and being adaptive in this way.

Another hypothesis is that the function of depression, and of low mood, is to make people accept unobtainable goals and so change those goals (Klinger, 1975). This may make sense for low mood, but not for severe depression. Another view, particularly in relation to postpartum depression, is that it is essentially a plea for help to the woman's partner in looking after the newborn child (Hagen, 1999). The social navigation hypothesis is that low mood and depression focuses resources and motivates partners to help (Watson and Andrews, 2002). Yet another approach is that varied situations can cause non-severe depression and that the symptoms serve related but distinguishable functions (Keller and Nesse, 2006). For example, sadness would result from loss, whereas crying may be a social signal, and fatigue reflects physical or mental weariness. But all these really deal with sadness at a low to moderately high level, and offer no evolutionary explanation for clinical and disabling depression (Nettle, 2004).

A different approach to depression is to view it as sadness having become excessive and out of control, in other words, malignant. Cancer is an example of a normal healthy process, cell multiplication, going wrong and becoming malignant. Cancer has its origin in a single cell with a small defect, which then goes through a series of stages that lead to malignancy. The same may be true for depression in the sense that there is a normal process that has become disordered. It may be that because sadness is a complex emotion it may increase to a malignant state due to loss of normal controls. The complexity of the processes involved may have prevented the evolution of adequate preventive mechanisms. Severe depression may result from the interaction of natural biological sadness and negative cognition – malignant sadness (Wolpert, 2001). There may be a positive feedback loop between the biological basis of sadness and the psychological basis that leads to severe depression. There is also a contribution by other factors, such as genetic disposition and cytokines produced by the immune system.

References

Hagen, E.H. (1999). The function of postpartum depression. *Evolution and Human Behavior,* **20**, 325–359.

Keller, M.C. and Nesse, R.M. (2006). The evolutionary significance of depressive symptoms: different adverse situations lead to different depressive symptom patterns. *Journal of Personality and Social Psychology*, **91**, 316–330.

Kleinman, A. (1988) *Rethinking Psychiatry: From Cultural Category to Personal Experience*. New York, Free Press.

Klinger, E. (1975). Consequences of commitment to and disengagement from incentives. *Psychological Review*, **82**, 1–25.

Mill, J.S. (1962). *On Bentham and Coleridge*. Smith Peter.

Nettle, D. (2004). Evolutionary origins of depression: a review and reformulation. *Journal of Affective Disorders*, **81**, 91–102.

Price, J., Sloman, L., Gardner, R., Gilbert, P., and Rohde, P. (1994). The social competition hypothesis of depression. *The British Journal of Psychiatry*, **164**, 309–315.

Raguram, R. et al. (1996). Stigma, depression, and somatization in South India. *The American Journal of Psychiatry*, **153**, 1043–1049.

Sexton, A. and Kumin, M. (1999). *The Complete Poems*. Anne Sexton, Mariner.

Styron, W. (1991). *Darkness visible*. Picador.

Watson, P.J. and Andrews, P.W. (2002). Toward a revised evolutionary adaptationist analysis of depression: the social navigation hypothesis. *Journal of Affective Disorders*, **72**, 1–14.

Wolpert, L. (2001). *Malignant Sadness: The Anatomy of Depression*. London, Faber & Faber.

Wolpert, L. (2008). Depression in an evolutionary context. *Philosophy, Ethics, and Humanities in Medicine*, **3**, 8.

Chapter 2

Depression in the medically ill

Monica Kelly Cowles, Carmine M. Pariante, and
Charles B. Nemeroff

Introduction

It is well accepted that depression is a risk factor for premature death. The most likely explanation of this observation is that depression is a risk factor for suicide, which is undoubtedly true. However, the impact of depression can be even more significant when it accompanies other serious medical illnesses. The impact of comorbid depression on medical disorders is multifaceted, and potentially devastating. The classical model for this association is that medical disorders increase the risk of depression – and of more severe forms of depression. For example, a recent study revealed a strong association between the cumulative number of illnesses and the estimated relative risk of suicide in elderly (66 years or older) patients with medical illness: a patient with three illnesses had about a threefold increased risk of suicide, and a patient with five illnesses had a fivefold increase (Juurlink et al. 2004). Although among such patients some commit suicide to escape pain rather than because of clinical depression, this is still an extremely dramatic clinical observation. Furthermore, a recent World Health Organization (WHO) World Health Survey (WHS) studied 245 404 adults from 60 countries from across all regions of the world, to obtain data for health, health-related outcomes, and their determinants. Participants with one or more chronic physical disease – angina, arthritis, asthma, and diabetes – had a significantly higher likelihood of comorbid depression (Moussavi et al. 2007). This chapter will concentrate on this model, by reviewing the evidence linking depression with a worse clinical outcome of medical illnesses. However, at least two other models are present, as discussed in several chapters in this book. First, depression may increase the risk, or worsen the outcome, of medical disorders: for example, by affecting the pathophysiological processes or the compliance to treatment. Second, both depression and medical disorders may be linked to a third common cause: for example, early life trauma may predispose to adverse mental and physical health in adulthood.

Epidemiology

The lifetime prevalence of depression in the general US population is 17.1%: higher in women (21%) than in men (13%). On the basis of the National Comorbidity Survey, the prevalence of depression within the 30 days prior to interview was approximately 5% (Blazer et al. 1994; Kessler et al. 1994). These rates increase with comorbid medical illness. There are associations with the type of comorbid medical illness (see Table 2.1), number of comorbid medical illnesses, and the acuity of illness (Brown et al. 1992; Bukberg et al. 1984; Burvill et al. 1995; Carney et al. 1987; Frasure-Smith et al. 1993; Goodnick et al. 1995; Greenwald et al. 1989; Hance et al. 1996; Joffe et al. 1986; Kathol et al. 1990; Robinson et al. 1984; Sano et al. 1989; Schleifer et al. 1989). The very clear association between depression and coronary heart disorder is discussed in Chapter 18 of

Table 2.1 Selected epidemiologic studies of depression associated with medical illness

Reference	Illness	Prevalence of depression (%)
Burvill et al. 1995	Cerebrovascular accident	23
Robinson et al. 1984	Cerebrovascular accident	27 (major depression)
		20 (minor depression)
Sano et al. 1989	Parkinson's disease	51
Greenwald et al. 1989	Alzheimer's disease	11
Schleifer et al. 1989	Myocardial infarction	18 (major depression)
		27 (minor depression)
Frasure-Smith et al. 1993	Myocardial infarction	16
Hance et al. 1996	Coronary artery disease	17
Carney et al. 1987	Coronary artery disease	18
Bukberg et al. 1984*	Cancer	42
Kathol et al. 1990*	Cancer	25–38
Joffe et al. 1986	Cancer	33
Goodnick et al. 1995	Diabetes Mellitus	8.5–27.3
Brown et al. 1992	Human immunodeficiency virus	5.6–12.2

Note: *Study involved hospitalized patients.

this book, while the impact of depression on mortality from medical illnesses is discussed in Chapter 20 of this book.

Kessler et al. (1997), using data from the National Comorbidity Survey, reported that within a 12-month period the number of chronic medical illnesses increases the rates of both minor and major depression when compared to those depressed patients without comorbid medical illness. In many, but not all, of the major medical disorders, the prevalence rate of major depression is inordinately high. The rate also increases with acuity of care with a low of 9% in the ambulatory setting and a high of 30% in the hospital setting (Katon and Sullivan, 1990).

Evaluating and diagnosing depression

Depression in the medically ill is under-diagnosed and under-treated. Even when the treating physician recognizes that a patient has multiple symptoms of depression, it is often regarded as a 'normal' psychological response to an emerging or chronic medical illness. Non-psychiatric physicians are often heard to say, 'after all the patient just had a heart attack' or 'was just diagnosed with cancer'. There are a myriad of reasons why this viewpoint is still unfortunately endorsed in some clinical settings. Adjustment disorder initially presents with many of the symptoms of depression. While adjustment (depressive) symptoms are not always abnormal or requiring immediate pharmacological treatment, certainly these symptoms cannot be overlooked and dismissed, because only some of these patients will recover without any treatment. When this does not occur and depression continues or even worsens, the 'adjustment disorder' has evolved into an autonomous major depression and its impact can be substantial. Predictors of major depression, such as a prior history of depression, family history, diagnostic criteria, and type and severity of medical illness contribute a great deal to the diagnostic evaluation and treatment plan.

When considering the diagnosis of depression in any patient population, it is essential to keep in mind the differential diagnoses illustrated in Table 2.2. For patients with comorbid medical illness there will most likely be multiple factors contributing to their mood disorder. First, one must consider the profound psychosocial disruption caused by the serious illness, and the associated inability to reach personal goals (as discussed also in Chapter 3). Second, there are untoward effects of medications and physiologic effects from their medical illness. Many medications have been implicated in causing depression. This list, as shown in Table 2.3, includes antihypertensives (β-blockers, reserpine, methyldopa, guanethidine, and clonidine), corticosteroids, antineoplastic agents, and interferon-α (Katon and Sullivan 1990; McDaniel et al. 1995; Newport and Nemeroff 1998; and Chapters 17 of this book). Many substances of abuse are also associated with depression and include alcohol, benzodiazepines, opiates, and cocaine.

As noted earlier, there are also numerous medical conditions which are directly associated with depression (refer to Table 2.4). When these specific medical conditions are treated, the depression generally resolves as well. This subtype of depression is different etiologically than either primary depression or depression secondary to a general medical condition. For the patients referred to

Table 2.2 Differential diagnosis

(1) Major depressive episode – Unipolar
(2) Bipolar I/II disorder, most recent episode depressed
(3) Adjustment disorder with depressed mood
(4) Dysthymic disorder
(5) Anxiety disorder with depressive symptoms
(6) Substance-induced mood disorder, iatrogenic versus otherwise
(7) Mood disorder due to a general medical condition
(8) Psychological factors affecting medical condition

Table 2.3 Chemotherapeutic and other pharmacologic agents linked to depression

Antineoplastic agents	Analgesics
♦ Alkylating agents	♦ Codeine
• Dacarbazine	♦ Indometacin
• Hexamethylamine	♦ Oxycodone
♦ Corticosteroids	
♦ Ciclosporin	Cardiovascular agents
♦ Cyproterone	♦ α-Methyldopa
♦ Interferon	♦ Reserpine
♦ L-Asparaginase	♦ Propranolol
♦ Methotrexate	♦ Calcium Channel Blockers
♦ Procarbazine	Neurological agents
♦ Tamoxifen	♦ Levodopa
♦ Vinblastine	♦ Phenobarbital
♦ Vincristine	
	Gastrointestinal agents
Corticosteroids	♦ Cimetidine
	Antifungals
	♦ Amphotericin B

psychiatrists, the etiology of their depression is likely multifactorial. A family history of mood disorders, previous episodes of depression, medications linked with depression, and illness linked with depression are all potential contributors to the current depressive episode. Optimal care requires cognizance of all contributing medical conditions and their respective treatment options in addition to a thorough psychiatric evaluation and treatment plan.

There has been much debate surrounding the diagnosis of depression in the medically ill. According to the Diagnostic and Statistical Manual of Mental Disorders (DSM-IV-TR), as shown in Table 2.5, a diagnosis of major depressive disorder (MDD) requires at least five of nine specified symptoms during a two-week period (American Psychiatric Association 2000). These symptoms are often divided into two groups, psychological and neurovegetative. The psychological symptoms include depressed mood, anhedonia, feelings of worthlessness or guilt, and recurrent thoughts of death. The neurovegetative symptoms include significant change in weight (gain or loss), change in sleep (insomnia or hypersomnia), psychomotor changes, fatigue or loss of energy, and a diminished ability to concentrate. These symptoms, in the absence of any other illness, are often extremely debilitating. In the presence of medical illness, they are not only debilitating, there can be, as mentioned previously, a significant impact on the patient's overall morbidity and mortality. It is therefore vitally important to determine if the symptoms arise from the medical illness, a depressive state or some combination of the two, thus allowing for the development of the most appropriate treatment plan.

It is widely acknowledged that the neurovegetative symptoms found in those with depression mirror 'sickness behavior': change in appetite, sleep, energy, concentration, and motivation.

Table 2.4 Medical conditions physiologically associated with depression

Endocrine disorders
◆ Hypothyroidism
◆ Hyperthyroidism
◆ Parathyroid disorders
◆ Cushing's syndrome
◆ Hyperprolactinemia

Neurologic disorders
◆ Cerebrovascular disease
◆ Central nervous system (CNS) lesions including tumours
◆ Neurosyphilis
◆ Multiple sclerosis
◆ Neurosarcoidosis
◆ CNS vasculitis
◆ HIV-associated CNS pathology
◆ Dementia
◆ Huntington's disease
◆ Parkinson's disease
◆ Traumatic brain injury

Other disorders
◆ Vitamin deficiencies (e.g. folate and vitamin B12)
◆ Anemia
◆ Hypoxia
◆ End-stage renal disease/uremia
◆ Systemic lupus erythematosus and other connective tissue diseases
◆ Occult malignancy (e.g. pancreatic cancer)

Table 2.5 DSM-IV-TR criteria for major depressive episode

A. Five (or more) of the following symptoms have been present during the same two-week period and represent a change from previous functioning; at least one of the symptoms is either (1) depressed mood or (2) loss of interest or pleasure.

(1) depressed mood most of the day, nearly every day, as indicated by either subjective report or observation made by others

(2) markedly diminished interest or pleasure in all, or almost all, activities most of the day, nearly every day

(3) significant weight loss when not dieting or weight gain, or decrease or increase in appetite nearly every day

(4) insomnia or hypersomnia nearly every day

(5) psychomotor agitation or retardation nearly every day

(6) fatigue or loss of energy nearly every day

(7) feelings of worthlessness or excessive or inappropriate guilt (which may be delusional) nearly every day

(8) diminished ability to concentrate, or indecisiveness, nearly every day

(9) recurrent thoughts of death (not just fear of dying), recurrent suicidal ideation without a specific plan, or a suicide attempt or specific plan for committing suicide

B. The symptoms do not meet criteria for a mixed episode.

C. The symptoms cause clinically significant distress or impairment in social, occupational, or other important areas of functioning.

D. The symptoms are not due to the direct physiologic effects of a substance or general medical condition.

E. The symptoms are not better accounted for by bereavement, i.e. after the loss of a loved one, the symptoms persist for longer than two months or are characterized by marked functional impairment, morbid preoccupation with worthlessness, suicidal ideation, psychotic symptoms, or psychomotor retardation.

Note: DSM-IV-TR *Diagnostic and Statistical Manual of Mental Disorders, Fourth Edition, Text Revision.Washington, DC, American Psychiatric Association, 2000.*

The DSM-IV states: 'do not include symptoms that are clearly due to a general medical condition'. The question then becomes how does the consultation-liaison (CL) psychiatrist best diagnose depression given these likely comorbid neurovegetative symptoms?

There have been many studies performed in an effort to develop reliable criteria for the diagnosis of depression in the medically ill. Cohen-Cole et al. (1993) proposed two systems of diagnosis: one best used in the clinical setting, the other for research purposes. The *exclusive* approach is most appropriate for research questions in that it exhibits a high degree of specificity. The symptoms associated with sickness behaviour previously described would not count towards a diagnosis of depression. Rather mood, anhedonia, feelings of guilt, worthlessness, and hopelessness and suicidality would be the primary indicators. The *inclusive* approach, however, is more appropriate for optimal patient care. If a patient meets the criteria for depression, whether it is for major depressive disorder or subsyndromal depression, treatment should be offered. The risk of over-diagnosis appears to be small, 1.5–8%, whereas missing an opportunity to treat depression can have serious consequences. Studies have shown that failure to treat even subsyndromal depression leads to increased morbidity, longer hospital stays, and increased pain, as well as an adverse effect on quality of life (Judd et al. 1996). Therefore, in the remainder of the chapter, the term *depression* unless otherwise noted includes MDD, dysthymic disorder, and subsyndromal depression.

As shown in Table 2.6, there are many screening instruments which can be useful tools for the clinical psychiatrist. As Krishnan et al. (2002) point out in their review of comorbidity of depression with medical illness in the elderly, many of these screening instruments include *distress scales,* the scores from which are not necessarily highly related to the diagnosis of a psychiatric disorder or highly specific for the psychiatric syndromes they are designed to assess'. Nonetheless they have utility given the latest evidence which suggests that a clinical threshold need not be crossed for there to be a deleterious outcome with respect to the comorbid illness. Chochinov et al. (1997) were able to show that simply asking 'Are you depressed?' was more sensitive and specific than a screening questionnaire or visual analogue scale in the detection of depression in a group of terminally ill patients. This simple question should be routinely asked of all patients with medical illness.

An obvious advantage of Chochinov's approach lies with its simplicity. Many clinicians contend that an in-depth, invasive interview may lead to the patient subjectively feeling worse. Not only is it difficult to ask a patient facing death about suicidal ideation and hopelessness, their answers

Table 2.6 Screening instruments for assessing depression in medical patients

Screening instrument	Abbreviation	Method of administration	Comments	Time requirement
Open interview		Clinician administered		variable
Structured clinical interview	SCID	Clinician administered	Diagnoses DSM disorders	1–2 hours
Hamilton Depression Rating scale	HAM-D	Clinician administered	Measures depression severity	15–20 min
Montgomery-Asberg Depression Rating scale	MADRS	Clinician administered	Measures depression severity	15–20 min
Symptom Check List-90-Revision	SCL-90-R	Self-report	Screens depression and other psychiatric morbidity	15–20 min
Brief-Symptom Inventory	BSI	Self-report	Abbreviated form of SCL-90-R	10–15 min
Illness Distress scale	IDS	Self-report	Measures physical and emotional distress	5–10 min
Psychological Distress Inventory	PDI	Self-report	Measures psychological distress	5 min
Carroll Depression Rating scale	CDRS	Self-report	Measures depression severity	5 min
Geriatric Depression Scale (Short Form)	GDS	Self-report	Measures depression severity	5 min
Zung Depression scale	Zung	Self-report	Measures depression severity	5 min
Beck Depression Inventory for Primary Care	BDI-PC	Self-report	Measures depression severity	5 min
Depression in the Medically Ill scale	DMI-10	Self-report	Detects presence of depression	5 min

may have different implications with respect to simply facing reality as opposed to being a result of depression. For these reasons, Parker et al. (2001) developed a 16-question self-report screening instrument, Depression in the Medically Ill scale, which utilizes a cognitive-based approach for the detection of depression. This approach was initially validated with the development and use of a modified Beck Depression Inventory, the Beck Depression Inventory for Primary Care, which excludes somatic symptoms (Parker et al. 2002; Steer et al. 1999). It was based in part on the findings of Clark et al. (1983) who determined that in the medically ill population, somatic symptoms are often non-discriminatory with respect to the accurate diagnosis of depression. Instead it is important to focus on cognitive symptoms such as a 'loss of interest, sense of failure, sense of punishment and suicidal thoughts'. The final screening tool was optimized and now consists of ten questions. Wilhelm et al. (2004) then examined the validity of this approach in a study evaluating 212 patients for the presence of depression with a variety of comorbid medical illnesses including neurological disorders, cardiopulmonary disease, malignancy, loss of mobility and renal disease. The Beck Depression Inventory for Primary Care was used as the comparison screening instrument and clinicians independently evaluated the patients for the presence of an affective disorder based on DSM-IV criteria. Both scales detected depression in 85% of the patients with a DSM-IV major depressive episode. Because the Depression in the Medically Ill scale is a short, self-report questionnaire its utility may lie in assisting the clinician with more efficiently diagnosing depression while at the same time minimizing the potential perceived adverse impact of undergoing a psychiatric evaluation.

Symptom amplification and functional disability

Patients with comorbid depression and medical illness have been shown to report more physical symptoms associated with their medical illness than their non-depressed counterparts (Katon et al. 2001). In addition, there is now a burgeoning database which suggests that pain is a core symptom of major depression (Ohayon and Schatzberg 2003; see also Chapter 19 in this book). The majority of patients with acute or chronic medical illness are able to adapt to the symptoms caused by their illness. However it appears that the presence of depression negatively affects the adaptation process and exacerbates the patient's perception of their own symptom severity and corresponding level of disability. There have been many studies addressing this concept with various comorbid illnesses including hepatitis C (Dwight et al. 2000), diabetes (Lustman et al. 1988), inflammatory bowel disease (Walker et al. 1996), head injury (Fann et al. 1995), and coronary artery disease (Sullivan et al. 2000). The presence of depression with comorbid medical illness has the potential of complicating the patient's own perception of their disease. If this occurs, patients tend to have increased generalized symptoms in addition to those specifically associated with their disease. This in turn often leads to limited functioning and increased disability when compared to their non-depressed counterparts with similar disease severity. According to the WHO 2005 estimates, depression is responsible for 10% of all disability-adjusted life-years (the sum of years lived with disability and years of life lost) by non-communicable diseases (Prince et al. 2007).

Treatment

Treatment of depression to remission is of paramount importance. Depression that is under-treated is un-treated depression. In the remainder of this chapter, as well as in subsequent system-specific chapters, treatment recommendations will be outlined. In brief, the same treatment modalities available for the general population are also available for the medically ill. There are, of course, important exceptions and these will be noted.

A treatment plan should be constructed with a multidisciplinary approach in mind as the medically ill population is likely to have a team of caregivers as opposed to a single physician. Indeed, a recent study evaluated a multifaceted psychiatric intervention targeted at rheumatology and diabetes patients, consisting of an intervention conducted by a psychiatric liaison nurse and/or referral to a consult-liaison psychiatrist, followed by advice to the treating physician or organization of a multidisciplinary case conference. This intervention led to an improvement in depression and quality of life, and a reduction in hospital admissions (Stiefel et al. 2008).

Different treatment modalities include pharmacologic therapy, psychotherapy (e.g. supportive, cognitive behavioural, interpersonal, psychodynamic, and group therapies), electroconvulsive therapy (ECT) and when necessary, psychiatric hospitalization. Whatever the course of treatment, appropriate follow-up is critical. It falls to the consult-liaison psychiatrist to not only evaluate the patient and formulate an assessment and treatment recommendations, but to also communicate with and educate both the primary treating physician and the patient to maximize implementation of the recommended treatment.

Conclusions

Historically, depression in the medically ill was often considered a natural and expected response to medical illness. In this context, treatment of depression was often considered secondary to treatment of the medical illness, if the depression was even treated at all. Today, this perspective can no longer be accepted. Furthermore, it should be considered negligent to ignore signs of depression in the medically ill. There now exists overwhelming evidence supporting the fact that the accurate diagnosis and appropriate treatment of depression in the medically ill improves quality of life, enhances the patient's ability to be actively engaged in their treatment, decreases symptom quantity and severity and decreases cost utilization. Most importantly it decreases morbidity and mortality. The effect of depression on the course of medical illness is multifaceted as there are systemic pathophysiologic implications as well as psychological and behavioural ramifications. There are many treatment options available including pharmacologic therapy, psychotherapy, electroconvulsive therapy and when necessary, psychiatric hospitalization. The consult-liaison psychiatrist should formulate a treatment plan, keeping in mind the specific comorbid medical illness and whatever limitations that illness may impose, and work closely with the patient, patient's family, and primary physician with regard to implementation of this plan. It cannot be overstated that for the depressed medically ill patient, treatment of their depression to remission is of paramount importance.

References

American Psychiatric Association (2000). *Diagnostic and Statistical Manual of Mental Disorders*. Fourth Edition, Text Revised Edition. Washington, DC , American Psychiatric Press.

Blazer, D.G., Kessler, R.C., McGonagle, K.A., and Swartz, M.S. (1994). The prevalence and distribution of major depression in a national community sample: the National Comorbidity Survey. *American Journal of Psychiatry*, **151**, 979–986.

Brown, G.R., Rundell, J.R., McManis, S.E., Kendall, S.N., Zachary, R., and Temoshok, L. (1992). Prevalence of psychiatric disorders in early stages of HIV infection. *Psychosomatic Medicine*, **54**, 588–601.

Bukberg, J., Penman, D., and Holland, J.C. (1984). Depression in hospitalized cancer patients. *Psychosomatic Medicine*, **46**, 199–212.

Burvill, P.W., Johnson, G.A., Jamrozik, K.D., Anderson, C.S., Stewart-Wynne, E.G., and Chakera, T.M. (1995). Prevalence of depression after stroke: the Perth Community Stroke Study. *British Journal of Psychiatry*, **166**, 320–327.

Carney, R.M., Rich, M.W., Tevelde, A., Saini, J., Clark, K., and Jaffe, A.S. (1987). Major depressive disorder in coronary artery disease. *American Journal of Cardiology*, **60**, 1273–1275.

Chochinov, H.M., Wilson, K.G., Enns, M., and Lander, S. (1997). 'Are you depressed?' Screening for depression in the terminally ill. *American Journal of Psychiatry*, **154**, 674–676.

Clark, D.C., vonAmmon, C.S., and Gibbons, R.D. (1983). The core symptoms of depression in medical and psychiatric patients. *Journal of Nervous and Mental Disease*, **171**, 705–713.

Cohen-Cole, S.A., Brown, F.W., and McDaniel, J.S. (1993). Assessment of depression and grief reactions in the medically ill. In Stoudemire, A. and Fogel, B.S. (ed.) *Psychiatric Care of the Medical Patient*, pp. 53–69. New York, Oxford University Press.

Dwight, M.M., Kowdley, K.V., Russo, J.E., Ciechanowski, P.S., Larson, A.M., and Katon, W.J. (2000). Depression, fatigue, and functional disability in patients with chronic hepatitis C. *Journal of Psychosomatic Research*, **49**, 311–317.

Fann, J.R., Katon, W.J., Uomoto, J.M., and Esselman, P.C. (1995). Psychiatric disorders and functional disability in outpatients with traumatic brain injuries. *American Journal of Psychiatry*, **152**, 1493–1499.

Frasure-Smith, N., Lesperance, F., and Talajic, M. (1993). Depression following myocardial infarction. Impact on 6-month survival. *JAMA*, **270**, 1819–1825.

Goodnick, P.J., Henry, J.H., and Buki, V.M. (1995). Treatment of depression in patients with diabetes mellitus. *Journal of Clinical Psychiatry*, **56**, 128–136.

Greenwald, B.S., Kramer-Ginsberg, E., Marin, D. B. et al. (1989). Dementia with coexistent major depression. *American Journal of Psychiatry*, **146**, 1472–1478.

Hance, M., Carney, R.M., Freedland, K.E., and Skala, J. (1996). Depression in patients with coronary heart disease. A 12-month follow-up. *General Hospital Psychiatry*, **18**, 61–65.

Joffe, R.T., Rubinow, D.R., Denicoff, K.D., Maher, M., and Sindelar, W.F. (1986). Depression and carcinoma of the pancreas. *General Hospital Psychiatry*, **8**, 241–245.

Judd, L.L., Paulus, M.P., Wells, K.B., and Rapaport, M.H. (1996). Socioeconomic burden of subsyndromal depressive symptoms and major depression in a sample of the general population. *American Journal of Psychiatry*, **153**, 1411–1417.

Juurlink, D.N., Herrmann, N., Szalai, J.P., Kopp, A., and Redelmeier, D.A. (2004). Medical illness and the risk of suicide in the elderly. *Archives of Internal Medicine*, **164**, 1179–1184.

Kathol, R.G., Mutgi, A., Williams, J., Clamon, G., and Noyes, R., Jr. (1990). Diagnosis of major depression in cancer patients according to four sets of criteria. *American Journal of Psychiatry*, **147**, 1021–1024.

Katon, W. and Sullivan, M.D. (1990). Depression and chronic medical illness. *Journal of Clinical Psychiatry*, **51 Suppl**, 3–11.

Katon, W., Sullivan, M., and Walker, E. (2001). Medical symptoms without identified pathology: relationship to psychiatric disorders, childhood and adult trauma, and personality traits. *Annals of Internal Medicine*, **134**, 917–925.

Kessler, R.C., McGonagle, K.A., Zhao, S. et al. (1994). Lifetime and 12-month prevalence of DSM-III-R psychiatric disorders in the United States. Results from the National Comorbidity Survey. *Archives of General Psychiatry*, **51**, 8–19.

Kessler, R.C., Zhao, S., Blazer, D.G., and Swartz, M. (1997). Prevalence, correlates, and course of minor depression and major depression in the National Comorbidity Survey. *Journal of Affective Disorders*, **45**, 19–30.

Krishnan, K.R., Delong, M., Kraemer, H. et al. (2002). Comorbidity of depression with other medical diseases in the elderly. *Biological Psychiatry*, **52**, 559–588.

Lustman, P.J., Clouse, R.E., and Carney, R.M. (1988). Depression and the reporting of diabetes symptoms. *International Journal of Psychiatry in Medicine*, **18**, 295–303.

McDaniel, J.S., Musselman, D.L., Porter, M.R., Reed, D.A., and Nemeroff, C.B. (1995). Depression in patients with cancer. Diagnosis, biology, and treatment. *Archives of General Psychiatry*, **52**, 89–99.

Moussavi, S., Chatterji, S., Verdes, E., Tandon, A., Patel, V., and Ustun, B. (2007). Depression, chronic diseases, and decrements in health: results from the World Health Surveys. *Lancet*, **370**, 851–858.

Newport, D.J. and Nemeroff, C.B. (1998). Assessment and treatment of depression in the cancer patient. *Journal of Psychosomatic Research*, **45**, 215–237.

Ohayon, M.M. and Schatzberg, A.F. (2003). Using chronic pain to predict depressive morbidity in the general population. *Archives of General Psychiatry*, **60**, 39–47.

Parker, G., Hilton, T., Hadzi-Pavlovic, D., and Bains, J. (2001). Screening for depression in the medically ill: the suggested utility of a cognitive-based approach. *Australian and New Zealand Journal of Psychiatry*, **35**, 474–480.

Parker, G., Hilton, T., Bains, J., and Hadzi-Pavlovic, D. (2002). Cognitive-based measures screening for depression in the medically ill: the DMI-10 and the DMI-18. *Acta Psychiatrica Scandinavica*, **105**, 419–426.

Prince, M., Patel, V., Saxena, S. et al. (2007). No health without mental health. *Lancet*, **370**, 859–877.

Robinson, R.G., Starr, L.B., and Price, T.R. (1984). A two year longitudinal study of mood disorders following stroke. Prevalence and duration at six months follow-up. *British Journal of Psychiatry*, **144**, 256–262.

Sano, M., Stern, Y., Williams, J., Cote, L., Rosenstein, R., and Mayeux, R. (1989). Coexisting dementia and depression in Parkinson's disease. *Archives of Neurology*, **46**, 1284–1286.

Schleifer, S.J., ari-Hinson, M.M., Coyle, D.A. et al. (1989). The nature and course of depression following myocardial infarction. *Archives of Internal Medicine*, **149**, 1785–1789.

Steer, R.A., Cavalieri, T.A., Leonard, D.M., and Beck, A.T. (1999). Use of the Beck Depression Inventory for Primary Care to screen for major depression disorders. *General Hospital Psychiatry*, **21**, 106–111.

Stiefel, F., Zdrojewski, C., Bel, H.F. et al. (2008). Effects of a multifaceted psychiatric intervention targeted for the complex medically ill: a randomized controlled trial. *Psychotherapy and Psychosomatics*, **77**, 247–256.

Sullivan, M.D., LaCroix, A.Z., Spertus, J.A., and Hecht, J. (2000). Five-year prospective study of the effects of anxiety and depression in patients with coronary artery disease. *American Journal of Cardiology*, **86**, 1135–1138, A6, A9.

Walker, E.A., Gelfand, M.D., Gelfand, A.N., Creed, F., and Katon, W.J. (1996). The relationship of current psychiatric disorder to functional disability and distress in patients with inflammatory bowel disease. *General Hospital Psychiatry*, **18**, 220–229.

Wilhelm, K., Kotze, B., Waterhouse, M., Hadzi-Pavlovic, D., and Parker, G. (2004). Screening for depression in the medically ill: a comparison of self-report measures, clinician judgment, and DSM-IV diagnoses. *Psychosomatics*, **45**, 461–469.

Chapter 3

Explaining depression: neuroscience is not enough, evolution is essential

Randolph M. Nesse

Neuroscience provides proximate explanations based on mechanisms, but a full biological explanation of depression also requires an evolutionary explanation of the origins and functions of the capacity for low mood. Failure to recognize that both are essential slows progress. Mood regulates patterns of investment as a function of environmental propitiousness. When investments are not resulting in progress towards a goal, low mood gives a fitness advantage. If a person cannot give up an unreachable goal, low mood can escalate to clinical depression. There are several evolutionary reasons why brain systems that regulate mood are vulnerable to dysfunction.

Introduction

In the course of research for a book on why natural selection has left humans so vulnerable to depression, I asked three leading neuroscientists why the capacity for depression exists at all. One suggested that groups with a mix of optimists and pessimists do better than other groups. A second said that negative mood is harmful while good mood gets people to want to have sex and do other things that increase fitness. A third said that depression results from neurotransmitter-receptor abnormalities.

These responses suggest that even some of the best neuroscientists are unfamiliar with evolutionary principles that long ago transformed behavioural biology. Evolutionary explanations based on benefits to the group have been recognized as problematic for 40 years (Williams, 1966). The belief that positive emotions are useful but negative emotions are harmful is an illusion (Nesse, 2004). Finally, reductionist explanations for why some individuals get depressed do not address the question of why depression exists (Kendler, 2005).

Perhaps more important than specific misunderstandings, however, is the larger problem of widespread failure to recognize that biological traits need both evolutionary and proximate explanations. Neuroscience can never provide a full biological explanation for depression, it can only explain mechanisms. Progress will speed up when we concurrently address the evolutionary question of why depression exists at all. This thesis is supported by considering how the application of how three simple evolutionary principles can advance depression research. The first principle is that proximate explanations based on brain mechanisms are insufficient; every trait also needs an evolutionary explanation. The second is that diseases do not have evolutionary explanations, however evolution can explain why some aspects of the body have been left vulnerable to failure. Third, many symptoms, such as pain, fever, cough, and negative emotions, are not usually the result of bodily defects, they are adaptive responses shaped by natural selection. The brain mechanisms that regulate these responses are vulnerable to dysregulation; we need to find out why.

Proximate and evolutionary questions

Asking evolutionary as well as proximate questions long ago transformed the study of animal behaviour (Alcock, 2005; Alcock and Sherman, 1994; Dewsbury, 1999; Krebs and Davies, 1984). The crucial advance was Tinbergen's (1963) observation that a full biological explanation of any trait requires answers to four questions: two proximate and two evolutionary (Box 3.1). Modern animal-behaviour texts begin with these four questions (Alcock, 1993; Beckhoff and Allen, 1995; Krebs and Davies, 1997), but with a few exceptions (Gazzaniga, 2004); neuroscience texts do not mention them.

As Tinbergen and Mayr emphasized (Dewsbury, 1999; Mayr, 1982; Tinbergen, 1963), proximate and evolutionary questions are not alternatives; answers to both are essential for any complete explanation. Proximate explanations describe the mechanistic details of a trait – its composition and structure at all levels, how the mechanism works, and how it arises in the course of ontogeny. Evolutionary explanations describe how a trait came to be the way it is – the historical sequence of previous traits and the evolutionary forces that shaped the trait. For instance, a proximate explanation for the human locus coeruleus includes the details of its anatomy, chemistry, connections, and its developmental origins. An evolutionary explanation describes its phylogeny, and how its functions give a selective advantage (presumably by regulating noradrenergic transmission and coordinating the emergency response).

Evolutionary hypotheses in neuroscience

Much neuroscience is devoted to studies of adaptive function, however only rarely are such studies recognized as tests of evolutionary hypotheses about how a trait influences fitness (Box 3.2). Instead, neural components are often presumed to have specific functions – as parts of the 'brain as a machine'. This approach has generated much knowledge, but it can be misleading (Childs, 1999; Nesse and Stearns, 2008). Machines have discrete parts engineered to serve one or a few functions. Organisms are products of sequential tiny changes over millions of generations that result in partially differentiated components that may serve many functions. They are hard to reverse engineer because they were not designed by an engineer. Far from implying that traits are perfect, an evolutionary approach shows why many of the body's 'design' are botched, at best (Crespi, 2000; Nesse, 2005b; Nesse and Williams, 1994; Williams, 1996; Williams and Nesse, 1991). An evolutionary view suggests that we should expect evolved brains to be jumbles of incompletely differentiated, jury-rigged parts with multiple overlapping functions.

One conclusion is that few brain structures should have only one or two specific clearly describable functions. Instead, multiple actions, which may or may not correspond to our notions of functions, are distributed across many cross-connected incompletely differentiated structures.

Box 3.1 Tinbergen's four questions (Tinbergen, 1963)

Two proximate questions (about mechanisms)
1. Mechanism – What are the trait's components and how do they work?
2. Ontogeny – What is the ontogeny of this trait?

Two evolutionary questions (about origins)
3. Phylogeny – What is the phylogeny of this trait?
4. Adaptive function – What selective advantages/costs and other evolutionary factors shaped this trait?

Box 3.2 Testing evolutionary hypotheses

Like other scientific hypotheses, proposals about a trait's evolutionary origins or functions can be easy, difficult, or temporarily impossible to test. A controversy that began with Gould and Lewontin's critique of 'adaptationist' thinking (1979) has been both helpful and harmful. The benefit is increased attention to all potential explanations, including genetic drift and other evolutionary factors other than natural selection (Pigliucci and Kaplan, 2000). The cost is a widespread misimpression that evolutionary hypotheses are untestable, 'just-so-stories'. This notion persists despite many effective rebuttals (Alcock, 1998; Borgia, 1994; Queller, 1995; Selzer, 1993)

The issue arises in large part because proximate scientists are unfamiliar with the methods used to test evolutionary hypotheses (Alcock, 2005; Mace et al. 2003; Mayr, 1983; Nesse, 1999d; Reeve and Sherman, 1993; Rose and Lauder, 1996; Stearns and Hoekstra, 2005;). When applicable, the comparative method is strong (Pagel, 1994). For instance, the shape and size of beaks in different species of finches correlates well with the kinds of foods available, and when only harder seeds are available, beaks become thicker in just a few generations (Grant, 1999). Only rarely do neuroscientists have access to data that allow such comparisons (Butler and Hodos, 1996; Glenn Northcutt and Kaas, 1995; Panksepp et al. 2002).

Extirpation is a mainstay for physiological studies of function; take out an organ and see what goes wrong. From the studies of patients with localized brain damage to knock-out mice or aspiration of brain structures, neuroscientists routinely test hypotheses about the adaptive functions of genes (Alcock, 2005; Mayr, 1983; Rose and Lauder, 1996b), neurotransmitters, receptors, and brain structures (Bloom, 1994; Gazzaniga, 1995; Kandel et al. 2000). Such studies are rarely recognized as tests of evolutionary hypotheses about adaptive functions.

Assessing form in relation to function is a mainstay in general biology, where its challenges are recognized. When the details of a trait exactly match those that would well serve a function, that is useful evidence. Stronger evidence is provided by predicting previously unobserved details. For behavioural traits, the situations that elicit the behaviour may provide the best available evidence.

The distributed regulation of motivation offers a good example (Berridge, 2004). Other chapters in this volume illustrate both the value and the difficulties of trying to localize functions. This is discouraging to the goal of fully understanding the brain, but it helps to explain why neuroscience is so difficult. It is not just because the systems are complex, but because the brain's components and connections do not have a coherent organization of the sort found in human-designed machines. Bodies are not irreducibly complex, but some aspects may be indescribably complex.

Many studies address the functions of neurotransmitters and receptors in depression and other disorders (Barnes and Sharp, 1999). Most propose one or a few functions for each transmitter or receptor, sometimes framed in terms of effects on other neural structures, and sometimes in terms of effects on cognition or behaviour. Dopamine, for instance, has long been said to mediate motivation and reward. On deeper analysis this turns out to be far too simple (Berridge, 2004; Salamone et al. 2005; Wise, 2004).

An evolutionary approach provides a different perspective on the origins of traits in conjunction with functions. For instance, duplication of receptor or transmitter genes can give advantages by allowing more exact control of different tissues (Fryxell, 1995; Roth et al. 1982). The proopiomelanocortin (POMC) gene was duplicated before the appearance of the jawed fish, thus paving the way for receptor differentiation and further transmitter specialization. Tissue-specific actions for POMC peptides now differ in different species (Takahashi and Kawauchi, 2006). Differentiation of function in different tissues gives the selective advantage that drives this process, however the functions that are served by different opiods and MSH's are multiple and hard to describe.

The animal behaviour literature contains extensive discussions about how to specify objects of evolutionary explanation, and how to pose and test specific hypotheses (Alcock, 2005; Reeve and Sherman, 1993; Rose and Lauder, 1996). Debates continue, but they are settling down, at least about core issues (Alcock, 2001; Rose and Lauder, 1996; Segerstråle, 2000). In neuroscience the topic is curiously neglected; I suspect this is because there is incomplete recognition that proximate and evolutionary questions are separate, and because some neuroscientists, having never been exposed to the methods for testing such hypotheses, proceed as if data on proximate mechanisms can answer such questions.

Evolutionary explanations for diseases

An evolutionary approach to depression does not mean proposing that depressive disorders are useful. Attempts to find direct evolutionary explanations for a disease are misguided because natural selection does not shape diseases. Selection and genetic drift can, however, explain aspects of the body that leave it vulnerable to a disease, such as wisdom teeth, a small birth canal, and a low anxiety threshold (Williams and Nesse, 1991). Asking and answering such questions has contributed to the rapid growth of evolutionary medicine (http://evmedreview.com, 2008; Nesse and Stearns, 2008; Nesse and Williams, 1994; Stearns and Ebert, 2001; Stearns and Koella, 2007; Stearns et al. 2007; Trevathan et al. 2008). Much progress has been made in discovering why aging occurs (Finch, 2007), why natural selection has not resulted in better protection against cancer (Frank, 2007; Greaves, 2002), and why we are so vulnerable to anxiety (McGuire and Troisi, 1998; Nesse, 1999a).

There are six evolutionary reasons why a trait may have 'design' features that leave bodies vulnerable to a disease (Box 3.3). For a list, see the text box below, for details, see primary sources (Evolution and Medicine Review, 2008; Nesse and Stearns, 2008; Nesse and Williams, 1994; Stearns and Ebert, 2001; Stearns and Koella, 2007; Stearns et al. 2007; Trevathan et al. 2008). The last item, adaptive responses, is not really a reason for vulnerability, but it belongs on the list because responses such as pain, cough, and fever are sometimes confused with diseases. They are responses useful in specific circumstances; selection has shaped systems that express the response when they detect cues associated with those circumstances. For instance, lipolysaccharide (LPS), whose presence is strongly correlated with a bacterial infection, arouses an inflammatory response.

Explaining vulnerability to one disease may require several kinds of explanations. For instance, vulnerability to atherosclerosis results from a combination of mismatch, pathogen evolution, constraints and tradeoffs and adaptive responses (Nesse and Weder, 2007).

The first task in an evolutionary analysis of a medical condition is to determine if it arises directly from a bodily defect or if it is an adaptive response to a more fundamental problem. For example, paralysis, seizures, hallucinations, and cancer are direct manifestations of bodily defects. They have no utility. In contrast, pain, fever, cough, and anxiety are not defects or diseases, they are adaptive responses to more fundamental problems (Nesse, 2005c).

Why are such reactions so aversive? Imagine if they were not. A few rare people have a congenital inability to experience pain. They are almost all dead by early adulthood (Rosemberg et al. 1994; Sternbach, 1963). The experience of pain means something is wrong, but the capacity for pain is an essential adaptation. What about anxiety? Patients with too much anxiety crowd clinics. Those with hypophobia don't complain, but some get into trouble and others die young (Lee et al. 2006).

Box 3.3 Six evolutionary explanations for vulnerability

1. Infection by agents that evolve faster than we do
2. Mismatch between our bodies and novel environments
3. Constraints on what selection can do
4. Tradeoffs that limit the perfection of any trait
5. Traits that increase reproduction at the expense of health
6. Protective responses such as pain, fever, cough, and anxiety

Like everything else in the body, the mechanisms that regulate protective responses can fail, causing conditions such as chronic pain and anxiety disorders. Even responses from intact regulation mechanisms can cause problems. For instance, fever can result in seizures, and diarrhoea can cause dehydration and death. These dire consequences seem to suggest that natural selection has done a poor job of shaping the regulation mechanisms. The relative safety of using drugs to block fever, cough, and diarrhoea further suggests that natural selection may not be able to shape effective regulation mechanisms.

However, false alarms are normal and inevitable for bodily defences. A full analysis of the optimal threshold for expressing a defence requires signal detection theory (Nesse, 2005c). In general, however, the cost of a false alarm is likely to be small compared to the cost of failing to activate the protective state when it is needed, so the optimal response threshold results in many false alarms. Fleeing in response to the sound of a breaking twig costs only a few calories. Not fleeing may be infinitely costly if the sound was made by a lion. False alarms are normal and common. This is the 'smoke detector principle' (Nesse, 2005c).

As with other diseases, serious depression is not an adaptation shaped by natural selection. It has no evolutionary explanation. However, we do need an evolutionary explanation for why natural selection has left us so vulnerable to a disease as common and devastating as depression. Some abnormal depression is related to normal low mood, so explaining the origins and functions of mood is an essential foundation for understanding depression.

The utility of emotions and mood

Emotions and moods give organisms a selective advantage by adjusting physiological and cognitive parameters to deal with situations that have repeatedly influenced fitness over the course of evolution (Ekman, 1992; Keltner et al. 2006; Nesse, 1990; Panksepp, 1998; Plutchik, 2003; Tooby and Cosmides, 1990). Moods are longer in duration and less tightly tied to specific cues than emotions, but both are special modes for coping with certain situations (Nesse, 1999c; 2006, Thayer, 1996). Single-celled organisms have two behaviours: move towards resources or away from danger (Adler, 1966; Larsen et al. 1974). From these primal origins, behavioural activation (BAS) and behavioural inhibition (BIS) brain systems developed; they increase fitness in situations characterized by opportunity/gain or threat/loss, respectively (Barrett, 2006; Gray, 1987; Watson et al. 1988).

Moods and emotions are almost all positive or negative because neutral situations do not influence fitness (Barrett, 2006; Nesse, 1990; 1999c). Natural selection has differentiated generic positive and negative states into more specialized emotions that are helpful (on average) in the specific situations that a species has encountered (Nesse, 2004; Plutchik, 1980). The so-called 'basic emotions' correspond to especially common well-defined situations, such as threat (for anxiety) and gaining valued resources (for joy).

Positive emotions seem more useful than negative ones because they are elicited in propitious situations. In situations involving threat or loss, negative moods and emotions are more useful. They adjust physiology, motivation, and behaviour to cope with such situations involving threats or losses (Nesse, 1990; 1999c; Plutchik, 2003; Tooby and Cosmides, 1990). For instance, Walter Cannon long ago recognized the utility of the emergency response in situations that required fight or flight (Cannon, 1914). This emergency system has false alarms; when recurrent, they are called panic disorder (Nesse, 1987).

Depression

Much neuroscience research proceeds on the assumption that 'depression is a brain disease'. This is certainly correct in the sense that all mood and behaviour is mediated by brain mechanisms (Kendler, 2005). In some cases, it is correct in the more specific sense that depression arises from primary brain abnormalities. The slogan has also helped the public to understand that depression is not a personal failing, but a treatable condition.

However, assuming that depression is a brain disease limits scientific progress in several ways (Kendler, 2005; Moncrieff, 2007). First, it implies that genetic and brain variations that predispose to depression are abnormalities, when they may be neutral, or even advantageous, in certain environments. Second, it neglects the role of life events and other causal factors that interact with brain variations to cause most depression. Third, it implies that depression symptoms are pathological, distracting attention from the task of finding the functions for normal low mood. Fourth, it implies that brain changes associated with depression are abnormalities, although they can equally well reflect the normal actions of mechanisms that mediate mood (Halbreich, 2006; Mayberg et al. 1999). Finally, diagnostic criteria based only on symptoms encourage studying major depression as if it is one condition with one aetiology, although it can have many different aetiologies (Antonijevic, 2006; Keller and Nesse, 2005; Kendler, 2005).

In contrast, an evolutionary perspective recognizes that depression symptoms can be normal or abnormal depending on the situation (Horwitz and Wakefield, 2007), that multiple factors may combine to cause a single case of depression, that etiological factors may differ markedly from case to case (Nesse, 2006), and that different depression symptoms may have been shaped to cope with different precipitating situations (Keller and Nesse, 2006a). Before even addressing aetiology – proximate explanations for why one person gets pathological depression and another does not – an evolutionary approach addresses the more fundamental questions of why the capacity for low mood exists at all, how it is normally regulated, and how it is related to some cases of depression.

Is mood an adaptation? General evidence

The hypothesis that the capacity for mood is normal and useful is supported by its universality, as contrasted with abnormal phenomena such as seizures and hallucinations that most people never experience. So many people now assume that 'depression' refers to an abnormal state that the phrases low mood and high mood are adopted here to describe the range from despair to elation without any implication of normality or abnormality.

Stronger evidence that the capacity for mood is an adaptation is provided by the close regulation of mood by the fitness implications of a situation. Fast progress towards a valued resource elicits positive mood; lack of progress lowers mood. Selection can shape regulation systems only for traits important to fitness, such as breathing and anxiety. The stimuli that influence mood are less tangible than those that regulate breathing, but there is no doubt that mood is carefully regulated (Brown and Harris, 1978; Larsen, 2000; Monroe and Simons, 1991; Thayer, 1996).

Direct evidence for the utility of a response is provided by individuals who lack the capacity. For instance, and as discussed above, individuals born with no capacity for pain experience accumulating damage that causes death by early adulthood (Rosemberg et al. 1994; Sternbach, 1963). It would be difficult to distinguish individuals who lack low mood from the merely fortunate. Nonetheless, if mood is useful, then individuals who lack a capacity for low mood have a disorder. If and when we discover drugs that reliably block low mood, this will make it possible to study the functions of low mood directly. In the meanwhile, insight comes from the problems caused by hypomania (Doran, 2008). Inability to experience low mood results not only in social complications, but also in tendencies to make impulsive decisions and to start too many projects. Whether it results in persisting too long in fruitless enterprises is yet to be conformed.

The evolutionary origins of low mood

The above background guides correct formulation of the core question: In what kinds of situations arising repeatedly over evolutionary history would individuals with a capacity for low mood get a fitness advantage? On the face of it, pessimism, lack of initiative, low self-worth, and fatigue seem worse than useless. However, in situations when all possible actions will bring costs greater than benefits, the best thing to do is . . . nothing.

A seminal article by Klinger (1975) initiated modern work on mood as an adaptation that regulates goal pursuit. He noted that rapid progress towards a goal arouses high mood that motivates continued effort and risk-taking. When efforts to reach a goal are failing, low mood motivates pulling back to conserve resources and reconsider options. If conditions do not improve and no other strategy is viable, low mood disengages motivation from the unreachable goal so efforts can be turned to more productive activities. If the individual persists in pursuing an unreachable goal, ordinary negative affect can escalate into pathological depression.

In a series of articles (1983; 1990) and a book (1998), Carver and Scheier outline a control theory model supported by experimental data showing that mood is influenced mainly, not by levels of resources or payoffs, but by the rate of approach to a goal. In a particularly important finding, negative mood is aroused more readily by obstacles encountered in pursuit of positive goals than it is by the inability to escape dangers (Carver, 2004). This challenges models for depression based only on stress and losses (Blanchard et al. 1993), and suggests deeper attention to personal goals and the BAS.

Many are now studying the exigencies that arise in the pursuit of personal goals (Emmons, 1999; Emmons and King, 1988; Little, 2000). Klinger calls these 'current concerns', Little calls them problems arising in 'personal projects' (Little, 2006), while others focus on 'possible selves' (Cantor, 1990; Oyserman and Markus, 1990). Studies of the life course document increasing distress as it becomes apparent that a goal, such as having children, will not be met. When the goal is finally given up, negative affect decreases abruptly (Heckhausen et al. 2001). Other studies show that the impact of a life event depends profoundly on an individual's values (Diener and Fujita, 1995), and life context (Brown and Harris, 1978; Finlay-Jones and Brown, 1981; Monroe and Simons, 1991).

Why do people persist in pursuing unreachable goals? Each of several reasons is a different pathway to depression. Extreme ambition may leave a person dissatisfied even with exceptional achievements. A wish to please everyone is a common unreachable goal, as is trying to reform an abusive or alcoholic partner. Anxiety can prevent taking the risks necessary to escape an untenable life situation. Even without these factors, many people find themselves trapped pursuing an unattainable goal. The word 'goal' suggests tangible things such as getting a job, but many of life's largest goals are more personal, such as getting a spouse to be affectionate, finding sexual satisfaction, pleasing a parent, becoming recognized as a poet, or helping a child to get off drugs. Giving up such goals can mean giving up what gives meaning to life and a social identity.

Individuals differ in their general ability to disengage from unreachable goals (Wrosch and Scheier, 2003). Those more capable of giving up are less prone to low mood, as are those who reengage more quickly after a loss (Wrosch et al. 2003). These findings challenge the conventional wisdom that persistence is always wise, and they suggest studies to determine whether depression remission often follows finding a new strategy or giving up a goal. Existing evidence finds depression much more prevalent in women who have experienced a 'fresh start' event (Brown et al. 1992).

The general idea that low mood arises when desires cannot be satisfied is by no means new (Nussbaum, 1994). What is new is trying to understand how the capacity for mood was shaped by its ability to increase fitness in certain situations. The most general answer is: *mood regulates patterns of resource investment as a function of propitiousness* (Nesse, 1991; 1999b; 2000). In a propitious environment, small investments offer big payoffs, so high mood and risk-taking increase fitness. In an unpropitious environment, costs and risks are greater than benefits, so low mood and anxiety increase fitness.

Payoffs vary across time and projects. As one activity continues, such as foraging, marginal benefits decline. When benefits from the current activity become lower than those for an alternative, behaviour shifts to the next activity. Charnov's marginal value theorem shows that the optimal time for an animal to quit foraging in one location and move to another is when the rate of return from the current patch declines below the average rate of return over several patches (1976). Scores of experiments show that even simple organisms make good decisions about when to move to a new patch (Real and Caraco, 1986; Stephens and Krebs, 1986). Related mechanisms regulate the decision to quit foraging altogether. As the evening air cools, bumblebees eventually spend more calories per minute than they gain. At that point, the best thing to do is to stop and wait for more propitious conditions (Heinrich, 1979).

Humans are more complicated. We pursue multiple long-term goals simultaneously. Success depends on judiciously allocating effort among diverse enterprises, including getting material resources, getting and keeping a partner, taking care of children, making and keeping friends, and gaining social status. They often conflict, so life is difficult. When a strategy is not working, low mood disengages effort and motivates consideration of other ways to reach the goal (Gut, 1989). If no strategy seems likely to work, motivation disengages from that enterprise, and shifts effort to another. If pursuit of an unreachable goal continues, ordinary low mood can escalate into severe depression (Gut, 1989; Klinger, 1975).

Note that low mood is elicited not by stress or losses, but by inability to make progress towards an important goal. After a loss, sadness can improve coping and prevent additional losses (Nesse, 2005a). Sadness and low mood are phenomenologically similar, and they are often associated because losses often disrupt strategies for getting crucial resources, but they correspond to different situations.

Anxiety and low mood are also highly comorbid. When loss is likely, anxiety is useful. Failing efforts to preserve a major life enterprise, such as a marriage or a job, are likely to arouse anxiety (because of the threat of loss) and low mood (because efforts to prevent the loss are failing). Comorbidity of depression and anxiety can also arise from the risks of leaving an intolerable job or marriage (Maser and Cloninger, 1990).

The above generic theory has several more domain-specific versions. One group, starting from ethological observations (Price, 1967), has emphasized an inability to yield in status competitions as the crucial situation that gives rise to depression (Gilbert, 1992; Gilbert and Allan, 1998; Price and Sloman, 1987; Price et al. 1994). They interpret depression as 'involuntary yielding behavior' that stops attacks by dominants. This makes important links with social competition (Price et al. 1994) and it helps to explain social aspects of depression symptoms, such as low self-esteem. It is also supported by reanalyses of life events data showing that depression is precipitated not by stress in general, but by events that involve being trapped or humiliated (Brown et al. 1995; Kendler et al. 2003). So far, we lack data on what percentage of depressions arise mainly from losing status competitions.

Watson and Andrews (2002) have suggested that depression guides 'social navigation' by manipulating others. They also suggest that depression can focus cognitive effort on solving social problems, an idea also proposed by Gut (1989) and Bibring (1953). Hagen argues that depression itself and even suicidal tendencies are adaptations to manipulate others to get resources at crucial times such as birth of a child (2002). Allen and Badcock (2003) argue that depression is useful in situations that involve high risk of exclusion from a social group, to signal submission and motivate actions that will make one accepted by the group. These views have been criticized by Nettle (2004) who argues, as I do, that serious depression is rarely useful. He instead emphasizes the vulnerability of any system that depends on many genes (Keller and Miller, 2006) and the possibility that tendencies to negative emotions may have been selected because they motivate high ambition (Ross et al. 2001).

The different subtypes of anxiety aroused by different dangers (Marks and Nesse, 1994) suggests that selection could also have shaped subtypes of depression to deal with problems in different domains. Data confirming this nonobvious prediction support the more general hypothesis that depression symptoms are adaptive. Two preliminary studies found significant differences in depression symptoms depending on the precipitant (Keller and Nesse, 2005; 2006b). Not only are the symptoms remarkably different depending on the cause, the patterns are congruent with functional expectations. In a larger replication, bereavement and romantic break-ups were associated with sadness, anhedonia, appetite loss, and guilt, while chronic stress and failures were associated with fatigue and hypersomnia (Keller et al. 2007b). If different depression symptoms have different functions, studying depression as a single syndrome may conceal more important phenomena.

Why so vulnerable?

Over 10% of people in the United States experience serious depression, many during early adulthood when other chronic diseases are rare (Kessler et al. 1997). Why has natural selection left the mood regulation system so vulnerable to failure? Each of the six categories from Darwinian medicine (Nesse and Williams, 1994) offers possible explanations (see text box 3.3).

Modern environments may increase the risk of depression, although no reliable data allow comparisons with hunter-gatherer populations (Cordain et al. 2002). Depressogenic situations may be especially common in modern life because goals are far larger and longer in duration than those the regulation mechanism was shaped for (Nesse, 2000). Physical factors such as artificial light, and changes in exercise and diet that can directly influence brain mechanisms also deserve consideration (Frasure-Smith et al. 2004).

Infectious causes are likely given the link between inflammatory cytokines and depression (Pollak and Yirmiya, 2002; Schiepers et al. 2005). A large literature documents the utility of 'sickness behavior' in animals (Hart, 1990). During an infection, effort and conflict are best avoided. Specific organisms are rarely identified, although Borna virus may cause a few cases (Bode and Ludwig, 2003). Another factor may be autoimmune reactions resulting from lack of childhood exposure to the diversity of pathogens found in more natural human environments (Rook and Lowry, 2008).

Constraints on what selection can accomplish are relevant. For instance, complex traits such as the ability to regulate mood, tend to have high variance that leaves some individuals at pathological extremes (Keller and Miller, 2006).

Tradeoffs are probably important. Low mood has costs, lost opportunities at the very least. Inappropriate high mood results in taking risks and wasting energy that may have been even more costly. Vulnerability to depression could also result if individuals who struggle especially hard to avoid failure tend, on average, to be especially successful (Nettle, 2004; Ross et al. 2001).

Finally, there is the possibility, emphasized here, that depression is prevalent because human social life routinely results in substantial numbers of individuals getting trapped pursuing unreachable goals. The proportion should vary substantially depending on cultural factors, and this variation may help to explain cultural differences in depression rates.

Why are some people more vulnerable to depression than others? This question at the centre of much neuroscience research, is entirely different from the question of why depression exists, but an evolutionary perspective may be useful nonetheless. One possibility is that differences in baseline mood, and differences in the gain setting for mood regulation systems, may have little influence on fitness. For instance, 5HT-related polymorphisms that increase the risk of depression in response to life events (Caspi et al. 2003), interferon (Kraus et al. 2007), and tryptophan depletion (Jans et al. 2006) may offer benefits in some circumstances; they should not be assumed to be defects (Barr et al. 2004). A polymorphism that is associated with decreased synthesis of IL-6 protects against depression caused by interferon treatment (Bull et al. 2008); one wonders if individuals with this polymorphism might be more vulnerable to infection.

Finally, there is the question of how to understand the effects of stressors on mood regulation mechanisms. They are usually interpreted as 'kindling' (Post and Weiss, 1998) or otherwise damaging the system. However, the body has many facultative adaptations that adapt individuals to their environments. For instance, early heat exposure increases the number of sweat glands. Each additional depression episode seems to reduce the threshold for further episodes (Kendler et al. 2000). This may well reflect damage of the same sort that causes chronic pain. It is conceivable, however, that it is related to a system that adapts the depression threshold based on experience in the social environment.

Bipolar disorder needs a separate analysis, but increasing evidence that many depressives have bipolar tendencies is clearly important (Akiskal, 2003). At the very least, it calls attention to the tight links between the BIS and BAS. A control theory approach suggests the existence of a feed-forward mechanism to prevent overshoot by dampening mood even as it rises, and increasing mood soon after it falls (Nesse, 2006). Failure of such a mechanism would explain many aspects of bipolar disorder. It is worth noting that this book dedicates three chapters to bipolar disorder, and in particular to the similarities and dissimilarities between unipolar and bipolar disorders (see Chapters 6, 21, and 22).

Practical implications

While we await stronger conclusions about the evolutionary origins and functions of low mood, an evolutionary approach has practical implications for depression research strategies.

Measure and analyse specific symptoms, not just depression

Diagnostic algorithms collapse multiple variables into a binary datum. Depression scales collapse multiple symptoms into a single continuous variable. If depression was unitary, these data reduction strategies would be sensible. However, different precipitants arouse different symptoms (Keller et al. 2007a), so analysing specific symptoms is essential, as is measuring the domain of the precipitant.

Study etiological subtypes of depression

It has been hard to define depression subtypes based on aetiology, although attempts are being made on the basis of patterns of neuroendocrine changes (Antonijevic, 2006). Basing subtypes on the category of precipitant is a strategy worth considering. Another is to define categories based on the several ways a defensive response can become dysregulated. As shown in the text box below (Box 3.4), a normal regulation mechanism does not guarantee that the response will be useful, and etiological subtypes of depression correspond to different mechanism abnormalities.

Put depression diagnostic criteria on a scientific foundation

The diagnosis of DSM-IV Major Depression ignores context, with the telling exception of grief (American Psychiatric Association, 1994). However, if low mood can be useful, then distinguishing normal from pathological responses requires considering context (Horwitz and Wakefield, 2007; Nesse and Jackson, 2006). Searching systematically for situations that could cause low mood would make the clinical evaluation of depression like that for other medical problems, such as pain, fever, and fatigue, that are investigated by considering what may be arousing the defence.

Gather data on motivational structure

The evidence that severe life events precipitate depression is overwhelming (Brown et al. 1988; Caspi et al. 2003; Finlay-Jones and Brown, 1981; Kessler, 1997; Monroe and Simons, 1991). Research has moved steadily from life event checklists to methods that take account of the individual's life context (Monroe and Simons, 1991; Paykel, 2001). This parallels recognition in psychology that emotions are elicited not just by cues, but by an individual's appraisal of what information means for ability to reach personal goals (Ellsworth, 1991; Scherer et al. 2001).

Behavioural ecology has well-established categories for the resources organisms need: somatic resources (personal health, attractiveness and ability, and material resources), reproductive resources (a mate and offspring), and social resources (allies and status) (Krebs and Davies, 1991). Mood is influenced by an individual's ability to get these resources, the gaps between resources and personal goals, and how individuals cope with these gaps. We need instruments to measure the motivational structure of individuals' lives. Such measures would have immediate applications. For instance, how do individuals trapped pursuing an unreachable goal compare to others on HPA axis abnormalities, agitated depression symptoms, and drug response?

Box 3.4 Etiological subtypes based on regulation mechanism status

1. Regulation mechanism is normal; low mood is useful in this specific instance
2. Regulation mechanism is normal; low mood is useless or harmful in this specific instance
3. Regulation mechanism threshold or gain is abnormal; depression symptoms are excessive or deficient
4. Regulation mechanism is fundamentally abnormal; depression symptoms arise without a precipitant, or in response to a situation that should not lower mood
5. Secondary complications of depression, such as complications of weight loss
6. Depression arising from mechanisms unrelated to those that normally regulate mood

Consider the many ways genes can influence vulnerability

About 40% of the vulnerability to depression can be attributed to genetic differences (Levinson, 2006; Sullivan et al. 2000), however, no locus accounts for more than a few percentage of the variation (Holmans et al. 2007). Epigenetics and heterogeneity offer possible explanations (Caspi et al. 2003; Levinson, 2006). However, thousands of genes influence the brain systems that regulate mood, so polymorphisms at many loci will influence depression vulnerability. Why none have major effects remains a good evolutionary question. One possible answer is that polymorphisms with large effects on mood may have been selected out.

A second implication is that genes may influence depression by complex indirect pathways. One comprehensive developmental model considers 64 pathways (Sullivan et al. 2000), however, other pathways may be even less direct. For instance, diet and exercise influence depression (Duman, 2005), so genetic variations that influence food or exercise preferences (Heller et al. 1988) should influence mood. Likewise, any polymorphism that increases the likelihood of becoming trapped in the pursuit of an unreachable life goal should contribute to depression.

Animal models

The Porsolt test uses rat swimming behaviour to identify promising new drugs; longer swimming is presumed to indicate delayed onset of helplessness (Petit-Demouliere et al. 2005). But when rats stop swimming they do not drown, they just float, a fine adaptive strategy. Rats on antidepressants swim more than is optimal; in a natural environment they would drown sooner (Nadeau, 1999). New strategies for drug discovery may emerge from animal models based on goal pursuit. Animal models of depression are discussed in several chapters of this book (see Chapters 7–12).

Study functional effects of antidepressants

Much research on antidepressants presumes that they normalize some aspect of neurochemistry (Barden et al. 1995). However, if some depression is an excessive response from a normal system, then antidepressants may act by blocking the low mood system at various loci in the same ways that analgesics block pain. Antidepressants usually do not cause euphoria for the same reason that aspirin does not lower body temperature below normal. The common phylogenetic origins of pain, anxiety, and low mood in the BIS may explain why antidepressants tend to be useful for blocking diverse defensive responses. The last chapter of this book (Chapter 27) illustrates the future directions for antidepressants research.

Conclusion

Mainstream research on the causes of depression has been making full use of only one half of biology. Asking evolutionary as well as proximate questions should speed progress, especially for disorders such as depression that can arise from dysregulation of useful responses. The above proposals about specific functions of low mood and its relationship to depression need much more work before they can be considered confirmed. The broad thesis of this article is not that we know why depression exists, it is that seeking the answer will bring major advances.

This perspective is prone to misunderstanding. The utility of some low mood does not imply that we should not treat depression. Quite the contrary. Much of general medicine consists of relieving suffering by blocking pain, cough, and other aversive symptoms even when they are normal responses to a problem whose source is still being sought. Furthermore, the utility of some low mood is fully compatible with the hypothesis that some clinical depression arises from abnormal brain mechanisms, and most arises from interactions of brain variations with environmental situations. There is nothing radical about an evolutionary approach to mood disorders, and the enterprise should not be viewed as controversial, although straightforward reasoning from well-established evolutionary principles can yield surprising conclusions. More important, it suggests specific new research that is badly needed.

Acknowledgements

Thanks to the Berlin Institute for Advanced Study for a Fellowship that made preparation of this chapter possible.

References

Adler, J. (1966). Chemotaxis in bacteria. *Science*, **153**, 708–716.

Akiskal, H.S. (2003). The evolutionary significance of affective temperaments. *American Psychiatric Association Annual Meeting*, San Francisco, May 17–22.

Alcock, J. (1993). *Animal Behavior: An Evolutionary Approach*. Sunderland, MA, Sinauer.

Alcock, J. (1998). Unpunctuated equilibrium in the natural history essays of Stephen Jay Gould. *Evolution and Human Behavior*, **19**, 321–336.

Alcock, J. (2001). *The Triumph of Sociobiology*. New York, Oxford University Press.

Alcock, J. (2005). *Animal Behavior: An Evolutionary Approach*. Sunderland, MA, Sinauer.

Alcock, J. and Sherman, P. (1994). The utility of the proximate-ultimate dichotomy in ethology. *Ethology*, **96**, 58–62.

Allen, N.B. and Badcock, P.B.T. (2003). The social risk hypothesis of depressed mood: evolutionary, psychosocial and neurobiological perspectives. *Psychological Bulletin*, **129**, 887–913.

American Psychiatric Association (1994). *Diagnostic and Statistical Manual of Mental Disorders*. Fourth Edition (DSM-IV). Washington, DC, APA Press.

Antonijevic, I.A. (2006). Depressive disorders – is it time to endorse different pathophysiologies? *Psychoneuroendocrinology*, **31**, 1–15.

Barden, N., Reul, J.M.H.M., and Holsboer, F. (1995). Do antidepressants stabilize mood through actions on the hypothalamic-pituitary-adrenocortical system? *Trends in Neurosciences*, **18**, 6–11.

Barnes, N.M. and Sharp, T. (1999). A review of central 5-HT receptors and their function. *Neuropharmacology*, **38**, 1083–1152.

Barr, C.S., Newman, T.K., Schwandt, M. et al. (2004). Sexual dichotomy of an interaction between early adversity and the serotonin transporter gene promoter variant in rhesus macaques. *Proceedings of the National Academy of Sciences, US A*, **101**, 12358–12363.

Barrett, L.F. (2006). Valence as a basic building block of emotional life. *Journal of Research in Personality*, **40**, 35–55.

Beckhoff, M. and Allen, C. (1995). Teleology, function, design and the evolution of animal behavior. *Trends in Ecology and Evolution*, **10**, 253–255.

Berridge, K.C. (2004). Motivation concepts in behavioral neuroscience. *Physiology and Behavior*, **81**, 179–209.

Bibring, E. (1953). The mechanisms of depression. In Greenacre, P. (ed.) *Affective Disorders*. New York, International Universities Press.

Blanchard, R.J., Yudko, E.B., Rodgers, R.J., and Blanchard, D.C. (1993). Defense system psychopharmacology: an ethological approach to the pharmacology of fear and anxiety. *Behavioural Brain Research*, **58**, 155–165.

Bode, L. and Ludwig, H. (2003). Borna disease virus infection, a human mental-health risk. *Clinical Microbiology Reviews*, **16**, 534–545.

Borgia, G. (1994). The scandals of San Marco. *The Quarterly Review of Biology*, **69**, 373–375.

Brown, G.W. and Harris, T. (1978). *Social Origins of Depression.* New York, The Free Press.

Brown, G., Adler, Z., and Bilfulco, A. (1988). Life events, difficulties and recovery from chronic depression. *British Journal of Psychiatry, 152,* 487–498.

Brown, G.W., Lemyre, L., and Bifulco, A. (1992). Social factors and recovery from anxiety and depressive disorders. A test of specificity. *British Journal of Psychiatry, 161,* 44–54.

Brown, G.W., Harris, T.O., and Hepworth, C. (1995). Loss, humiliation and entrapment among women developing depression: a patient and non-patient comparison. *Psychological Medicine, 25,* 7–21.

Bull, S.J., Huezo-Diaz, P., Binder, E.B . et al. (2008). Functional polymorphisms in the interleukin-6 and serotonin transporter genes, and depression and fatigue induced by interferon-alpha and ribavirin treatment . *Molecular Psychiatry,* epub Pay 6, doi: 10.1038/mp2008.48.

Butler, A.B. and Hodos, W. (1996). *Comparative Vertebrate Neuroanatomy.* New York, John Wiley and Sons.

Cannon, W.B. (1914). The emergency function of the adrenal medulla in pain and the major emotions. *American Journal of Physiology, 33,* 356–372.

Cantor, N. (1990). From thought to behavior: 'Having' and 'doing' in the study of personality and cognition. *American Psychologist, 45,* 735–750.

Carver, C.S. and Scheier, M.F. (1983). *Attention and Self-Regulation: A Control Theory Approach to Human Behavior.* New York, Springer-Verlag.

Carver, C.S. and Scheier, M.F. (1990). Origins and functions of positive and negative affect: a control-process view. *Psychological Review, 97,* 19–35.

Carver, C.S. and Scheier, M. (1998). *On the Self-Regulation of Behavior.* Cambridge and New York, Cambridge University Press.

Carver, C.S. (2004). Negative affects deriving from the behavioral approach system. *Emotion, 4,* 3–22.

Caspi, A., Sugden, K., Moffitt, T.E . et al. (2003). Influence of life stress on depression: moderation by a polymorphism in the 5-HTT gene. *Science, 301,* 386–389.

Charnov, E.L. (1976). Optimal foraging: the marginal value theorem. *Theoretical and Population Biology, 9,* 129–136.

Childs, B. (1999). *Genetic Medicine: A Logic of Disease.* Baltimore, MD, Johns Hopkins University Press.

Cordain, L., Eaton, S.B., Miller, J.B., Mann, N., and Hill, K. (2002). The paradoxical nature of hunter-gatherer diets: meat-based, yet non-atherogenic. *European Journal of Clinical Nutrition, 56,* S42–S52.

Crespi, B.J. (2000). The evolution of maladaptation. *Heredity, 84* (Pt 6), 623–629.

Dewsbury, D.A. (1999). The proximate and the ultimate: past, present and future. *Behavioural Process, 46,* 189–199.

Diener, E. and Fujita, F. (1995). Resources, personal strivings, and subjective well-being: a nomothetic ideographic approach. *Journal of Personality and Social Psychology, 68,* 926–935.

Doran, C.M. (2008). *The Hypomania Handbook: The Challenge of Elevated Mood.* Philadelphia., Wolters Kluwer Health/Lippincott Williams and Wilkins.

Duman, R.S. (2005). Neurotrophic factors and regulation of mood: role of exercise, diet and metabolism. *Neurobiology of Aging, 26,* 88–93.

Ekman, P. (1992). An argument for basic emotions. *Cognition and Emotion, 6,* 169–200.

Ellsworth, P. (1991). Some implications for cognitive appraisal theories of emotion. In Strongman, K.T. (ed.) *International Review of Studies of Emotion.* Chishester, Wiley.

Emmons, R.A. (1999). *The Psychology of Ultimate Concerns: Motivation and Spirituality in Personality.* New York, Guilford Press.

Emmons, R.A. and King, L.A. (1988). Conflict among personal strivings: immediate and long-term implications for psychological and physical well-being. *Journal of Personality and Social Psychology, 54,* 1040–1048.

Finch, C.E. (2007). *The Biology of Human Longevity: Inflammation, Nutrition, and Aging in the Evolution of Lifespans.* Burlington, MA, Academic Press.

Finlay-Jones, R. and Brown, G. (1981). Types of stressful life events and the onset of anxiety and depression. *Psychological Medicine,* **11**, 803–815.

Frank, S.A. (2007). *Dynamics of Cancer: Incidence, Inheritance, and Evolution.* Princeton, NJ, Princeton University Press.

Frasure-Smith, N., Lesperance, F., and Julien, P. (2004). Major depression is associated with lower omega-3 fatty acid levels in patients with recent acute coronary syndromes. *Biological Psychiatry,* **55**, 891–896.

Fryxell, K. (1995). The evolutionary divergence of neurotransmitter receptors and second-messenger pathways. *Journal of Molecular Evolution,* **41**, 85–97.

Gazzaniga, M.S. (ed.) (1995). *The Cognitive Neurosciences.* Cambridge, MA., Bradford, MIT Press.

Gazzaniga, M.S. (2004). *The Cognitive Neurosciences III.* Bradford Book .

Gilbert, P. (1992). *Depression: The Evolution of Powerlessness.* New York, Guilford.

Gilbert, P. and Allan, S. (1998). The role of defeat and entrapment (arrested flight) in depression: an exploration of an evolutionary view. *Psychological Medicine,* **28**, 585–598.

Glenn, N.R. and Kaas, J.H. (1995). The emergence and evolution of mammalian neocortex. *Trends in Neurosciences,* **18**, 373–379.

Gould, S.J. and Lewontin, R.C. (1979). The spandrels of San Marco and the Panglossian paradigm: a critique of the adaptationist programme. *Proceedings of the Royal Society London,* **205**, 581–598.

Grant, P.R. (1999). *Ecology and Evolution of Darwin's Finches.* Princeton, NJ, Princeton University Press.

Gray, J.A. (1987). *Fear and Stress.* Cambridge, Cambridge University Press.

Greaves, M. (2002). Cancer causation: the Darwinian downside of past success? *Lancet Oncology,* **3**, 244–251.

Gut, E. (1989). *Productive and Unproductive Depression.* New York, Basic Books.

Hagen, E.H. (2002). Depression as bargaining: the case postpartum. *Evolution and Human Behavior,* **23**, 323–336.

Halbreich, U. (2006). Major depression is not a diagnosis, it is a departure point to differential diagnosis – clinical and hormonal considerations: (A commentary and elaboration on Antonejevic's paper). *Psychoneuroendocrinology,* **31**, 16–22.

Hart, B.L. (1990). Behavioral adaptations to pathogens and parasites: five strategies. *Neuroscience and Biobehavioral Reviews,* **14**, 273–294.

Heckhausen, J., Wrosch, C., and Fleeson, W. (2001). Developmental regulation before and after a developmental deadline: the sample case of 'biological clock' for childbearing. *Psychology of Aging,* **16**, 400–413.

Heinrich, B. (1979). *Bumblebee Economics.,* Cambridge, Harvard University Press.

Heller, R.F., O'connell, D.L., Roberts, D.C. et al. (1988). Lifestyle factors in monozygotic and dizygotic twins. *Genetic Epidemiology,* **5**, 311–321.

Holmans, P., Weissman, M.M., Zubenko, G.S. et al. (2007). Genetics of recurrent early-onset major depression (GenRED): final genome scan report. *American Journal of Psychiatry,* **164**, 248–258.

Horwitz, A.V. and Wakefield, J.C. (2007). *The Loss of Sadness: How Psychiatry Transformed Normal Sorrow into Depressive Disorder.* New York, Oxford University Press. http://evmedreview.com (2008).

Jans, L.A.W., Riedel, W.J., Markus, C.R., and Blokland, A. (2007). Serotonergic vulnerability and depression: assumptions, experimental evidence and implications. *Molecular Psychiatry,* **12**, 522–543.

Kandel, E.R., Schwartz, J.H., and Jessell, T.M. (2000). *Principles of Neural Science.* New York, McGraw-Hill, Health Professions Division.

Keller, M.C. and Miller, G. (2006). Resolving the paradox of common, harmful, heritable mental disorders: which evolutionary genetic models work best? *Behavioral and Brain Sciences,* **29**, 385–404.

Keller, M.C. and Nesse, R.M. (2005). Is low mood an adaptation? Evidence for subtypes with symptoms that match precipitants. *Journal of Affective Disorders, 86*, 27–35.

Keller, M.C. and Nesse, R.M. (2006a). The evolutionary significance of depressive symptoms: different adverse situations lead to different depressive symptom patterns. *Journal of Personality and Social Psychology, 91*, 316–330.

Keller, M.C. and Nesse, R.M. (2006b). The evolutionary significance of depressive symptoms: different adverse situations lead to different depressive symptom patterns. *Journal of Personality and Social Psychology, 91*, 316–330.

Keller, M.C., Neale, M.C., and Kendler, K.S. (2007a). Association of different adverse life events with distinct patterns of depressive symptoms. *The American Journal of Psychiatry, 164*, 1521–1529.

Keller, M.C., Neale, M.C., and Kendler, K.S. (2007b). Association of different adverse life events with distinct patterns of depressive symptoms. *American Journal of Psychiatry, 164*, 1521.

Keltner, D., Oatley, K., and Jenkins, J.M. (2006). *Understanding Emotions.* Oxford, UK, Blackwell Publishing.

Kendler, K.S., Hettema, J.M., Butera, F., Gardner, C.O., and Prescott, C.A. (2003). Life event dimensions of loss, humiliation, entrapment, and danger in the prediction of onsets of major depression and generalized anxiety. *Archives of General Psychiatry, 60*, 789–796.

Kendler, K.S., Thornton, L.M., and Gardner, C.O. (2000). Stressful life events and previous episodes in the etiology of major depression in women: an evaluation of the 'kindling' hypothesis. *American Journal of Psychiatry, 157*, 1243–1251.

Kendler, K.S. (2005). Toward a philosophical structure for psychiatry. *American Journal of Psychiatry, 162*, 433–440.

Kessler, R.C. (1997). The effects of stressful life events on depression. *Annual Review of Psychology, 48*, 191–214.

Kessler, R.C., Zhao, S., Blazer, D.G., and Swartz, M. (1997). Prevalence, correlates, and course of minor depression and major depression in the National Comorbidity Survey. *Journal of Affective Disorders, 45*, 19–30.

Klinger, E. (1975). Consequences of commitment to and disengagement from incentives. *Psychological Review, 82*, 1–25.

Kraus, M.R., Al-Taie, O., Schafer, A., Pfersdorff, M., Lesch, K.-P., and Scheurlen, M. (2007). Serotonin-1A receptor gene HTR1A variation predicts interferon-induced depression in chronic Hepatitis C. *Gastroenterology, 132*, 1279–1286.

Krebs, J. and Davies, N. (1991). *Behavioral Ecology: An Evolutionary Approach.* Oxford, Blackwell.

Krebs, J.R. and Davies, N.B. (eds) (1984). *Behavioural Ecology: An Evolutionary Approach.* Sunderland, MA, Sunderland.

Krebs, J.R. and Davies, N.B. (1997). *Behavioural Ecology: An Evolutionary Approach.* Oxford, Blackwell Science.

Larsen, R.J. (2000). Toward a science of mood regulation. *Psychological Inquiry, 11*, 129–141.

Larsen, S.H., Reader, R.W., Kort, E.N., Tso, W.-W., and Adler, J. (1974). Change in direction of flagellar rotation is the basis of the chemotactic response in Escherichia coli. *Nature, 249*, 74–77.

Lee, W.E., Wadsworth, M.E.J., and Hotopf, M. (2006). The protective role of trait anxiety: a longitudinal cohort study. *Psychological Medicine, 36*, 345–351.

Levinson, D.F. (2006). The genetics of depression: a review. *Biological Psychiatry, 60*, 84–92.

Little, B.R. (2000). Persons, contexts, and personal projects: assumptive themes of a methodological transactionalism. In Wapner, S. (ed.) *Theoretical Perspectives in Environment Behavior Research: Underlying Assumptions, Research Problems, and Methodologies.* New York, NY, Kluwer Academic/Plenum Publishers.

Little, B.R. (2006). Personality science and self-regulation: personal projects as integrative units. *Applied Psychology, 55*, 419–427.

Mace, R., Jordan, F., and Holden, C. (2003). Testing evolutionary hypotheses about human biological adaptation using cross-cultural comparison. *Comparative Biochemistry and Physiology. Part A, Molecular & Integrative Physiology,* **136**, 85–94.

Marks, I.M. and Nesse, R.M. (1994). Fear and fitness: an evolutionary analysis of anxiety disorders. *Ethology and Sociobiology,* **15**, 247–261.

Maser, J. and Cloninger, R. (eds) (1990). *Comorbidity of Mood and Anxiety Disorders.* Washington, D.C, American Psychiatric Press.

Mayberg, H.S., Liotti, M., Brannan, S.K. et al. (1999). Reciprocal limbic-cortical function and negative mood: converging PET findings in depression and normal sadness. *American Journal of Psychiatry,* **156**, 675–682.

Mayr, E. (1982). *The Growth of Biological Thought: Diversity, Evolution, and Inheritance.* Cambridge, MA, The Belknap Press of Harvard University Press.

Mayr, E. (1983). How to carry out the adaptationist program? *American Naturalist,* **121**, 324–333.

Mcguire, M.T. and Troisi, A. (1998). *Darwinian Psychiatry* Cambridge, MA, . Harvard University Press.

Moncrieff, J. (2007). Rebuttal: depression is not a brain disease. *Canadian Journal of Psychiatry,* **52**, 100.

Monroe, S.M. and Simons, A.D. (1991). Diathesis-stress theories in the context of life stress research: implications for the depressive disorders. *Psychological Bulletin,* **110**, 406–425.

Nadeau, B. (1999). The forced swim test: an empirical and rational analysis of immobility and its reduction by antidepressants. *Department of Psychology.* Vancouver, BC, Simon Fraser University.

Nesse, R.M. (1987). An evolutionary perspective on panic disorder and agoraphobia. *Ethology and Sociobiology,* **8**, 73–83.

Nesse, R.M. (1990). Evolutionary explanations of emotions. *Human Nature,* **1**, 261–289.

Nesse, R.M. (1991). What is mood for? *Psycholoquy,* **2**.

Nesse, R . (1999a). Proximate and evolutionary studies of anxiety, stress and depression: synergy at the interface. *Neuroscience and Biobehavioral Reviews,* **23**, 895–903.

Nesse, R.M. (1999b). The evolution of hope and despair. *Journal of Social Issues,* **66**, 429–469.

Nesse, R.M. (1999c). Proximate and evolutionary studies of anxiety, stress, and depression: synergy at the interface. *Neuroscience and Biobehavioral Reviews,* **23**, 895–903.

Nesse, R.M. (1999d). Testing evolutionary hypotheses about mental disorders. In Stearns, S. (ed.) *Evolution in Health and Disease.* New York, Oxford University Press.

Nesse, R.M. (2000). Is depression an adaptation? *Archives of General Psychiatry,* **57**, 14–20.

Nesse, R.M. (2004). Natural selection and the elusiveness of happiness. *Philosophical Transactions of the Royal Society of London. Series B, Biological Sciences,* **359**, 1333–1347.

Nesse, R.M. (2005a). An evolutionary framework for understanding grief. In Carr, D., Nesse, R., and Wortman, C.B. (eds.) *Late Life Widowhood in the United States.* New York, Springer.

Nesse, R.M. (2005b). Maladaptation and natural selection. *The Quarterly Review of Biology,* **80**, 62–70.

Nesse, R.M. (2005c). Natural selection and the regulation of defenses: a signal detection analysis of the smoke detector principle. *Evolution and Human Behavior,* **26**, 88–105.

Nesse, R.M. (2006). Evolutionary explanations for mood and mood disorders. In Stein, D.J., Kupfer, D.J., and Schatzberg, A.F. (eds.) *The American Psychiatric Publishing Textbook of Mood Disorders.* Washington, D.C, American Psychiatric Publishing.

Nesse, R.M. and Jackson, E.D. (2006). Evolution: psychiatric nosology's missing biological foundation. *Clinical Neuropsychiatry,* **3**, 121–131.

Nesse, R.M. and Stearns, S.C. (2008). The great opportunity: evolutionary applications to medicine and public health. *Evolutionary Applications,* **1**, 28–48.

Nesse, R.M. and Weder, A. (2007). Darwinian medicine: what evolutionary medicine offers to endothelium researchers. In Aird, W. (ed.) *Endothelial Biomedicine.* Cambridge, Cambridge University Press.

Nesse, R.M. and Williams, G.C. (1994). *Why We Get Sick: The New Science of Darwinian Medicine.* New York, Vintage Books.

Nettle, D. (2004). Evolutionary origins of depression: a review and reformulation. *Journal of Affective Disorders,* **81,** 91–102.

Nussbaum, M.C. (1994). *The Therapy of Desire: Theory and Practice in Hellenistic Ethics.* Princeton, Princeton University Press.

Oyserman, D. and Markus, H. (1990). Possible selves and delinquency. *Journal of Personality and Social Psychology,* **59,** 112–125.

Pagel, M. (1994). Detecting correlated evolution on phylogenies: a general method for the comparative analysis of discrete characters. *Proceedings: Biological Sciences,* **255,** 37–45.

Panksepp, J. (1998). *Affective Neuroscience: The Foundations of Human and Animal Emotions.* London, Oxford University Press.

Panksepp, J., Moskal, J., Panksepp, J.B., and Kroes, R. (2002). Comparative approaches in evolutionary psychology: molecular neuroscience meets the mind. *Neuroendocrinology Letters,* 23, 105–115.

Paykel, E.S. (2001). The evolution of life events research in psychiatry. *Journal of Affective Disorders,* **62,** 141–149.

Petit-Demouliere, B., Chenu, F., and Bourin, M. (2005). Forced swimming test in mice: a review of antidepressant activity. *Psychopharmacology,* **177,** 245–255.

Pigliucci, M. and Kaplan, J. (2000). The fall and rise of Dr Pangloss: adaptationism and the Spandrels paper 20 years later. *Trends in Ecology and Evolution,* **15,** 66–70.

Plutchik, R. (1980). *Emotion: A Psychoevolutionary Synthesis.* New York, Harper and Row.

Plutchik, R. (2003). *Emotions and Life: Perspectives from Psychology, Biology, and Evolution.* Washington, DC, American Psychological Association.

Pollak, Y. and Yirmiya, R. (2002). Cytokine-induced changes in mood and behaviour: implications for 'depression due to a general medical condition', immunotherapy and antidepressive treatment. *The International Journal of Neuropsychopharmacology,* **5,** 389–399.

Post, R.M. and Weiss, S.R. (1998). Sensitization and kindling phenomena in mood, anxiety, and obsessive-compulsive disorders: the role of serotonergic mechanisms in illness progression. *Biological Psychiatry,* **44,** 193–206.

Price, J., Sloman, L., Gardner, R., Gilbert, P., and Al, E. (1994). The social competition hypothesis of depression. *British Journal of Psychiatry,* **164,** 309–315.

Price, J.S. (1967). The dominance hierarchy and the evolution of mental illness. *Lancet,* 2, 243–246.

Price, J.S. and Sloman, L. (1987). Depression as yielding behavior: an animal model based on Schyelderup-Ebbe's pecking order. *Ethology and Sociobiology,* **8,** 85s–98s.

Queller, D.C. (1995). The spaniels of St. Marx and the panglossian paradox: a critique of a rhetorical programme. *The Quarterly Review of Biology,* **70,** 485–489.

Real, L. and Caraco, T. (1986). Risk and foraging in stochastic environments. *Annual Review of Ecology and Systematics,* **17,** 371–390.

Reeve, H.K. and Sherman, P.W. (1993). Adaptation and the goals of evolutionary research. *The Quarterly Review of Biology,* **68,** 1–32.

Rook, G.A.W. and Lowry, C.A. (2008). The hygiene hypothesis and psychiatric disorders. *Trends in Immunology,* **29,** 150–158.

Rose, M.R. and Lauder, G.V. (eds.) (1996). *Adaptation.* San Diego, Academic Press.

Rosemberg, S., Marie, S.K., and Kliemann, S. (1994). Congenital insensitivity to pain with anhidrosis (hereditary sensory and autonomic neuropathy type IV). *Pediatric Neurology,* **11,** 50–56.

Ross, S.R., Stewart, J., Mugge, M., and Fultz, B. (2001). The imposter phenomenon, achievement dispositions, and the five factor model. *Personality and Individual Differences,* **31,** 1347–1355.

Roth, J., Leroith, D., Shiloach, J., Rosenzweig, J.L., Lesniak, M.A., and Havrankova, J. (1982). The evolutionary origins of hormones, neurotransmitters, and other extracellular chemical messengers. *Seminars in Medicine of the Beth Israel Hospital, Boston,* **306,** 523–527.

Salamone, J.D., Correa, M., Mingote, S.M., and Weber, S.M. (2005). Beyond the reward hypothesis: alternative functions of nucleus accumbens dopamine. *Current Opinion in Pharmacology,* **5**, 34–41.

Scherer, K.R., Schorr, A., and Johnstone, T. (2001). *Appraisal Processes in Emotion: Theory, Methods, Research.* New York, Oxford University Press.

Schiepers, O.J.G., Wichers, M.C., and Maes, M. (2005). Cytokines and major depression. *Progress in Neuro-Psychopharmacology and Biological Psychiatry,* **29**, 201–217.

Segerstråle, U.C.O. (2000). *Defenders of the Truth: The Battle for Science in the Sociobiology Debate and Beyond.* New York, Oxford University Press.

Selzer, J. (ed.) (1993). *Understanding Scientific Prose.* Madison, University of Wisconsin.

Stearns, S.C. and Ebert, D. (2001). Evolution in health and disease. *Quarterly Review of Biology,* **76**, 417–432.

Stearns, S.C. and Hoekstra, R.F. (2005). *Evolution: An Introduction.* Oxford [England], New York, Oxford University Press.

Stearns, S.C. and Koella, J.K. (eds.) (2007) *Evolution in Health and Disease.* Second Edition, Oxford, Oxford University Press.

Stearns, S.C., Nesse, R.M., and Haig, D. (2007). Introducing evolutionary thinking to medicine. In Stearns, S.C. and Koella, J.K. (eds.) *Evolution in Health and Disease.* Second Edition. Oxford, Oxford University Press.

Stephens, D.W. and Krebs, J.R. (1986). *Foraging Theory.* Princeton, NJ, Princeton University Press.

Sternbach, R.A. (1963). Congenital insensitivity to pain. *Psychological Bulletin,* **60**, 252–264.

Sullivan, P.F., Neale, M.C., and Kendler, K.S. (2000). Genetic epidemiology of major depression: review and meta-analysis. *American Journal of Psychiatry,* **157**, 1552–1562.

Takahashi, A. and Kawauchi, H. (2006). Evolution of melanocortin systems in fish. *General and Comparative Endocrinology,* **148**, 85–94.

Thayer, R.E. (1996). *The Origin of Everyday Moods.* New York, Oxford University Press.

Tinbergen, N. (1963). On the aims and methods of ethology. *Zeitschrift für Tierpsychologie,* **20**, 410–463.

Tooby, J. and Cosmides, L. (1990). The past explains the present: emotional adaptations and the structure of ancestral environments. *Ethology and Sociobiology,* **11**, 375–424.

Trevathan, W.R., Mckenna, J.J. and Smith, E.O. (eds) (2008). *Evolutionary Medicine.* Second Edition. New York, Oxford University Press.

Watson, D., Clark, L.A., and Carey, G. (1988). Positive and negative affect and their relation to anxiety and depressive disorders. *Journal of Abnormal Psychology,* **97**, 346–353.

Watson, P.J. and Andrews, P.W. (2002). Toward a revised evolutionary adaptationist analysis of depression: the social navigation hypothesis. *Journal of Affective Disorders,* **72**, 1–14.

Williams, G.C. (1966). *Adaptation and Natural Selection: A Critique of Some Current Evolutionary Thought.* Princeton, N.J, Princeton University Press.

Williams, G.C. (1996). *Plan and Purpose in Nature.* London, Weidenfeld and Nicolson.

Williams, G.C. and Nesse, R.M. (1991). The dawn of Darwinian medicine. *Quarterly Review of Biology,* **66**, 1–22.

Wise, R.A. (2004). Dopamine, learning and motivation. *Nature Reviews Neuroscience,* **5**, 483–494.

Wrosch, C. and Scheier, M.F. (2003). Personality and quality of life: the importance of optimism and goal adjustment. *Quality of Life Research,* **12 Suppl 1**, 59–72.

Wrosch, C., Scheier, M.F., Miller, G.E., Schulz, R., and Carver, C.S. (2003). Adaptive self-regulation of unattainable goals: goal disengagement, goal re-engagement, and subjective well-being. *Personality and Social Psychology Bulletin of the Menninger Clinic,* **29**, 1494–1508.

Chapter 4

Evolutionary genetics of affective disorders

Bernard J. Crespi

I review evolutionary-genetic models for the generation, maintenance, and loss of allelic variation underlying polygenic disease, in the context of affective disorders and related conditions. Genetically based liability to these disorders appears to be due to some combination of mutation-selection balance involving common, small-effect variants and rare, large-effect variants, and natural selection involving antagonistic pleiotropy and balancing selection. At present, the primary usefulness of evolutionary genetics in the study of affective disorders is that it provides important insights into choices of genes, alleles, and haplotypes for analysis via genome scan and association studies, and motivates a focus on the potential for pleiotropic, beneficial effects of alleles and genotypes that also influence disease risk.

Introduction

Most evolutionary approaches to the analysis of human cognitive function, affective states, and mental disorders have focused on the potential adaptive significance of the phenotypes involved, in ancestral or modern environments (e.g. Nesse, 1999; Nettle, 2001; 2004; and Chapter 3 of this book). According to such evolutionary hypotheses, natural selection has optimized human mental phenotypes in the context of functions that are related to reproductive success, and mental disorders have been inferred to represent either unavoidable, maladaptive by-products of such selection (e.g. Burns, 2006), tails of continuous distributions of genetically based cognitive-affective functional abilities (e.g. Nesse, 2004), or manifestations of associations between enhanced abilities in some domain of performance, such as creativity, emotional sensitivity, or propensity to strive for success, and increased risk of mental illness (e.g. Nettle, 2001; 2004; 2006a). In this context, major depression and bipolar disorder can be interpreted as forms of dysregulation of adaptive mental systems that regulate mood, where low mood and high mood are normally adaptive states that contextually regulate physiology, cognition, and behaviour to maximize fitness (Johnson, 2005; Nesse, 2000; Nettle, 2004; Wolpert, 2008).

Hypotheses for the adaptive significance of human mental traits are extremely difficult to evaluate rigorously, as such tests require quantification of cognitive, affective, and behavioural phenotypes in relation to some measures of performance or fitness that are relevant in the context of human evolutionary history. Hypotheses of maladaptation are even more challenging to test, as they require information on genetic, physiological, or developmental mechanisms that allows exclusion of hypotheses based on adaptation or adaptive tradeoffs (Crespi, 2000; Nesse, 2005). Moreover, even when analyses of the functional design and adaptive nature of cognitive and emotional phenotypes yield results consistent with optimization (e.g. Keller and Nesse, 2005; 2006), the implications of such evolutionary, ultimate-level findings for proximate-level analyses of the aetiologies of mental disorders, or treatment strategies, often remain unclear (Nesse, 1999).

As a result, most workers studying or treating affective disorders do so in the absence of evolutionary perspectives, which are viewed as either highly speculative or largely irrelevant.

Adaptive significance is not just a function of phenotypes – it is also a property of the genetic, genomic, and epigenetic variation that underlies observed variation in mental traits or other phenotypes. Thus, just as a phenotype may be adaptive or maladaptive in some environmental context, an allele or haplotype may have increased or decreased in frequency as a result of selection over evolutionary time, or it may be maintained at some intermediate frequency. For evolutionary analyses of mental disorders, a focus at the level of alleles and haplotypes offers a number of useful analytic properties, such as the ability to infer the action of population-genetic processes, including selection for advantageous alleles, selection against deleterious alleles, or genetic drift, from data collected in extant populations (e.g. Biswas and Akey, 2006; Boyko et al. 2008; Sabeti et al. 2006). Such evolutionary-genetic analyses permit rigorous quantification of how natural selection, drift, mutation, and other processes have influenced genetic liability to affective disorders, which in turn provides direct insights into the proximate genetic, physiological and developmental underpinnings of mental disorders, and the role of optimization by selection in ultimate-level studies of adaptive significance (Crespi et al. 2007).

In this chapter, I provide an overview of the evolutionary genetics of affective disorders. My main goal is to integrate results from recent studies of the phenotypic structure and genetic basis of affective and related mental disorders with evolutionary models of the genetic, genomic, and epigenetic bases of polygenic human disease. I first define the cognitive-affective phenotypes and psychiatric conditions under consideration, to elucidate their phenotypic architecture, and I review the connections of phenotypic architecture, and formal diagnostic categories, with variation at the genetic level. Second, I attempt to square our knowledge of the genetic basis of affective and other mental disorders with current evolutionary, population-genetic models for the bases of human polygenic disease risk, to assess how well the 'genetics' meets the 'evolution' of mental disorders. Finally, on the basis of the results of these analyses, I suggest how molecular-evolutionary analyses can be applied to further our understanding of the aetiologies of affective disorders at both the proximate and ultimate levels.

Phenotypic and genetic architecture of psychotic-affective disorders

Major depression, bipolar disorder, and schizophrenia exhibit broad partial overlap in their constituent behavioural, cognitive, affective, and neurological phenotypes, with gradations between them characterized in terms of schizoaffective disorder, or depression (bipolar or unipolar) with psychotic features (Baethge et al. 2005; Boks et al. 2007a; Kempf et al. 2005; Lin and Mitchell, 2008; Smoller et al. 2008). Discussion of the nature of psychological variation between and within these conditions is beyond the scope of this article. However, on the basis of several criteria including patterns of shared phenotypes between disorders, patterns of inheritance within families, and the incidence of these disorders in neurogenetic syndromes (Boks et al. 2007b; Gothelf, 2007; Lin and Mitchell, 2008), depression, bipolar disorder, and schizophrenia can usefully be characterized as encompassing a 'schizophrenia spectrum', 'psychotic spectrum', or, as described here, 'psychotic-affective spectrum' (Crespi and Badcock, 2008; Ivleva et al. 2008; Marneros and Akiskal, 2006). These three conditions also partially overlap in their genetic underpinnings (Craddock and Forty, 2006; Blackwood et al. 2007; Farmer et al. 2007; Goes et al. 2008; López-León et al. 2007; Owen et al. 2007; Potash, 2006; and Chapter 6 of this book), with some genes, such as DISC1 and G72, now known to harbour allelic variants that affect susceptibility to all three disorders (Chubb et al. 2008; Rietschel et al. 2008). Such patterns of partial phenotypic and genetic overlap in psychotic-affective disorders have motivated the hypothesis that major depression, bipolar disorder, and schizophrenia share some genetic risk factors, but are also underlain by genetic variants that are more or less specific to one or two of the disorders (Craddock and Forty, 2006; Craddock et al. 2006; Hamshere et al. 2006). The presence of a psychotic-affective spectrum, analogous to the autistic spectrum, indicates that analyses of the evolutionary genetics of affective disorders cannot be easily parsed from analyses of disorders that involve strong elements of psychotic features, mainly schizophrenia.

Conditions on the psychotic-affective spectrum also apparently grade more or less smoothly into normality in non-clinical populations, with schizophrenia grading into schizotypy (Claridge, 1997; Fanous et al. 2007; Stefanis et al. 2007), major depression grading into neuroticism (Fullerton et al. 2003; Shifman et al. 2008), and mania in bipolar disorder grading into hypomania and normality (Chapters 21 and 22 in this book). Such continuous variation in phenotypes is indicative of polygenic underpinnings, with many genes, each of small effect, mediating expression (e.g. Craddock et al. 2008; Rapoport et al. 2005; Shifman et al. 2008; Tamminga and Holcomb, 2005), and it suggests that genetic liability to psychotic-affective spectrum conditions forms a continuous spectrum with variation in human personality traits (Fanous and Kendler, 2004; Nettle, 2006a), with important implications for the population-genetic factors that generate, maintain, and remove variation that affects disease risk and phenotypic variation. However, the interface of personality with psychiatric genetics has yet to be sufficiently developed to allow firm inferences to be drawn regarding the nature of associations between normal versus more-or-less pathological cognitive-affective traits; for example, genetically mediated personality traits may modulate the clinical presentation of affective disorders, rather than representing direct causal influences on the disorders themselves (Serretti et al. 2006), and depressive personality disorder appears to be at least partially distinct from major depression itself (Ørstavik et al. 2007).

Psychotic-affective spectrum conditions may be caused not just by apparent cumulative and interactive effects of allelic variation with relatively small effects, but also by *de novo* genetic variations of relatively large effect, either at a genetic scale, such as breakpoints in the DISC1 gene leading to major depression and schizophrenia (Muir et al. 2008), or at a genomic scale, such as gene copy-number variation due to duplications or deletions of regions that contain multiple genes. Genomic alterations include, for example, velocardiofacial syndrome as a result of deletions at 22q11.2, which involves an over-twentyfold increase in the incidence of schizophrenia, bipolar disorder, and major depression (Gothelf, 2007), and Klinefelter syndrome, caused by one or more 'extra' X chromosomes in males, which involves a four- to tenfold increased risk of these psychotic-affective spectrum conditions (Boks et al. 2007b). The degree to which such large-scale genomic alterations represent the high end of a continuum of genomic copy-number variants, that grade into smaller, cumulative effects on liability that segregate in populations (rather than arise sporadically, *de novo*), remains to be determined. However, recent findings that up to 7–10% of cases of schizophrenia (Walsh et al. 2008; Xu et al. 2008), and autism (Marshall et al. 2008; Sebat et al. 2007; Stefansson et al. 2008), may be associated with copy-number variants suggest that this source of genetic variability contributes substantially to the general incidence of mental disorders.

A third important cause of gene-level variation affecting liability of psychotic-affective conditions, in addition to genetic variants and genomic copy-number variants of large or small effect, is epigenetic variation (Mill and Petronis, 2007), especially in genes subject to genomic imprinting (Crespi, 2008a; Crespi and Badcock, 2008). Imprinted genes, which are selectively expressed according to their parent of origin (Haig, 2004; Tycko and Morison, 2002), comprise only a small proportion of the human genome, but they are disproportionately involved in brain development and function (Davies et al. 2008), and they can be dysregulated in more ways than non-imprinted genes, due to: (1) functional haploidy, such that all allelic variants can have immediate phenotypic effects; (2) alterations in methylation status or histone modifications, in addition to heritable changes in nucleotide sequence affecting expression and function; and (3) the differential involvement of imprinted genes in highly pleiotropic developmental systems mediated in part by antagonistic 'tugs-of-war' between maternally derived genes and paternally derived genes (Haig, 2004; Charalambous et al. 2007; Smits and Kelsey, 2006; Smith et al. 2006; Ubeda and Wilkins, 2008). In accordance with these properties of imprinted genes, they exert highly disproportionate effects on disease risk and progression in, for example, placentation (Fowden et al. 2006) and carcinogenesis (Jelinic and Shaw, 2007). The degree to which segregating variation, or *de novo* alterations, in imprinted genes affect susceptibility to psychotic-affective disorders remains to be determined (Crespi, 2008a; Crespi and Badcock, 2008). However, Prader-Willi syndrome due to uniparental disomy of chromosome 15, which is due to alterations to imprinted gene expression, is the most-penetrant cause of psychotic-affective disorders known to date (Soni et al. 2007; 2008), the imprinted LRRTM1 gene, associated with schizophrenia and schizoaffective disorder, underlies one of the strongest genome-scan linkages to schizophrenia (Francks et al. 2007), and a recent linkage study of anxiety (Middledorp et al. 2008) implicated the imprinted gene cluster at 14q32.2. Crow (2008) has also suggested that epigenetic variation of large effect underlies psychotic-affective disorders, a hypothesis that remains tenable to the degree that genetic and genomic variants continue to explain only a relatively small proportion of inherited or *de novo* risk.

Genetic, genomic, and epigenetic variation exerts its effects on liability to affective-psychotic conditions via alterations to more or less 'normal' neurocognitive architecture. In humans, a primary axis of such architecture is sex, with males and females differing quantitatively in a large suite of neurodevelopmental, neuroanatomical, psychological, and other traits (Baron-Cohen, 2003; Geary, 1998). Sex-specific associations of alleles with some psychotic-affective conditions (e.g. Pickard et al. 2007), and the higher incidence of major depression in females than males (Marcus et al. 2008; Smith et al. 2008), notably implicate sex as an important causal factor in the evolutionary genetics of mental disorders. Crespi and Badcock (2008) suggest that genomic-imprinting effects generate a second axis of human cognitive variation, whereby a canalized neurodevelopmental continuum stretches from a bias towards relative effects of maternally expressed imprinted genes, to dynamically balanced normality, to a bias towards effects of paternally expressed imprinted genes. Considered jointly with the axis of male–female variation, variation along such a genomic-imprinting effects axis helps to explain several of the strong observed sex biases in the prevalence and severity of both psychotic-affective and autistic-spectrum conditions (Crespi and Badcock, 2008), such as the overall male bias to autism, more severe autism in females, the overall female bias to depression, and more severe schizophrenia in males. This model points to genes underlying sex differences in neurodevelopment, and imprinting effects, as important factors in the expression of psychotic-affective conditions, in part via modification of the penetrance of allelic effects (e.g. Zhao et al. 2007); it also suggests that epistatic interactions between imprinted genes and non-imprinted genes involved in sex differentiation, as apparently found in Turner syndrome (Crespi, 2008b) may play important roles in human development.

Evolutionary-genetic models of psychotic-affective conditions

The relatively high heritabilities of neurodevelopmental conditions such as schizophrenia and autism have been considered to pose an evolutionary paradox, given that allelic variants increasing the risk of such conditions should be strongly selected against, resulting in low levels of additive genetic variation maintained in populations (Keller and Miller, 2006). Three main categories of evolutionary-genetic model have been proposed thus far to explain such an apparent paradox in the maintenance of alleles for polygenic disease risk (Table 4.1):

1. models based on a large number of slightly deleterious variants, most of small effect, subject to inputs via mutation across many loci, maintenance by drift under sufficiently weak selection or small population size, and removal via purifying selection (Bodmer and Bonilla, 2008; Hughes et al. 2003; Kryukov et al. 2007);

2. models based on the effects of rare, more highly deleterious genetic or genomic variants, with common variants of small effect exerting a relatively small influence on overall disease risk (Bodmer and Bonilla, 2008; Fearnhead et al. 2004; Walsh et al. 2008; Zhao et al. 2007); and

3. models based on evolutionary advantages, now or in the past, of alleles that also increase disease risk (Kryukov et al. 2007).

The first model corresponds to the common disease-common variants hypothesis (Lohmueller et al. 2003), whereby polygenic disease is due to cumulative and interactive combinations of many deleterious alleles, each of small effect, in the context of the myriad mutational targets provided by large numbers of genes, large mutation-prone genes, and complex pathways (e.g. Smith et al. 2006); by contrast, under the second model, segregating genetic variation in disease risk has minor effects compared to larger effect, *de novo* variants. Variation is maintained under the third model by any of a number of selective processes, such as balancing selection or antagonistic pleiotropy, that can maintain risk alleles at non-trivial frequencies (Keller and Miller, 2006; Kryukov et al. 2007). These models are not mutually exclusive, and the first two models may grade into one another given continuous distributions of frequencies for disease risk alleles across loci, effect sizes, and levels of penetrance (Boyko et al. 2008). Moreover, effects of genetic drift may interact with effects of purifying selection, by generating increases in the frequencies of more-deleterious variants in relatively small groups, such as human founder populations (e.g. Boyko et al. 2008; Fearnhead et al. 2004; Lohmueller et al. 2008;). How well do these models fit with the available data, and what are the implications for elucidating the genetic bases of neuro-developmental disorders?

Table 4.1 Three non-exclusive evolutionary-genetic models may help to explain the role of different population-genetic forces in the origin, maintenance, and loss of genetic variation that underlies susceptibility to affective disorders, and each of these models has important implications for future analyses

Evolutionary-genetic model	Population-genetic forces	Implications for future studies
Many variants, each of small effect; variants rare or common	Weak purifying selection on de novo and segregating variants	Target alleles apparently subject to weak purifying selection; analyse variants common and rare in association and genome scan studies
Rare variants, each of large effect	Strong purifying selection, mainly on de novo variants	Most known risk variants of small effect are more or less irrelevant; systematically target copy-number variants and rare alleles
Common variants, each of small to moderate effect	Positive selection, antagonistic pleiotropy, balancing selection	Target alleles and haplotypes apparently subject to selection test for beneficial effects of risk and protective variants

(a) Common or rare alleles subject to purifying selection

Slightly deleterious alleles can be maintained at appreciable frequencies, across many loci, when mutations to such alleles are common across the genome and purifying selection is relatively weak. If risk alleles exhibit appreciable allele frequencies and small effect sizes, then the common variant – common disease paradigm described for schizophrenia, bipolar disorder, and other diseases by Lohmueller et al. (2003) holds, but if disease is mediated predominantly by rare alleles, then current molecular-psychiatric strategies for identifying disease loci, such as whole-genome scans that probe relatively common variants, will be largely ineffective (Bodmer and Bonilla, 2008; Boyko et al. 2008; Hughes, 2007). Kryukov et al. (2007) integrated information from known human disease mutations, human-chimp divergences, and human genetic variation to show that up to 70% of low-frequency missense mutations are deleterious, which implies that mutation-selection balance of low-frequency alleles is a feasible population-genetic mechanism for the maintenance of common human polygenic diseases (see also Fay et al. 2001). For psychotic-affective disorders, these inferences are consistent with results from five recent studies: (1) a higher frequency of rare variants, for six schizophrenia-associated genes, in patients than in controls (Winantea et al. 2006); (2) the presence of rare variants of the SYNGR1 gene in schizophrenia patients but not controls (Cheng and Chen, 2007); (3) the observation that over 60% of cases of schizophrenia in Daghestan genetic isolates were offspring of consanguineous marriages (Bulayeva et al. 2005); (4) a significantly higher incidence of rare, large-haplotype, recessive genotypes in schizophrenia patients than controls (Lencz et al. 2007); and (5) the presence of rare, high-risk allelic variants detected in a study of the role of DISC1 alleles in schizophrenia risk (Song et al. 2008). These convergent findings should motivate genotyping strategies that detect a higher proportion of low-frequency variants, given their potential cumulative role in disease risk, and the resultant data sets will also allow robust estimation of Tajima's D-statistic (e.g. Winantea et al. 2006), whereby evidence for purifying selection, balancing selection, and positive selection can be inferred from the distribution of allele-frequency variation (Bamshad and Wooding, 2003; Biswas and Akey, 2006).

Regardless of the spectrum of allele frequencies for risk alleles, there is now considerable population-genetic evidence for the presence of abundant, slightly deleterious variants in humans, many of which are apparently subject to purifying selection (Bustamante et al. 2005; Hughes, 2007; Hughes et al. 2003; Lohmueller et al. 2008; Yampolsky et al. 2005). Such purifying selection has been detected, for example, via quantification of global reductions in human among-population differentiation for amino-acid altering mutational sites, especially for disease-related genes (Barreiro et al. 2008). Perhaps the most important implication of these findings is that identification of sites that are likely subject to purifying selection provides a strong clue to functional significance, allowing efficient, evolutionarily informed choices of SNPs and other variants for linkage or association studies (Hughes, 2007). Such studies will in turn determine the degree to which mutation-selection balance across many loci can cumulatively account for a substantial proportion of disease risk, for common diseases in general and psychotic-affective disorders in particular.

(b) Rare genomic alterations subject to strong purifying selection

An important role for individually rare, highly deleterious genomic variants is provided by Stefansson et al. (2008), Walsh et al. (2008), and Xu et al. (2008), who reported notably higher frequencies of rare, high-penetrance structural genomic changes (duplications and deletions) in schizophrenia cases than in controls (e.g. 15–20% vs. 5% in Walsh et al. 2008). These findings concord with recent studies of autism reporting similarly increased frequencies of copy-number variants in patients (Marshall et al. 2008; Sebat et al. 2007), with a stronger advanced paternal-age effect in sporadic than familial schizophrenia (Sipos et al. 2004), and with a recent genetic model of autism that posits a high incidence of *de novo* large-effect mutations with higher penetrance in males than females (Zhao et al. 2007). By this model, most of the genes thus far implicated in neurodevelopmental disorders via association or linkage studies have been suggested to represent modifier loci of small effect that are largely irrelevant to the overall risk of disease (Walsh et al. 2008; Zhao et al. 2007). An important corollary of this model is that alleles of relatively large effect and penetrance more readily result in familial concentration of disease cases (Bodmer and Bonilla, 2008), a pattern commonly found in psychotic-affective disorders (e.g. Potash et al. 2001; Schurhoff et al. 2003); this pattern may be interpreted as broadly concordant with the rare, large-effect deleterious-allele model for genes or copy-number variants, or as evidence that other population-genetic factors are involved.

These recent studies are of considerable importance in revealing that gene copy-number variation mediates a considerable proportion of the risk for neurodevelopmental disorders (Cantor and Geschwind, 2008), although bipolar disorder and major depression have yet to be studied in this context. Such analyses have, however, focused on relatively severe cases (such as childhood onset schizophrenia, and Kanner autism), such that the expected role of copy-number variants in less-severe conditions, such as high-functioning autism, bipolar II, or mild unipolar depression, remains unclear. More generally, the effects of relatively common copy-number variants in modulating dimensional variation in neurodevelopmental conditions and cognitive phenotypes have yet to be assessed. Evidence for functional, adaptive effects of such variants comes from Sharp et al. (2005), who show that genomic copy-number polymorphisms are common in humans and likely mediate normal variation as well as disease, and from Hahn et al. (2007) and Jiang et al. (2007), who describe evidence for an accelerated rate of evolution in gene copy number among primates and along the human lineage, driven in part by positive selection on brain-related genes.

(c) Common alleles subject to positive selection or balancing selection

Alleles or genotypes that increase susceptibility to affective disorders may be maintained in human populations because they are, or have been, advantageous in some context other than disease. The primary models based on effects of positive selection (selection 'for' particular genetic variants, that arise and sweep through populations to some frequency; Sabeti et al. 2006; Hughes, 2007) that have been proposed include: (1) changing selection pressures, such that common alleles that were advantageous in ancestral environments (e.g. 'thrifty' genes affecting the regulation of metabolism) are now deleterious, and derived alleles are selected for (Di Rienzo, 2006; Di Rienzo and Hudson, 2005), (2) balancing selection, whereby individuals with heterozygous genotypes are favoured, resulting in the maintenance at high frequency of deleterious homozygotes, and (3) antagonistic pleiotropy, whereby selected alleles exert positive effects in one context, or early in the lifespan, that are stronger than, or balanced by, negative effects expressed in some other context or later in life (Keller and Miller, 2006; Kryukov et al. 2007).

The ancestral-susceptibility model has been supported by data from molecular evolutionary, geographic and physiological analyses of genes involved in risk of hypertension, type 2 diabetes, and several other common human diseases (e.g. Di Rienzo and Hudson, 2005; Helgason et al. 2007; Young et al. 2005). Lo et al. (2007) describe evidence that this model may apply in the context of schizophrenia-protective haplotypes of the GABRB2 gene being subject to recent positive selection, although in this case the causes and context of selection remain to be elucidated. More generally, an ancestral-susceptibility model for mental disorders must posit and evaluate roles for specific environmental or epistatic effects that mediate large-scale shifts in how specific alleles influence disease risk. The most obvious difference between ancestral and modern human environments, as regards susceptibility to affective disorders, is the social environment shifting away from villages and extended families towards the novel, large social groups of cities and the novel, small groupings of more or less isolated nuclear families. However, reductions in the strength of social support networks might be expected to simply increase depression risk in modern environments, rather than change the direction or nature of gene by environment inter-actions. Alternatively, the human social environment may have qualitatively changed, in ways related to increased levels of stress and complexity. A discussion of the genetic of stress response is offered in Chapter 5.

Evidence for balancing selection among genotypes, for genes whose variants influence susceptibility of psychotic-affective disorders, is limited to studies that show effects of heterosis for such genes as DRD2, DRD3, DRD4, HTR2A, SLC6A4, and TPH1, in some physiological and behavioural contexts (e.g. Comings and MacMurray, 2000; Reuter and Hennig, 2005). The gen-eral paucity of population-genetic evidence for balancing selection on genes underling mental disorders may arise in part from ascertainment bias in SNP-based scans for selection, such that high-frequency variants are differentially detected (Kelley and Swanson, 2008). At the phenotypic and epidemiological levels, psychotic-affective cognition or disorders have been associated with measures of enhanced creativity (Nettle, 2001; Burch et al. 2006), mating success (Nettle and Clegg, 2006), socio-economic achievement (Jamison, 1996; Johnson, 2005) and, in several stud-ies, higher fertility of first-order relatives (reviewed in Crespi and Badcock, 2008; Crespi et al. 2007), compared to controls. These findings are consistent with evolutionary benefits of alleles and genotypes underlying such disorders but they do not directly or quantitatively address any particular model on the basis of positive or balancing selection.

Clear evidence for antagonistic pleiotropy of alleles underlying psychotic-affective disorders has been reported for APOE genotypes, such that the E4 allele, linked with higher risk of major depression (Yen et al. 2007) and bipolar disorder (Bellivier et al. 1997) is also associated with enhanced verbal skills in childhood and other potential early life benefits (Alexander et al. 2007). Similarly, the schizophrenia-risk haplotype of DAOA, a gene additionally linked with bipolar disorder (Prata et al. 2008), is also associated with enhanced semantic fluency (Opgen-Rhein et al. 2008), and the schizophrenia-risk haplotype of the PPP1R1B is associated with measures of enhanced frontostriatal function (Meyer-Lindenberg et al. 2007). The generality of a role for antagonistic pleiotropy in psychotic-affective conditions remains unclear, primarily because of the lack of study of this mechanism outside the context of senescence theory (e.g. Capri et al. 2006). Pleiotropy itself is a virtually universal mode of gene action (e.g. Barriero et al. 2008; Knight et al. 2006), and most of the genes involved in neurodevelopment and neurological func-tion are known to be fundamentally involved in other processes as well (Kendler, 2005), such as mediation of tumour suppression by the APC and TP53 genes, both of which have been impli-cated in risk of psychotic-affective disorders (Cui et al. 2005; Ni et al. 2005) and have also apparently been subject to positive selection in the human lineage (Crespi et al. 2007; Voight et al. 2006). Another example of pleiotropic effects in 'neuronal' genes is testicular functions in males, given strong patterns of gene co-expression in brain and testis (Guo et al. 2005) that are apparently underlain by shared receptor functions such as exocytosis (Meizel, 2004). Genes differentially expressed in testis exhibit notably enhanced signatures of positive selection in humans (Nielsen et al. 2005), selection that may generate negative pleiotropic effects in the context of neuronal activities (Qin et al. 2007).

The primary evidence congruent with a hypothesis of positive selection having some role in the evolutionary-genetic basis of psychotic-affective disorders, either in increasing, maintaining, or reducing levels of genetic variation, is that a considerable number of the genes that have been linked with schizophrenia, bipolar disorder, major depression, and other diseases (Barriero et al. 2008), show evidence of positive selection in recent human evolution. These include some of the best-supported candidate genes for affective disorders (Table 4.2), and for schizophrenia (Crespi et al. 2007), such as DTNBP1, NRG1, and SLC6A4, and schizophrenia-associated genes show a statistically stronger signal of positive selection than a control set of genes involved in neuronal activities (Crespi et al. 2007). A variety of hypotheses may potentially explain the phenotypic basis of this molecular-evolutionary pattern, including: (1) positive selection for alleles protective against mental disorders or reduced cognitive-affective function (e.g. Weiss et al. 2007); (2) antagonistic pleiotropy, such that advantageous effects of selected alleles or genotypes in some context, such as creativity or social-emotional cognition, are not outweighed by an increased risk of mental disorders conferred by these same alleles, across evolutionary time (Burns, 2006; Crespi et al. 2007; Nettle, 2001); or (3) positive selection in contexts unrelated to mental disorders, given the highly pleiotropic nature of most of the genes involved. These hypotheses can be evaluated in two main ways:

1. Genes, alleles, and haplotypes inferred as being subject to positive selection in humans can be chosen as markers to evaluate their potential associations with the risk of psychotic-affective or other polygenic disorders (Crespi et al. 2007; Thomas and Kejariwal, 2004). The beauty of this approach is that alleles subject to positive selection are predicted to be functional (McVean and Spencer, 2006), which should increase the likelihood that associations will be ascertained (Biswas and Akey, 2006). Such studies can also be conducted in the framework of which haplotypes are ancestral versus derived in humans ancestry, to infer the validity of the ancestral-susceptibility model in the context of mental diseases (e.g. Weiss et al. 2007).

2. Positively selected SNPs and haplotypes, and disease-associated alleles, can each be tested in relation to multiple cognitive-affective phenotypes (e.g. Comings et al. 2003; Meyer-Lindenberg et al. 2007) including those that may be beneficial, rather than focusing exclusively on deficits and potential disease endophenotypes. For example, two recent studies have indeed shown that schizophrenia-risk alleles (for the SLC6A4 and TPH1 genes) were pleiotropically associated with measures of increased creativity (Bachner-Melman et al. 2005; Reuter et al. 2006). Such studies allow testing of the idea that having some moderate number of alleles associated with risk of psychotic-affective disorders, across many loci, leads to enhancements in some cognitive domains, while having 'too many' such alleles increases risk of disease (Nesse, 2004).

Table 4.2 Evidence of positive selection is available for each of a large suite of genes that harbour variants implicated in bipolar disorder, major depression, and schizoaffective disorder

Gene	Evidence for positive selection in humans
ALG9	Voight et al. (2006)
APOE	Crespi et al. (2007, Table 4)
BRD1	Voight et al. (2006)
CABIN1	Voight et al. (2006)
CAPON	Voight et al. (2006)

(Continued)

Table 4.2 (Continued) Evidence of positive selection is available for each of a large suite of genes that harbour variants implicated in bipolar disorder, major depression, and schizoaffective disorder

Gene	Evidence for positive selection in humans
CLOCK	Voight et al. (2006)
DISC1	Crespi et al. (2007) (human-chimp lineage)
DOCK9	Voight et al. (2006)(p = 0.0504)
DRD4	Crespi et al. (2007, Table 4)
DTNBP1	Voight et al. (2006), Crespi et al. (2007, Table 4)
GABRA1	Voight et al. (2006)
GRM3	Voight et al. (2006), Crespi et al. (2007, Table 4)
HMG2L1	Voight et al. (2006)
IMPA2	Voight et al. (2006)
LRRTM1	Voight et al. (2006), Francks et al. (2007)
MAOA	Crespi et al. (2007, Table 4)
NPAS3	Crespi et al. (2007, Table 4)
NR3C1	Bustamante et al. (2005)
NR3C2	Bustamante et al. (2005) (p = 0.068)
NRG1	Crespi et al. (2007)
PAX1	Bustamante et al. (2005)
PDE11A	Voight et al. (2006)
PDLIM5	Crespi et al. 2007, Table 4), Voight et al. (2006) (selected SNPs, not gene-wide significant)
PIK3C3	Voight et al. (2006)
PLCG1	Voight et al. (2006)
RFX4	Voight et al. (2006)
SLC12A6	Voight et al. (2006)
SLC6A3	Bustamante et al. (2005)(p = 0.06)
SLC6A4	Bustamante et al. (2005), Voight et al. (2006)
SYNGR1	Voight et al. (2006)
SYNJ1	Voight et al. (2006)
TOM1	Voight et al. (2006)
TPH1	Bustamante et al. (2005)(p = 0.06)

Notes: Details of Voight et al. (2006) results are available in the Haplotter web interface, and Crespi et al. (2007, Table 4) collates relevant information on positive selection from previous studies. Most of the genetic-association citations are available in Carter (2007) and Crespi et al. (2007); additional citations are available upon request. Genes in boldface exhibit especially well-replicated associations, and many of the genes have also been associated with schizophrenia risk. Alleles or haplotypes that have been inferred as subject to positive selection in humans are especially likely to exhibit functional effects on affect and cognition, and so may be especially useful targets for molecular-psychiatric analyses.

A key consideration regarding the evaluation of alternative yet non-exclusive models for the evolutionary-genetic forces affecting human disease-related genes is that formal models for the maintenance of variation generally assume equilibria between opposing population-genetic processes (Di Rienzo, 2006), yet there is no good reason to expect that modern human populations are in equilibrium (Lohmueller et al. 2008). Indeed, Hawks et al. (2007) describe population-genomic evidence that humans are currently undergoing an acceleration of adaptive evolution, due to a combination of larger population sizes (creating more potential targets for adaptive mutation), expanding populations (which increase the fixation probabilities of adaptive mutations), and more rapid environmental change (which generates stronger selection itself). To the extent that such environmental change involves aspects of human social and emotional cognition that mediate reproductive success, positive selection on genes affecting liability to mental disorders is an expected consequence. It is also of critical importance to avoid a false dichotomy between models on the basis of positive or balancing selection, and models invoking mutation-selection balance (Nettle, 2006b), because the processes are not incompatible and studies conducted to date provide clear evidence for both (Barriero et al. 2008; Bustamante et al. 2005; Crespi et al. 2007; Fay et al. 2001; Keller and Miller, 2006).

Conclusions

The fields of molecular-genetic psychiatry and human evolutionary genetics have burgeoned over the past ten years but continue to develop in virtual isolation. Study of the evolutionary genetics of psychotic-affective disorders is thus in its infancy, but it holds enormous promise for future progress in both domains. At present, the primary usefulness of evolutionary-genetic tools for elucidation of the aetiologies of such disorders is that they provide windows into the expected functionality of specific genetic variants as either positively selected, subject to balancing selection, or subject to weak purifying selection. They also provide a temporal dimension to the distribution of human disease-related genetic variation, and insights into which methods are most likely to efficiently detect loci and alleles underlying disease. As firm evidence accumulates regarding the set of genes and alleles mediating the expression of mental disorders, functional information in particular becomes increasingly important in forging links from genetic, genomic, and epigenetic variation to physiology, neurodevelopment, cognition, and behaviour (Kelley and Swanson, 2008). Evidence regarding the adaptive significance of genetic variants underlying susceptibility to psychotic-affective disorders will also allow much more robust evaluation of hypotheses that posit selective benefits to phenotypes associated, in less extreme form, with disorders of cognition and affect.

Acknowledgements

I am grateful to NSERC and the Canada Council for the Arts for financial support, and to R. Nesse and C. Pariante for motivating and supporting my work on affective disorders.

References

Alexander, D.M., Williams, L.M., Gatt, J.M. et al. (2007). The contribution of apolipoprotein E alleles on cognitive performance and dynamic neural activity over six decades. *Biological Psychology*, **75**, 229–238.

Bachner-Melman, R., Dina, C., Zohar, A.H. et al. (2005). AVPR1a and SLC6A4 gene polymorphisms are associated with creative dance performance. *PLoS Genetics*, **1**, e42.

Baethge, C., Baldessarini, R.J., Freudenthal, K., Streeruwitz, A., Bauer, M., and Bschor, T. (2005). Hallucinations in bipolar disorder: characteristics and comparison to unipolar depression and schizophrenia. *Bipolar Disorder*, **7**, 136–145.

Bamshad, M. and Wooding, S.P. (2003). Signatures of natural selection in the human genome. *Nature Reviews Genetics*, **4**, 99–111.

Baron-Cohen, S. (2003). *The Essential Difference: The Truth about the Male and Female Brain.* New York, Basic Books/Penguin.

Barreiro, L.B., Laval, G., Quach, H., Patin, E., and Quintana-Murci, L. (2008). Natural selection has driven population differentiation in modern humans. *Nature Genetics*, **40**, 340–345.

Bellivier, F., Laplanche, J.L., Schürhoff, F. et al. (1997). Apolipoprotein E gene polymorphism in early and late onset bipolar patients. *Neuroscience Letters*, **233**, 45–48.

Biswas, S. and Akey, J.M. (2006). Genomic insights into positive selection. *Trends in Genetics*, **22**, 437–446.

Blackwood, D.H., Pickard, B.J., Thomson, P.A., Evans, K.L., Porteous, D.J., and Muir, W.J. (2007). Are some genetic risk factors common to schizophrenia, bipolar disorder and depression? Evidence from DISC1, GRIK4 and NRG1. *Neurotoxicity Research*, **11**, 73–83.

Bodmer, W. and Bonilla, C. (2008). Common and rare variants in multifactorial susceptibility to common diseases. *Nature Genetics*, **40**, 695–701.

Boks, M.P., Leask, S., Vermunt, J.K., and Kahn, R.S. (2007a). The structure of psychosis revisited: the role of mood symptoms. *Schizophrenia Research*, **93**, 178–185.

Boks, M.P., de Vette, M.H., Sommer, I.E. et al. (2007b). Psychiatric morbidity and X-chromosomal origin in a Klinefelter sample. *Schizophrenia Research*, **93**, 399–402.

Boyko, A.R., Williamson, S.H., Indap, A.R. et al. (2008). Assessing the evolutionary impact of amino acid mutations in the human genome. *PLoS Genetics*, **4**, e1000083.

Bulayeva, K.B., Leal, S.M., Pavlova, T.A. et al. (2005). Mapping genes of complex psychiatric diseases in Daghestan genetic isolates. *American Journal of Medical Genetics Part B Neuropsychiatric Genetics*, **132**, 76–84.

Burch, G.S., Pavelis, C., Hemsley, D.R., and Corr, P.J. (2006). Schizotypy and creativity in visual artists. *British Journal of Psychology*, **97**, 177–190.

Burns, J.K. (2006). Psychosis: a costly by-product of social brain evolution in Homo sapiens. *Progress in Neuro-Psychopharmacology and Biological Psychiatry*, **30**, 797–814.

Bustamante, C.D., Fledel-Alon, A., Williamson, S. et al. (2005). Natural selection on protein-coding genes in the human genome. *Nature*, **437**, 1153–1157.

Cantor, R.M. and Geschwind, D.H. (2008). Schizophrenia: genome, interrupted. *Neuron*, **58**, 165–167.

Capri, M., Salvioli, S., Sevini, F. et al. (2006). The genetics of human longevity. *Annals of the New York Academy of Sciences*, **1067**, 252–263.

Carter, C.J. (2007). Multiple genes and factors associated with bipolar disorder converge on growth factor and stress activated kinase pathways controlling translation initiation: implications for oligodendrocyte viability. *Neurochemistry International*, **50**, 461–490.

Charalambous, M., da Rocha, S.T., and Ferguson-Smith, A.C. (2007). Genomic imprinting, growth control and the allocation of nutritional resources: consequences for postnatal life. *Current Opinions in Endocrinology, Diabetes and Obesity*, **14**, 3–12.

Cheng, M.C. and Chen, C.H. (2007). Identification of rare mutations of synaptogyrin 1 gene in patients with schizophrenia. *Journal of Psychiatric Research*, **41**, 1027–1031.

Chubb, J.E., Bradshaw, N.J., Soares, D.C., Porteous, D.J., and Millar, J.K. (2008). The DISC locus in psychiatric illness. *Molecular Psychiatry*, **13**, 36–64.

Claridge, G. (ed.) (1997). *Schizotypy: Implications for Illness and Health.* Oxford., Oxford University Press.

Comings, D.E., Gonzalez, N.S., Cheng Li, S.C., and MacMurray, J. (2003). A 'line item' approach to the identification of genes involved in polygenic behavioral disorders: the adrenergic alpha2A (ADRA2A) gene. *American Journal of Medical Genetics. Part B, Neuropsychiatric Genetics*, **118**, 110–114.

Comings, D.E. and MacMurray, J.P. (2000). Molecular heterosis: a review. *Molecular Genetics and Metabolism*, **71**, 19–31.

Craddock, N. and Forty, L. (2006). Genetics of affective (mood) disorders. *European Journal of Human Genetics*, **14**, 660–668.

Craddock, N., O'Donovan, M.C., and Owen, M.J. (2006). Genes for schizophrenia and bipolar disorder? Implications for psychiatric nosology. *Schizophrenia Bulletin*, **32**, 9–16.

Craddock, N., O'Donovan, M.C., and Owen, M.J. (2008). Genome-wide association studies in psychiatry: lessons from early studies of non-psychiatric and psychiatric phenotypes. *Molecular Psychiatry*, **13**, 649–653.

Crespi, B. (2000). The evolution of maladaptation. *Heredity*, **84**, 623–639.

Crespi, B. (2008a). Genomic imprinting in the development and evolution of psychosis. *Biological Reviews*, **83**, 441–493.

Crespi, B. (2008b). Turner syndrome and the evolution of human sexual dimorphism. *Evolutionary Applications*, **1**, 449–461.

Crespi, B. and Badcock, C. (2008) Psychosis and autism as diametrical disorders of the social brain. *Behavioral and Brain Sciences*, **31**, 241–261.

Crespi, B., Summers, K., and Dorus, S. (2007). Adaptive evolution of genes underlying schizophrenia. *Proceedings of the Royal Society of London Series B, Biological Sciences*, **274**, 2801–2810.

Crow, T.J. (2008). Craddock and Owen vs Kraepelin: 85 years late, mesmerised by 'polygenes'. *Schizophrenia Research*, **103**, 156–160.

Cui, D.H., Jiang, K.D., Jiang, S.D., Xu, Y.F., and Yao, H. (2005). The tumor suppressor adenomatous polyposis coli gene is associated with susceptibility to schizophrenia. *Molecular Psychiatry*, **10**, 669–677.

Davies, W., Isles, A.R., Humby, T., and Wilkinson, L.S. (2008). What are imprinted genes doing in the brain? *Epigenetics*, **2**, 201–206.

Di Rienzo, A. (2006). Population genetics models of common diseases. *Current Opinion in Genetics & Development*, **16**, 630–6.

Di Rienzo, A. and Hudson, R.R. (2005). An evolutionary framework for common diseases: the ancestral-susceptibility model. *Trends in Genetics*, **21**, 596–601.

Fanous, A.H. and Kendler, K.S. (2004). The genetic relationship of personality to major depression and schizophrenia. *Neurotoxicity Research*, **6**, 43–50.

Fanous, A.H., Neale, M.C., Gardner, C.O. et al. (2007). Significant correlation in linkage signals from genome-wide scans of schizophrenia and schizotypy. *Molecular Psychiatry*, **12**, 958–965.

Farmer, A., Elkin, A., and McGuffin, P. (2007). The genetics of bipolar affective disorder. *Current Opinion in Psychiatry*, **20**, 8–12.

Fay, J.C., Wyckoff, G.J., and Wu, C.I. (2001). Positive and negative selection on the human genome. *Genetics*, **158**, 1227–1234.

Fearnhead, N.S., Wilding, J.L., Winney, B. et al. (2004). Multiple rare variants in different genes account for multifactorial inherited susceptibility to colorectal adenomas. *Proceedings of the National Academy of Sciences, USA*, **101**, 15992–15997.

Fowden, A.L., Sibley, C., Reik, W., and Constancia, M. (2006). Imprinted genes, placental development and fetal growth. *Hormone Research*, **65 Suppl 3**, 50–58.

Francks, C., Maegawa, S., Laurén, J. et al. (2007). LRRTM1 on chromosome 2p12 is a maternally suppressed gene that is associated paternally with handedness and schizophrenia. *Molecular Psychiatry*, **12**, 1129–1139.

Fullerton, J., Cubin, M., Tiwari, H. et al. (2003). Linkage analysis of extremely discordant and concordant sibling pairs identifies quantitative-trait loci that influence variation in the human personality trait neuroticism. *American Journal of Human Genetics*, **72**, 879–890.

Geary, D.C. (1998). *Male, Female: The Evolution of Human Sex Differences*. Washington, DC, American Psychological Association.

Goes, F.S., Sanders, L.L., and Potash, J.B. (2008). The genetics of psychotic bipolar disorder. *Current Psychiatry Reports*, **10**, 178–189.

Gothelf, D. (2007). Velocardiofacial syndrome. *Child and Adolescent Psychiatric Clinics of North America*, **16**, 677–693.

Guo, J.H., Huang, Q., Studholme, D.J., Wu, C.Q., and Zhao, Z. (2005). Transcriptomic analyses support the similarity of gene expression between brain and testis in human as well as mouse. *Cytogenetic and Genome Research*, **111**, 107–109.

Hahn, M.W., Demuth, J.P., and Han, S.G. (2007). Accelerated rate of gene gain and loss in primates. *Genetics*, **177**, 1941–1949.

Haig, D. (2004). Genomic imprinting and kinship: how good is the evidence? *Annual Reviews of Genetics*, **38**, 553–585.

Hamshere, M.L., Williams, N.M., Norton, N. et al. (2006). Genome wide significant linkage in schizophrenia conditioning on occurrence of depressive episodes. *Journal of Medical Genetics*, **43**, 563–567.

Hawks, J., Wang, E.T., Cochran, G.M., Harpending, H.C., and Moyzis, R.K. (2007). Recent acceleration of human adaptive evolution. *Proceedings of the National Academy of Sciences USA*, **104**, 20753–20758.

Helgason, A., Pálsson, S., Thorleifsson, G. et al. (2007). Refining the impact of TCF7L2 gene variants on type 2 diabetes and adaptive evolution. *Nature Genetics*, **39**, 218–225.

Hughes, A.L. (2007). Looking for Darwin in all the wrong places: the misguided quest for positive selection at the nucleotide sequence level. *Heredity*, **99**, 364–373.

Hughes, A.L., Packer, B., Welch, R., Bergen, A.W., Chanock, S.J., and Yeager, M. (2003). Widespread purifying selection at polymorphic sites in human protein-coding loci. *Proceedings of the National Academy of Sciences USA*, **100**, 15754–15757.

Ivleva, E., Thaker, G., and Tamminga C.A. (2008). Comparing genes and phenomenology in the major psychoses: schizophrenia and bipolar 1 disorder. *Schizophrenia Bulletin*, **34**, 734–742.

Jamison, K.R. (1996). *Touched with Fire: Manic-Depressive Illness and the Artistic Temperament*. New York, The Free Press.

Jelinic, P. and Shaw, P. (2007). Loss of imprinting and cancer. *Journal of Pathology*, **211**, 261–268.

Jiang, Z., Tang, H., Ventura, M. et al. (2007). Ancestral reconstruction of segmental duplications reveals punctuated cores of human genome evolution. *Nature Genetics*, **39**, 1361–1368.

Johnson, S.L. (2005). Mania and dysregulation in goal pursuit: a review. *Clinical Psychology Review*, **25**, 241–262.

Kelley, J.L. and Swanson, W.J. (2008). Positive selection in the human genome: from genome scans to biological significance. *Annual Review of Genomics and Human Genetics*, **9**, 143–160.

Keller, M.C. and Miller, G. (2006). Resolving the paradox of common, harmful, heritable mental disorders: which evolutionary genetic models work best? *Behavioral and Brain Sciences*, **29**, 385–404.

Keller, M.C. and Nesse, R.M. (2005). Is low mood an adaptation? Evidence for subtypes with symptoms that match precipitants. *Journal of Affective Disorders*, **86**, 27–35.

Keller, M.C. and Nesse, R.M. (2006). The evolutionary significance of depressive symptoms: different adverse situations lead to different depressive symptom patterns. *Journal of Personality and Social Psychology*, **91**, 316–330.

Kempf, L., Hussain, N., and Potash, J.B. (2005). Mood disorder with psychotic features, schizoaffective disorder, and schizophrenia with mood features: trouble at the borders. *International Review of Psychiatry*, **17**, 9–19.

Kendler, K.S. (2005). 'A gene for . . .': the nature of gene action in psychiatric disorders. *The American Journal of Psychiatry*, **162**, 1243–1252.

Knight, C.G., Zitzmann, N., Prabhakar, S. et al. (2006). Unraveling adaptive evolution: how a single point mutation affects the protein coregulation network. *Nature Genetics*, **38**, 1015–1022.

Kryukov, G.V., Pennacchio, L.A., and Sunyaev, S.R. (2007). Most rare missense alleles are deleterious in humans: implications for complex disease and association studies. *American Journal of Human Genetics*, **80**, 727–739.

Lencz, T., Lambert, C., DeRosse, P. et al. (2007). Runs of homozygosity reveal highly penetrant recessive loci in schizophrenia. *Proceedings of the National Academy of Sciences USA*, **104**, 19942–19947.

Lin, P.I. and Mitchell, B.D. (2008). Approaches for unraveling the joint genetic determinants of schizophrenia and bipolar disorder. *Schizophrenia Bulletin*, **34**, 791–797.

Lo, W.S., Xu, Z., Yu, Z. et al. (2007). Positive selection within the schizophrenia-associated GABA(A) receptor beta2 gene. *PLoS ONE*, **2**, e462.

Lohmueller, K.E., Pearce, C.L., Pike, M., Lander, E.S., and Hirschhorn, J.N. (2003). Meta-analysis of genetic association studies supports a contribution of common variants to susceptibility to common disease. *Nature Genetics*, **33**, 177–182.

Lohmueller, K.E., Indap, A.R, Schmidt, S. et al. (2008). Proportionally more deleterious genetic variation in European than in African populations. *Nature*, **451**, 994–997.

López-León, S., Janssens, A.C., González-Zuloeta Ladd, A.M. et al. (2007). Meta-analyses of genetic studies on major depressive disorder. *Molecular Psychiatry*, **13**, 772–785.

Marcus, S.M., Kerber, K.B., Rush, A.J. et al. (2008). Sex differences in depression symptoms in treatment-seeking adults: confirmatory analyses from the Sequenced Treatment Alternatives to Relieve Depression study. *Comprehensive Psychiatry*, **49**, 238–246.

Marneros, A. and Akiskal, H.S. (eds.) (2006). *The Overlap of Affective and Schizophrenic Spectra*. New York, Cambridge University Press.

Marshall, C.R., Noor, A., Vincent, J.B. et al. (2008). Structural variation of chromosomes in autism spectrum disorder. *American Journal of Human Genetics*, **82**, 477–488.

McVean, G. and Spencer, C.C. (2006). Scanning the human genome for signals of selection. *Current Opinion in Genetics & Development*, **16**, 624–629.

Meizel, S. (2004). The sperm, a neuron with a tail: 'neuronal' receptors in mammalian sperm. *Biological Reviews Cambridge Philosophical Society*, **79**, 713–732.

Meyer-Lindenberg, A., Straub, R.E., Lipska, B.K. et al. (2007). Genetic evidence implicating DARPP-32 in human frontostriatal structure, function, and cognition. *Journal of Clinical Investigation*, **117**, 672–682.

Middeldorp, C.M., Hottenga, J.J., Slagboom, P.E. et al. (2008). Linkage on chromosome 14 in a genome-wide linkage study of a broad anxiety phenotype. *Molecular Psychiatry*, **13**, 84–89.

Mill, J. and Petronis, A. (2007). Molecular studies of major depressive disorder: the epigenetic perspective. *Molecular Psychiatry*, **12**, 799–814.

Muir, W.J., Pickard, B.S., and Blackwood, D.H. (2008). Disrupted-in-Schizophrenia-1. *Current Psychiatry Reports*, **10**, 140–147.

Nesse, R.M. (1999). Proximate and evolutionary studies of anxiety, stress and depression: synergy at the interface. *Neuroscience and Biobehavioral Reviews*, **23**, 895–903.

Nesse, R.M. (2000). Is depression an adaptation? *Archives of General Psychiatry*, **57**, 14–20.

Nesse, R.M. (2004). Cliff-edged fitness functions and the persistence of schizophrenia. *Behavioral and Brain Sciences*, **27**, 862–863.

Nesse, R.M. (2005). Maladaptation and natural selection. *The Quarterly Review of Biology*, **80**, 62–70.

Nettle, D. (2001). *Strong Imagination: Madness, Creativity and Human Nature*. Oxford, Oxford University Press.

Nettle, D. (2004). Evolutionary origins of depression: a review and reformulation. *Journal of Affective Disorders*, **81**, 91–102.

Nettle, D. (2006a). The evolution of personality variation in humans and other animals. *American Psychologist*, **61**, 622–631.

Nettle, D. (2006b). Reconciling the mutation–selection balance model with the schizotypy–creativity connection. *Behavioral and Brain Sciences*, **29**, 418.

Nettle, D. and Clegg, H. (2006). Schizotypy, creativity and mating success in humans. *Proceedings of the Royal Society of London Series B, Biological Sciences*, **273**, 611–615.

Ni, X., Trakalo, J., Valente, J. et al. (2005). Human p53 tumor suppressor gene (TP53) and schizophrenia: case-control and family studies. *Neuroscience Letters*, **388**, 173–178.

Nielsen, R., Bustamante, C., Clark, A.G. et al. (2005). A scan for positively selected genes in the genomes of humans and chimpanzees. *PLoS Biology*, **3**, e170.

Ørstavik, R.E., Kendler, K.S., Czajkowski, N., Tambs, K., and Reichborn-Kjennerud, T. (2007). The relationship between depressive personality disorder and major depressive disorder: a population-based twin study. *American Journal of Psychiatry*, **164**, 1866–1872.

Opgen-Rhein, C., Lencz, T., Burdick, K.E. et al. (2008). Genetic variation in the DAOA gene complex: impact on susceptibility for schizophrenia and on cognitive performance. *Schizophrenia Research*, **103**, 169–177.

Owen, M.J., Craddock, N., and Jablensky, A. (2007). The genetic deconstruction of psychosis. *Schizophrenia Bulletin*, **33**, 905–911.

Pickard, B.S., Thomson, P.A., Christoforou, A. et al. (2007). The PDE4B gene confers sex-specific protection against schizophrenia. *Psychiatric Genetics*, **17**, 129–133.

Potash, J.B. (2006). Carving chaos: genetics and the classification of mood and psychotic syndromes. *Harvard Review of Psychiatry*, **14**, 47–63.

Potash, J.B., Wilour, V.L., Chiu, Y.F. et al. (2001). The familial aggregation of psychotic symptoms in bipolar disorder pedigrees. *American Journal of Psychiatry*, **158**, 1258–1264.

Prata, D., Breen, G., Osborne, S., Munro, J., St Clair, D., and Collier, D. (2008). Association of DAO and G72(DAOA)/G30 genes with bipolar affective disorder. *American Journal of Medical Genetics Part B Neuropsychiatric Genetics* , **147**, 144–147.

Qin, J., Calabrese, P., Tiemann-Boege, I. et al. (2007). The molecular anatomy of spontaneous germline mutations in human testes. *PLoS Biology*, **5**, e224.

Rapoport, J.L., Addington, A.M., and Frangou, S. (2005). The neurodevelopmental model of schizophrenia: update 2005. *Molecular Psychiatry*, **10**, 434–449.

Reuter, M. and Hennig, J. (2005). Pleiotropic effect of the TPH A779C polymorphism on nicotine dependence and personality. *American Journal of Medical Genetics. Part B, Neuropsychiatric Genetics*, **134**, 20–24.

Reuter, M., Roth, S., Holve, K., and Hennig, J. (2006). Identification of first candidate genes for creativity: a pilot study. *Brain Research*, **1069**, 190–197.

Rietschel, M., Beckmann, L., Strohmaier, J. et al. (2008). G72 and its association with major depression and neuroticism in large population-based groups from Germany. *American Journal of Psychiatry*, **165**, 753–762.

Sabeti, P.C., Schaffner, S.F., Fry, B. et al. (2006). Positive natural selection in the human lineage. *Science*, **312**, 1614–1620.

Schürhoff, F., Szöke, A., Méary, A. et al. (2003). Familial aggregation of delusional proneness in schizophrenia and bipolar pedigrees. *American Journal of Psychiatry*, **160**, 1313–1319.

Sebat, J., Lakshmi, B., Malhotra, D. et al. (2007). Strong association of de novo copy number mutations with autism. *Science*, **316**, 445–449.

Serretti, A., Mandelli, L., Lorenzi, C. et al. (2006). Temperament and character in mood disorders: influence of DRD4, SERTPR, TPH and MAO-A polymorphisms. *Neuropsychobiology*, **53**, 9–16.

Sharp, A.J., Locke, D.P., McGrath, S.D. et al. (2005). Segmental duplications and copy-number variation in the human genome. *American Journal of Human Genetics*, **77**, 78–88.

Shifman, S., Bhomra, A., Smiley, S. et al. (2008). A whole genome association study of neuroticism using DNA pooling. *Molecular Psychiatry*, **13**, 302–312.

Sipos, A., Rasmussen, F., Harrison, G. et al. (2004). Paternal age and schizophrenia: a population based cohort study. *British Medical Journal*, **329**, 1070.

Smith, F.M., Garfield, A.S., and Ward, A. (2006). Regulation of growth and metabolism by imprinted genes. *Cytogenetic and Genome Research*, **113**, 279–291.

Smits, G. and Kelsey, G. (2006). Imprinting weaves its web. *Developmental Cell*, **11**, 598–599.

Smith, D.J., Kyle, S., Forty, L. et al. (2008). Differences in depressive symptom profile between males and females. *Journal of Affective Disorders*, **108**, 279–284.

Smith, D.I., Zhu, Y., McAvoy, S., and Kuhn, R. (2006). Common fragile sites, extremely large genes, neural development and cancer. *Cancer Letters*, **232**, 48–57.

Smoller, J.W., Gardner-Schuster, E., and Misiaszek M. (2008). Genetics of anxiety: would the genome recognize the DSM? *Depression and Anxiety*, **25**, 368–377.

Song, W., Li, W., Feng, J., Heston, L.L., Scaringe, W.A., and Sommer, S.S. (2008). Identification of high risk DISC1 structural variants with a 2% attributable risk for schizophrenia. *Biochemical and Biophysical Research Communications*, **367**, 700–706.

Soni, S., Whittington, J., Holland, A.J. et al. (2007). The course and outcome of psychiatric illness in people with Prader-Willi syndrome: implications for management and treatment. *Journal of Intellectual Disability Research*, **51**, 32–42.

Soni, S., Whittington, J., Holland, A.J. et al. (2008). The phenomenology and diagnosis of psychiatric illness in people with Prader-Willi syndrome. *Psychological Medicine*, **4**, 1–10.

Stefanis, N.C., Trikalinos, T.A., Avramopoulos, D. et al. (2007). Impact of schizophrenia candidate genes on schizotypy and cognitive endophenotypes at the population level. *Biological Psychiatry*, **62**, 784–792.

Stefansson, H., Rujescu, D., Cichon, S., et al. (2008) Large recurrent microdeletions associated with schizophrenia. *Nature*, **455**, 232–236.

Tamminga, C.A. and Holcomb, H.H. (2005). Phenotype of schizophrenia: a review and formulation. *Molecular Psychiatry*, **10**, 27–39.

Thomas, P.D. and Kejariwal, A. (2004). Coding single-nucleotide polymorphisms associated with complex vs. Mendelian disease: evolutionary evidence for differences in molecular effects. *Proceedings of the National Academy of Sciences, USA,* **101**, 15398–15403.

Tycko, B. and Morison, I.M. (2002). Physiological functions of imprinted genes. *Journal of Cell Physiology*, **192**, 245–258.

Ubeda, F. and Wilkins, J.F. (2008). Imprinted genes and human disease: an evolutionary perspective. *Advances in Experimental Medicinal Biology*, **626**, 101–115.

Voight, B.F., Kudaravalli, S., Wen, X., and Pritchard, J.K. (2006). A map of recent positive selection in the human genome. *PLoS Biology*, **4**, e72.

Walsh, T., McClellan, J.M., McCarthy, S.E. et al. (2008). Rare structural variants disrupt multiple genes in neurodevelopmental pathways in schizophrenia. *Science*, **320**, 539–543.

Weiss, L.A., Purcell, S., Waggoner, S. et al. (2007). Identification of EFHC2 as a quantitative trait locus for fear recognition in Turner syndrome. *Human Molecular Genetics*, **16**, 107–113.

Winantea, J., Hoang, M.N., Ohlraun, S. et al. (2006). A summary statistic approach to sequence variation in noncoding regions of six schizophrenia-associated gene loci. *European Journal of Human Genetics*, **14**, 1037–1043.

Wolpert, L. (2008). Depression in an evolutionary context. *Philosophy, Ethics, and Humanities in Medicine*, **3**, 8.

Xu, B., Roos, J.L., Levy, S. et al. (2008). Strong association of de novo copy number mutations with sporadic schizophrenia. *Nature Genetics*, **40**, 880–885.

Yampolsky, L.Y., Kondrashov, F.A., and Kondrashov, A.S. (2005). Distribution of the strength of selection against amino acid replacements in human proteins. *Human Molecular Genetics*, **14**, 3191–3201.

Yen, Y.C., Rebok, G.W., Gallo, J.J., Yang, M.J., Lung, F.W., and Shih, C.H. (2007). ApoE4 allele is associated with late-life depression: a population-based study. *American Journal of Geriatric Psychiatry*, **15**, 858–868.

Young, J.H., Chang, Y.P., Kim, J.D. et al. (2005). Differential susceptibility to hypertension is due to selection during the out-of-Africa expansion. *PLoS Genetics*, **1**, e82.

Zhao, X., Leotta, A., Kustanovich, V. et al. (2007). A unified genetic theory for sporadic and inherited autism. *Proceedings of the National Academy of Sciences USA*, **104**, 12831–12836.

Chapter 5

Genetic factors in stress and major depression

Stephan Claes, Elisabeth B. Binder, and Charles B. Nemeroff

Introduction

A large number of family and twin studies have revealed the importance of genetic factors in the vulnerability for major depressive disorder (MDD). In first-degree family members of MDD patients, the risk to develop the disorder is increased by a factor of almost three (Sullivan et al. 2000). A meta-analysis of twin studies indicated that about 40% of the liability to develop major depression is accounted for by additive genetic factors (Kendler et al. 2006). These heritability estimates are higher in women compared to men, implying that some of the genes for major depression could be sex-specific in their effect. The role of these genetic factors within an evolutionary perspective is discussed in Chapters 3 and 4 of this book, while the genetics of bipolar disorder is specifically discussed in Chapter 6. The pharmacogenetics of antidepressants response – that is, looking at genes influencing clinical response to drugs rather than pathophysiological mechanisms – is discussed in Chapter 23. More information of the genetic regulation of the stress response is also presented in Chapter 14.

The same research group published a large study comprising more than 15,000 Swedish twins (Hettema et al. 2006), in an attempt to uncover the genetic contributions to major depression, a number of anxiety disorders, and neuroticism as a personality trait. They identified a set of common genes increasing the vulnerability for high neuroticism, depression and anxiety disorders. Another set of genes was involved in the risk for MDD and anxiety, but not high neuroticism. These results may imply that there are no genetic factors that solely increase the risk for major depression, but instead we should search for genes increasing the risk for both MDD and anxiety disorders, with neuroticism as a potential endophenotype. The search for such genes should take into account impaired stress coping mechanisms in MDD pathogenesis.

First, clinically, different forms of stress, including acute stress (negative life events), chronic stress, and early life stress have been shown to precipitate MDD. The majority of first episodes of MDD are preceded by an acute stressful experience or adverse life event (Mazure et al. 2000), although the importance of life events diminishes as the number of depressive episodes increases. Chronic stress, especially when associated with a psychological dimension of 'entrapment' or humiliation is reported to be particularly depressogenic (Kendler et al. 2003). Third, severe adverse experiences in early life (early life stress, ELS), such as child abuse and neglect, increase the vulnerability for MDD and for a number of anxiety disorders later in life (Duncan et al. 1996). Mullen et al. (1988) found that 20% of women who had been exposed to sexual abuse as a child had psychiatric disorders, predominantly depressive in type, compared with 6.3% of the non-abused population.

Second, dysfunction of stress response systems such as the corticotrophin-releasing factor (CRF) system and the hypothalamic-pituitary-adrenal (HPA) axis are thought to be important factors in the neurobiology of MDD. The concentration of cortisol, the end product of the HPA axis, is increased in blood and urine of major depressive patients (Gold et al. 2002; Sachar et al. 1970). The concentration of CRF is increased in the cerebrospinal fluid (CSF) of depressed patients as compared to controls (Nemeroff et al.1988). Post-mortem brain studies showed that CRF mRNA expression and peptide concentration is increased in MDD patients in critical brain regions such as the locus coeruleus, the raphe nuclei, and the hypothalamus (Austin et al. 2003, Bissette et al. 2003; Merali et al. 2006; Raadsheer et al. 1994), and this is paralleled by a down regulation of CRF receptors, all pointing to an overactive CRF system in depression. Finally, numerous studies initiated in the 1960s have indicated that negative feedback in the HPA axis system is deficient in MDD, as exemplified by the Dexamethasone Suppression Test (DST), or the more sensitive combined Dexamethasone/CRF stimulation test (Holsboer, 2000; Holsboer-Trachsler et al. 1991). The role of the HPA axis in affective disorders and other stress-related conditions is discussed in several other Chapters of this book (Chapters 7–9, 11, 15, 16, 19, 21, and 26).

Basal HPA axis function, independent of disease status, is determined by both environmental and genetic factors. Stressors such as child abuse can produce lifelong disturbances in HPA axis function (Heim et al. 2000; 2008; Tyrka et al. 2008), which in part represents one of the mechanisms by which such stressors lead to an increased risk for MDD and related disorders later in life. However, genetic variations are crucial as well. In a review, Bartels et al. (2003) concluded that the heritability of basal cortisol secretion is quite high, around 60%, indicating that genes are important in regulating basal HPA axis function. The heritability of the HPA axis response to specific stressors, such as the Trier Social Stress Test, has been less well established, and seems to be context dependent (Federenko et al. 2004). The perception of chronic stress is moderately heritable, depending on the clinical instrument (Federenko et al. 2006). Some of the HPA axis abnormalities observed in MDD might have a genetic background. Holsboer et al. (1995) reported that the HPA feedback disturbance observed among patients with depression was also present in otherwise healthy individuals with a first-degree relative with an affective illness. Moreover, this disturbance was shown to be stable over a five-year period (Modell et al. 1998).

As a consequence, genes that play a role in the regulation of the stress response, the HPA axis and CRF secretion and function are of interest as candidate genes for abnormal stress coping and the development of MDD, PTSD, and other anxiety disorders. Theoretically, numerous functional candidate genes could be involved, as several biological systems, including immune activation, cortisol transport across the membrane, serotonin and norepinephrine pathways, interact with HPA axis function. This chapter will focus on genes directly influencing the function of CRF, Arginine Vasopressin (AVP), and cortisol, and, more specifically, on four genes that have been most extensively studied up to date: genes encoding the CRF1 receptor (CRHR1), the Arginine Vasopressin 1b receptor (AVPR1B), the glucocorticoid receptor (NR3C1), and the co-chaperone protein FKBP5 (FKBP5). For each of these genes, animal and human studies concerning their role in stress response regulation and in the vulnerability for MDD and other stress-related disorders will be discussed.

The CRF receptor 1 (CRHR1) gene

Two receptors have been identified within the CRF system, CRF1 and CRF2, encoded by the CRHR1 gene on chromosome 17 and the CRHR2 gene on chromosome 5, respectively. However, the CRF1 receptor appears to be more directly involved in HPA axis regulation and depression and anxiety-related phenotypes (Nemeroff and Vale, 2005; Reul and Holsboer, 2002).

Even though the CRF1 receptor shares 70% sequence identity with the CRF2 receptor, it has much higher affinity for CRF. The CRF1 receptor is highly expressed in rodents, non-human primates, and humans in the anterior pituitary, neocortex, hippocampus, amygdala, and cerebellum (see Hauger et al. 2003 for review)

In animal studies, evidence for a potential role of CRHR1 in the stress response and related disorders was found. Transgenic mice lacking the gene encoding the CRF1 receptor showed a reduction of the stress induced release of ACTH and corticosterone (CORT), and reduced anxiety-related behaviour (Timpl et al. 1998). The results demonstrated a key role of the CRF1 receptor in mediating the stress response and anxiety-related behaviour. In a more complex model, Müller et al. (2003) knocked out the CRHR1 gene postnatally in the limbic system and not at the level of the pituitary. These transgenic animals showed normal HPA axis activity in basal circumstances and after stress exposure due to the intact pituitary CRF system. However, anxiety-related behaviour was reduced, indicating that the role of CRF in anxiety regulation is independent of its HPA axis related function. Furthermore, the elevation of CORT and ACTH secretion after stress was prolonged in these transgenic mice, suggesting a role of CRF1 in negative feedback regulation of the HPA axis.

Only recently association studies examining CRHR1 gene variants in MDD have been published. In a small study in Mexican-American MDD patients (Licinio et al. 2004), an increased response to antidepressants in highly anxious patients homozygous for a specific CRHR1 haplotype was found. In Han Chinese populations, evidence for the association of one of three CRHR1 SNPs with liability to develop MDD (Liu et al. 2006), as well with the response to antidepressant drugs (Liu et al. 2007) has been reported. More recently, Bradley et al. (2008) performed an association study examining gene x environment interactions to determine the effects of 15 CRHR1 SNPs and measures of child abuse on adult depressive symptoms. The authors studied a sample of 422 individuals at high risk for childhood trauma and a second independent sample of 199 individuals, and found significant gene x environment interactions with multiple individual SNPs as well as with a common haplotype spanning intron 1 of the CRHR1 gene in both samples. This led to the conclusion that specific CRHR1 polymorphisms modulate the effect of ELS on the risk for adult depressive symptoms. Interaction of CRHR1 polymorphisms with negative life events on suicide attempts and alcohol abuse have also been reported, supporting the moderating effect of CRF1 activity on stress-related psychiatric phenotypes (Blomeyer et al. 2008; Wasserman et al. 2008).

Taken together, these data suggest that CRHR1 genetic variation modulates the risk for MDD by interacting with the effect of ELS and possibly other stress exposures.

The AVP receptor 1b gene

A role for AVP in modulating stress response is supported by its known synergism with the CRF system. Several subtypes of AVP receptors have been identified. The ACTH releasing properties of AVP are mediated by the AVP 1b receptor 1B (AVPR1b) subtype. In situ hybridization studies revealed that AVPR1b mRNA is expressed in the pituitary, but also in multiple other brain regions, and in a number of peripheral tissues and moreover, there is an overlapping expression pattern with the CRF1 receptor, especially in limbic brain regions (Grazzini et al. 1996; Lolait et al. 1995; see also Chapter 16 in this book).

Animal models targeting the AVPR1b gene have yielded discordant results. In a study by Tanoue et al. (2004) circulating concentrations of ACTH and CORT were lower in Avpr1b knockout (KO) mice compared with wild-type (WT) mice under resting conditions. Furthermore, the increase in ACTH after a forced swim stress was significantly suppressed in these animals. However, in another study Avprb1 deficient mice were not different regarding basal plasma levels of ACTH and CORT (Lolait et al. 2007). Acute restraint stress increased plasma ACTH and CORT to a similar extent in both the Avpr1b mutant and WT mice. However, in the Avpr1b KO group subjected to 14 sessions of daily restraint stress, plasma ACTH concentrations were decreased when compared with WT mice. In contrast, the CORT elevations induced by restraint did not adapt in either the Avpr1b KO or WT mice. This converges with other lines of evidence indicating that AVP is especially important in the regulation of chronic stress.

In a genetic association study, van West et al. (2004) constructed a gene-based SNP map of the AVPR1b receptor gene and studied association with MDD in a population from northern Sweden and in a Belgian population. In both groups, a highly significant difference in global haplotype distribution was found. This was caused by the overrepresentation of the same SNP haplotype in controls, thus suggesting a protective effect of this haplotype in both populations. More recently, Dempster et al. (2007) genotyped SNPs across the AVPR1B gene in a family-based sample of 382 Hungarian families with childhood-onset mood disorders. Two of the AVPR1B SNPs showed individual associations, and haplotype analysis demonstrated significant overtransmission of the most frequent haplotype. In both the van West and Dempster studies, stratifying the sample by sex established that the association was predominantly in affected females, pointing to gender differences in AVP function. Recently, Keck et al. (2008) have also published an association of a combined risk genotype of SNPs with AVPR1B and CRHR1 with panic disorder in two independent German samples, underlining the synergistic effects of these two neuropeptide transmitter systems in anxiety and depression.

The glucocorticoid receptor gene

For several reasons, the gene (NR3C1) encoding the glucocorticoid receptor (GR) is a prime candidate for mediating vulnerability to develop MDD. First, the HPA axis negative feedback is mainly regulated by this protein, especially under conditions of high cortisol secretion. Impairment of the HPA axis negative feedback is one of the main neurobiological findings in MDD. Second, a number of studies have shown a reduction of GR function in depressed patients in in vitro studies. Third, treatment with antidepressants leads to an increase of both the expression and the activity of the GR (Pariante and Miller, 2001). Finally, rodents that have been subjected to early neglect develop a depression-like phenotype that is associated with decreased GR expression in the hippocampus (Ladd et al. 2004).

Strong evidence for the potential importance of GR gene variations in mediating stress response impairment and stress-related clinical disorders is derived from animal models. Complete absence of functional GR is incompatible with life (Reichard et al. 1998). However, a number of partial and conditional KT mice models for the GR gene have been produced. Ridder et al. (2005) produced a mouse strain with a 50% reduction of GR expression. Although these mice exhibited normal basal activity of the HPA axis and reacted normally to anxiety tests, they exhibited a disinhibited HPA axis with impaired negative feedback, and developed more severe helplessness in animal models for depression. Interestingly, this study also found that these animals displayed a reduction in brain-derived neurotrophic factor (BDNF) expression, also reported in humans with depression. Boyle et al. (2005) generated a line of mice with time-dependent, forebrain-specific disruption of GR. These animals showed HPA axis hyperactivity, impaired negative feedback, increased depression-like behaviour in models such as the forced swim test and the tail suspension test and decreased pleasure seeking. Importantly, a number of these abnormalities were normalized by chronic treatment with the tricyclic antidepressant imipramine. These studies indicate that partial or conditional knockouts of the GR gene yield an animal model for depression with good face, construct, and predictive validity (see also Chapter 9).

In humans, several studies have identified genetic polymorphisms in the GR gene (for a review, see De Rijk et al. 2002). The gene encodes three protein domains: the immunogenic domain, the DNA domain, and the ligand-binding domain. A number of mutations have been described in the ligand-binding domain. These mutations are very rare, mostly only found in a single family and result in a marked reduction of the sensitivity of the receptor. This leads to a combination of serious endocrinological dysfunctions summarized as 'glucocorticoid resistance syndrome'. For our purposes, SNPs in the region encoding the immunogenic domain, leading to more subtle changes in GR function, are more relevant. Several such SNPs have been identified, such as R23K (allele frequency: 3%), N363S (4%), BclI (37%), and A3669G (15%), all of which have been found to alter the function of GR (DeRijk and De Kloet, 2008). The R23K mutation leads to a relative decrease in the sensitivity of GRs (Van Rossum et al. 2002) and would therefore be a logical candidate for increasing the risk for MDD. The N363S and BclI mutation leads to an increased sensitivity of the HPA negative feedback. Several of these SNPs seem to influence HPA axis reactivity to social stress (Kumsta et al. 2007; van West et al. submitted), increasing their potential interest in relation to MDD.

In an early small study, five missense variants in the amino-terminal domain of the GR gene showed no association with puerperal psychosis or schizophrenia (Feng et al. 2000). More recently, a genetic association study in 314 MDD patients and 354 control individuals from two populations found evidence for association with a SNP in the promoter region in the Belgian population and with R23K in the Swedish population (van West et al. 2006). Eleven percent of the Swedish MDD patients carried the mutant G-allele, compared to four percent of the control individuals. Almost simultaneously, another association study in German MDD patients found evidence for a potential role of the R23K mutation as well. They found a frequency of the mutation of 4% in control individuals, compared to 6% in depressive patients, and 8% in patients with recurrent major depression (van Rossum et al. 2006). In a smaller study of premenopausal women, Krishnamurthy et al. (2008) found an increase of the G/G genotype of the Bcl1 polymorphism in women with major depression. This study did not include the R23K mutation. The same overrepresentation of BclI G/G in major depression was also reported by van Rossum et al. (2006). Clearly, R23K and BclI polymorphisms are just two of the SNPs that could influence GR function and susceptibility to major depression. Putatively, SNPs in the GR promoter region that influence expression might also be relevant. According to Wüst et al. (2007), the R23K mutation is actually in linkage disequilibrium with a polymorphism in the promoter region that diminishes GR expression, which would offer an alternative explanation for the positive association findings. Finally, it should be emphasized that also epigenetic mechanisms such as DNA methylation diminish GR function and potentially increase the risk for MDD. These epigenetic alterations in GR responsiveness can be induced by known risk factors for depression, such as early life stress (Meaney and Szyf, 2005).

The FKBP5 gene

FK506 binding protein 5 (FKBP5) regulates GR sensitivity. It directly interacts with heat shock protein 90 (hsp90), which binds to the GR, allowing it to form the mature GR heterocomplex. Once cortisol binds to the complex, FKBP5 is replaced by FKBP4, and translocation of GR to the nucleus is initiated (Grad and Picard, 2007; Pratt and Toft, 2003). By regulating GR sensitivity, FKBP5 is an excellent candidate for the genetic regulation of the stress response and vulnerability for stress-related disorders.

Mice lacking a functional FKBP5 gene have been studied. These animals show a normal phenotype and reproductive behaviour, and no abnormalities in androgen receptor function (Yong et al. 2007). However, data on GR function, HPA axis activity after stress exposure and depression-related behaviour in animal models are not yet available.

The potential role of the FKBP5 gene in MDD was highlighted when significant associations of response to antidepressants and the recurrence of depressive episodes were found with FKBP5 SNPs in two independent samples of patients with MDD, bipolar disorder, or dysthymia (Binder et al. 2004). Interestingly, the alleles associated with poor treatment response were also associated with increased intracellular FKBP5 protein expression, increased induction of FKBP5 mRNA by cortisol, and reduced HPA axis dysregulation in the Dex-CRH test upon inpatient admission. Association with treatment response were not replicated in small Chinese (Tsai et al. 2007) and Spanish samples (Papiol et al. 2007), with both studies only investigating one of the associated SNPs, rs1360780. However, in a large study of 1523 MDD patients who participated in the Sequenced Treatment Alternatives to Relieve Depression (STAR*D) study, Lekman et al. (2008) demonstrated an association with antidepressant treatment outcome and a promoter FKBP5 SNP also as observed by Binder et al. (2004). In this study they also reported an association between SNP rs1360780 and MDD, but no association with the number of depressive episodes. Interestingly, a large family-based association study in two bipolar disorder samples, totalling 317 families with 554 children, found significant evidence for the involvement of several FKBP5 SNPs in bipolar disorder (Willour et al. 2008). Association with mood disorder per se were not observed by Binder et al. 2004 and in a second German study investigating 248 depressive episode patients, of which 77% suffered from bipolar disorder (Gawlik et al. 2006). Finally, in 762 individuals with significant childhood abuse, as well as non-child abuse trauma, Binder et al. (2008) found that 4 SNPs in the FKBP5 locus significantly interacted with the severity of child abuse to predict the magnitude of adult PTSD symptoms. They further observed a functional effect of these SNPs on dexamethasone-induced suppression of the HPA axis, with the direction of this effect being opposite in PTSD patients compared to individuals not suffering from PTSD.

Figure 5.1 offers a graphical representation of the genomic location of the FKBP5 gene polymorphisms that have been considered in the available studies. The cited studies converge to indicate that genetic variation of the FKBP5 gene contributes to the vulnerability and the treatment response in MDD and bipolar disorder, and may moderate the effect of childhood abuse.

Discussion

Several strategies are being pursued in the search for genes relevant to mood disorders. Systematic genome wide association approaches are underway, and the first results regarding bipolar disorder have been published recently (Baum et al. 2008; Sklar et al. 2008; WTCCC 2007). Although such studies are of great interest, a systematic scrutiny of genes involved in key neurobiological systems is necessary as well. One of the advantages of the latter approach is that the focus is not primarily on finding genes for a DSM-defined disease entity, but rather to investigate the impact of genetic variation in disease-relevant systems on the physiologic control of this system and on the shared vulnerability for several related diseases. This could be termed a systematic hypothesis-based candidate gene approach. It should be noted that one of the most reproducible findings in psychiatric genetics, which is the involvement of the serotonin transporter promoter length polymorphism in MDD vulnerability after childhood adversity (Caspi et al. 2003), is a result of this strategy.

Clearly, the CRF system and the stress response pathways in general are of great interest, given the fact that mood and anxiety disorders are stress-related to varying degrees. This chapter presents an overview of the current data on four major functional candidate genes within this system. The focus is not only on whether variation in these genes contributes to specific DSM diagnoses, but also how it affects stress responsivity in general, and which variants interact with which stressors in order to generate neurobiological dysfunctions that in turn increase the vulnerability to develop psychiatric disorders, e.g. MDD or PTSD.

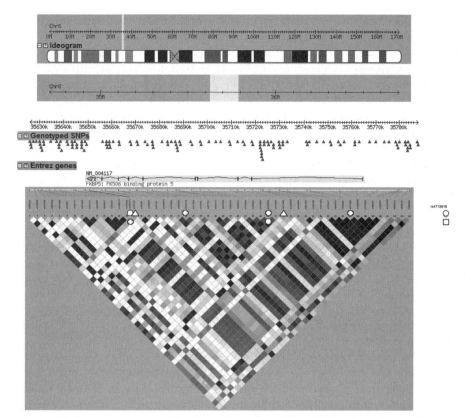

Fig. 5.1 Graphical representation of the genomic location of the FKBP5 gene polymorphisms

Note: This figure represents the chromosomal position of FKBP5 on chromosome 6p as well as the exon intron structure as shown on www.hapmap.org. The 5′ end of the gene is located on the right side of the panel.

All SNPs with a minor allele frequency of 5% or higher in the Caucasian sample of the HapMap project (CEU) were included in the linkage disequilibrium (LD) plot using Haploview software. LD is represented by r-squared. Black squares indicate complete LD and an r-squared = 1 between the connected SNPs and white no LD and an r-squared of 0.

Symbols mark the SNPs with strongest association in the studies described.

Circles: Binder et al., 2004, squares: Lekman et al 2008, triangles: Willour et al, 2008 and crosses: Binder et al., 2008

There is increasing evidence for an important role of each of those four genes. For the CRHR1, AVPR1b, and GR genes, animal models clearly demonstrate their role in regulating the stress response. For the GR and FKBP5 genes, the influence of SNPs on HPA axis function in humans has been demonstrated as well. Finally, for all four genes there are two or more independent reports indicating a role in the vulnerability for MDD or anxiety disorders. At this stage the evidence is probably strongest for FKBP5, as it is confirmed by four large studies. Particularly interesting are the studies available for CRHR1 and FKBP5 that have scrutinized interactions between specific stressors and disease vulnerability.

Clearly, this is only the beginning. For the four genes discussed here, the full scope of genetic variation still needs to be clarified, together with a systematic study of the effect of these SNPs on CRF and HPA axis function (both basal and in response to specific stressors), and finally a further assessment of allele frequencies in different axis I disorder patient groups. Multicentre studies will be necessary in order to create samples large enough to assess the combined effects of genetic variations in different HPA axis related genes. Finally these findings will have to be compared to the outcome of genome wide association approaches in order to allow an overall appreciation of the relative contribution of these genes to psychopathological vulnerability.

Acknowledgments

Stephan Claes is a Senior Clinical Investigator of the Fund for Scientific Research – Flanders (FWO-Vlaanderen), Belgium
Charles B. Nemeroff is supported by NIH MH-42088, MH-58922, MH-69056, MH-77083, and RR-25008.

References

Austin, M.C., Janosky, J.E. and Murphy, H.A. (2003). Increased corticotropin-releasing hormone immunoreactivity in monoamine-containing pontine nuclei of depressed suicide men. *Molecular Psychiatry*, **8**, 324–332.

Bartels, M., Van den Berg, M., Sluyter, F., Boomsma, D.I., and de Geus, E.J. (2003). Heritability of cortisol levels: Review and simultaneous analysis of twin studies. *Psychoneuroendocrinology*, **28**, 121–137.

Baum, A.E., Akula, N., Cabanero, M., et al. (2008). A genome-wide association study implicates diacylglycerol kinase eta (DGKH) and several other genes in the etiology of bipolar disorder. *Molecular Psychiatry*, **13**, 197–207.

Binder, E.B., Salyakina, D., Lichtner, P., et al. (2004). Polymorphisms in FKBP5 are associated with increased recurrence of depressive episodes and rapid response to antidepressant treatment. *Nature Genetics*, **36**, 1319–1325.

Binder, E.B., Bradley, R.G., Liu, W., et al. (2008). Association of FKBP5 polymorphisms and childhood abuse with risk of posttraumatic stress disorder symptoms in adults. *JAMA*, **299**, 1291–1305.

Bissette, G., Klimek, V., Pan, J., Stockmeier, C., and Ordway G. (2003). Elevated concentrations of CRF in the locus coeruleus of depressed subjects. *Neuropsychopharmacology*, **28**, 1328–1335.

Blomeyer, D., Treutlein, J., Esser, G., Schmidt, M.H., Schumann, G., and Laucht, M. (2007). Interaction between CRHR1 Gene and stressful life events predicts adolescent heavy alcohol use. *Biological Psychiatry*, **63**, 146–151

Boyle, M.P., Brewer, J.A., Funatsu, M., et al. (2005). Acquired deficit of forebrain glucocorticoid receptor produces depression-like changes in adrenal axis regulation and behavior. *Proceedings of the National Academy of Sciences of the United States of America*, **102**, 473–478.

Bradley, R.G., Binder, E.B., Epstein, M.P., et al. (2008). Influence of child abuse on adult depression: moderation by the corticotropin-releasing hormone receptor gene. *Archives of General Psychiatry*, **65**, 190–200.

Caspi, A., Sugden, K., Moffitt, T.E., et al. (2003). Influence of life stress on depression: moderation by a polymorphism in the 5-HTT gene. *Science*, **301**, 386–389.

De Rijk, R.H., Schaaf, M., and de Kloet, E. R. (2002). Glucocorticoid receptor variants: clinical implications. *The Journal of Steroid Biochemistry and Molecular Biology*, **81**, 103–122.

De Rijk, R.H. and de Kloet ER. (2008). Corticosteroid receptor polymorphisms: determinants of vulnerability and resilience. *European Journal of Pharmacology*, **583**, 303–311.

Dempster, E.L., Burcescu, I., Wigg, K., et al. (2007). Evidence of an association between the vasopressin V1b receptor gene (AVPR1B) and childhood-onset mood disorders. *Archives of General Psychiatry*, **64**, 1189–1195.

Duncan, R.D., Saunders, B.E., Kilpatrick, D.G., Hanson, R.F., and Resnick, H.S. (1996). Childhood physical assault as a risk factor for PTSD, depression, and substance abuse: findings from a national survey. *The American Journal of Orthopsychiatry*, **66**, 437–448.

Federenko, I.S., Schlotz, W., Kirschbaum, C., Bartels, M., Hellhammer, D.H., and Wüst, S. (2006). The heritability of perceived stress. *Psychological Medicine*, **36**, 375–385.

Federenko, I.S., Nagamine, M., Hellhammer, D.H., Wadhwa, P.D., and Wüst, S. (2004). The heritability of hypothalamus pituitary adrenal axis responses to psychosocial stress is context dependent. *The Journal of Clinical Endocrinology and Metabolism*, **89**, 6244–6250.

Feng, J., Zheng, J., Bennett, W.P., et al. (2000). Five missense variants in the amino-terminal domain of the glucocorticoid receptor: no association with puerperal psychosis or schizophrenia. *American Journal of Medical Genetics*, **96**, 412–417.

Gawlik, M., Moller-Ehrlich, K., Mende, M., et al. (2006). Is FKBP5 a genetic marker of affective psychosis? A case control study and analysis of disease related traits. *BMC Psychiatry*, **6**, 52.

Gold, P.W., Drevets, W.C., and Charney, D.S. (2002). New insights into the role of cortisol and the glucocorticoid receptor in severe depression. *Biological Psychiatry*, **52**, 381–385.

Grad, I. and Picard, D. (2007). The glucocorticoid responses are shaped by molecular chaperones. *Molecular and Cellular Endocrinology*, **275**, 2–12.

Grazzini, E., Lodboerer, A.M., Perez-Martin, A., Joubert, D., and Guillon, G. (1996). Molecular and functional characterization of V1b vasopressin receptor in rat adrenal medulla. *Endocrinology*, **137**, 3906–3914.

Hauger, R.L., Grigoriadis, D.E., Dallman, M.F., Plotsky, P.M., Vale, W.W., and Dautzenberg, F.M. (2003). International union of pharmacology. XXXVI. Current status of the nomenclature for receptors for corticotropin-releasing factor and their ligands. *Pharmacological Reviews*, **55**, 21–26.

Heim, C., Mletzko, T., Purselle, D., Musselman, D.L., and Nemeroff, C.B. (2008). The dexamethasone/corticotropin-releasing factor test in men with major depression: role of childhood trauma. *Biological Psychiatry*, **63**, 398–405.

Heim, C., Newport, D.J., Heit, S., et al. (2000). Pituitary-adrenal and autonomic responses to stress in women after sexual and physical abuse in childhood. *JAMA*, **284**, 592–597.

Hettema, J.M., Neale, M.C., Myers, J.M., Prescott, C.A., and Kendler, K.S. (2006). A population-based twin study of the relationship between neuroticism and internalizing disorders. *The American Journal of Psychiatry*, **163**, 857–864.

Holsboer, F. (2000). The corticosteroid receptor hypothesis of depression. *Neuropsychopharmacology*, **23**, 477–501.

Holsboer, F., Lauer, C.J., Schreiber, W., and Krieg, J.C. (1995). Altered hypothalamic-pituitary-adrenocortical regulation in healthy subjects at high familial risk for affective disorders. *Neuroendocrinology*, **62**, 340–347.

Holsboer-Trachsler, E., Stohler, R., and Hatzinger, M. (1991). Repeated administration of the combined dexamethasone-human corticotropin releasing hormone stimulation test during treatment of depression. *Psychiatry Research*, **38**, 163–171.

Keck, M.E., Kern, N., Erhardt, A., et al. (2008). Combined effects of exonic polymorphisms in CRHR1 and AVPR1B genes in a case/control study for panic disorder. *American Journal of Medical Genetics. Part B, Neuropsychiatric Genetics*, April 2. [Epub ahead of print].

Kendler, K.S., Gatz M, Gardner, C.O., and Pedersen NL. (2006). A Swedish national twin study of lifetime major depression. *The American Journal of Psychiatry*, **163**, 109–114.

Kendler, K.S., Hettema, J.M., Butera, F., Gardner, C.O., and Prescott, C.A. (2003). Life event dimensions of loss, humiliation, entrapment, and danger in the prediction of onsets of major depression and generalized anxiety. *Archives of General Psychiatry*, **60**, 789–796.

Krishnamurthy, P., Romagni, P., Torvik, S., et al. (2008). P.O.W.E.R. (Premenopausal, Osteoporosis Women, Alendronate, Depression) Study Group.Glucocorticoid receptor gene polymorphisms in premenopausal women with major depression. *Hormone and Metabolic Research*, **40**, 194–198.

Kumsta, R., Entringer, S., Koper, J.W., van Rossum, E.F., Hellhammer, D.H., and Wüst, S. (2007). Sex specific associations between common glucocorticoid receptor gene variants and hypothalamus-pituitary-adrenal axis responses to psychosocial stress. *Biological Psychiatry*, **62**, 863–869.

Ladd, C.O., Huot, R.L., Thrivikraman, K.V., Nemeroff, C.B., and Plotsky, P.M. (2004). Long-term adaptations in glucocorticoid receptor and mineralocorticoid receptor mRNA and negative feedback on the hypothalamo-pituitary-adrenal axis following neonatal maternal separation. *Biological Psychiatry*, **55**, 367–375.

Lekman, M., Laje, G., Charney, D., et al. (2008). The FKBP5-gene in depression and treatment response-an association study in the Sequenced Treatment Alternatives to Relieve Depression (STAR*D) Cohort. *Biological Psychiatry*, January 10. [Epub ahead of print].

Licinio, J., O'Kirwan, F., Irizarry, K., et al. (2004). Association of a corticotropin-releasing hormone receptor 1 haplotype and antidepressant treatment response in Mexican-Americans. *Molecular Psychiatry*, **9**, 1075–1082.

Liu, Z., Zhu, F., Wang, G., et al. (2006). Association of corticotropin-releasing hormone receptor1 gene SNP and haplotype with major depression. *Neuroscience Letters*, **404**, 358–362.

Liu, Z., Zhu, F., Wang, G., et al. (2007). Association study of corticotropin-releasing hormone receptor1 gene polymorphisms and antidepressant response in major depressive disorders. *Neuroscience Letters*, **414**, 155–158.

Lolait, S.J., O'Carroll, A.M., Mahan, L.C., et al. (1995). Extrapituitary expression of the rat V1b vasopressin receptor gene. *Proceedings of the National Academy of Sciences of the United States of America*, **92**, 6783–6787.

Lolait, S.J., Stewart, L.Q., Jessop, D.S., Young, W.S. III, and O'Carroll, A.M. (2007). The hypothalamic-pituitary-adrenal axis response to stress in mice lacking functional vasopressin V1b receptors. *Endocrinology*, **148**, 849–856.

Mazure, C.M., Bruce, M.L., Maciejewski, P.K., and Jacobs, S.C. (2000). Adverse life events and cognitive-personality characteristics in the prediction of major depression and antidepressant response. *The American Journal of Psychiatry*, **157**, 896–903.

Meaney, M.J. and Szyf, M. (2005). Environmental programming of stress responses through DNA methylation: Life at the interface between a dynamic environment and a fixed genome. *Dialogues in Clinical Neuroscience*, **7**, 103–123.

Merali, Z., Kent, P., Du, L., et al. (2005). Corticotropin-releasing hormone, Arginine Vasopressin, Gastrin-releasing peptide, and neuromedin B alterations in stress-relevant brain regions of suicides and control subjects. *Biological Psychiatry*, **59**, 594–602.

Modell, S., Lauer, C.J., Schreiber, W., Huber, J., Krieg, J.C., and Holsboer, F. (1998). Hormonal response pattern in the combined DEX-CRH test is stable over time in subjects at high familial risk for affective disorders. *Neuropsychopharmacology*, **18**, 253–262.

Mullen, P.E., Romans-Clarkson, S.E., Walton, V.A., and Herbison, G.P. (1988). Impact of sexual and physical abuse on women's mental health. *Lancet*, **1**, 841–845.

Müller, M.B., Zimmermann, S., Sillaber, I., et al. (2003). Limbic corticotropin-releasing hormone receptor1 mediates anxiety-related behavior and hormonal adaptation to stress. *Nature Neuroscience*, **6**, 1100–1107.

Nemeroff, C.B., Owens, M.J., Bissette, G., Andorn, A.C., and Stanley, M. (1988). Reduced corticotropin releasing factor binding sites in the frontal cortex of suicide victims. *Archives of General Psychiatry*, **45**, 577–579.

Nemeroff, C.B. and Vale, W.W. (2005). The neurobiology of depression: inroads to treatment and new drug discovery. *The Journal of Clinical Psychiatry*, **66 Suppl 7**, 5–13.

Papiol, S., Arias, B., Gasto, C., Gutierrez, B., Catalan, R., and Fananas, L. (2007). Genetic variability at HPA axis in major depression and clinical response to antidepressant treatment. *Journal of Affective Disorders*, **104**, 83–90.

Pariante, C.M. and Miller, A.H. (2001). Glucocorticoid receptors in major depression: relevance to pathophysiology and treatment. *Biological Psychiatry*, **49**, 391–404.

Pratt, W.B. and Toft, D.O. (2003). Regulation of signaling protein function and trafficking by the hsp90/hsp70-based chaperone machinery. *Experimental Biology And Medicine (Maywood, N.J.)*, **228**, 111–133.

Raadsheer, F.C., Hoogendijk, W.J., Stam, F.C., Tilders, F.J., and Swaab, D.F. (1994). Increased numbers of corticotropin-releasing hormone expressing neurons in the hypothalamic paraventricular nucleus of depressed patients. *Neuroendocrinology*, **60**, 436–444.

Reichardt, H.M., Kaestner, K.H., Tuckermann, J., et al. (1998). DNA binding of the glucocorticoid receptor is not essential for survival. *Cell*, **93**, 531–541.

Ridder, S., Chourbaji, S., Hellweg, R., et al. (2005). Mice with genetically altered glucocorticoid receptor expression show altered sensitivity for stress-induced depressive reactions. *The Journal of Neuroscience: The Official Journal of the Society for Neuroscience*, **25**, 6243–6250.

Reul, J.M. and Holsboer, F. (2002). Corticotropin-releasing factor receptors 1 and 2 in anxiety and depression. *Current Opinion in Pharmacology*, **2**, 23–33.

Pariante, C.M. (2004). Glucocorticoid receptor function in vitro in patients with major depression. *Stress*, **7**, 209–19.

Sachar, E.J., Hellman, L., Fukushima, D.K., and Gallagher, T.F. (1970). Cortisol production in depressive illness. A clinical and biochemical clarification. *Archives of General Psychiatry*, **23**, 289–298.

Sklar, P., Smoller, J.W., Fan, J., et al. (2008). Whole-genome association study of bipolar disorder. *Molecular Psychiatry*, March 4. [Epub ahead of print].

Sullivan, P.F., Neale, M.C., and Kendler, K.S. (2000). Genetic epidemiology of major depression: review and meta-analysis. *The American Journal of Psychiatry*, **157**, 1552–1562.

Tanoue, A., Ito, S., Honda, K., et al. (2004). The vasopressin V1b receptor critically regulates hypothalamic-pituitary-adrenal axis activity under both stress and resting conditions. *The Journal of Clinical Investigation*, **113**, 302–309.

Timpl, P., Spanagel, R., Sillaber, I., et al. (1998). Impaired stress response and reduced anxiety in mice lacking a functional corticotropin-releasing hormone receptor 1. *Nature Genetics*, **19**, 162–166.

Tsai, S.J., Hong, C.J., Chen, T.J., and Yu, Y.W. (2007). Lack of supporting evidence for a genetic association of the FKBP5 polymorphism and response to antidepressant treatment. *American Journal of Medical Genetics. Part B, Neuropsychiatric Genetics*, **144**, 1097–1098.

Tyrka, A.R., Wier, L., Price, L.H. et al. (2008). Childhood parental loss and adult hypothalamic-pituitary-adrenal function. *Biological Psychiatry*, March 11. [Epub ahead of print].

van Rossum, E.F., Koper, J.W., Huizenga, N.A. et al. (2002). A polymorphism in the glucocorticoid receptor gene, which decreases sensitivity to glucocorticoids in vivo, is associated with low insulin and cholesterol levels. *Diabetes*, **51**, 3128–3134.

van Rossum, E.F., Binder, E.B., Majer, M. et al. (2006). Polymorphisms of the glucocorticoid receptor gene and major depression. *Biological Psychiatry*, **59**, 681–688.

van West, D., Del-Favero, J., Aulchenko, Y. et al. (2004). A major SNP haplotype of the arginine vasopressin 1B receptor protects against recurrent major depression. *Molecular Psychiatry*, **9**, 287–292

van West, D., Van Den Eede, F., Del-Favero, J. et al. (2006). Glucocorticoid receptor gene-based SNP analysis in patients with recurrent major depression. *Neuropsychopharmacology*, **31**, 620–627.

van West, D., Claes, S., Del-Favero, J., Van Broeckhoven, C., Sulon, J., and Deboutte, D. The R23K mutation in the GR gene changes the HPA axis response to psychosocial stress in prepubertal children. (submitted)

Wasserman, D., Sokolowski, M., Rozanov, V., and Wasserman, J. (2008). The CRHR1 gene: a marker for suicidality in depressed males exposed to low stress. *Genes, brain, and behavior*, **7**, 14–19.

Willour, V.L., Chen, H., Toolan, J. *et al.* (2008). Family-based association of FKBP5 in bipolar disorder. *Molecular Psychiatry*, January 8. [Epub ahead of print].

Wellcome Trust Case Control Consortium. (2007). Genome-wide association study of 14,000 cases of seven common diseases and 3,000 shared controls. *Nature*, **447**, 661–678.

Wüst S. (2007). Presentation at the Second Meeting of West European Societies of Biological Psychiatry, 13–15 December 2007, France, Strasbourg.

Yong, W., Yang, Z., Periyasamy, S. et al. (2007). Essential role for Co-chaperone Fkbp52 but not Fkbp51 in androgen receptor-mediated signaling and physiology. *The Journal of Biological Chemistry*, **282**, 5026–5036.

Chapter 6

Bipolar disorder and unipolar depression: what is the genetic relationship?

Daniel J. Smith, Michael J. Owen, and Nick Craddock

Introduction

In this chapter we consider the complex question of the genetic relationship between unipolar depression and bipolar affective disorder. Several areas are addressed, including a discussion of difficulties with phenotype definition, issues of classification and diagnosis, and a summary of genetic findings to date. We also consider three potential models of the genetic relationship between these diagnoses and end with a discussion of future directions for genetic research in this area. This is the third of four chapters in this book that discuss the genetics of affective disorders, together with Chapter 4, 5, and 23. This is also the first chapter to discuss the differences and similarities between depression and bipolar disorder, together with Chapter 21, 22, and 26.

Defining the phenotype for genetic studies of depression and bipolar disorder

Although genetic research is currently producing significant findings for mood disorders, for many years the field had been hampered by limitations which are inherent within our current phenotypic definitions of depression and bipolar disorder.

Diagnostic classifications are not aetiologically driven

Depression and bipolar disorder are complex conditions caused by the dynamic interaction of multiple genetic and environmental risk factors. Although the diagnostic criteria for these disorders outlined in the Diagnostic and Statistical Manual (DSM-IV; American Psychiatric Association 1994) and the International Classification of Diseases (ICD-10; World Health Organisation, 1992) have undoubtedly been useful, a major limitation for their use in genetic studies has been that these diagnoses are based on arbitrarily agreed thresholds of symptoms rather than on an understanding of etiological or pathophysiological factors. There is also insufficient recognition of recent evidence suggesting that the phenotypes of unipolar and bipolar depression are different (Forty et al. 2008; and Chapters 21 and 22 of this book) .

Clinical and genetic heterogeneity within DSM-IV and ICD-10 diagnoses

Formal categorical diagnoses such as those within DSM and ICD probably encompass a wide range of depressive and bipolar conditions which, although falling within the same general diagnostic category, may share very different biological and environmental aetiologies. For example, it seems likely that a young woman in her twenties presenting with a DSM-IV defined major depressive episode (MDE) in the context of a strong family history of bipolar disorder may have aetiological factors which differ substantially from an elderly man with cerebrovascular disease who presents with a similarly defined MDE. Lumping such cases together in a genetic study obviously has implications for the likelihood of reliably identifying genetic risk factors for depression (Angst, 2007).

Categories and dimensions

There is currently a great deal of debate about the boundaries of DSM-IV and ICD-10 criteria for depression and bipolar disorder. These diagnoses are almost exclusively categorical and take very little account of important dimensional aspects of mood symptoms and temperament. In recent years it has been increasingly recognized that the boundary between recurrent major depression and bipolar disorder is far from clear-cut and that this has important implications for research and treatment (Smith et al. 2008). Similarly, the boundary between extremes of affective temperament (such as dysthymic or cyclothymic traits) and clinical caseness is unclear and greater recognition of this may be very important in future genetic studies of mood disorders.

Genetic findings to date on depression and bipolar disorder

Classical genetic epidemiological studies of depression and bipolar disorder (family, twin, and adoption studies) have established that both conditions are substantially heritable. Most heritability estimates are between 33% and 42% for depression and 80% and 90% for bipolar disorder (Craddock and Forty, 2006). Although (for bipolar disorder particularly) it was originally hoped that these high heritability estimates would lead to the discovery of single gene mutations, this has not proven to be the case. The reality has been that many candidate genes have not been replicated and those that have are of only a small effect. As with many other psychiatric conditions, the most likely model of inheritance is one of multiple genes of relatively small effect interacting with each other and with environmental factors to confer susceptibility to the illness (Zandi et al. 2007).

Linkage studies of depression

Compared to bipolar disorder and schizophrenia, relatively few genetic linkage studies of depression have been conducted, perhaps because of a widespread view that depression is 'less genetic' than these other conditions. Holmans and colleagues recently reported the final stage of a whole genome linkage scan of 656 families from the Genetics of Recurrent Early-Onset Major Depression (GenRED) study (Holmans et al. 2007). Regions of chromosomes 15q, 17p, and 8p were identified as likely to include susceptibility genes for depression. It was of interest to learn that 15q had also been identified as a linkage region in two other independent samples, including a study from Utah (Camp et al. 2005) and in the collaborative European–US Depression Network (DeNT) study (McGuffin et al. 2005).

Association studies of depression

As with linkage studies, relatively few large-scale association studies with major depression as the principal phenotype have been conducted. Perhaps the most interesting finding to emerge has been the report of an interaction between a functional variant of the serotonin transporter gene-linked polymorphic region (5HTTLPR) and life events in early adulthood (Caspi et al. 2003), although not all studies have replicated this finding (Zammit and Owen, 2006) and this variant has not shown significance overall with MDD (Levinson et al. 2006). Nonetheless, large-scale association studies are currently in progress and it is hoped that these will deliver new candidate gene abnormalities which are involved in major depression.

Linkage studies of bipolar disorder

Although several chromosomal locations have been implicated in individual linkage studies of bipolar disorder, only a few regions have been consistently identified in meta-analyses. Modest support for regions on 9q, 10q, 14q, and regions of chromosome 18 were obtained in one meta-analysis (Segurado et al. 2003) and for 13q and 22q in another (Badner and Gershon, 2002). Since these meta-analyses were published, several more recent genome-wide linkage scans have identified strong support for the 6q region (which had not been implicated in the previous meta-analyses) (McQueen et al. 2005). Similarly, the 12q region has been implicated in two genome-wide linkage scans (Ewald et al. 2002; Shink et al. 2005) and it is interesting to note that this region has also been implicated in two linkage studies of unipolar depression (Abkevich et al. 2003; McGuffin et al. 2005).

Association studies of bipolar disorder

A large number of association studies for functional candidate genes for bipolar disorder (including the serotonin transporter (5HTT), monoamine oxidase inhibitor (MAOA), catechol-o-methyl transferase (COMT), brain derived neurotrophic factor (BDNF), tyrosine hydroxylase (TH), D-amnio acid oxidase activator (DAOA), neuregulin (NRG1), and the disrupted in schizophrenia genes 1 and 2 (DISC-1 and DISC-2) have been conducted. Overall, these studies suggest modest support for MAOA, COMT, 5HTT, and DAOA (Craddock and Forty, 2006). Findings for BDNF have been both positive and negative but there is recent evidence that this gene may be associated with a rapid-cycling sub-phenotype of bipolar disorder (Green et al. 2006). Several of these genes (particularly DAOA, DISC-1, and NRG1) have also been implicated for schizophrenia.

Genome-wide association studies of bipolar disorder

Recent technological advances now permit large numbers of single nucleotide polymorphisms (SNPs) to be examined across whole regions of interest and within the last 12 months three genome-wide association (GWA) studies of bipolar disorder have been published. In the first, the Welcome Trust Case Control Consortium (WTCCC) reported GWA results for almost 2000 bipolar cases and 3000 controls. The strongest was with rs420259 at chromosome 16p12. Several genes at this locus could have pathological relevance to bipolar disorder, including: PALB2, which is involved in the stability of key nuclear structures including chromatin and the nuclear matrix; NDUFAB1, which encodes a subunit of complex I of the mitochondrial respiratory chain; and DCTN5, which codes for a protein involved in intracellular transport that is known to interact with the gene 'disrupted in schizophrenia 1' (DISC1). A number of other regions of interest were identified, including genes involved in ion channel function (KCNC2), voltage-dependant calcium channel function (CACNA1C), GABA neurotransmission (GABRB1), glutamate neurotransmission (GRM7), and synaptic function (SYN3).

In the second published GWA study of bipolar disorder, Sklar and colleagues studied almost 1500 patients with BP-I and 2000 controls drawn from the Systematic Treatment Enhancement Program for Bipolar Disorder (STEP-BD) combined with UK samples (Sklar et al. 2008). They found support for myosin5B (MYO5B), tetraspanin-8 (TSPAN8), and the epidermal growth factor receptor (EGFR). A comparison of the strongest associations from this study with findings from the WTCCC study indicated concordant signals for SNPs within the voltage-gated calcium channel, L-type, alpha 1C subunit (*CACNA1C*) gene.

In the third bipolar GWA study, using DNA pooling on two independent case-control samples of European ancestry, Baum and colleagues identified that 88 SNPs representing 80 different genes were replicated for association in both samples (Baum et al. 2008). A number of these SNPs were selected for individual genotyping and the strongest association signal was for a marker within the gene coding for diacylglycerol kinase eta (*DGKH*) which codes for a key protein in the lithium-sensitive phosphatydil inositol pathway.

Overall, these landmark GWA studies suggest that this approach holds considerable promise for the identification of novel genetic risk factors for bipolar disorder (and, by extension, depression). It is likely that the value of these studies will be extended by much greater sample sizes and by employing alternative approaches to phenotype definition, such as the use of symptom dimensions (Craddock et al. 2004).

The possible genetic relationship between depression and bipolar disorder

Mood disorders, in common with most psychiatric diagnoses, are complex phenotypes resulting from the interaction of complicated genetics with an equally complex environment. It is therefore unsurprising that we do not as yet have models of genetic inheritance that adequately explain the relationship between depression and bipolar disorder. However, three hypotheses about this relationship are possible. In the first, depression and bipolar disorder are distinct syndromes which do not share any genetic risk factors. In the second, depression and bipolar disorder are essentially phenotypic expressions of the same disorder, with bipolar disorder representing a less common but more severe sub-type (and depression a more common but less severe subtype). The third hypothesis holds that both of these scenarios may be correct, with both depression and bipolar disorder having genetic risk factors which are shared, as well as sets of genes which may be specific to each diagnosis.

Depression and bipolar disorder as genetically distinct syndromes

The view that depression and bipolar disorder are distinct in terms of genetic risk was first suggested in the 1950s by the family studies of Leonard, who observed from his cohort of patients with recurrent depression that those who also had a history of mania tended to report more mania in their families than those who experienced only depressive episodes (Goodwin and Jamison, 2007). In the 1960s, Angst and Perris provided independent family history data to support this and several additional lines of evidence subsequently supported the concept of a unipolar/bipolar division: twice as many women as men experienced depression (whereas the ratio in bipolar disorder was 1:1); bipolar disorder tended to have a much earlier age of onset; and mortality (mostly through suicide) was consistently higher in the bipolar group (Goodwin and Jamison, 2007). This dichotomous conceptualization has survived for many years and has been enshrined within ICD-10 and DSM-IV.

However, subsequent family, twin, and adoption studies have not wholly supported this distinction and clinicians have long been aware that bipolar disorder and depression do not generally 'breed true' within families. For example, the morbid risk of depression in the first degree relatives of bipolar probands is estimated at 11.4% compared to a morbid risk of bipolar disorder of 7.8% (McGuffin and Katz, 1989). In brief, there is little evidence to suggest that depression and bipolar disorder are genetically separate and this view is supported by the evidence reviewed above of shared regions of the genome for both diagnoses (Abkevich et al. 2003; McGuffin et al. 2005).

Depression and bipolar disorder as points on a broad bipolar spectrum

It has been suggested that the bipolar spectrum can be viewed as a quantitative phenotype, with bipolar individuals carrying more risk alleles for mood disorder and therefore suffering from a more severe (but less common) illness, whereas individuals with unipolar depression would have fewer risk alleles but be more prevalent (Fig. 6.1) (Kelsoe, 2003).

A quantitative trait model of the bipolar spectrum would predict that there would be a ranking of severity; for example, with schizoaffective disorder the most severe and least common; followed by bipolar disorder, type I; followed by bipolar disorder, type II; followed by recurrent unipolar depression, single episode unipolar depression, and finally dysthymia/cyclothymia. Epidemiological studies lend some support to this, with several identifying that severe forms of bipolar disorder have a lifetime prevalence of around 1% with less severe forms (such as bipolar disorder, type II) affecting up to 5% of the population, and dysthymia and cyclothymia occurring in up to 10% (Judd et al. 2003; Kessler et al. 1994; Smith et al. 1992).

The proposition that the bipolar spectrum is a quantitative trait also implies that the genes involved in mood disorders will have an effect on affective temperaments within non-clinical populations. For example, it might be expected that the non-affectively ill relatives of bipolar or depressed probands would have evidence of sub-clinical abnormalities of affective temperament. Few studies to date have examined this in a satisfactory way but recent preliminary data suggest that this may be the case. Evans and colleagues used the Temperament Evaluation of Memphis, Pisa and San Diego (TEMPS-A) to assess five affective dimensions (dysthymia, hyperthymia, cyclothymia, irritability, and anxiety) in 220 relatives of 86 bipolar probands and 53 controls and found that unaffected relatives had significantly higher scores on the dysthymia and cyclothymia dimensions (Evans et al. 2005).

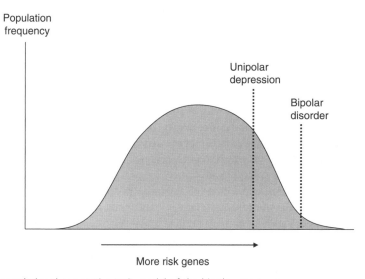

Fig. 6.1 Isocorrelational quantative trait model of the bipolar spectrum.

Genetic influences on depression and bipolar are both shared and specific

In order to assess whether bipolar disorder and unipolar depression are genetically separate or part of genetic continuum, Winokur and colleagues performed a detailed family study where they compared rates of mania, depression, and psychosis in the relatives of three groups: probands with bipolar I disorder; probands with unipolar depression; and controls (Winokur et al. 1995). They found that mania was more frequent in the families of patients with bipolar disorder than in controls or families of patients with unipolar depression (and that the unipolar group and controls had similar rates of mania within their relatives). This suggests that bipolar disorder may be a separate illness from unipolar depression because of an increase in familial mania. These investigators also divided bipolar patients into two groups based on history of psychotic symptoms and these groups did not differ from each other in terms of risk for familial mania or depression. This lack of an increase in familial illness according to severity of bipolar disorder argues against an affective continuum (Winokur et al. 1995).

A more recent study from the Maudsley Twin Register used structural equation model-fitting methods on a sample of 67 twin pairs (30 monozygotic and 37 dizygotic) where one of the twins had DSM-IV defined bipolar disorder to examine the genetic overlap between bipolar disorder and unipolar depression (McGuffin et al. 2003). Although there were substantial genetic and nonfamilial correlations between mania and depression (0.65 and 0.59, respectively), approximately 71% of the genetic variance for mania was not shared with depression. In other words, although bipolar disorder and unipolar depression in this study were not genetically distinct, bipolar disorder probably has an additional set of risk genes which are relatively specific to the manic syndrome. This study also failed to support the model whereby BP is seen as simply a more severe form of UP.

A three-dimensional model of mood-psychosis disorders

In the same way that unipolar depression and bipolar disorder have both shared and specific genetic risks, a significant degree of overlap also exists with regard to bipolar disorder and schizophrenia (Craddock and Owen, 2005). Evidence from family studies, twin studies, genome-wide linkage studies, and association studies all now suggest that the traditional diagnostic separation of bipolar disorder from schizophrenia is not supported by findings from genetic epidemiology (for a comprehensive review see Craddock et al. 2005). On the basis of these findings, for the purposes of both research and treatment, it may be that unipolar depression, bipolar disorder, and schizophrenia are best considered as part of an over-lapping, three-dimensional model which might include such diagnoses as 'psychosis-spectrum illness' or 'mood–reality disorder' (Craddock and Owen, 2005) (Fig. 6.2).

The potential utility of this approach was illustrated by recent findings with the D-amino-acid oxidase (DAO) activator (*DAOA*; formerly known as G72) and the putative gene referred to as *G30 (DAOA/G30)* gene. Variation at this locus had previously been found to be associated with both schizophrenia and bipolar disorder (Williams et al. 2006). Williams and colleagues tested the hypothesis that association at *DAOA/G30* might identify an underlying domain of psychopathology that would cut across traditional diagnostic categories by testing for the association of polymorphisms within the *DAOA/G30* locus with a 'psychosis domain' and a 'mood domain' in a large sample of patients with DSM-IV schizophrenia ($n = 709$), bipolar disorder type I ($n = 706$), and controls ($n = 1416$) (Williams et al. 2006). There was significant association with bipolar disorder but no association with schizophrenia and analyses across the diagnostic categories revealed significant evidence for association within the subset of cases ($n = 818$) in which episodes

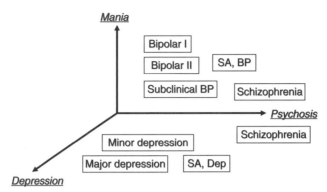

Fig 6.2 Three-dimensional model of mood-psychosis disorders.

of major mood disorder had occurred. A similar pattern of association was evident in bipolar and in schizophrenia cases in which individuals had experienced major mood disorder but there was no evidence for association within the subset of cases ($n = 1153$) in which psychotic features occurred. These findings suggest that variation at the *DAOA/G30* locus does not primarily increase susceptibility for prototypical schizophrenia per se but rather influences susceptibility to episodes of mood disorder.

Future research

To some degree, genetic studies of depression and bipolar disorder have been hindered by an overly rigid adherence to formal DSM-IV and ICD-10 diagnostic categories and future studies will require innovative approaches to defining phenotypes. As noted above, such studies will need to cut across traditional diagnostic boundaries, as well as taking account of gene-environment interactions. In recent years, several promising sub-phenotypes of bipolar disorder have been tested, including: early age-at-onset (Faraone et al. 2006; Holmans et al. 2007); lithium responsiveness (Alda et al. 2005); rapid-cycling bipolar disorder (Green et al. 2006); puerperal psychosis (Jones and Craddock 2002); and the presence of psychotic symptoms within bipolar disorder (Potash et al. 2003).

Alternative approaches may include the use of new diagnostic criteria, for example, 'bipolar spectrum' definitions (Angst, 2003; Ghaemi et al. 2002), as well dimensional assessments of bipolar symptoms and temperament (Goodwin and Jamison, 2007). A few early studies along these lines suggest that these are promising strategies (Craddock et al. 2004; Rybakowski et al. 2005; Sharma et al. 2005; Smith et al. 2005). In our own work, we are developing affective temperament scores, as measured by the TEMPS-A, as novel phenotypes in genetic association studies for mood disorder (Akiskal et al. 2005). An example hypothesis of this approach would be that the Val66Met polymorphism of BDNF – known to be associated with *rapid-cycling* BP disorder (Green et al. 2006) – will be associated with extreme scores on 'cyclothymia', irrespective of DSM-IV diagnosis.

Although there is growing interest in a potential role for copy number variations (CNVs) in the identification of genetic risk factors for schizophrenia, very little work on CNVs has so far been conducted for unipolar depression and bipolar disorder. From the schizophrenia CNV research, it is already clear that certain caveats will apply: CNVs will likely have small population effect sizes, even if individually associated with higher risk than common SNPs, and they will often involve many genes and will not therefore necessarily help to elucidate simple mechanisms.

Similarly, although the phenomenon of epigenetic imprinting has been suggested as another potentially important avenue, there is as yet very little direct evidence for the involvement of imprinting in the transgenerational transmission of phenotypes in mammals, in contrast to polygenic inheritance which is common across the animal and plant kingdoms (Crespi et al. 2008; Davies et al. 2007).

The feasibility and considerable promise of unbiased genome-wide association studies in future genetic studies of depression, bipolar disorder, and schizophrenia has been discussed above. It is unlikely that specific loci with effects in excess of 10% will be identified; rather, we are likely to identify multiple (interacting) genes of small effect. It is hoped that advances in bioinformatics will be able to identify combinations of genes with stronger effects.

The future challenge for the field of mood disorder genetics is to combine advances in bioinformatics and molecular genetic technologies with equally important developments in our understanding of the nosology of mood syndromes, with a long-term view to improving diagnosis and developing treatments for patients which are more closely targeted at biologically relevant clusters of symptoms, rather than somewhat heterogeneous diagnostic categories.

References

Abkevich, V., Camp, N., Hensel, C. et al. (2003). Predisposition locus for major depression on chromosome 12q22-12q23.2. *American Journal of Human Genetics*, **73**, 1271–1281.

Akiskal, H.S., Mendlowicz, M.V., Jean-Louis, G. et al. (2005). TEMPS-A: validation of a short version of a self-rated instrument designed to measure variations in temperament. *Journal of Affective Disorders*, **85**, 45–52.

Alda, M., Grof, P., Rouleau, G.A. et al. (2005). Investigating responders to lithium prophylaxis as a strategy for mapping susceptibility genes for bipolar disorder. *Progress in Neuro-Psychopharmacology and Biological Psychiatry*, **29**, 1038–1045.

Angst, J. (2007). Psychiatric diagnoses: the weak component of modern research. *World Psychiatry*, **6**, 94–95.

Angst, J., Gamma, A., Bennazzi, F., Ajdacic, V., Eich, D., and Rossler, W. (2003). Toward a re-definition of subthreshold bipolarity: epidemiology and proposed criteria for bipolar-II, minor bipolar disorders and hypomania. Journal of Affective Disorders, **73**, 133–146.

American Psychiatric Association. (1994). Diagnostic and Statistical Manual of Mental Disorders (4th edn). Washington, D.C.

Badner, J. and Gershon, E. (2002). Meta-analysis of whole-genome linkage scans of bipolar disorder and schizophrenia. *Molecular Psychiatry*, **7**, 405–411.

Baum, A.E., Akula, N., Cabanero, M. et al. (2008). A genome-wide association study implicates diacylglycerol kinase eta (DGKH) and several other genes in the etiology of bipolar disorder. *Molecular Psychiatry*, **13**, 197–207.

Camp, N.J., Lowry, M.R., Richards, R.L. et al. (2005). Genome-wide linkage analyses of extended Utah pedigrees identifies loci that influence recurrent, early-onset major depression and anxiety disorders. American Journal of Medical Genetics Part B: *Neuropsychiatric Genetics*, **135B**, 85–93.

Caspi, A., Sugden, K., Moffitt, T.E. et al. (2003). Influence of life stress on depression: moderation by a polymorphism in the 5-HTT gene. Science, **301**, 386–389.

Craddock, N. and Forty, L. (2006). Genetics of affective (mood) disorders. *European Journal of Human Genetics*, **14**, 660–668.

Craddock, N., Jones, I., Kirov, G., and Jones, L. (2004) The Bipolar Affective Disorder Dimension Scale (BADDS) – a dimensional scale for rating lifetime psychopathology in Bipolar spectrum disorders. *BMC Psychiatry*, **4**, 19.

Craddock, N., O'Donovan, M.C., and Owen, M.J. (2005). The genetics of schizophrenia and bipolar disorder: dissecting psychosis. *Journal of Medical Genetics*, **42**, 193–204.

Craddock, N. and Owen, M.J. (2005). The beginning of the end for the Kraepelinian dichotomy. *British Journal of Psychiatry*, **186**, 364–366.

Crespi, B. and Badcock C. (2008). The evolutionary social brain: from genes to psychiatric conditions. *Behavioural Brian Science*, **31**, 284–320.

Davies, W., Isles, A.R., Humby, T., and Wilkinson, L.S. (2007). What are imprinted genes doing in the brain? *Epigenetics*, **2**, 201–206.

Evans, L., Akiskal, H.S., Keck, P.E. et al. (2005). Familiarity of temperament in bipolar disorder: support for a genetic spectrum. *Journal of Affective Disorders*, **85**, 153–168.

Ewald, H., Flint, T., Kruse, T.A., and Mors, C. (2002). A genome-wide scan shows significant linkage between bipolar disorder and chromosome 12q24.3 and suggestive linkage to chromosomes 1p22-21, 4p16, 6q14-21, 10q26 and 16p13.3. *Molecular Psychiatry*, **7**, 734–744.

Faraone, S.V., Lasky-Su, J., Glatt, S.J. et al. (2006). Early onset bipolar disorder: possible linkage to chromosome 9q34. *Bipolar Disorders*, **8**, 144–151.

Forty, L., Smith, D., Jones, L. et al. (2008). Clinical differences between bipolar and unipolar depression. *The British Journal of Psychiatry*, **192**, 388–389.

Ghaemi, S.N., Ko, J.Y., and Goodwin, F.K. (2002) Cade's disease and beyond: misdiagnosis, antidepressant use and a proposed definition for bipolar spectrum disorder. *Canadian Journal of Psychiatry*, **47**, 125–134.

Goodwin, F.K. and Jamison, K.R. (2007) Manic-Depressive Illness: Bipolar Disorders and Recurrent Depression. (2nd edn). New York, Oxford University Press.

Green, E.K., Raybould, R., Macgregor, S. et al. (2006). Genetic variation of brain-derived neurotrophic factor (BDNF) in bipolar disorder: case-control study of over 3000 individuals from the UK. *British Journal of Psychiatry*, **188**, 21–25.

Holmans, P., Weissman, M.M., Zubenko, G.S. et al. (2007). Genetics of Recurrent Early-Onset Major Depression (GenRED): final genome scan report. *American Journal of Psychiatry*, **164**, 248–258.

Jones, I. and Craddock, N. (2002). Do puerperal psychotic episodes identify a more familial sub-type of bipolar disorder? Results of a family history study. *Psychiatric Genetics*, **12**, 177–180.

Judd, L., Angst, J., Akiskal, H.S. et al. (2003). The prevalence and disability of bipolar spectrum disorders in the US population: re-analysis of the ECA database taking into account subthreshold cases. *Journal of Affective Disorders*, **73**, 123–131.

Kelsoe, J.R. (2003). Arguments for the genetic basis of the bipolar spectrum. *Journal of Affective Disorders*, **73**, 183–197.

Kessler, R., McGonagle, K.A., Zhao, S. et al. (1994). Life-time and 12-month prevalence of DSM-III-R psychiatric disorders in the United States. *Archives of General Psychiatry*, **51**, 8–19.

Levinson, D.F. (2006). The genetics of depression: a review. *Biological Psychiatry*, 60, 84–92.

McGuffin, P. and Katz, R. (1989) The genetics of depression and manic depressive disorder. *British Journal of Psychiatry*, **155**.

McGuffin, P., Rijsdijk, F., Andrew, M., Sham, P., Katz, R., and Cardno, A. (2003). The heritability of bipolar affective disorder and the genetic relationship to unipolar depression. *Archives of General Psychiatry*, **60**, 497–502.

McGuffin, P., Knight, J., Breen, G. et al. (2005). Whole genome linkage scan of recurrent depressive disorder from the depression network study. *Human Molecular Genetics*, **14**, 3337–3345.

McQueen, M.B., Devlin, B., Faraone, S.V. et al. (2005). Combined analysis from eleven linkage studies of bipolar disorder provides strong evidence of susceptibility loci on chromosomes 6q and 8q. *American Journal of Human Genetics*, **77**, 582–595.

Potash, J.B., Zandi, P.P., Willour, V.L. et al. (2003). Suggestive linkage to chromosomal regions 13q31 and 22q12 in families with psychotic bipolar disorder. *American Journal of Psychiatry*, **160**, 680–686.

Rybakowski, J.K., Suwalska, A., Lojko, D., Rymaszewska, J., and Kiejna, A. (2005). Bipolar mood disorders among Polish psychiatric outpatients treated for major depression. *Journal of Affective Disorders*, **84**, 141–147.

Segurado, R.D.S., Levinson, D.F., Lewis, C.M. et al. (2003). Genome scan meta-analysis of schizophrenia and bipolar disorder, part III: bipolar disorder. *American Journal of Human Genetics*, **73**, 49–62.

Sharma, V., Khan, M., and Smith, A. (2005). A closer look at treatment resistant depression: is it due to a bipolar diathesis? *Journal of Affective Disorders*, **84**, 251–257.

Shink, E., Morissette, J., Sherrington, R. et al. (2005). A genome-wide scan points to a susceptibility locus for bipolar disorder on chromosome 12. *Molecular Psychiatry*, **10**, 545–552.

Sklar, P., Smoller, J.W., Fan, J., et al. (2008). Whole-genome association study of bipolar disorder. *Molecular Psychiatry*.

Smith, A.L. and Weissman, M.M. (1992). 'Epidemiology', in E.S. Paykel (ed.) *Handbook of Affective Disorders*. Edinburgh, Churchill Livingstone.

Smith, D.J., Harrison, N., Muir, W. et al. (2005). The high prevalence of bipolar spectrum disorders in young adults with recurrent depression: toward an innovative diagnostic framework. *Journal of Affective Disorders*, **84**, 167–178.

Smith, D.J., Ghaemi, S.N., and Craddock, N. (2008). The broad clinical spectrum of bipolar disorder: implications for research and practice. *Journal of Psychopharmacol*, **22**, 397–400.

Williams, N.M., Green, E.K., Macgregor, S. et al. (2006). Variation at the DAOA/G30 locus influences susceptibility to major mood episodes but not psychosis in schizophrenia and bipolar disorder. *Archives of General Psychiatry*, **63**, 366–373.

Winokur, G., Coryell, W., Keller, M. et al.(1995). A family study of manic-depressive (bipolar I) disease. Is it a distinct illness separable from primary unipolar depression? *Archives of General Psychiatry*, **52**, 367–373.

World Health Organisation (1992). *The ICD-10 classification of mental and behavioural disorders*. Geneva, WHO.

Zammit, S. and Owen, M.J. (2006). Stressful life events, 5-HTT genotype and risk of depression. *British Journal of Psychiatry*, **188**, 199–201.

Zandi, P.P., Badner, B.J., Steele, J., Willour, V.L. et al. (2007). Genome-wide linkage scan of 98 bipolar pedigrees and analysis of clinical covariates. *Molecular Psychiatry*, **12**, 630–639.

Chapter 7

The significance of dysregulated basal glucocorticoid pulsatility in affective disorders

Becky L. Conway-Campbell, Crispin C. Wiles, and Stafford L. Lightman

Depressive illness is characterized by changes in the basal set-point of the hypothalamic-pituitary-adrenal (HPA) axis, resulting in altered regulation of glucocorticoid secretory activity (Holsboer 2000). This is the first of five chapters in this book that present not only clinical data but also experimental evidence from animal models relevant to the role of the HPA in affective disorders, together with Chapters 8, 9, 11, and 26.

The neuroendocrine HPA axis is under the control of neural circuits in the CNS and has actions on many peripheral systems throughout the body. The principle signal arises from activation of parvocellular neurones of the hypothalamic paraventricular nucleus (PVN), which synthesize and secrete corticotrophin-releasing factor (CRF), and/or arginine vasopressin (AVP). These peptides then act synergistically on corticotropes of the anterior pituitary gland, to release adrenocorticotrophic hormone (ACTH) which amplifies the neuroendocrine signal. ACTH acts directly at the adrenal cortex to increase the rate of synthesis and release of adrenal corticosteroids which function as effector hormones. Secretory activity can be modulated at both the pituitary and adrenal levels, but it is primarily the hypothalamic neuroendocrine signal which governs the pattern of HPA activity via a complex pattern of neural inputs, gene expression, and feedback control.

One of the classic identifying features of adrenal corticosteroids (cortisol in man and corticosterone in rodents) is the intrinsic rhythm of its secretion (Lightman et al. 2000; Young et al. 2004). Over the last decade, we have used an automated blood sampling system to define corticosterone pulsatility in free-running rats in their home cages. These studies have revealed a complex ultradian rhythm of endogenous corticosterone, with discrete peaks occurring at approximately hourly intervals. Modulation of the amplitude of these pulses generates the well-characterized circadian profile. This pulsatility has also been reported in numerous species including rat (Atkinson et al. 2006; Jasper and Engeland, 1991; 1994; Windle et al. 1998a), rhesus monkey (Sarnyai et al. 1995; Tapp et al. 1984), Syrian hamster (Loudon et al. 1994; Lucas et al. 1999), horse (Cudd et al. 1995), sheep (Engler et al. 1989a, b), and goat (Carnes et al. 1990;1992). In man, an ultradian pattern of cortisol release is also evident and forms the basis of the typical diurnal rhythm (Hellman et al. 1970; Veldhuis et al. 1990; Weitzman et al. 1971; Young et al. 2004; see also Chapter 15 in this book). We have recently developed an automated sampling system for use in humans, allowing more frequent sampling than has been possible before (Henley et al. 2009). A typical 24-hour cortisol profile taken from a healthy female volunteer is shown in Fig. 7.1. It is likely that the peaks and troughs of free cortisol in human plasma will be even greater than those of total cortisol as cortisol-binding globulin (CBG) will re-equilibrate with free cortisol in the minutes after each

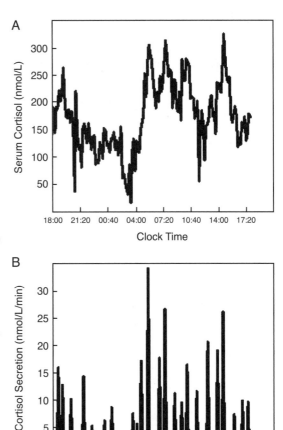

Fig. 7.1 Ultradian cortisol rhythm in a healthy human female volunteer. Reprinted with permission from the European Journal of Pharmacology, The significance of glucocorticoid pulsatility, S. Lightman et al., © 2008 Elsevier BV.

Note: A: Serum cortisol concentrations obtained utilizing a human automated blood sampling system at 10-min intervals reveals the ultradian pattern underlying a circadian profile (unpublished results). B: Deconvolution analysis technique estimates 24 secretory events with mean secretion pulse height 15.3 nmol/L/min, pulse mass 115.1 nmol/L/min and interpulse interval 59.2 min.

secretory episode. Interestingly, the ultradian pattern shows marked sexual diergism (Seale et al. 2004a, b), and is remarkably plastic, with changes seen during lactation and ageing (Lightman et al. 2000), the presence of, or susceptibility to disease (Windle et al. 1998a; 2001), and early life programming (Shanks and Lightman, 2001).

Despite the highly conserved nature of glucocorticoid pulsatility among different species, and the long-standing associations between changes in HPA axis activity and disease (Gibbons, 1964; Young et al. 2004), there has been relatively little research into the significance of the glucocorticoid ultradian rhythm. The universal phenomenon of ultradian patterns of circulating hormones acting as a means of signalling within mammalian systems is well established. Pulsatile release of gonadotrophin releasing hormone (GnRH) is essential for normal reproductive function (Belchetz et al. 1978), and the sexually dimorphic differences in the pattern of pulsatile growth hormone (GH) secretion results in differential expression of liver enzymes and IGF-1 dependent growth responses (Clark et al. 1987; Waxman et al. 1995). Indeed, the importance of the ultradian pattern of presentation of these hormones is clearly recognized, and has led to the introduction of a novel type of clinical therapy where manipulation of the temporal pattern of ligand exposure to their cognate receptors results in therapeutic benefits (Amato et al. 2000; Kesrouani et al. 2001).

Basal glucocorticoid pulsatility and stress

There are powerful and dynamic interactions between basal glucocorticoid pulsatility and normal HPA axis function, thus determining an individual's ability to cope with a stressful situation, either real or imagined. It has been demonstrated (Windle et al. 1998b) that the time of onset of a stressor in relation to the phase of an endogenous basal pulse can determine the physiological response. Female Sprague-Dawley rats undergoing automated blood sampling were exposed to the mild stressor of white noise at 114 dB for ten minutes. Subsequent examination of the hormone profiles identified two separate groups of animals – responders and non-responders (Fig. 7.2).

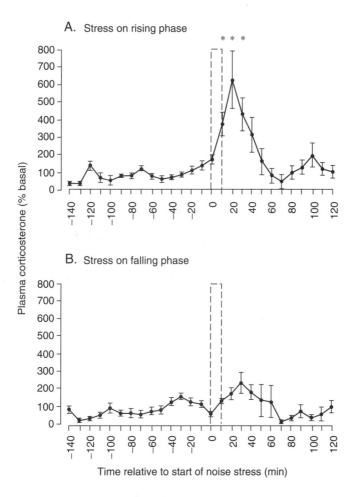

Fig. 7.2 Mean profiles from 'responder' and 'non-responder' groups indicate the differential response to noise stress depending on the relative timing of noise-stress onset with endogenous basal pulsatility. Reprinted with permission from Endocrinology, Ultradian rhythm of basal corticosterone release, R J Windle et al. 139, 443–450. © 1998 The Endocrine Society. Reprinted with permission from the European Journal of Pharmacology, The significance of glucocorticoid pulsatility, S. Lightman et al., © 2008 Elsevier BV.

Note: The dotted rectangle indicates the time of onset and offset of the noise stressor (Windle et al. 1998b).

Those animals which had rising endogenous basal corticosterone levels immediately prior to the onset of the stressor responded with an additional release of corticosterone. Those in which basal corticosterone levels were falling at the time of onset of the stressor showed little or no corticosterone response. A subsequent experiment (Windle et al. 1998a) showed that pituitary responsiveness to exogenous CRH is not affected by pulse phase. Thus the regulation of glucocorticoid pulsatility seems to be a result of rapidly alternating periods of activity and inhibition within the HPA axis, controlled at a supra-pituitary site. These data strongly indicate that basal glucocorticoid pulsatility regulates the ability of an animal to mount a stress response. The acute stress response maximizes the ability of the body to mobilize fuel to escape a predator (or other stressful situation) and reassert equilibrium once the damage has passed.

HPA axis feedback and pulsatility

Glucocorticoid feedback operates at multiple time domains and involves both the recently described rapid non-genomic responses as well as the classical genomic responses (Hinz and Hirschelmann, 2000; Keller-Wood and Dallman, 1984). Although the precise mechanisms of non-genomic glucocorticoid feedback have proved elusive (Di et al. 2003; Karst et al. 2005) the existence of fast rate-sensitive feedback has long been recognized (Dallman and Yates, 1969). When a rat is exposed to a rapidly increasing concentration of exogenous steroids, it has limited capacity to mount a HPA response to stress (Dallman, 2005). Using our automated blood sampling system, we have been able to show that administration of an intravenous bolus of steroid (which results in increasing steroid concentrations) can rapidly inhibit basal HPA activity in conscious animals (Fig. 7.3). Circulating concentrations of endogenous corticosterone are significantly lower within 30 minutes of exogenous steroid injection and considering that the half life for corticosterone clearance is approximately ten minutes (Glenister and Yates, 1961; Woodward et al. 1991), the fast feedback signal generated by the steroid bolus is presumably non-genomic. We propose that because this effect is rapid enough to function within the timespan of ultradian pulsatility it may explain why pulses are composed of alternating phases of activation and inhibition. Thus, during the secretory phase of a pulse the rapid rise in corticosterone causes a fast feedback signal that results in the inhibitory phase of the pulse where corticosterone is cleared according to its half life. This inhibitory phase is short in duration thus allowing a new

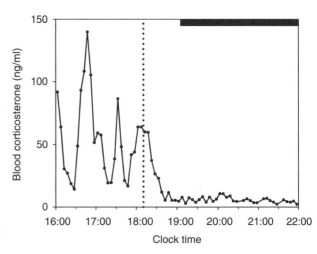

Fig. 7.3 Rapid feedback of endogenous corticosterone by methylprednisolone. Reprinted with permission from the European Journal of Pharmacology, The significance of glucocorticoid pulsatility, S. Lightman et al., © 2008 Elsevier BV.

Note: Blood samples were collected around the diurnal peak at 5-min intervals using an automated blood-sampling system. Within half an hour of an intravenous bolus of methylprednisolone (250 μg; vertical line), endogenous corticosterone concentrations are low and pulsatility is shut off.

pulse to soon be initiated. We also have evidence to show that this fast rate-sensitive feedback of basal HPA activity can be blocked by a selective MR antagonist (Atkinson et al. 2008) but not by GR antagonists (Spiga et al. 2007).

Cellular responsiveness

The cellular response to glucocorticoid treatment in cell culture systems has been well studied, however our understanding of the in vivo cellular signalling systems responsible for dynamic responses to rapidly fluctuating hormone levels is less complete. We hypothesize that any perturbation within this highly dynamic system may potentially underlie the pathophysiology associated with affective disorders. It is well established that the genomic effects of glucocorticoids are mediated through two cognate receptors, the type I high-affinity mineralocorticoid receptor (MR) and the type II low-affinity glucocorticoid receptor (GR) (de Kloet et al. 1990). Both MR and GR are members of the nuclear receptor superfamily, one of the most abundant classes of transcriptional regulators in vertebrates (Mangelsdorf et al. 1995). The primary function of these receptors is to act as ligand activated transcription factors, able to detect circulating steroid levels and transmit that information into intranuclear transcriptional responses in target cells. To date, there has been relatively little information about how endogenous basal pulsatile glucocorticoid exposure affects target organs in vivo.

An important glucocorticoid target is the hippocampal formation, a brain structure which plays a major role in stress-related memory and learning. The hippocampus is considered by some to be a primary target for damage during major recurrent depressive illness (Bremner et al. 2000; Holsboer, 2000; Sheline, 1996; Sheline et al. 1999; 1996). The altered cortisol secretion in depressive patients has been found to be correlated with both morphological changes in the hippocampus and significant impairment of cognitive function. Furthermore, these studies have indicated that recurring major depression is associated with hippocampal volume loss, with the degree of change determined by the duration of illness. The phenomenon of decreased hippocampal size has also been associated with other physiological conditions, such as chronic stress (McEwen, 2005) and aging (Lupien et al. 1998) where the basal cortisol profile is altered, thus potentially implicating the aberrant circulating GC profile in a causal role. There is also robust evidence that the pattern of glucocorticoids is important for hippocampal function with particular relevance to depression. Several studies identify a flattening of the diurnal rhythm of cortisol secretion in patients with depression (Deuschle et al. 1997; Gibbons, 1964; Wong et al. 2000; Yehuda et al. 1996). This lack of diurnal variation during constant glucocorticoid replacement can itself attenuate serotonin (5-HT) receptor (5-HT1a) function (Leitch et al. 2003), and reduce the effectiveness of selective serotonin reuptake inhibitor (SSRI) treatment for elevating forebrain 5-HT levels (Gartside et al. 2003). Finally, the diurnal rhythm of corticosterone appears to be necessary for neurogenesis in the hippocampus (Huang and Herbert, 2006). This leads on to the question of how glucocorticoids have these dramatic effects in the hippocampus. Glucocorticoids can readily enter the brain, and can be measured at significant levels in rat hippocampal extracellular fluid (ECF) by microdialysis (Linthorst et al. 1994). Furthermore, a recent elegant study has shown that corticosterone exhibits an ultradian rhythmicity in the ECF within discrete brain structures including the hippocampus (HC) as measured by microdialysis in the brains of freely behaving rats (Droste et al. 2008). Although similar studies are not possible in the human brain, we can extrapolate some very useful information from this study. In man, the major circulating glucocorticoid is cortisol which, unlike corticosterone, is a very good substrate for the multi-drug resistance (MDR) pump which will actively remove cortisol from the brain. This mechanism could account for a reduction in the half-life of cortisol in the brain and effectively sharpen the pulses that the hippocampus is being exposed to.

Upon gaining access to the ECF within the brain, the glucocorticoid ligand is then able to diffuse freely into cells, bind and activate cytoplasmic GR and MR, and initiate translocation into the nucleus and binding to glucocorticoid regulatory elements (GREs) in the promoters of target genes to regulate gene expression. Interestingly, we have found that GR and MR, which are both abundantly co-expressed in the hippocampus, respond in a defined and distinct manner depending on the pattern of pulsatile presentation (Conway-Campbell et al. 2007). We have been able to measure receptor activation, nuclear translocation and DNA binding kinetics of both GR and MR after different corticosterone administration protocols in adrenalectomized rats. We have compared a corticosterone profile similar to that seen following an acute stress with a temporal profile more similar to an endogenous corticosterone pulse. Hippocampal GR and MR were rapidly activated following both the acute pulse (Fig. 7.4) and the more prolonged 'stress' increase (Fig. 7.5) in corticosterone. Following the longer duration increase in corticosterone during a 'stress' mimicking pulse, both MR and GR levels remained associated with DNA for the duration of the increased plasma corticosteroid levels. What was extraordinary however, was the response to the rapid pulse of corticosterone. After activation, GR associated with, then dissociated from the DNA extremely swiftly, returning to baseline levels by 60 minutes after each pulse, as depicted in the representative schematic (Fig. 7.6). Interestingly, MR did not dissociate from the DNA so rapidly, with association remaining high up to 60 minutes after each pulse. This timing is coincident with the duration of the physiological interpulse interval. We were therefore able to demonstrate that, in the hippocampus, the pulsatile exposure to corticosterone is a sufficient stimulus to retain the high affinity MR in association with target genes, while the lower affinity GR dissociates in parallel with rapidly dropping steroid levels. The differential DNA binding kinetics of both receptors may explain the dual action of corticosterone in the hippocampus, with MR preventing disturbance of homeostasis and GR promoting recovery following stress (de Kloet et al. 1998).

Molecular mechanisms

At the molecular level, differential rates for dissociation from DNA by hippocampal GR and MR may simply reflect their different affinities for the ligand (Reul and de Kloet, 1985). While GR dissociates from glucocorticoid quite rapidly ($t_{1/2}$ = 5 min for hGR binding to cortisol), MR remains bound for significantly longer ($t_{1/2}$ = 45 min for hMR binding to cortisol). This raises the possibility that increased ligand affinity may also confer increased DNA-binding stability of MR compared to GR, effectively prolonging the MR signal. Evidence in support of this theory exists in the literature. Stavreva and colleagues have shown in a series of elegant cell culture experiments that the stability of GR on a target promoter was dependent on GR's affinity for ligand (Stavreva et al. 2004). Although not investigating MR, GR dynamics were examined with either corticosterone or the high-affinity synthetic agonist dexamethasone using live cell imaging with a green fluorescent protein tagged GR (GFP-GR). This study was performed in a cell line engineered to stably integrate an array of multiple copies of GREs in the murine mammary tumour virus (MMTV) promoter, so that fluorescence confocal microscopy was able to detect this array of GREs as two bright spots within the nucleus. The recruitment of GFP-GR to the array was observed after five minutes of treatment with either corticosterone or dexamethasone. Interestingly, after a stringent wash over a five-minute period to remove all the ligand from the culture medium, transcription from the MMTV promoter was completely abolished in the case of corticosterone, but continued at 50% of maximal levels in the case of dexamethasone. Conversely, Meijsing and colleagues concluded that ligand dissociation was not required for GR

A
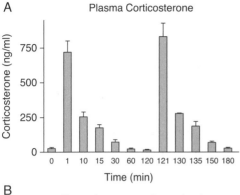

B
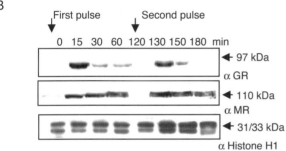

C
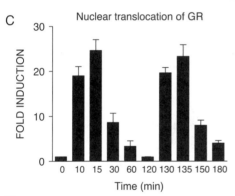

D
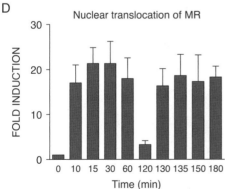

Fig. 7.4 IV injection of corticosterone results in brief elevation of circulating corticosterone and differential nuclear retention patterns of hippocampal GR and MR. Reprinted with permission from Endocrinology, Proteasome-dependent down-regulation of activated nuclear hippocampal glucocorticoid receptors determines dynamic responses to corticosterone, B L Conway-Campbell. 148, 5470-7. © 2007 The Endocrine Society.

Note: A. Plasma corticosterone levels were undetectable in the ADX rats before corticosterone injection (time 0 min) and rose to a maximal value 1 min after injection, then cleared according to the approximately 10 min half life of corticosterone in blood. A second injection at 120 min exhibited a similar profile to the first. B. Nuclear translocation of both hippocampal GR (upper panel) and MR (middle panel) was rapidly induced following the rise in circulating corticosterone. Both GR and MR were detected in the nucleus as early as 10 min after each pulse. Nuclear retention time for GR was extremely brief with clearance evident at 30 min post injection and returning to near basal levels by 60 min. Nuclear retention time for MR was longer in duration with levels remaining high up to 60 min. C. Summary graph of fold inductions of nuclear translocation for the entire timecourse for GR. D. Summary graph of fold inductions of nuclear translocation for the entire timecourse for MR. GR and MR both exhibit similar rapid kinetics in the initial induction of nuclear translocation in response to each pulse of corticosterone. The clearance rate for GR is significantly more rapid than for MR. Nuclear GR levels decline to baseline by 60 min post injection, but MR still remains maximally elevated at 60 min post injection. Nuclear GR levels at 60 min are not significantly different to basal levels ($p = 0.1331$). Nuclear MR levels are significantly different to basal levels ($p = 0.0207$) and not significantly different to maximal levels ($p = 0.9249$) (Conway-Campbell et al. 2007).

Fig. 7.5 IP injection of corticosterone results in prolonged elevation of circulating corticosterone and prolonged nuclear retention of hippocampal GR and MR. Reprinted with permission from Endocrinology, Proteasome-dependent down-regulation of activated nuclear hippocampal glucocorticoid receptors determines dynamic responses to corticosterone, B L Conway-Campbell. 148, 5470-7. © 2007 The Endocrine Society.

Note: A. Plasma corticosterone levels were undetectable in the ADX rats before corticosterone injection (time 0 min) and rose to a maximal value 30 min after injection, remaining elevated at 60 min and reducing to near baseline levels at 120 min. B. Nuclear translocation of both hippocampal GR (upper panel) and MR (middle panel) was induced in parallel with the rise in circulating corticosterone at 30 min post injection. Nuclear levels remained elevated at 60 min, decreasing towards baseline levels by 120 min. Histone H1 (lower panel) indicates loading control for each sample. C. Summary graph of fold inductions of nuclear translocation of GR for $n = 6$/timepoint. D. Summary graph of fold inductions of nuclear translocation of MR for $n = 6$/timepoint. There is no significant difference between GR and MR for either the initial induction of nuclear translocation (ns, $p = 0.8738$) or the nuclear retention levels at 120 min (ns, $p = 0.9739$) (Conway-Campbell et al. 2007).

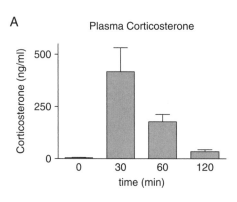

A — Plasma Corticosterone

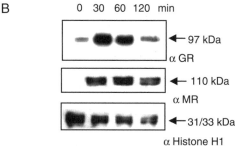

B

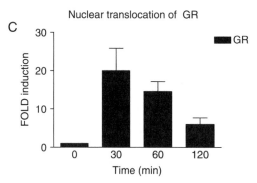

C — Nuclear translocation of GR

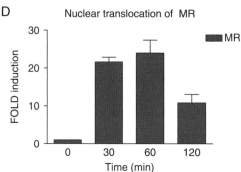

D — Nuclear translocation of MR

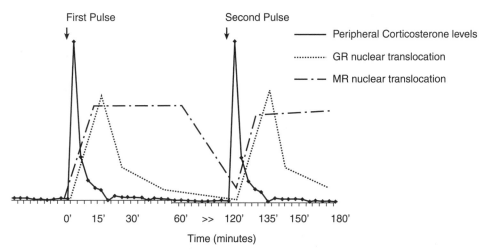

Fig. 7.6 Schematic representation of GR and MR nuclear translocation and retention kinetics after two bolus IV injections at times 0 and 120 min. Reprinted with permission from the European Journal of Pharmacology, The significance of glucocorticoid pulsatility, S Lightman et al, © 2008 Elsevier B V.

Note: The peripheral corticosterone levels measured by automated sampling at 5-min intervals show a rapid spike of corticosterone into the circulation after each IV bolus injection. This is followed by a rapid clearance consistent with the approximate 10 min half life of corticosterone in blood. The consequent activation and nuclear translocation kinetics of GR and MR are traced over the profile. GR exhibits rapid nuclear translocation, then clearance after each bolus IV injection. In contrast, nuclear MR levels remain high for 60 min after each bolus IV injection.

dissociation from GREs, based on mobility after photobleaching (FRAP) experiments using dexamethasone modified to bind covalently to GR (Meijsing et al. 2007). They concluded however, that the ligand-binding domain (LBD) was important, as LBD deletion constructs of GR dissociated faster from the GRE. It remains to be seen how relevant these covalently bound ligands and GR mutants are to endogenous corticosterone-induced transcriptional activity, but certainly the GR LBD appears to play a critical role.

We should therefore like to put forward a putative model describing our hypothesis that dissociation of ligand from GR but not MR (or alternatively a non-ligand LBD related mechanism) is the first step in destabilizing the complex from its association with the GRE on target promoters (as depicted in Fig. 7.7). The functional significance of this rapid turnover of activated GR on the regulatory elements of DNA may be to allow dynamic and continuous responses to the highly fluctuating hormone levels observed in pulsatile glucocorticoid secretion, while MR maintains a continuous basal level of homeostasis. This mechanism may underlie the dual action of corticosterone via its two receptors.

Importantly, our study shows that during endogenous pulsatility in a normal healthy animal, GR is not constantly activated but instead periodically activated in synchronization with rising and falling ligand levels. It is perhaps reasonable then to hypothesize that this is the ideal pattern as it is associated with younger animals, both stress-free and in good health. Changes from this normal pattern are associated with aging, disease, and affective disorders, and can therefore be assumed to be sub-optimal. On the basis of our findings, we hypothesize that changes in glucocorticoid exposure, even subtle changes in the basal ultradian rhythm, such as an increase in the frequency of the pulses throughout the 24-hour diurnal profile will have profound effects on GR, especially those in the hippocampus. The constant drive of GR signalling via abnormal increases in glucocorticoid pulse frequency may potentially have deleterious effects on the function of hippocampal neurons, leading to the functional and morphological changes

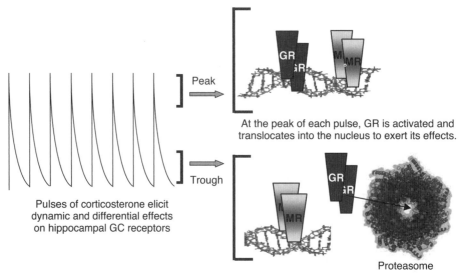

Fig. 7.7 Proposed model of pulsatile corticosterone regulation of glucocorticoid receptors in the hippocampus. Reprinted with permission from Endocrinology, Proteasome-dependent down-regulation of activated nuclear hippocampal glucocorticoid receptors determines dynamic responses to corticosterone, B L Conway-Campbell. 148, 5470-7. © 2007 The Endocrine Society. Reprinted with permission from the European Journal of Pharmacology. The significance of glucocorticoid pulsatility, S. Lightman et al., © 2008 Elsevier B V. See colour plate section for colour version.

Note: Schematic depiction of circulating corticosterone pulsatility, showing how the peak and trough of each pulse differentially affects GR and MR. During the peak of each pulse, both GR and MR are maximally activated and localized to the nuclear compartment where they are known to bind to GREs in the promoters of GC target genes in the genome. Then during the trough of each pulse, nuclear GR is specifically downregulated while MR is retained in the nucleus. This mechanism allows nuclear GR to be constantly and rapidly cleared ensuring dynamic interaction with fluctuating GC levels.

observed in major recurrent depression (although this is still a controversial area: see Chapter 11 in this book).

Glucocorticoid replacement paradigms

We have devised a novel infusion system, designed to mimic the pattern observed in depressive illness, for the purpose of a systematic study to assess the effect on hippocampal function and behaviour in an animal model. As no extant corticosterone replacement paradigms mimic the physiological ultradian rhythm of corticosterone secretion we have therefore addressed this problem by developing an infusion protocol with which we are able to selectively replace corticosterone with pulsatile characteristics of our own choice into adrenalectomized animals. In order to achieve this, we use corticosterone solubilized in a cyclodextrin vehicle, which is infused into the femoral vein and is controlled by a computer-driven infusion pump. This allows us to reproduce

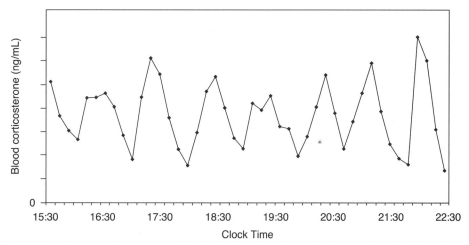

Fig. 7.8 Seven-hour corticosterone profile of a single adrenalectomized rat undergoing infused pulsatile corticosterone replacement during the automated blood sampling procedure. Reprinted with permission from the European Journal of Pharmacology, The significance of glucocorticoid pulsatility, S Lightman et al, © 2008 Elsevier B V.

Note: Both the frequency and amplitude of these pulses mimic those seen in an adrenal-intact animal (Wiles et al. unpublished data).

physiological corticosterone pulses at a rate and amplitude similar to those found in adrenal intact animals. Combining our automated infusion system with automated blood sampling directly from the jugular vein every ten minutes, we have been able to verify the infusion pattern (Fig. 7.8). This infusion system gives us a novel way to directly compare the effects of different patterns of corticosterone administration on a slew of physiological and behavioural variables, and should be able to provide us with critical insights into how this striking endogenous glucocorticoid pulsatility regulates hippocampal function, and how alterations in the pattern lead to hippocampal impairment, cognitive deficits and potential development of affective disorders.

References

Amato, G., Mazziotti, G., Di Somma, C. et al. (2000). Recombinant growth hormone (GH) therapy in GH-deficient adults: a long-term controlled study on daily versus thrice weekly injections. *J Clin Endocrinol Metab.*, **85**, 3720–3725.

Atkinson, H.C., Wood, S.A., Castrique, E.S., Kershaw, Y.M., Wiles, C.C., and Lightman, S. (2008). Corticosteroids mediate fast feedback of the rat hypothalamic-pituitary-adrenal axis via the mineralo-corticoid receptor. *American Journal of Physiology*, **294**, E1011–1012.

Atkinson, H.C., Wood, S.A., Kershaw, Y.M., Bate, E., and Lightman, S.L. (2006). Diurnal variation in the responsiveness of the hypothalamic-pituitary-adrenal axis of the male rat to noise stress. *J Neuroendocrinol.*, **18**, 526–533.

Belchetz, P.E., Plant, T.M., Nakai, Y., Keogh, E.J., and Knobil, E. (1978). Hypophysial responses to continuous and intermittent delivery of hypopthalamic gonadotropin-releasing hormone. *Science*, **202**, 631–633.

Bremner, J.D., Narayan, M., Anderson, E.R., Staib, L.H., Miller, H.L., and Charney, D.S. (2000). Hippocampal volume reduction in major depression. *Am J Psychiatry*, **157**, 115–118.

Carnes, M., Lent, S.J., Goodman, B., Mueller, C., Saydoff, J., and Erisman, S. (1990). Effects of immunone-utralization of corticotropin-releasing hormone on ultradian rhythms of plasma adrenocorticotropin. *Endocrinology*, **126**, 1904–1913.

Carnes, M., Brownfield, M., Lent, S.J., Nichols, K., and Schuler, L. (1992). Pulsatile ACTH and cortisol in goats: effects of insulin-induced hypoglycemia and dexamethasone. *Neuroendocrinology*, **55**, 97–104.

Clark, R.G., Carlsson, L.M., and Robinson, I.C. (1987) Growth hormone secretory profiles in conscious female rats. *J.Endocrinol.*, **114**, 399–407.

Conway-Campbell, B.L., McKenna, M.A., Wiles, C.C., Atkinson, H.C., de Kloet, E.R., and Lightman, S. L. (2007). Proteasome-dependent down-regulation of activated nuclear hippocampal glucocorticoid receptors determines dynamic responses to corticosterone. *Endocrinology*, **148**, 5470–5477.

Cudd, T.A., LeBlanc, M., Silver, M. et al. (1995). Ontogeny and ultradian rhythms of adrenocorticotropin and cortisol in the late-gestation fetal horse. *J Endocrinol.*, **144**, 271–283.

Dallman, M.F. (2005). Fast glucocorticoid actions on brain: Back to the future. *Front Neuroendocrinol.*, **26**, 103–108.

Dallman, M.F. and Yates, F.E. (1969). Dynamic asymmetries in the corticosteroid feedback path and distribution-metabolism-binding elements of the adrenocortical system. *Ann N Y Acad Sci.*, **156**, 696–721.

de Kloet, E.R., Reul, J.M., and Sutanto, W. (1990). Corticosteroids and the brain. *J Steroid Biochem Mol Biol.*, **37**, 387–394.

de Kloet, E.R., Vreugdenhil, E., Oitzl, M.S., and Joels, M. (1998). Brain corticosteroid receptor balance in health and disease. *Endocr Rev.*, **19**, 269–301.

Deuschle, M., Schweiger, U., Weber, B. et al. (1997). Diurnal activity and pulsatility of the hypothalamus-pituitary-adrenal system in male depressed patients and healthy controls. *J Clin Endocrinol Metab.*, **82**, 234–238.

Di, S., Malcher-Lopes, R., Halmos, K.C., and Tasker, J.G. (2003). Nongenomic glucocorticoid inhibition via endocannabinoid release in the hypothalamus: a fast feedback mechanism. *J Neurosci.*, **23**, 4850–4857.

Droste, S.K., de Groote, L., Atkinson, H.C., Lightman, S.L., Reul, J.M., and Linthorst, A.C. (2008). Corticosterone levels in the brain show a distinct ultradian rhythm but a delayed response to forced swim stress. *Endocrinology.*

Engler, D., Pham, T., Fullerton, M.J., Clarke, I.J., and Funder, J.W. (1989a). Evidence for an ultradian secretion of adrenocorticotropin, beta-endorphin and alpha-melanocyte-stimulating hormone by the ovine anterior and intermediate pituitary. *Neuroendocrinology*, **49**, 349–360.

Engler, D., Pham, T., Fullerton, M.J., Ooi, G., Funder, J.W., and Clarke, I.J. (1989b). Studies of the secretion of corticotropin-releasing factor and arginine vasopressin into the hypophysial-portal circulation of the conscious sheep. I. Effect of an audiovisual stimulus and insulin-induced hypoglycemia. *Neuroendocrinology*, **49**, 367–381.

Gartside, S.E., Leitch, M.M., and Young, A.H. (2003). Altered glucocorticoid rhythm attenuates the ability of a chronic SSRI to elevate forebrain 5-HT: implications for the treatment of depression. *Neuropsychopharmacology*, **28**, 1572–1578.

Gibbons, J.L. (1964). Cortisol secretion rate in depressive illness. *Arch Gen Psychiatry*, **10**, 572–575.

Glenister, D.W. and Yates, F.E. (1961). Sex difference in the rate of disappearance of corticosterone-4-C14 from plasma of intact rats: further evidence for the influence of hepatic Delta4-steroid hydrogenase activity on adrenal cortical function. *Endocrinology*, **68**, 747–758.

Hellman, L., Nakada, F., Curti, J. et al. (1970). Cortisol is secreted episodically by normal man. *J Clin Endocrinol Metab.*, **30**, 411–22.

Henley, D., Leendertz, J., Russell, G. et al. (2009). Development of an automated blood sampling system for use in humans. *J Med Eng Technol.*, **33**, 1–10.

Hinz, B. and Hirschelmann, R. (2000). Rapid non-genomic feedback effects of glucocorticoids on CRF-induced ACTH secretion in rats. *Pharm Res*, **17**, 1273–7.

Holsboer, F. (2000) The corticosteroid receptor hypothesis of depression. *Neuropsychopharmacology*, **23**, 477–501.

Huang, G.J. and Herbert, J. (2006). Stimulation of neurogenesis in the hippocampus of the adult rat by fluoxetine requires rhythmic change in corticosterone. *Biol Psychiatry.*, **59**, 619–624.

Jasper, M.S. and Engeland, W.C. (1991). Synchronous ultradian rhythms in adrenocortical secretion detected by microdialysis in awake rats. *AJP – Regulatory, Integrative and Comparative Physiology*, **261**, R1257–R1268.

Jasper, M.S. and Engeland, W.C. (1994). Splanchnic neural activity modulates ultradian and circadian rhythms in adrenocortical secretion in awake rats. *Neuroendocrinology*, **59**, 97–109.

Karst, H., Berger, S., Turiault, M., Tronche, F., Schutz, G., and Joels, M. (2005). Mineralocorticoid receptors are indispensable for nongenomic modulation of hippocampal glutamate transmission by corticosterone. *Proc Natl Acad Sci USA*, **102**, 19204–19207.

Keller-Wood, M.E. and Dallman, M.F. (1984). Corticosteroid inhibition of ACTH secretion. *Endocr. Rev.*, **5**, 1–24.

Kesrouani, A., Abdallah, M.A., Attieh, E., Abboud, J., Atallah, D., and Makhoul, C. (2001). Gonadotropin-releasing hormone for infertility in women with primary hypothalamic amenorrhea. Toward a more-interventional approach. *J Reprod Med.*, **46**, 23–28.

Leitch, M.M., Ingram, C.D., Young, A.H., McQuade, R., and Gartside, S.E. (2003). Flattening the corticosterone rhythm attenuates 5-HT1A autoreceptor function in the rat: relevance for depression. *Neuropsychopharmacology*, **28**, 119–125.

Lightman, S.L., Windle, R.J., Julian, M.D. et al. (2000). Significance of pulsatility in the HPA axis. In Novartis, F. (ed.) *Mechanisms and Biological Significance of Pulsatile Hormone Secretion*. Wiley.

Lightman, S.L., Wiles, C.C., Atkinson, H.C. et al. (2008). The significance of glucocorticoid pulsatility. *European Journal of Pharmacology*, **583**, 255–262.

Linthorst, A.C., Flachskamm, C., Holsboer, F., and Reul, J.M. (1994). Local administration of recombinant human interleukin-1 beta in the rat hippocampus increases serotonergic neurotransmission, hypothalamic-pituitary-adrenocortical axis activity, and body temperature. *Endocrinology*, **135**, 520–532.

Loudon, A.S., Wayne, N.L., Krieg, R., Iranmanesh, A., Veldhuis, J.D., and Menaker, M. (1994). Ultradian endocrine rhythms are altered by a circadian mutation in the Syrian hamster. *Endocrinology*, **135**, 712–718.

Lucas, R.J., Stirland, J.A., Darrow, J.M., Menaker, M., and Loudon, A.S. (1999). Free running circadian rhythms of melatonin, luteinizing hormone, and cortisol in Syrian hamsters bearing the circadian tau mutation. *Endocrinology*, **140**, 758–764.

Lupien, S.J., de Leon, M., de Santi, S., Convit, A., Tarshish, C., and Nair, N. (1998). Cortisol levels during human aging predict hippocampal atrophy and memory deficits. *Nat Neurosci.*, **1**, 69–73.

Mangelsdorf, D.J., Thummel, C., Beato, M. et al. (1995). The nuclear receptor superfamily: the second decade. *Cell*, **83**, 835–839.

McEwen, B.S. (2005). Glucocorticoids, depression, and mood disorders: structural remodeling in the brain. *Metabolism*, **54**, 20–23.

Meijsing, S.H., Elbi, C., Luecke, H.F., Hager, G.L., and Yamamoto, K.R. (2007). The ligand binding domain controls glucocorticoid receptor dynamics independent of ligand release. *Mol Cell Biol.*, **27**, 2442–2451.

Reul, J.M. and de Kloet, E.R. (1985). Two receptor systems for corticosterone in rat brain: microdistribution and differential occupation. *Endocrinology*, **117**, 2505–2511.

Sarnyai, Z., Veldhuis, J.D., Mello, N.K. et al. (1995). The concordance of pulsatile ultradian release of adrenocorticotropin and cortisol in male rhesus monkeys. *J Clin Endocrinol Metab.*, **80**, 54–59.

Seale, J.V., Wood, S.A., Atkinson, H.C. et al. C.D. (2004a). Gonadectomy reverses the sexually diergic patterns of circadian and stress-induced hypothalamic-pituitary-adrenal axis activity in male and female rats. *J Neuroendocrinol*, **16**, 516–524.

Seale, J.V., Wood, S.A., Atkinson, H.C., Harbuz, M.S., and Lightman, S.L. (2004b). Gonadal steroid replacement reverses gonadectomy-induced changes in the corticosterone pulse profile and stress-induced hypotha-lamic-pituitary-adrenal axis activity of male and female rats. *J.Neuroendocrinol.*, **16**, 989–998.

Shanks, N. and Lightman, S.L. (2001). The maternal-neonatal neuro-immune interface: Are there long-term implications for inflammatory or stress-related disease? *J Clin Invest.*, **108**, 1567–1573.

Sheline, Y.I. (1996). Hippocampal atrophy in major depression: a result of depression-induced neurotoxicity? *Mol Psychiatry*, **1**, 298–299.

Sheline, Y.I., Sanghavi, M., Mintun, MA., and Gado, M.H. (1999). Depression duration but not age predicts hippocampal volume loss in medically healthy women with recurrent major depression. *J Neurosci.*, **19**, 5034–5043.

Sheline, Y.I., Wang, P.W., Gado, M.H., Csernansky, J.G., and Vannier, M.W. (1996). Hippocampal atrophy in recurrent major depression. *Proc Natl Acad Sci USA*, **93**, 3908–3913.

Spiga, F., Harrison, L.R., Wood, S.A. et al. (2007). Effect of the glucocorticoid receptor antagonist Org 34850 on basal and stress-induced corticosterone secretion. *J Neuroendocrinol.*, **19**, 891–900.

Stavreva, D.A., Muller, W.G., Hager, G.L., Smith, C.L., and McNally, J.G. (2004). Rapid glucocorticoid receptor exchange at a promoter is coupled to transcription and regulated by chaperones and proteasomes. *Mol Cell Biol.*, **24**, 2682–2697.

Tapp, W.N., Holaday, J.W., and Natelson, B.H. (1984). Ultradian glucocorticoid rhythms in monkeys and rats continue during stress. *AJP – Legacy*, **247**, R866–R871.

Veldhuis, J.D., Iranmanesh, A., Johnson, M.L., and Lizarralde, G. (1990). Amplitude, but not frequency, modulation of adrenocorticotropin secretory bursts gives rise to the nyctohemeral rhythm of the corticotropic axis in man. *J Clin Endocrinol Metab.*, **71**, 452–463.

Waxman, D.J., Ram, P.A., Pampori, N.A., and Shapiro, B.H. (1995). Growth hormone regulation of male-specific rat liver P450s 2A2 and 3A2: induction by intermittent growth hormone pulses in male but not female rats rendered growth hormone deficient by neonatal monosodium glutamate. *Mol Pharmacol.*, **48**, 790–797.

Weitzman, E.D., Fukushima, D., Nogeire, C., Roffwarg, H., Gallagher, T.F., and Hellman, L. (1971). Twenty-four hour pattern of the episodic secretion of cortisol in normal subjects. *J Clin Endocrinol Metab.*, **33**, 14–22.

Windle, R.J., Wood, S.A., Lightman, S.L., and Ingram, C.D. (1998a). The pulsatile characteristics of hypothalamo-pituitary-adrenal activity in female Lewis and Fischer 344 rats and its relationship to differential stress responses. *Endocrinology*, **139**, 4044–4052.

Windle, R.J., Wood, S.A., Shanks, N., Lightman, S.L., and Ingram, C.D. (1998b). Ultradian rhythm of basal corticosterone release in the female rat: dynamic interaction with the response to acute stress. *Endocrinology*, **139**, 443–450.

Windle, R.J., Wood, S.A., Kershaw, Y.M., Lightman, S.L., Ingram, C.D., and Harbuz, M.S. (2001). Increased corticosterone pulse frequency during adjuvant-induced arthritis and its relationship to alterations in stress responsiveness. *J Neuroendocrinol.*, **13**, 905–911.

Wong, M.L., Kling, M.A., Munson, P. J. et al. (2000). Pronounced and sustained central hypernoradrenergic function in major depression with melancholic features: relation to hypercortisolism and corticotropin-releasing hormone. *Proc Natl Acad Sci USA*, **97**, 325–330.

Woodward, C.J., Hervey, G.R., Oakey, R.E., and Whitaker, E.M. (1991). The effects of fasting on plasma corticosterone kinetics in rats. *Br J Nutr.*, **66**, 117–127.

Yehuda, R., Teicher, M.H., Trestman, R.L., Levengood, R.A., and Siever, L.J. (1996). Cortisol regulation in posttraumatic stress disorder and major depression: a chronobiological analysis. *Biol Psychiatry*, **40**, 79–88.

Young, E.A., Abelson, J., and Lightman, S.L. (2004). Cortisol pulsatility and its role in stress regulation and health. *Front Neuroendocrinol.*, **25**, 69–76.

Chapter 8

Early life programming of affective function

Caitlin S. Wyrwoll, Megan C. Holmes, and Jonathan R. Seckl

Introduction

It seems obvious that factors influencing development will have persisting effects throughout the individual's lifespan. Yet, with the exception of teratogenesis, this concept has been largely overlooked in the heat of the genomic revolution and its accompanying trend to explain adult variation in terms of individual SNPs and haplotypes, merely amplified by the adult environment. However, starting with the pioneering work of Waddington and colleagues in Edinburgh (Waddington, 1940), and more recently the plethora of epidemiological data indicating early life antecedents of common cardiometabolic disorders (Barker et al. 1993a, b, c; 1989a, b; Hales et al. 1991), the role of developmental environmental factors in subsequent structure, physiology, function, and pathology has been reawakened. Of course, nothing is new on earth and even in the nineteenth century, Weismann had noted that the temperature at which genetically identical insect pupae were incubated determined the adult phenotype (Weismann, 1892). Moreover, neuroscience has long been replete with examples of perinatal environmental factors having persisting organizational and functional effects. A fine example is perinatal exposure of songbirds and rodents to androgens which, only at this time, permanently determine hypothalamic anatomy, chemistry and function, and associated sexual behaviour irrespective of the ostensible genetic sex of the individual (for a review see Breedlove, 1992). Indeed, the vertebrate brain appears exquisitely sensitive to developmental programming, perhaps a reflection of its limited scope for plasticity in terms of cellular number and structure after developmental cell expansion, differentiation, wiring and pruning are complete. Here we address the emerging biology, concerning developmental programming by stress and its glucocorticoid hormonal mediators of the CNS and affective function. This is the second of five chapters in this book that present not only clinical data but also experimental evidence from animal models relevant to the role of the hypothalamic-pituitary-adrenal (HPA) in affective disorders, together with Chapters 7, 9, 11, and 26.

Developmental programming

A plethora of studies in both humans and animal models have indicated that environmental events in early life are important determinants of common human disorders in adulthood. Thus, data from populations in Europe, Asia, Africa, Australia, and North America have shown that low birth weight (assumed to be a marker of an adverse intrauterine environment) predisposes affected individuals to hypertension, dyslipidemia, insulin resistance, type 2 diabetes, obesity, and death from ischemic heart disease in adulthood (for a review see Barker, 2004). Importantly, this association between low birth weight and adult disease is largely independent of adult lifestyle risk factors (smoking, obesity, social class, alcohol excess, lack of exercise), which are additive to the effects of birth weight. This association is, moreover, continuous as it affects birth weights within the normal range, rather than those of severely undersized, multiple, or premature babies. The correlation between birth weight and disease in adult life has been ascribed to developmental programming, whereby environmental factors act during specific developmental periods to affect the development and subsequent organization of sensitive tissues, producing alterations in structure and function that persist throughout life. The individual organ system affected by the environmental factor is determined by its vulnerability to that factor, which depends on the timing of exposure and on the susceptibility of the developing cells and tissues to its influence. Additionally, post-natal catch-up growth amplifies the risk of adult cardiovascular disease (Barker 1991; Bavdekar et al. 1999; Forsen et al. 1997; Law et al. 2002; Leon et al. 1996; Levine et al. 1994; Osmond et al. 1993). The environmental mechanisms of developmental programming identified so far can be simplified into two major groups: foetal glucocorticoid exposure (Benediktsson et al. 1993; Seckl and Holmes, 2007), which is the main focus of this chapter, and maternal-foetal nutrition (Barker et al. 1993c).

Glucocorticoids and developmental programming

Glucocorticoids are a group of steroid hormones synthesized by the adrenal cortex and released in response to stress. In humans, the principle glucocorticoid is cortisol while in rodents it is corticosterone. Glucocorticoid production by the adrenal cortex is under control of the HPA axis. Corticotrophin-releasing hormone (CRH) and arginine vasopressin (AVP) are secreted by the parvocellular neurons in the paraventricular nucleus (PVN) hypothalamus in response to a diurnal circadian rhythm, stress, and other stimuli. CRH and AVP are then released into the hypothalamic-hypophyseal portal system to stimulate release of adrenocorticotrophic hormone (ACTH) in the anterior pituitary (Plotsky et al. 1993). In turn, circulating ACTH stimulates glucocorticoid production from the zona fasciculata of the adrenal cortex. The hypothalamic and pituitary components of the HPA axis are then subject to negative feedback control by glucocorticoids via the glucocorticoid receptor (GR) and mineralocorticoid receptor (MR) in the hippocampus and GR at the hypothalamic PVN and anterior pituitary (de Kloet 1997; de Kloet et al. 2005; Plotsky et al. 1993). However, this classic feedback model for glucocorticoid action is now becoming increasingly complex, with emerging evidence for acute non-genomic effects of glucocorticoids on the brain (Karst et al. 2005), in addition to feed-forward actions (Dallman et al. 2007). The feed-forward actions of glucocorticoids occur after persistent stress, whereby the direct action of glucocorticoids on the brain is actually stimulatory, and there is a signal from abdominal energy stores that elicit HPA axis inhibition (Akana and Dallman, 1997; Dallman et al. 2007).

Glucocorticoids are highly lipophilic, readily diffusing through the plasma membrane into the cytoplasm and binding to the intracytoplasmic receptors GR and MR (Funder, 1997). While GR is expressed ubiquitously, MR is particularly concentrated in mineralocorticoid target tissues such as the distal nephron and colon, where the mineralocorticoid, aldosterone, binds to the MR to increase transepithelial sodium transport (Funder, 1997). Additionally, glucocorticoids bind to both GR and MR and thus, active glucocorticoids must be metabolized in mineralocorticoid target tissues to ensure aldosterone specific activation of the MR.

Intracellular levels of bioactive glucocorticoid can be modified by the enzyme 11β-hydroxysteroid dehydrogenase (11β-HSD) which interconverts the active glucocorticoids cortisol and corticosterone with their biologically inactive forms, cortisone and 11-dehydrocorticosterone (DHC), respectively. There are two distinct forms of 11β-HSD, 11β-HSD1, and 11β-HSD2. 11β-HSD1 is a lower affinity, NADP(H)-dependent bidirectional enzyme (Agarwal et al. 1989), although in vivo it acts predominantly as an 11β-oxoreductase to enhance glucocorticoid activity (Seckl and Walker, 2001). 11β-HSD2 is a high affinity NAD-dependent enzyme which exhibits exclusive 11β-dehydrogenase activity (conversion of active cortisol and corticosterone to inert cortisone and 11-DHC, respectively) to abrogate intracellular glucocorticoid action (Agarwal et al. 1995).

Prenatally, glucocorticoids are important in the structural development and functional matura-tion of foetal organs. Glucocorticoids cause tissue to change from a proliferative state to one that is more mature and functionally differentiated (Celsi et al. 1998). Therefore, the size and cellular configuration of a glucocorticoid sensitive organ can be influenced by the developmental pattern of glucocorticoid exposure (Celsi et al. 1998). Overexposure of the foetus to glucocorticoids can, however, be detrimental through retardation of foetal growth. In humans, clinical administration of repeated doses of synthetic glucocorticoids is common in women at risk of preterm delivery (Anonymous, 1995). In such cases, glucocorticoid administration serves to advance foetal lung maturation thereby reducing neonatal morbidity and mortality (Anonymous, 1995). The long-term effects of this treatment are not fully elucidated although there are suggestions that foetal growth and subsequent development may be impaired (Sloboda et al. 2005). Potentially, because excess glucocorticoids affect foetal growth and organ development, this could impact not only on immediate health, but also extend well into adult life.

Placental 11β-HSD2

Given the importance of glucocorticoids in foetal development, transfer of glucocorticoids between the mother and foetus needs to be closely regulated. This is achieved by the placental glucocorticoid barrier, which involves glucocorticoid inactivation within the placenta by 11β-HSD2. 11β-HSD2 is highly expressed in the placenta and is located at the interface between maternal and foetal circulations, in the syncytiotrophoblast in humans (Brown et al. 1996b) and the labyrinthine zone in rodent placentas (Waddell and Atkinson, 1994; Waddell et al. 1998). In the rat, 11β-HSD2 expression within the labyrinth zone of the placenta falls during late gestation, which may facilitate glucocorticoid passage to the foetus before parturition and thus promote lung maturation (Burton et al. 1996).

It has been hypothesized that relative deficiency of placental 11β-HSD2 may underpin aspects of developmental programming by allowing excess glucocorticoid passage from the 'high' gluco-corticoid maternal circulation to the 'low' glucocorticoid foetal environment (Edwards et al. 1993). Indeed, 11β-HSD2 activity within the rat and human placenta correlates positively with offspring birth weight (Benediktsson et al. 1993; Murphy et al. 2002; Stewart et al. 1995a), suggesting that normal variation in foetal exposure to maternal glucocorticoids impact on foetal growth. Accordingly, disruption of the placental glucocorticoid barrier has ramifications for foetal growth and development. Specifically, reduced expression of 11β-HSD2 in human placentas result in low birth weight babies (Shams et al. 1998; Stewart et al. 1995a), as does pharmacological inhibition of 11β-HSD2 by carbenoxolone in rats (Lindsay et al. 1996a). Additionally, mice homozygous for deleterious mutations in the gene encoding 11β-HSD2 (11β-HSD2$^{-/-}$ mice) have a lower birth weight than congenic wild-type mice (Holmes et al. 2006a). Furthermore, administration of dex-amethasone, a synthetic glucocorticoid which is a poor substrate for inactivation by 11β-HSD2, reduces maternal weight gain and offspring birth weight (Burton and Waddell, 1994; Benediktsson et al. 1993; Smith and Waddell, 2000). In contrast, treatment with metyrapone, an 11β-hydroxylase inhibitor, during late pregnancy decreases endogenous glucocorticoid synthesis and increases foetal and placental weights by day 22 of gestation (Burton and Waddell, 1994). Interestingly, the timing of prenatal glucocorticoid exposure is important, with a greater birth weight reduction if glucocorticoids are administered in the later stages of pregnancy (Nyirenda et al. 1998).

Very similar 'small baby' cardiometabolic phenotypes occur in offspring of animals subjected to maternal malnutrition (Hales et al. 1991; Langley and Jackson, 1994; Langley-Evans et al. 1996a; Woodall et al. 1996). Crucially, at least in programming models involving maternal low-protein diets, this is accompanied by an increase in both maternal and foetal glucocorticoid levels (Guzman et al. 2006; Lesage et al. 2001). Low-protein diets are also associated with a decrease in placental 11β-HSD2 activity (Langley-Evans et al. 1996b), which increases access of maternal glucocorticoids to the foetus. Moreover, dexamethasone administration during pregnancy decreases maternal food intake (Woods and Weeks, 2005). Interestingly, in the maternal protein restriction model, offspring hypertension can be prevented by treating the pregnant dam with glucocorticoid synthesis inhibitors, and can be recreated by replacement of corticosterone, at least in female offspring (Langley-Evans, 1997). Consequently, the mechanisms by which maternal undernutrition and foetal glucocorticoid overexposure programme the foetus are likely to be interrelated (Langley-Evans et al. 1996b).

Potentially, because excess glucocorticoids affect foetal growth and organ development, this could impact not only on immediate health, but also extend into adult life. Thus prenatal dexamethasone, stress or 11ß-HSD2 inhibition programmes higher adult blood pressure, glucose and insulin levels in rats, sheep and other models species (Benediktsson et al. 1993; Dodic et al. 1998; 1999; 2002a, b; Gatford et al. 2000; Jensen et al. 2002; Lindsay et al. 1996a, b; Levitt et al. 1996a; Sugden et al. 2001). While all such models show that a variety of maternal insults exert remarkably similar, though not identical, effects upon offspring physiology, extrapolation to humans has remained moot, particularly because of species differences in placental anatomy and the detailed ontogeny of 11β-HSD2 expression (Brown et al. 1996a; Stewart et al. 1995b). Crucially, recent work in singleton-bearing non-human primates has shown that dexamethasone exposure in late gestation causes adverse cardiometabolic and neuroendocrine sequellae in the juvenile offspring (de Vries et al. 2007). Furthermore, animal studies have provided substantial evidence that excess glucocorticoid exposure in utero programmes the HPA axis as well as behaviour (Cratty et al. 1995; Holmes et al. 2006a; O'Regan et al. 2004; Sloboda et al. 2002; Welberg et al. 2001). As levels of glucocorticoids are key to the stress response, these steroids have become clear candidate factors responsible for programming of the HPA axis and behaviour (Seckl, 2008). Thus, the effects of early developmental exposure to glucocorticoids on programming HPA axis function and behaviour are the main focus of this chapter.

Glucocorticoids and CNS development

The developing brain is extremely sensitive to prenatal exposure to glucocorticoids, which are critical for normal maturation in most regions of the developing CNS (Korte, 2001; Meaney et al. 1996). Thus glucocorticoids initiate terminal maturation, remodel axons and dendrites and determine programmed cell death (Meyer, 1983). In sheep, prenatal glucocorticoid administration retards brain weight at birth (Huang et al. 1999), delaying maturation of neurons, myelination, glia, and vasculature (Huang et al. 2001a, b). The perinatal hippocampus is especially sensitive to glucocorticoids with consequences for subsequent memory and behaviour (Bremner et al. 1995; Stein et al. 1997; Sheline et al. 1996). Thus, antenatal treatment of rhesus monkeys with dexamethasone causes dose-associated degeneration of hippocampal neurones and reduced hippocampal volume which persists at 20 months of age (Uno et al. 1990). Prenatal stress (induced by repeated restraint of the pregnant rodent in the last week of pregnancy) reduces actively proliferating hippocampal cells and appears to feminize sexually dimorphic parameters of the adult hippocampus (Mandyam et al. 2008). The controversies around this area are the focus of another chapter in this book, Chapter 11.

The importance of glucocorticoids in neural development is reflected by the high expression of GR and MR in the developing brain (Diaz et al. 1998; Fuxe et al. 1985; Kitraki et al. 1997). However, the abundance of 11β-HSD2 in the CNS until midgestation presumably protects the developing brain from premature glucocorticoid exposure (Brown et al. 1996a; Diaz et al. 1998; Robson et al. 1998). After midgestation, 11β-HSD2 expression declines and this coincides with the terminal stage of neurogenesis (Brown et al. 1996a; Diaz et al. 1998). Similar patterns of expression occur in the human foetal brain with 11β-HSD2 silenced between gestational weeks 19–26 (Stewart et al. 1994). Unusually, 11β-HSD2 is expressed in the cerebellum until weaning and is sensitive in the early post-natal period to glucocorticoid-induced remodelling (Robson et al. 1998). Thus, cerebellar size is reduced in 11β-HSD2$^{-/-}$ mice in early post-natal life due to a decrease in size of both the molecular and internal granule layers (Holmes et al. 2006b). This associates with a delay in attainment of neurodevelopmental landmarks such as negative geotaxis and eye opening (Holmes et al. 2006b). Thus, the timing of exposure of the developing brain to glucocorticoids seems to be tightly regulated, notably by the presence of local 11β-HSD2.

Glucocorticoid programming and the HPA axis

Studies in numerous animal models have revealed that the HPA axis is acutely sensitive to prenatal glucocorticoid exposure. HPA axis activity is altered in models of excess maternal glucocorticoids and prenatal stress, with maternal dexamethasone treatment increasing corticosterone and ACTH levels in the adult offspring, although interestingly, mostly in males (Levitt et al. 1996b; Muneoka et al. 1997; O'Regan et al. 2004; Welberg et al. 2001). These effects seem to reflect a change in the feedback of the HPA axis at the level of the hypothalamus, since CRH mRNA increased in the PVN whereas hippocampal MR and GR both decreased (Cratty et al. 1995; Welberg et al. 2000). Moreover, tissue glucocorticoid action is likely further increased by elevations in hepatic and visceral adipose tissue GR expression (Cleasby et al. 2003; Nyirenda et al. 1998). Furthermore, the normal HPA axis period of hyporesponsiveness in early post-natal life is abolished in adult rats exposed to prenatal stress (Maccari and Morley-Fletcher, 2007), while normal age-related HPA-axis dysfunction is accelerated by prenatal stress (Pardon and Rattray, 2008). In sheep, a single injection of betamethasone, a synthetic glucocorticoid, on gestational day 104 altered HPA function in offspring at one year of age, with elevated basal and stimulated plasma cortisol concentrations (Sloboda et al. 2002). In primates, offspring of mothers treated with dexamethasone during late pregnancy have elevated basal and stress-stimulated cortisol levels (de Vries et al. 2007; Uno et al. 1994).

In rats, maternal protein restriction blunted the typical diurnal pattern of ACTH secretion in the offspring but plasma corticosterone levels remained normal (Langley-Evans et al. 1996a). Elevated expression of GR mRNA and decreased 11β-HSD2 expression was also observed in the kidney of adult rat offspring from protein restricted mothers (Bertram et al. 2001), which would potentially heighten tissue glucocorticoid action, causing hypertension.

Prenatal stress and glucocorticoid programming of behaviour

Prenatal stress in rodents induces anxiogenic and depressive-like behaviour as well as enhancing susceptibility to drug abuse (Archer and Blackman, 1971; Fride and Weinstock, 1988; Fride et al. 1986; Maccari and Morley-Fletcher, 2007; Thompson, 1957; Weinstock, 2005). At a cellular level, limbic neurons of offspring of prenatally stressed pregnancies show reduced plasticity in response to anxiogenic stimuli (Mairesse et al. 2007; Viltart et al. 2006). Prenatal stress also accelerates normal age-related cognitive decline which may be due to exacerbation of the age-related decrease in neurogenesis (Pardon and Rattray, 2008). These effects appear conserved, since prenatal stress in rhesus monkeys induces behavioural sensitization in the offspring (Schneider et al. 2008). Gratifyingly, prenatal exposure to glucocorticoids, the major hormonal mediators of chronic stress, has similar effects on the offspring. Thus, late gestational dexamethasone exposure in rats impairs the offspring's 'coping' behaviours in aversive situations later in life as exemplified by reduced exploration in the open field test and elevated plus maze (Welberg et al. 2001). Such increase in anxiety-like behaviour is evident as early as post-natal week 10 in rats prenatally exposed to dexamethasone (Nagano et al. 2008). Moreover, 11β-HSD2 appears important in these events since either treatment of pregnant rats with an 11β-HSD inhibitor or gene deletion in mice produces offspring with enhanced anxiety-related behaviours (Holmes et al. 2006a; Welberg et al. 2000). Interestingly, despite increased anxiety, the HPA axis activity of the 11β-HSD2$^{-/-}$ offspring appears unaffected, perhaps a reflection of the additional effects of attenuated HPA axis reactivity due to reduced glucocorticoid clearance with absence of renal 11β-HSD2 (Holmes et al. 2006a).

Behavioural changes in adults exposed prenatally to glucocorticoids appear associated with altered functioning of the amygdala – the key structure involved in the expression of fear and anxiety; with amygdala CRH levels implicated in fear-related behaviours. Prenatal glucocorticoid exposure increases adult CRH levels specifically in the central nucleus of the amygdala and therefore may be responsible for the increase in anxiety-like behaviour observed in these animals. Prenatal stress similarly programmes increased anxiety-related behaviours with elevated CRH in the amygdala (Cratty et al. 1995). Moreover, corticosteroids facilitate CRH mRNA expression in this nucleus (Hsu et al. 1998) and increase GR and/or MR in the amygdala (Welberg et al. 2000; 2001). A direct relationship between brain corticosteroid receptor levels and anxiety-like behaviour is supported by the phenotype of transgenic mice with selective loss of GR gene expression in the brain, which show markedly reduced anxiety (Boyle et al. 2006; Tronche et al. 1999; and Chapter 9 in this book). However, in human depression and schizophrenia, decreases in GR expression in specific brain regions such as the amygdala and hippocampus have been reported (Perlman et al. 2004; Webster et al. 2002). Interestingly, forebrain-specific MR-overexpressing transgenic mice exhibit reduced anxiety and altered behavioural response to novelty (Lai et al. 2007). It is unclear however, how depression and anxiety relate and whether they represent different disorders or have similar underlying dysfunction. Regardless, alterations in brain GR and MR appear critical for affective dysfunction.

CNS programming mechanisms

Locus of action: the mother the placenta and/or the foetus?

While the effects of maternal stress or glucocorticoids – or indeed anything else that impacts upon the mother for that matter – might act indirectly via alterations in maternal physiology or behaviour (reduced food intake, altered metabolism, hormones, and so on), a recent study in mice heterozygous for mutations of the 11β-HSD2 gene has indicated that at least in this setting, it is the placental and foetal glucocorticoid exposure that is key. Thus, 11β-HSD2$^{-/-}$ offspring from 11β-HSD2+/− matings have lower birth weight and as adults exhibit greater anxiety than their 11β-HSD2$^{+/+}$ (wild-type) littermates (Holmes et al. 2006a). Since in these studies the same mother gives rise to foetuses either lacking or having 11β-HSD2, these data underline the crucial role for feto-placental 11β-HSD2 in prenatal glucocorticoid programming (Holmes et al. 2006a). Given that foetal growth and development is dependent upon placental nutrient delivery it is possible that glucocorticoids may alter this process by direct effects upon the placenta. Indeed, amino acid and glucose placental transport are perturbed in placentas from 11β-HSD2$^{-/-}$ foetuses generated by heterozygous matings (Wyrwoll, Seckl and Holmes, unpublished observations). Further work is required, however, to ascertain whether aberrations in placental function as a consequence of excess prenatal glucocorticoids impact on foetal CNS development.

Mechanisms of glucocorticoid programming of the brain

It is unclear how prenatal glucocorticoids affect CNS development but several mechanisms have been proposed. The GR, while unlikely to be the only factor involved, has been heavily implicated in early life programming. This hypothesis is particularly appealing given the fundamental and widespread role of the GR as a transcription factor. Epigenetic modifications of the GR is one potential mechanism by which the GR is altered by early life programming. Epigenetic inheritance is the transmission of non DNA-encoded information either from cell to daughter cell or from generation to generation. Within the cell, DNA is packaged into nucleosomes, in which it is wrapped around a core of histone proteins. It is the density of supercoiling of the histone-DNA complex that plays a role in the regulation of gene expression and this can be affected by epigenetic modifications (Fig. 8.1). Epigenetic inheritance can therefore be transmitted by modification of the methylation status of DNA and/or modification of histones by acetylation of their tails (for a review see Morgan et al. 2005). Generally, DNA methylation also represses gene expression by decreasing accessibility to the gene promoter, although stimulation of gene expression can result if methylation blocks binding of a suppressor. DNA methylation is involved in genomic imprinting and X-chromosome inactivation, and has also been linked with pathological states including cancer, birth defects, diabetes, heart disease, and neurological disorders. The usual targets for DNA methylation are CpG islands, groups of CG dinucleotide repeats within the DNA, the majority of which are located within or near the promoters or first exons of genes (Antequera and Bird, 1993). Histone acetylation is negatively regulated by histone deacetylases which block histone acetylation, remove existing acetyl groups from histones and consequently suppress gene expression (Grunstein, 1997).

The GR promoter is complex, with multiple tissue-specific alternate untranslated first exons in mouse, rat, and human (Hollenberg et al. 1985; McCormick et al. 2000; Strahle et al. 1992), most within a transcriptionally active CpG island. All the GR mRNA species give rise to the same receptor protein encoded by exons 2–9. Tissue-specific exon 1 usage is regulated by perinatal environment manipulations. Neonatal handling, which increases aspects of maternal behaviour to her pups, notably licking and grooming, permanently programmes increased expression of only one of the six alternate first exons (exon 1_7) utilized in the hippocampus (McCormick et al. 2000). Exon 1_7 contains a site that binds the neuronal transcription factor inducible growth factor A (NGFI-A). Interestingly, discrete perinatal events may permanently alter gene expression as selective methylation/demethylation of specific CpG dinucleotides of the GR gene occurs, notably around the putative NGFI-A site of exon 1_7. These sites are subject to differential and permanent demethylation, just after the time of birth, in association with the level of maternal care. Thus transcription from this brain-enriched promoter is reduced with lower density maternal care (Weaver et al. 2004). Such changes affect NGFI-A binding to the promoter, which appears to initiate demethylation of the 5'CpG site (Weaver et al. 2007). Additionally, this causes epigenetic reprogramming of the promoter which enables increased affinity for NGFI-A and stable activation (Weaver et al. 2007). Indeed, GR under some circumstances can mediate differential demethylation of target gene promoters which persists after steroid withdrawal, at least in liver-derived cells (Thomassin et al. 2001). This work highlights the possibility that early life environmental events permanently determine the set point of gene control throughout life. Indeed, prenatal

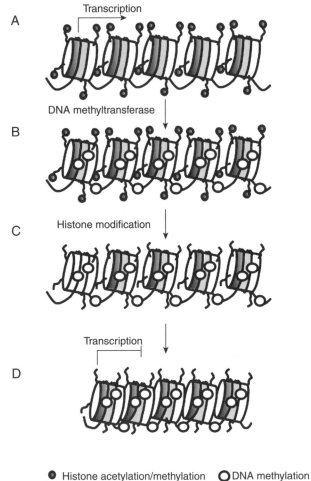

Fig. 8.1 DNA methylation and histone deacetylation act in conjunction to repress transcription.

Note: Transcriptionally active chromatin (A) is predominantly unmethylated and has high levels of acetylated histone tails. DNA methylation is catalysed by DNA methyltrans-ferases (B) and this can repress gene transcription via displacement of transcription factors that normally bind to the DNA. Further modifica-tion of histones via deacetylation or methylation (C) cause transcriptional silencing due to chromatin compaction (D).

administration of dexamethasone affects not only the metabolic parameters of the immediate off-spring as adults, but also their own offspring (Drake et al. 2005). The relevance of developmentally programmed epigenetic changes to human populations is, however, currently uncertain.

During development, serotonin (5-HT) alters transcription of hippocampal GR mRNA via the 5-HT$_7$ receptor. Exposure of foetal hippocampal neurons to 5-HT in vitro results in upregu-lation of GR mRNA but not MR mRNA (Erdeljan et al. 2001). Furthermore, studies in the rat have revealed that the upregulation of GR by 5-HT are mediated by NGFI-A (Meaney et al. 2000). Moreover in the guinea pig, the rapid elevation in hippocampal NFGI-A expression near term correlates with the increase in foetal plasma cortisol concentrations and this elevation can be brought about prematurely by foetal glucocorticoid exposure (Andrews et al. 2004). Interestingly, in the rat, dexamethasone treatment over the final third of pregnancy increases 5-HT transporter expression in the brain (Fumagalli et al. 1996; Slotkin et al. 1996), which could potentially reduce 5-HT bioavailability in the hippocampus and elsewhere and thus may induce a fall in GR and MR. Furthermore, prenatal stress increases 5-HT1A receptors, 5-HT2 recep-tors, as well as increased acetylcholine release in the hippocampus after mild stress (Maccari and Morley-Fletcher, 2007).

Evidence of developmental programming in humans

While birth weight is a crude measure of adverse prenatal environments there does appear to be a link between birth weight and behavioural disorders. Thus, birth weight is associated with schizophrenia, vulnerability to post-traumatic stress disorder (PTSD) and affective disorders in adults and children independent of maternal mental health (Alati et al. 2007; Cannon et al. 2002; Costello et al. 2007; Famularo and Fenton, 1994; Jones et al. 1998; Thompson et al. 2001; Wiles et al. 2005).

Maternal stress in pregnancy has been linked to emotional problems, decreased sociability, hyperactivity, attention deficits, and Tourette's syndrome in children (Leckman et al. 1990; Meijer, 1985; Linnet et al. 2003; Minde et al. 1968; O'Connor et al. 2003). Furthermore, in adults, prenatal stress has been correlated with schizophrenia, depression and drug abuse (Hultman et al. 1999; Huttunen and Niskanen, 1978; Imamura et al. 1999; Watson et al. 1999). Children with attention-deficit hyperactivity disorder tend to develop more severe symptoms if their mothers were exposed to either moderate or severe stress during pregnancy (Grizenko et al. 2008). Stressful events in the second trimester of human pregnancy associate with an increased incidence of offspring schizophrenia (Koenig et al. 2002). Implicated in this are the effects of pre-natal glucocorticoid exposure on the developing dopaminergic system which is associated with schizo-affective, attention-deficit hyperactivity and extrapyramidal disorders. Indeed, prenatal stress reduces cerebral asymmetry and dopamine turnover, consistent with schizophrenic humans (Weinstock, 2001). The offspring of mothers surviving a period of starvation in the Dutch hunger winter of 1944–45 and the Chinese famine of 1959–61 have substantially increased rates of major psychiatric disorders (Susser et al. 1996; St Clair et al. 2005; Susser and Lin, 1992). Furthermore, early malnutrition reduces brain DNA content, lowers IQ scores, and affects behaviour and emotionality in children (Galler and Ramsey, 1989; Galler et al. 1983a, b; Winick, 1971). The role of stress and glucocorticoids in these historic effects is unknown, but may be considerable.

Studies of trauma survivors diagnosed with PTSD reveal reduced urinary, plasma, and salivary cortisol levels (Yehuda, 2002), perhaps reflecting the increased tissue sensitivity to glucocorticoids in PTSD (Yehuda et al. 2004) and hence enhanced feedback. Recently, lower levels of salivary cortisol were reported in mothers who developed PTSD after being present at or near to the World Trade centre atrocity on 11 September 2001 in New York than in mothers who did not develop PTSD. Importantly, the one-year-old offspring of mothers with PTSD also had reduced salivary cortisol levels (Yehuda et al. 2005). These changes were most apparent in babies born to mothers who were in the last three months of their pregnancies when the trauma occurred, a time window also found to be crucial in the equivalent gestational period in rodents (Nyirenda et al. 1998). Intriguingly there was no effect on birth weight, though the incidence of intrauterine growth retardation was increased (Berkowitz et al. 2003) and head circumference reduced (Engel et al. 2005). The findings implicate the *in utero* environment as a major contributor to a possible biological risk factor for PTSD. Such effects may transmit into subsequent generations, since healthy adult children of Holocaust survivors with PTSD (and therefore lower plasma cortisol levels) themselves have lower cortisol levels though no PTSD (Yehuda et al. 2007). This appears to be confined to the children of Holocaust-exposed mothers with PTSD (Yehuda et al. 2007). The implication is that the marker of altered HPA axis functioning, itself perhaps a vulnerability factor, is transmitted into a subsequent generation, suggesting epigenetic 'inheritance' across at least one generation, as seen in rodent models (Drake et al. 2005).

In humans, clinical administration of repeated doses of synthetic glucocorticoids is common in women at risk of preterm delivery. In such cases, glucocorticoid administration serves to advance foetal lung maturation thereby reducing neonatal morbidity and mortality (Bolt et al. 2001).

The long-term effects of this treatment are not fully elucidated although there are suggestions that foetal growth and subsequent development may be impaired (for a review see Bolt et al. 2001). Glucocorticoid treatment during pregnancy reduces birth weight (for a review see Sloboda et al. 2005), but there is a lack of long-term follow-up studies addressing later effects of prenatal glucocorticoid exposure. Antenatal glucocorticoid administration has been linked with higher blood pressure in adolescence (Doyle et al. 2000). A number of studies aimed at establishing the long-term neurological and developmental effects of antenatal glucocorticoid exposure have been complicated by the fact that most of the children studied were born before term and were therefore already at risk of delayed neurological development. In a group of six-year-old children, antenatal glucocorticoid exposure was associated with subtle effects on neurological function, including reduced visual closure and visual memory (MacArthur et al. 1982). Some studies have demonstrated that children exposed to dexamethasone in early pregnancy because they were at risk of congenital adrenal hyperplasia, and who were born at term, showed increased emotionality, unsociability, decreased verbal working memory, avoidance and behavioural problems (Hirvikoski et al. 2007; Trautman et al. 1995), albeit not in all (Meyer-Bahlburg et al. 2004). Furthermore, multiple doses of antenatal glucocorticoids given to women at risk of preterm delivery were associated with reduced birth weight and head circumference in the offspring (French et al. 1999). There are also effects on behaviour; three or more courses of glucocorticoids associate with an increased risk of externalizing behaviour problems, distractibility and inattention (Yeh et al. 2004). Moreover, a controlled trial of post-natal dexamethasone in premature babies showed associations with lower subsequent IQ and decrements of other cortical functions (French et al. 1999).

As with animal models, the human HPA axis appears to be programmed by the early life environment. Higher plasma and urinary glucocorticoid levels are found in children and adults who were of lower birth weight (Clark et al. 1996; Phillips et al. 1998). This appears to occur in disparate populations (Phillips et al. 2000) and may precede overt adult disease (Levitt et al. 2000), at least in a socially disadvantaged South African population. Additionally, adult HPA responses to ACTH stimulation are exaggerated in those of low birth weight (Levitt et al. 2000; Reynolds et al. 2001; 2005), reflecting the stress axis biology elucidated in animal models. The HPA axis activation is associated with higher blood pressure, insulin resistance, glucose intolerance, and hyperlipidaemia (Reynolds et al. 2001). In contrast, adults prenatally exposed to the Dutch famine did not exhibit altered HPA axis activity or an altered HPA response to psychological stress in adult life (de Rooij et al. 2006).

Modification of the programmed phenotype by the post-natal environment

Importantly, developmental programming effects can be attenuated by modifications such as diet and pharmacological treatment. Thus, altered methylation status of the hippocampal GR gene and behavioural response to stress as a result of poor maternal care can be reversed by central infusion of L-methionine, a methyl donor, at three months of age (Weaver et al. 2005). A maternal diet low in protein also alters gene methylation status, and this too is apparently reversed by supplementation of the maternal low protein diet with folic acid, another methyl donor (Lillycrop et al. 2005). Furthermore, a post-natal diet enriched with omega-3 fatty acids attenuates the adverse effects of excess glucocorticoid exposure in utero on subsequent adult health in rats (Wyrwoll et al. 2006; 2007). Treatment with IGF-1 in adult life attenuates insulin and leptin resistance and reduces obesity, hyperphagia, and hypertension programmed in rats by maternal undernutrition (Vickers et al. 2001) while adult growth hormone treatment has similar effects

(Vickers et al. 2002). Leptin dynamics also appear to be crucial for determining developmental programming outcomes. Thus, programmed obesity and insulin resistance following maternal protein restriction is prevented by leptin supplementation during pregnancy and lactation (Stocker et al. 2004). Furthermore, neonatal leptin administration from post-natal day 3–13 in the rat normalizes caloric intake, locomotor activity, body weight, fat mass, and fasting plasma glucose, insulin and leptin in the offspring from protein restricted dams (Vickers et al. 2005). The vast majority of these studies however, have focused upon attenuation of adverse programmed metabolic outcomes and thus, the implications for these interventions on programmed changes in behaviour remain uncertain.

Overview

Clearly, an adverse perinatal environment exerts permanent effects on structure, physiology, or metabolism. Data from both animal models and humans advocate that events in early life profoundly impact upon neural development and consequent behaviour in adulthood. One of the key underlying mechanisms to these phenomena is alterations in expression of the GR gene, although the MR and other genes are also implicated. Further studies are required to fully comprehend the mechanisms, however, which will aid in the development of rational interventions for adverse programming outcomes.

References

Agarwal, A.K., Monder, C., Eckstein, B., and White, P.C. (1989). Cloning and expression of rat cDNA encoding corticosteroid 11 beta-dehydrogenase. *J Biol Chem.*, **264**, 18939–18943.

Agarwal, A.K., Rogerson, F.M., Mune, T., and White, P.C. (1995). Analysis of the human gene encoding the kidney isozyme of 11 beta-hydroxysteroid dehydrogenase. *J Steroid Biochem Mol Biol.*, **55**, 473–479.

Akana, S.F. and Dallman, M.F. (1997). Chronic cold in adrenalectomized, corticosterone (B)-treated rats: facilitated corticotropin responses to acute restraint emerge as B increases. *Endocrinology*, **138**, 3249–3258.

Alati, R., Lawlor, D.A., Mamun, A.A. et al. (2007). Is there a fetal origin of depression? Evidence from the Mater University Study of Pregnancy and its outcomes. *Am J Epidemiol.*, **165**, 575–582.

Andrews, M.H., Kostaki, A., Setiawan, E. et al. (2004). Developmental regulation of the 5-HT7 serotonin receptor and transcription factor NGFI-A in the fetal guinea-pig limbic system: influence of GCs. *J Physiol.*, **555**, 659–670.

Anonymous (1995). Effect of corticosteroids for fetal maturation on perinatal outcomes. NIH consensus development panel on the effect of corticosteroids for fetal maturation on perinatal outcomes. *JAMA.*, **273**, 413–418.

Antequera, F. and Bird, A. (1993). Number of CpG islands and genes in human and mouse. *Proc Natl Acad Sci USA*, **90**, 11995–11999.

Archer, J.E. and Blackman, D.E. (1971). Prenatal psychological stress and offspring behavior in rats and mice. *Dev Psychobiol.*, **4**, 193–248.

Barker, D.J., Osmond, C., Golding, J., Kuh, D., and Wadsworth, M.E. (1989a). Growth in utero, blood pressure in childhood and adult life, and mortality from cardiovascular disease. *BMJ*, **298**, 564–567.

Barker, D.J., Winter, P.D., Osmond, C., Margetts, B., and Simmonds, S.J. (1989b). Weight in infancy and death from ischaemic heart disease. *Lancet*, **2**, 577–580.

Barker, D.J.P. (1991). *Fetal and Infant Origins of Adult Disease.* London, BMJ.

Barker, D.J., Hales, C.N., Fall, C.H., Osmond, C., Phipps, K., and Clark, P.M. (1993a). Type 2 (non-insulin-dependent) diabetes mellitus, hypertension and hyperlipidaemia (syndrome X): relation to reduced fetal growth. *Diabetologia.*, **36**, 62–67.

Barker, D.J., Martyn, C.N., Osmond, C., Hales, C.N., and Fall, C.H. (1993b). Growth in utero and serum cholesterol concentrations in adult life. *BMJ*, **307**, 1524–1527.

Barker, D.J., Osmond, C., Simmonds, S.J., and Wield, G.A. (1993c). The relation of small head circumference and thinness at birth to death from cardiovascular disease in adult life. *BMJ*, **306**, 422–426.

Barker, D.J. (2004). The developmental origins of adult disease. *J Am Coll Nutr.*, **23**, 588S–595S.

Bavdekar, A., Yajnik, C.S., Fall, C.H. et al. (1999). Insulin resistance syndrome in 8-year-old Indian children: small at birth, big at 8 years, or both? *Diabetes*, **48**, 2422–2429.

Benediktsson, R., Lindsay, R.S., Noble, J., Seckl, J.R., and Edwards, C.R. (1993). Glucocorticoid exposure in utero: new model for adult hypertension. *Lancet*, **341**, 339–341.

Berkowitz, G.S., Wolff, M.S., Janevic, T.M., Holzman, I.R., Yehuda, R., and Landrigan, P.J. (2003). The World Trade Center disaster and intrauterine growth restriction. *Jama-Journal Of The American Medical Association*, **290**, 595–596.

Bertram, C., Trowern, A.R., Copin, N., Jackson, A.A., and Whorwood, C.B. (2001). The maternal diet during pregnancy programs altered expression of the glucocorticoid receptor and type 2 11beta-hydroxysteroid dehydrogenase: potential molecular mechanisms underlying the programming of hypertension in utero. *Endocrinology*, **142**, 2841–2853.

Bolt, R.J., van Weissenbruch, M.M., Lafeber, H.N., and Delemarre-van de Waal, H.A. (2001). Glucocorticoids and lung development in the fetus and preterm infant. *Pediatr Pulmonol.*, **32**, 76–91.

Boyle, M.P., Kolber, B.J., Vogt, S.K., Wozniak, D.F., and Muglia, L.J. (2006). Forebrain glucocorticoid receptors modulate anxiety-associated locomotor activation and adrenal responsiveness. *J Neurosci.*, **26**, 1971–1978.

Breedlove, S.M. (1992). Sexual dimorphism in the vertebrate nervous system. *J Neurosci.*, **12**, 4133–4142.

Bremner, J.D., Randall, P., Scott, T.M. et al. (1995). MRI-based measurement of hippocampal volume in patients with combat-related posttraumatic stress disorder.[comment]. *American Journal of Psychiatry*, **152**, 973–981.

Brown, R.W., Diaz, R., Robson, A.C. et al. (1996a). The ontogeny of 11 beta-hydroxysteroid dehydrogenase type 2 and mineralocorticoid receptor gene expression reveal intricate control of glucocorticoid action in development. *Endocrinology*, **137**, 794–797.

Burton, P.J. and Waddell, B.J. (1994). 11 β-Hydroxysteroid dehydrogenase in the rat placenta: developmental changes and the effects of altered glucocorticoid exposure. *J Endocrinol.*, **143**, 505–513.

Brown, R.W., Kotolevtsev, Y., Leckie, C. et al. (1996b). Isolation and cloning of human placental 11β-hydroxysteroid dehydrogenase-2 cDNA. *Biochem J.*, **313**, 1007–1017.

Burton, P.J., Smith, R.E., Krozowski, Z.S., and Waddell, B.J. (1996). Zonal distribution of 11 beta-hydroxysteroid dehydrogenase types 1 and 2 messenger ribonucleic acid expression in the rat placenta and decidua during late pregnancy. *Biol Reprod.*, **55**, 1023–1028.

Cannon, M., Jones, P.B., and Murray, R.M. (2002). Obstetric complications and schizophrenia: historical and meta-analytic review. *Am J Psychiatry*, **159**, 1080–1092.

Celsi, G., Kistner, A., Aizman, R. et al. (1998). Prenatal dexamethasone causes oligonephronia, sodium retention, and higher blood pressure in the offspring. *Pediatr Res.*, **44**, 317–322.

Clark, P.M., Hindmarsh, P.C., Shiell, A.W., Law, C.M., Honour, J.W., and Barker, D.J.P. (1996). Size at birth and adrenocortical function in childhood. *Clinical Endocrinology*, **45**, 721–726.

Cleasby, M.E., Kelly, P.A.T., Walker, B.R., and Seckl, J.R. (2003). Programming of rat muscle and fat metabolism by in utero overexposure to glucocorticoids. *Endocrinology*, **144**, 999–1007.

Costello, E.J., Worthman, C., Erkanli, A., and Angold, A. (2007). Prediction from low birth weight to female adolescent depression: a test of competing hypotheses. *Arch Gen Psychiatry.*, **64**, 338–344.

Cratty, M.S., Ward, H.E., Johnson, E.A., Azzaro, A.J., and Birkle, D.L. (1995). Prenatal stress increases corticotropin-releasing factor (Crf) content and release in rat amygdala minces. *Brain Research*, **675**, 297–302.

Dallman, M.F., Warne, J.P., Foster, M.T., and Pecoraro, N.C. (2007). Glucocorticoids and insulin both modulate caloric intake through actions on the brain. *J Physiol.*, **583**, 431–436.

de Kloet, E.R. (1997). Why dexamethasone poorly penetrates in brain. *Stress*, **2**, 1320.

de Kloet, E.R., Joels, M., and Holsboer, F. (2005). Stress and the brain: from adaptation to disease. *Nat Rev Neurosci.*, **6**, 463–475.

de Rooij, S.R., Painter, R.C., Phillips, D.I. et al. (2006). Hypothalamic-pituitary-adrenal axis activity in adults who were prenatally exposed to the Dutch famine. *Eur J Endocrinol.*, **155**, 153–160.

de Vries, A., Holmes, M., Heijnis, A. et al. (2007). Prenatal dexamethasone exposure induces changes in offspring cardio-metabolic and hypothalamic–pituitary-adrenal axis function without alteration of birth weight in a non-human primate, the African vervet, Chlorocebus aethiops. *J Clin Invest.*, **117**, 1058–1067.

Diaz, R., Brown, R.W., and Seckl, J.R. (1998). Distinct ontogeny of glucocorticoid and mineralocorticoid receptor and 11beta-hydroxysteroid dehydrogenase types I and II mRNAs in the fetal rat brain suggest a complex control of glucocorticoid actions. *J Neurosci.*, **18**, 2570–2580.

Dodic, M., May, C.N., Wintour, E.M., and Coghlan, J.P. (1998). An early prenatal exposure to excess glucocorticoid leads to hypertensive offspring in sheep. *Clin Sci.*, **94**, 149–155.

Dodic, M., Peers, A., Coghlan, J. et al. (1999). Altered cardiovascular haemodynamics and baroreceptor-heart rate reflex in adult sheep after prenatal exposure to dexamethasone. *Clin Sci.*, **97**, 103–109.

Dodic, M., Hantzis, V., Duncan, J. et al. (2002a). Programming effects of short prenatal exposure to cortisol. *Faseb Journal.*, **16**, 1017–1026.

Dodic, M., Moritz, K., Koukoulas, I., and Wintour, E.M. (2002b). Programmed hypertension: kidney, brain or both? *Trends in Endocrinology and Metabolism*, **13**, 403–408.

Doyle, L.W., Ford, G.W., Davis, N.M., and Callanan, C. (2000). Antenatal corticosteroid therapy and blood pressure at 14 years of age in preterm children. *Clin Sci.*, **98**, 137–142.

Drake, A.J., Walker, B.R., and Seckl, J.R. (2005). Intergenerational consequences of fetal programming by in utero exposure to glucocorticoids in rats. *Am J Physiol Regulatory Integrative Comp Physiol.*, **288**, R34–R38.

Edwards, C.R., Benediktsson, R., Lindsay, R.S., and Seckl, J.R. (1993). Dysfunction of placental glucocorticoid barrier: link between fetal environment and adult hypertension? *Lancet*, **341**, 355–357.

Engel, S.M., Berkowitz, G.S., Wolff, M.S., and Yehuda, R. (2005). Psychological trauma associated with the World Trade Center attacks and its effect on pregnancy outcome. *Paediatric And Perinatal Epidemiology*, **19**, 334–341.

Erdeljan, P., MacDonald, J.F., and Matthews, S.G. (2001). Glucocorticoids and serotonin alter glucocorticoid receptor (GR) but not mineralocorticoid receptor (MR) mRNA levels in fetal mouse hippocampal neurons, in vitro. *Brain Res.*, **896**, 130–136.

Famularo, R. and Fenton, T. (1994). Early developmental history and pediatric posttraumatic stress disorder. *Arch Pediatr Adolesc Med.*, **148**, 1032–1038.

Forsen, T., Eriksson, J.G., Tuomilehto, J., Teramo, K., Osmond, C., and Barker, D.J.P. (1997). Mother's weight in pregnancy and coronary heart disease in a cohort of Finnish men: follow up study. *British Medical Journal*, **315**, 837–840.

French, N.P., Hagan, R., Evans, S.F., Godfrey, M., and Newnham, J.P. (1999). Repeated antenatal corticosteroids: size at birth and subsequent development. *American Journal of Obstetrics & Gynecology*, **180**, 114–121.

Fride, E., Dan, Y., Feldon, J., Halevy, G., and Weinstock, M. (1986). Effects of prenatal stress on vulnerability to stress in prepubertal and adult rats. *Physiol Behav.*, **37**, 681–687.

Fride, E. and Weinstock, M. (1988). Prenatal stress increases anxiety related behavior and alters cerebral lateralization of dopamine activity. *Life Sci*, **42**, 1059–1065.

Fumagalli, F., Jones, S.R., Caron, M.G., Seidler, F.J., and Slotkin, T.A. (1996). Expression of mRNA coding for the serotonin transporter in aged vs. young rat brain: differential effects of glucocorticoids. *Brain Res.*, **719**, 225–228.

Funder, J.W. (1997). Glucocorticoid and mineralocorticoid receptors: biology and clinical relevance. *Annu Rev Med.*, **48**, 231–240.

Fuxe, K., Wikstrom, A.C., Okret, S. et al. (1985). Mapping of glucocorticoid receptor immunoreactive neurons in the rat tel- and diencephalon using a monoclonal antibody against rat liver glucocorticoid receptor. *Endocrinology.*, **117**, 1803–1812.

Galler, J.R., Ramsey, F., Solimano, G., and Lowell, W.E. (1983a). The influence of early malnutrition on subsequent behavioral development. II. Classroom behavior. *J Am Acad Child Psychiatry*, **22**, 16–22.

Galler, J.R., Ramsey, F., Solimano, G., Lowell, W.E., and Mason, E. (1983b). The influence of early malnutrition on subsequent behavioral development. I. Degree of impairment in intellectual performance. *J Am Acad Child Psychiatry*, **22**, 815.

Galler, J.R. and Ramsey, F. (1989). A follow-up study of the influence of early malnutrition on development: behavior at home and at school. *J Am Acad Child Adolesc Psychiatry*, **28**, 254–261.

Gatford, K.L., Wintour, E.M., de Blasio, M.J., Owens, J.A., and Dodic, M. (2000). Differential timing for programming of glucose homoeostasis, sensitivity to insulin and blood pressure by in utero exposure to dexamethasone in sheep. *Clin Sci.*, **98**, 553–560.

Grizenko, N., Shayan, Y.R., Polotskaia, A., Ter-Stepanian, M., and Joober, R. (2008). Relation of maternal stress during pregnancy to symptom severity and response to treatment in children with ADHD. *J Psychiatry Neurosci*, **33**, 10–16.

Grunstein, M. (1997). Histone acetylation in chromatin structure and transcription. *Nature*, **389**, 349–352.

Guzman, C., Cabrera, R., Cardenas, M., Larrea, F., Nathanielsz, P.W., and Zambrano, E. (2006). Protein restriction during fetal and neonatal development in the rat alters reproductive function and accelerates reproductive ageing in female progeny. *J Physiol.*, **572**, 97–108.

Hales, C.N., Barker, D.J., Clark, P.M. et al. (1991). Fetal and infant growth and impaired glucose tolerance at age 64. *British Medical Journal*, **303**, 1019–1022.

Hirvikoski, T., Nordenstrom, A., Lindholm, T. et al. (2007). Cognitive functions in children at risk for congenital adrenal hyperplasia treated prenatally with dexamethasone. *J Clin Endocrinol Metab.*, **92**, 542–548.

Hollenberg, S.M., Weinberger, C., Ong, E.S. et al. (1985). Primary structure and expression of a functional human glucocorticoid receptor cDNA. *Nature*, **318**, 635–641.

Holmes, M.C., Abrahamsen, C.T., French, K.L., Paterson, J.M., Mullins, J.J., and Seckl, J.R. (2006a). The mother or the fetus? 11beta-hydroxysteroid dehydrogenase type 2 null mice provide evidence for direct fetal programming of behavior by endogenous glucocorticoids. *J Neurosci.*, **26**, 3840–3844.

Holmes, M.C., Sangra, M., French, K.L. et al. (2006b). 11beta-Hydroxysteroid dehydrogenase type 2 protects the neonatal cerebellum from deleterious effects of glucocorticoids. *Neuroscience*, **137**, 865–873.

Hsu, D., Chen, F., Takahashi, L., and Kalin, N. (1998). Rapid stress-induced elevations in corticotropin-releasing hormone mRNA in rat central amygdala nucleus and hypothalamic paraventricular nucleus: an in situ hybridization analysis. *Brain Res.*, **788**, 305–310.

Huang, W.L., Beazley, L.D., Quinlivan, J.A., Evans, S.F., Newnham, J.P., and Dunlop, S.A. (1999). Effect of corticosteroids on brain growth in fetal sheep. *Obstetrics and Gynecology*, **94**, 213–218.

Huang, W.L., Harper, C.G., Evans, S.F., Newnham, J.P., and Dunlop, S.A. (2001a). Repeated prenatal corticosteroid administration delays astrocyte and capillary tight junction maturation in fetal sheep. *International Journal of Developmental Neuroscience*, **19**, 487–493.

Huang, W.L., Harper, C.G., Evans, S.F., Newnham, J.P., and Dunlop, S.A. (2001b). Repeated prenatal corticosteroid administration delays myelination of the corpus callosum in fetal sheep. *International Journal of Developmental Neuroscience*, **19**, 415–425.

Hultman, C.M., Sparen, P., Takei, N., Murray, R.M., and Cnattingius, S. (1999). Prenatal and perinatal risk factors for schizophrenia, affective psychosis, and reactive psychosis of early onset: case-control study. *Brit Med J.*, **318**, 421–426.

Huttunen, M.O. and Niskanen, P. (1978). Prenatal loss of father and psychiatric disorders. *Arch Gen Psychiatry*, **35**, 429–431.

Imamura, Y., Nakane, Y., Ohta, Y., and Kondo, H. (1999). Lifetime prevalence of schizophrenia among individuals prenatally exposed to atomic bomb radiation in Nagasaki City. *Acta Psychiatr Scand.*, **100**, 344–349.

Jensen, E.C., Gallaher, B.W., Breier, B.H., and Harding, J.E. (2002). The effect of a chronic maternal cortisol infusion on the late-gestation fetal sheep. *Journal of Endocrinology*, **174**, 27–36.

Jones, P.B., Rantakallio, P., Hartikainen, A.L., Isohanni, M., and Sipila, P. (1998). Schizophrenia as a long-term outcome of pregnancy, delivery, and perinatal complications: a 28-year follow-up of the 1966 north Finland general population birth cohort. *Am J Psychiatry*, **155**, 355–364.

Karst, H., Berger, S., Turiault, M., Tronche, F., Schutz, G., and Joels, M. (2005). Mineralocorticoid receptors are indispensable for nongenomic modulation of hippocampal glutamate transmission by corticosterone. *Proc Natl Acad Sci USA*, **102**, 19204–19207.

Kitraki, E., Kittas, C., and Stylianopoulou, F. (1997). Glucocorticoid receptor gene expression during rat embryogenesis. An in situ hybridization study. *Differentiation*, **62**, 21–31.

Koenig, J.I., Kirkpatrick, B., and Lee, P. (2002). Glucocorticoid hormones and early brain development in schizophrenia. *Neuropsychopharmacology*, **27**, 309–318.

Korte, S.M. (2001). Corticosteroids in relation to fear, anxiety and psychopathology. *Neuroscience and Biobehavioral Reviews*, **25**, 117–142.

Lai, M., Horsburgh, K., Bae, S.E. et al. (2007). Forebrain mineralocorticoid receptor overexpression enhances memory, reduces anxiety and attenuates neuronal loss in cerebral ischaemia. *Eur J Neurosci.*, **25**, 1832–1842.

Langley, S.C. and Jackson, A.A. (1994). Increased systolic blood pressure in adult rats induced by fetal exposure to maternal low protein diets. *Clin Sci (Lond).*, **86**, 217–222; discussion 121.

Langley-Evans, S.C. (1997). Hypertension induced by foetal exposure to a maternal low-protein diet, in the rat, is prevented by pharmacological blockade of maternal glucocorticoid synthesis. *Journal of Hypertension*, **15**, 537–544.

Langley-Evans, S.C., Gardner, D.S., and Jackson, A.A. (1996a). Maternal protein restriction influences the programming of the rat hypothalamic-pituitary-adrenal axis. *J Nutr.*, **126**, 1578–1585.

Langley-Evans, S.C., Phillips, G.J., Benediktsson, R. et al. (1996b). Protein intake in pregnancy, placental glucocorticoid metabolism and the programming of hypertension in the rat. *Placenta*, **17**, 169–172.

Law, C.M., Shiell, A.W., Newsome, C.A. et al. (2002). Fetal, infant, and childhood growth and adult blood pressure: a longitudinal study from birth to 22 years of age. *Circulation*, **105**, 1088–1092.

Leckman, J.F., Dolnansky, E.S., Hardin, M.T. et al. (1990). Perinatal factors in the expression of Tourette's syndrome: an exploratory study. *J Am Acad Child Adolesc Psychiatry*, **29**, 220–226.

Leon, D.A., Koupilova, I., Lithell, H.O. et al. (1996). Failure to realise growth potential in utero and adult obesity in relation to blood pressure in 50 year old Swedish men. *British Medical Journal*, **312**, 401–406.

Lesage, J., Blondeau, B., Grino, M., Breant, B., and Dupouy, J.P. (2001). Maternal undernutrition during late gestation induces fetal overexposure to glucocorticoids and intrauterine growth retardation, and disturbs the hypothalamo-pituitary adrenal axis in the newborn rat. *Endocrinology*, **142**, 1692–1702.

Levine, R.S., Hennekens, C.H., and Jesse, M.J. (1994). Blood pressure in prospective population based cohort of newborn and infant twins. *British Medical Journal*, **308**, 298–302.

Levitt, N., Lindsay, R.S., Holmes, M.C., and Seckl, J.R. (1996a). Dexamethasone in the last week of pregnancy attenuates hippocampal glucocorticoid receptor gene expression and elevates blood pressure in the adult offspring in the rat. *Neuroendocrinology*, **64**, 412–418.

Levitt, N.S., Lindsay, R.S., Holmes, M.C., and Seckl, J.R. (1996b). Dexamethasone in the last week of pregnancy attenuates hippocampal glucocorticoid receptor gene expression and elevates blood pressure in the adult offspring in the rat. *Neuroendocrinology*, **64**, 412–418.

Levitt, N.S., Lambert, E.V., Woods, D., Hales, C.N., Andrew, R., and Seckl, J.R. (2000). Impaired glucose tolerance and elevated blood pressure in low birth weight, non-obese young South African adults: early programming of the cortisol axis. *J Clin Endocrinol Metab.*, **85**, 4611–4618.

Lillycrop, K.A., Phillips, E.S., Jackson, A.A., Hanson, M.A., and Burdge, G.C. (2005). Dietary protein restriction of pregnant rats induces and folic acid supplementation prevents epigenetic modification of hepatic gene expression in the offspring. *J Nutr.*, **135**, 1382–1386.

Lindsay, R.S., Lindsay, R.M., Edwards, C.R., and Seckl, J.R. (1996a). Inhibition of 11-beta-hydroxysteroid dehydrogenase in pregnant rats and the programming of blood pressure in the offspring. *Hypertension*, **27**, 1200–1204.

Lindsay, R.S., Lindsay, R.M., Edwards, C.R.W., and Seckl, J.R. (1996b). Inhibition of 11ß-hydroxysteroid dehydrogenase in pregnant rats and the programming of blood pressure in the offspring. *Hypertension*, **27**, 1200–1204.

Linnet, K.M., Dalsgaard, S., Obel, C. et al. (2003). Maternal lifestyle factors in pregnancy risk of attention deficit hyperactivity disorder and associated behaviors: review of the current evidence. *Am J Psychiatry*, **160**, 1028–1040.

MacArthur, B.A., Howie, R.N., Dezoete, J.A., and Elkins, J. (1982). School progress and cognitive development of 6-year-old children whose mothers were treated antenatally with betamethasone. *Pediatrics*, **70**, 99–105.

Maccari, S. and Morley-Fletcher, S. (2007). Effects of prenatal restraint stress on the hypothalamus-pituitary-adrenal axis and related behavioural and neurobiological alterations. *Psychoneuroendocrinology*, **32** Suppl 1, S10–15.

Mairesse, J., Viltart, O., Salome, N. et al. (2007). Prenatal stress alters the negative correlation between neuronal activation in limbic regions and behavioral responses in rats exposed to high and low anxiogenic environments. *Psychoneuroendocrinology*, **32**, 765–776.

Mandyam, C.D., Crawford, E.F., Eisch, A.J., Rivier, C.L., and Richardson, H.N. (2008). Stress experienced in utero reduces sexual dichotomies in neurogenesis, microenvironment, and cell death in the adult rat hippocampus. *Dev Neurobiol.*, **68**, 575–589.

McCormick, J., Lyons, V., Jacobson, M. et al. (2000). 5'-heterogeneity of glucocorticoid receptor mRNA is tissue-specific; differential regulation of variant promoters by early life events. *Molec Endocrinol.*, **14**, 506–517.

Meaney, M.J., Diorio, J., Francis, D. et al. (2000). Postnatal handling increases the expression of cAMP-inducible transcription factors in the rat hippocampus: the effects of thyroid hormones and serotonin. *J Neurosci.*, **20**, 3926–3935.

Meaney, M.J., Diorio, J., Francis, D. et al. (1996). Early environmental regulation of forebrain glucocorticoid receptor gene expression: implications for adrenocortical responses to stress. *Developmental Neuroscience*, **18**, 49–72.

Meijer, A. (1985). Child psychiatric sequelae of maternal war stress. *Acta Psychiatr Scand.*, **72**, 505–511.

Meyer, J.S. (1983). Early adrenalectomy stimulates subsequent growth and development of the rat brain. *Exp Neurol.*, **82**, 432–446.

Meyer-Bahlburg, H.F., Dolezal, C., Baker, S.W., Carlson, A.D., Obeid, J.S., and New, M.I. (2004). Cognitive and motor development of children with and without congenital adrenal hyperplasia after early-prenatal dexamethasone. *J Clin Endocrinol Metab.*, **89**, 610–614.

Minde, K., Webb, G., and Sykes, D. (1968). Studies on the hyperactive child. VI. Prenatal and paranatal factors associated with hyperactivity. *Dev Med Child Neurol.*, **10**, 355–363.

Morgan, H.D., Santos, F., Green, K., Dean, W., and Reik, W. (2005). Epigenetic reprogramming in mammals. *Hum Mol Genet.*, 14 Spec No 1, R47–58.

Muneoka, K., Mikuni, M., Ogawa, T. et al. (1997). Prenatal dexamethasone exposure alters brain monoamine metabolism and adrenocortical response in rat offspring. *Am J Physiol*, **273**, R1669–1675.

Murphy, V.E., Zakar, T., Smith, R., Giles, W.B., Gibson, P.G., and Clifton, V.L. (2002). Reduced 11beta-hydroxysteroid dehydrogenase type 2 activity is associated with decreased birth weight centile in pregnancies complicated by asthma. *J Clin Endocrinol Metab.*, **87**, 1660–1668.

Nagano, M., Ozawa, H., and Suzuki, H. (2008). Prenatal dexamethasone exposure affects anxiety-like behaviour and neuroendocrine systems in an age-dependent manner. *Neurosci Res.*, **60**, 364–371.

Nyirenda, M.J., Lindsay, R.S., Kenyon, C.J., Burchell, A., and Seckl, J.R. (1998). Glucocorticoid exposure in late gestation permanently programs rat hepatic phosphoenolpyruvate carboxykinase and glucocorticoid receptor expression and causes glucose intolerance in adult offspring. *J Clin Invest.*, **101**, 2174–2181.

O'Connor, T.G., Heron, J., Golding, J., and Glover, V. (2003). Maternal antenatal anxiety and behavioural/emotional problems in children: a test of a programming hypothesis. *J Child Psychol Psychiatry.*, **44**, 1025–1036.

O'Regan, D., Kenyon, C.J., Seckl, J.R., and Holmes, M.C. (2004). Glucocorticoid exposure in late gestation in the rat permanently programs gender-specific differences in adult cardiovascular and metabolic physiology. *Am J Physiol Endocrinol Metab.*, **287**, E863–70.

Osmond, C., Barker, D.J.P., Winter, P.D., Fall, C.H.D., and Simmonds, S.J. (1993). Early growth and death from cardiovascular disease in women. *British Medical Journal*, **307**, 1524–1527.

Pardon, M.C. and Rattray, I. (2008). What do we know about the long-term consequences of stress on ageing and the progression of age-related neurodegenerative disorders? *Neurosci Biobehav Rev.*

Perlman, W.R., Webster, M.J., Kleinman, J.E., and Weickert, C.S. (2004). Reduced glucocorticoid and estrogen receptor alpha messenger ribonucleic acid levels in the amygdala of patients with major mental illness. *Biol Psychiatry*, **56**, 844–852.

Phillips, D.I., Fall, C.H.D., Whorwood, C.B. et al. (1998). Elevated plasma cortisol concentrations: an explanation for the relationship between low birthweight and adult cardiovascular risk factors. *J Clin Endocrinol Metab.*, **83**, 757–760.

Phillips, D.I.W., Walker, B.R., Reynolds, R.M. et al. (2000). Low birth weight predicts elevated plasma cortisol concentrations in adults from 3 populations. *Hypertension*, **35**, 1301-1306.

Plotsky, P.M., Thrivikraman, K.V., and Meaney, M.J. (1993). Central and feedback regulation of hypothalamic corticotropin-releasing factor secretion. *Ciba Found Symp.*, **172**, 59–75; discussion 75–84.

Reynolds, R.M., Walker, B.R., Syddall, H.E. et al. (2001). Altered control of cortisol secretion in adult men with low birth weight and cardiovascular risk factors. *J Clin Endocrinol Metab.*, **86**, 245–250.

Reynolds, R.M., Walker, B.R., Syddall, H.E., Andrew, R., Wood, P.J., and Phillips, D.I. (2005). Is there a gender difference in the associations of birthweight and adult hypothalamic-pituitary-adrenal axis activity? *Eur J Endocrinol.*, **152**, 249–253.

Robson, A.C., Leckie, C.M., Seckl, J.R., and Holmes, M.C. (1998). 11 Beta-hydroxysteroid dehydrogenase type 2 in the postnatal and adult rat brain. *Brain Res Mol Brain Res.*, **61**, 1–10.

Schneider, M.L., Moore, C.F., Gajewski, L.L. et al. (2008). Sensory processing disorder in a primate model: evidence from a longitudinal study of prenatal alcohol and prenatal stress effects. *Child Dev.*, **79**, 100–113.

Seckl, J.R. and Walker, B.R. (2001). Minireview: 11beta-hydroxysteroid dehydrogenase type 1-a tissue-specific amplifier of glucocorticoid action. *Endocrinology*, **142**, 1371–1376.

Seckl, J.R. and Holmes, M.C. (2007). Mechanisms of disease: glucocorticoids, their placental metabolism and fetal 'programming' of adult pathophysiology. *Nat Clin Pract Endocrinol Metab.*, **3**, 479–488.

Seckl, J.R. (2008). Glucocorticoids, developmental 'programming' and the risk of affective dysfunction. *Prog Brain Res.*, **167**, 17–4.

Shams, M., Kilby, M.D., Somerset, D.A. et al. (1998). 11Beta-hydroxysteroid dehydrogenase type 2 in human pregnancy and reduced expression in intrauterine growth restriction. *Hum Reprod.*, **13**, 799–804.

Sheline, Y.I., Wang, P.W., Gado, M.H., Csernansky, J.G., and Vannier, M.W. (1996). Hippocampal atrophy in recurrent major depression. *Proceedings of the National Academy of Sciences of the United States of America*, **93**, 3908–3913.

Sloboda, D.M., Moss, T.J., Gurrin, L.C., Newnham, J.P., and Challis, J.R. (2002). The effect of prenatal betamethasone administration on postnatal ovine hypothalamic-pituitary-adrenal function. *J Endocrinol.*, **172**, 71–81.

Sloboda, D.M., Challis, J.R., Moss, T.J., and Newnham, J.P. (2005). Synthetic glucocorticoids: antenatal administration and long-term implications. *Curr Pharm Des.*, **11**, 1459–1472.

Slotkin, T.A., Barnes, G.A., McCook, E.C., and Seidler, F.J. (1996). Programming of brainstem serotonin transporter development by prenatal glucocorticoids. *Brain Res Dev Brain Res*, **93**, 155–161.

Smith, J.T. and Waddell, B.J. (2000). Increased fetal glucocorticoid exposure delays puberty onset in postnatal life. *Endocrinology.*, **141**, 2422–2428.

St Clair, D., Xu, M.Q., Wang, P. et al. (2005). Rates of adult schizophrenia following prenatal exposure to the Chinese famine of 1959-1961. *Jama-Journal Of The American Medical Association*, **294**, 557–562.

Stein, M.B., Koverola, C., Hanna, C., Torchia, M.G., and McClarty, B. (1997). Hippocampal volume in women victimized by childhood sexual abuse. *Psychological Medicine*, **27**, 951–959.

Stewart, P.M., Murry, B.A., and Mason, J.I. (1994). Type 2 11 beta-hydroxysteroid dehydrogenase in human fetal tissues. *J Clin Endocrinol Metab.*, **78**, 1529–1532.

Stewart, P.M., Rogerson, F.M., and Mason, J.I. (1995a). Type 2 11 beta-hydroxysteroid dehydrogenase messenger ribonucleic acid and activity in human placenta and fetal membranes: its relationship to birth weight and putative role in fetal adrenal steroidogenesis. *J Clin Endocrinol Metab.*, **80**, 885–890.

Stewart, P.M., Whorwood, C.B., and Mason, J.I. (1995b). Type 2 11 beta-hydroxysteroid dehydrogenase in foetal and adult life. *J Steroid Biochem Mol Biol.*, **55**, 465–471.

Stocker, C., O'Dowd, J., Morton, N.M. et al. (2004). Modulation of susceptibility to weight gain and insulin resistance in low birthweight rats by treatment of their mothers with leptin during pregnancy and lactation. *Int J Obes Relat Metab Disord.*, **28**, 129–136.

Strahle, U., Schmidt, A., Kelsey, G. et al. (1992). At least three promoters direct expression of the mouse glucocorticoid receptor gene. *Proc Natl Acad Sci USA*, **89**, 6731–6735.

Sugden, M.C., Langdown, M.L., Munns, M.J., and Holness, M.J. (2001). Maternal glucocorticoid treatment modulates placental leptin and leptin receptor expression and materno-fetal leptin physiology during late pregnancy, and elicits hypertension associated with hyperleptinaemia in the early-growth-retarded adult offspring. *European Journal of Endocrinology*, **145**, 529–539.

Susser, E.S. and Lin, S.P. (1992). Schizophrenia after prenatal exposure to the Dutch Hunger Winter of 1944-1945. *Archives of General Psychiatry*, **49**, 983–988.

Susser, E., Neugebauer, R., Hoek, H.W. et al. (1996). Schizophrenia after prenatal famine. *Arch Gen Psychiat.*, **53**, 25–31.

Thomassin, H., Flavin, M., Espinas, M., and Grange, T. (2001). Glucocorticoid-induced DNA demethylation and gene memory during development. *Embo J.*, **20**, 1974–1983.

Thompson, W.R. (1957). Influence of prenatal maternal anxiety on emotionality in young rats. *Science*, **125**, 698–699.

Thompson, C., Syddall, H., Rodin, I., Osmond, C., and Barker, D.J. (2001). Birth weight and the risk of depressive disorder in late life. *Br J Psychiatry*, **179**, 450–455.

Trautman, P.D., Meyer-Bahlburg, H.F.L., Postelnek, J., and New, M.I. (1995). Effects of early prenatal dexamethasone on the cognitive and behavioral development of young children: results of a pilot study. *Psychoneuroendocrinology*, **20**, 439–449.

Tronche, F., Kellendonk, C., Kretz, O. et al. (1999). Disruption of the glucocorticoid receptor gene in the nervous system results in reduced anxiety. *Nature Genetics*, **23**, 99–103.

Uno, H., Lohmiller, L., Thieme, C. et al. (1990). Brain damage induced by prenatal exposure to dexamethasone in fetal rhesus macaques. I. hippocampus. *Developmental Brain Res.*, **53**, 157–167.

Uno, H., Eisele, S., Sakai, A. et al. (1994). Neurotoxicity of glucocorticoids in the primate brain. *Hormones and Behavior*, **28**, 336–348.

Vickers, M.H., Ikenasio, B.A., and Breier, B.H. (2001). IGF-I treatment reduces hyperphagia, obesity, and hypertension in metabolic disorders induced by fetal programming. *Endocrinology*, **142**, 3964–3973.

Vickers, M.H., Ikenasio, B.A., and Breier, B.H. (2002). Adult growth hormone treatment reduces hypertension and obesity induced by an adverse prenatal environment. *J Endocrinol.*, **175**, 615–623.

Vickers, M.H., Gluckman, P.D., Coveny, A.H. et al. (2005). Neonatal leptin treatment reverses developmental programming. *Endocrinology*, **146**, 4211–4216.

Viltart, O., Mairesse, J., Darnaudery, M. et al. (2006). Prenatal stress alters Fos protein expression in hippocampus and locus coeruleus stress-related brain structures. *Psychoneuroendocrinology*, **31**, 769–780.

Waddell, B., Benediktsson, R., Brown, R., and Seckl, J.R. (1998). Tissue-specific mRNA expression of 11β-hydroxysteroid dehydrogenase types 1 and 2 and the glucocorticoid receptor within rat placenta suggest exquisite local control of glucocorticoid action. *Endocrinology*, **139**, 1517–1523.

Waddell, B.J. and Atkinson, H.C. (1994). Production rate, metabolic clearance rate and uterine extraction of corticosterone during rat pregnancy. *Journal of Endocrinology*, **143**, 183–190.

Waddington, C.H. (1940). *Organisers and Genes*. Cambridge University Press.

Watson, J.B., Mednick, S.A., Huttunen, M., and Wang, X. (1999). Prenatal teratogens and the development of adult mental illness. *Dev Psychopathol.*, **11**, 457–466.

Weaver, I., Cervoni, N., Champagne, F. et al. (2004). Epigenetic programming by maternal behavior. *Nature Neurosci.*, **7**, 847–854.

Weaver, I.C., Champagne, F.A., Brown, S.E. et al. (2005). Reversal of maternal programming of stress responses in adult offspring through methyl supplementation: altering epigenetic marking later in life. *J Neurosci.*, **25**, 11045–11054.

Weaver, I.C., D'Alessio, A.C., Brown, S.E. et al. (2007). The transcription factor nerve growth factor-inducible protein a mediates epigenetic programming: altering epigenetic marks by immediate-early genes. *J Neurosci.*, **27**, 1756–1768.

Webster, M.J., Knable, M.B., O'Grady, J., Orthmann, J., and Weickert, C.S. (2002). Regional specificity of brain glucocorticoid receptor mRNA alterations in subjects with schizophrenia and mood disorders. *Mol Psychiatry*, **7**, 985–994, 924.

Weinstock, M. (2001). Alterations induced by gestational stress in brain morphology and behaviour of the offspring. *Prog Neurobiol.*, **65**, 427–451.

Weinstock, M. (2005). The potential influence of maternal stress hormones on development and mental health of the offspring. *Brain Behav Immun.*, **19**, 296–308.

Weismann, A. (1892). *Das Keimplasma. Eine Theorie der Vererbung,* Jena, Germany, Fischer.

Welberg, L.A., Seckl, J.R., and Holmes, M.C. (2000). Inhibition of 11beta-hydroxysteroid dehydrogenase, the foeto-placental barrier to maternal glucocorticoids, permanently programs amygdala GR mRNA expression and anxiety-like behaviour in the offspring. *Eur J Neurosci.*, **12**, 1047–1054.

Welberg, L.A., Seckl, J.R., and Holmes, M.C. (2001). Prenatal glucocorticoid programming of brain corticosteroid receptors and corticotrophin-releasing hormone: possible implications for behaviour. *Neuroscience.*, **104**, 71–79.

Wiles, N.J., Peters, T.J., Leon, D.A., and Lewis, G. (2005). Birth weight and psychological distress at age 45–51 years: results from the Aberdeen Children of the 1950s cohort study. *Br J Psychiatry*, **187**, 21–28.

Winick, M. (1971). Cellular growth during early malnutrition. *Pediatrics*, **47**, 969–978.

Woodall, S.M., Johnston, B.M., Breier, B.H., and Gluckman, P.D. (1996). Chronic maternal undernutrition in the rat leads to delayed postnatal growth and elevated blood pressure of offspring. *Pediatr Res.*, **40**, 438–443.

Woods, L.L. and Weeks, D.A. (2005). Prenatal programming of adult blood pressure: role of maternal corticosteroids. *Am J Physiol Regul Integr Comp Physiol.*, **289**, R955–962.

Wyrwoll, C.S., Mark, P.J., Mori, T.A., Puddey, I.B., and Waddell, B.J. (2006). Prevention of programmed hyperleptinemia and hypertension by postnatal dietary omega-3 fatty acids. *Endocrinology*, **147**, 599–606.

Wyrwoll, C.S., Mark, P.J., and Waddell, B.J. (2007). Developmental programming of renal glucocorticoid sensitivity and the renin-angiotensin system. *Hypertension*, **50**, 579–584.

Yeh, T., Lin, Y., Lin, H. et al. (2004). Outcomes at School Age after Postnatal Dexamethasone Therapy for Lung Disease of Prematurity. *New Engl J Med.*, **350**, 1304–1313.

Yehuda, R. (2002). Current concepts – Post-traumatic stress disorder. *New England Journal Of Medicine*, **346**, 108–114.

Yehuda, R., Golier, J.A., Yang, R.K., and Tischler, L. (2004). Enhanced sensitivity to glucocorticoids in peripheral mononuclear leukocytes in posttraumatic stress disorder. *Biological Psychiatry*, **55**, 1110–1116.

Yehuda, R., Engel, S.M., Brand, S.R., Seckl, J., Marcus, S.M., and Berkowitz, G.S. (2005). Transgenerational effects of posttraumatic stress disorder in babies of mothers exposed to the world trade center attacks during pregnancy. *Journal of Clinical Endocrinology and Metabolism*, **90**, 4115–4118.

Yehuda, R., Teicher, M.H., Seckl, J.R., Grossman, R.A., Morris, A., and Bierer, L.M. (2007). Parental posttraumatic stress disorder as a vulnerability factor for low cortisol trait in offspring of holocaust survivors. *Arch Gen Psychiatry*, **64**, 1040–1048.

Chapter 9

Modelling depression by GR mutant animals?

Sabine Chourbaji and Peter Gass

Background

Mutant mice represent important tools for the investigation of pathogenetic and therapeutic aspects of specific diseases. Taking into consideration the continuous progress in gene targeting, the focus on specific candidate genes, which may be manipulated and thereby analysed in various ways, became a promising scientific approach. Since not only the availability of such a target gene itself, but also the quality and quantity regarding temporal and region-specific expression represents a central aspect, it is important to consider, apply, and combine such facets by the use of respective techniques. With regard to depression the glucocorticoid receptor (GR) is thought to be a crucial factor, and animals carrying mutations of this receptor show alterations in the hypothalamic-pituitary-adrenal (HPA) system, which are comparable to morbid changes observed in depressed patients. Moreover, similarities that may model the human disease have been described in these mice on the behavioural and neurochemical level, which enhances the impact for clinical questions, such as the investigation of the effectiveness of GR antagonists or comparable medical approaches. The book chapter on hand summarizes different transgenic approaches used to alter or eliminate GR expression and function, and discusses the relevance of such mutants as models for depression in general or distinct aspects, respectively. This is the third of five chapters in this book that presents not only clinical data but also experimental evidence from animal models relevant to the role of the HPA in affective disorders, together with Chapters 7, 8, 11, and 26.

The relevance of the GR in depression

The HPA system controls the production, release, and feedback of the major stress hormone secreted by the adrenal gland, that is, cortisol in humans and corticosterone in rodents, which is effective by two types of intracellular corticosteroid receptors, revealing high genetic homology between many species: (i) the high-affinity mineralocorticoid receptor (MR); and (ii) the low-affinity glucocorticoid receptor (GR) (Beato et al. 1995; de Kloet et al. 1998). Both receptors are ligand-activated transcription factors that reside in the cytoplasm, dimerize upon ligand binding and translocate to the nucleus, where they exert transcriptional control in a positive or negative way. GR and MR belong to the same nuclear hormone receptor superfamily (Beato et al. 1995; Tronche et al. 1998) and modulate a variety of neural functions including stress responsiveness and cognition (de Kloet et al. 1998; Holsboer, 2000; Reul et al. 2000). With their different affinity for corticosterone they are differentially activated during the circadian rhythm and periods of stress: while the MR is thought to be responsible for the regulation of circadian glucocorticoid variations, the GR has been postulated to be involved in the modulation of stress effects (e.g. high levels of glucocorticoids during depression) (Holsboer, 2000). Nonetheless, one of the most important factors for the maintenance of homeostasis and to keep the allostatic load in balance is a stable MR/GR system. Current concepts suggest the GR as a potential pharmacological target for a new class of antidepressants, that is, GR antagonists, to treat special subtypes of depression, such as psychotic depression, and there in particular the psychotic and cognitive features (Schatzberg, 2008; and Chapter 26 in this book).

A fairly congruent biological finding in severely depressed patients represents a hyperactivity of the HPA-system, which is postulated to be caused by decreased glucocorticoid signalling leading to disturbances of the negative feedback at the level of the hypothalamus (Heuser et al. 1996; Holsboer and Barden, 1996; van Rossum et al. 2006; Zobel et al. 2001). The described HPA hyperactivity is often reflected by a basal hypercortisolemia. However, this abnormality and its causal pathophysiology can also be masked and may become only evident when the HPA-system is challenged by specific external stressors such as tense surroundings or characteristic pharmacological stimulation tests. In such clinical tests, dexamethasone (a synthetic glucocorticoid) is given to challenge the negative feedback of the HPA-system, which usually leads to a suppression of cortisol plasma levels in healthy control persons (Barden et al. 1997). While basal elevated plasma cortisol levels are less reliable in depressive patients, a typical non-suppression of cortisol levels after dexamethasone treatment, as well as an increased adrenocorticotropic hormone (ACTH) and cortisol release in the combined DEX/corticotropin releasing hormone (CRH) test, occur more frequently (Heuser et al. 1994; von Bardeleben and Holsboer, 1991).

Besides numerous stress-related molecules, which have been implicated in the vulnerability to psychiatric diseases such as depression, dysregulations and dysfunctions of corticosteroid receptors take up an important part in the pathogenesis of depression and post-traumatic stress disorder (Arborelius et al. 1999; Biondi and Picardi, 1999; Brown et al. 1999; de Kloet et al. 1998; Holsboer, 2000; Yehuda, 2001). However, it is yet uncertain whether these corticosteroid receptor disturbances are causative or result from affective disorders.

Current animal models mimic distinct aspects of depression

An important target of behavioural animal models of depression is to understand the interplay of diverse factors, such as neurotrophic circuits, the role of the stress-responsive HPA axis, and the beneficial effects of antidepressive treatments (e.g. antidepressants, electroconvulsive therapy [ECT]) or enriched environment (Chourbaji et al. 2005b), which have been shown to affect the course of the disease. Hereby one has to keep in mind that several restrictions (features that cannot be modelled i.e. suicidal ideation, feelings of guilt, delusions etc.) may not allow a complete illustration of a distinct disease, but only specific aspects, which may still be very informative. Considering such conditions, there is an increasing demand to develop and improve animal models of depression, in which several facets of the disease can be investigated as accurately as possible, including the analysis of brain tissues at timepoints of interest. Such animal models should preferably mimic specific features of the human condition with regard to its aetiology (*Construct Validity*), symptomatology (*Face Validity*), treatment or biological/pathophysiological basis (*Predictive Validity*). In this respect and against the background of a multifactorial derivation, the progress in developing and improving animal models constitutes a major scientific challenge, which is faced by many laboratories more and more successfully.

According to the 'Stress Hypothesis of Depression' (see Fig. 9.1), particularly mice with genetic alterations of the GR system would be expected to display changes of emotional behaviour and demonstrate depression-like states (Urani et al. 2003). However, only a few of several mouse strains carrying mutations of the GR have displayed depressive-like characteristics, which are presented in the following.

The Stress Hypothesis of Depression

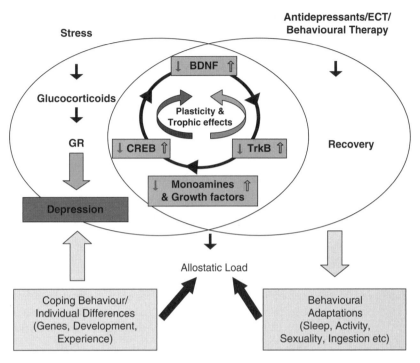

Fig. 9.1 The Stress Hypothesis of Depression postulates that stress – associated with intense release of glucocorticoids – evokes a depressive state by over-activation of GR which leads to dysregulations of homeostasis in terms of impaired monoaminergic functioning, reduced synaptic plasticity and disturbances of the neurotophin cycle, i.e. a downregulation of the brain derived neurotrophic factor BDNF, its tyrosine kinase receptor TrkB as well as the transcription factor CREB. All these changes are dependent on characteristic features (e.g. genetic makeup, development, life experiences) that modify the coping style of an individual and maybe reversed in a beneficial way by antidepressive treatments (including ECT), which aim at a reversal of molecular imbalances and at a restoration of a regular allostatic load, finally resulting in recovery from depression. The red arrows indicate the consequences of chronic stress, the green arrows show the effects of various antidepressive measurements.

Evaluation of the 'Stress Hypothesis of Depression' by targeted mutations of the GR

The 'Stress Hypothesis of Depression' postulates, that GR mediated functions (related with high levels of circulating glucocorticoids and reduction of neurotrophins and respective pathways) are disturbed in depressive patients. In experiments with animals it was furthermore shown, that stress, besides characteristic neuroendocrinological alterations such as increased corticosterone levels, leads to a reduction of GR and MR mRNA levels in the hippocampus (Sterlemann et al. 2008).

The animal models described below were designed to resemble the requirements of a depressive-like state as valid as possible and especially refer to such mice that over- or underexpress GR only to a certain extent (due to a gene dosage alteration), which may mimic the situation of patients with affective disorders more closely. Several research groups have investigated transgenic animal models focussing on the effects of altered GR expression and function. Their actual relevance will be discussed below.

GR$^{-/-}$ mice fail to represent a valid animal model of depression

The accessibility of classical homozygous GR mutant mice is restricted, since these animals die early caused by an impairment of the lung development. The little fraction of mice that survive to adulthood and which can be analysed, exhibit extreme elevations in plasma-ACTH (15-fold) and corticosterone (2.5-fold) (Cole et al. 1995; 2001). Since the molecular cause of survival might include alternative splice mechanisms resulting in uncontrollable residual GR activity, these animals have not been analysed behaviourally.

GR^{dim} mice display increased corticosterone levels

Glucocorticoid receptors control the expression of respective genes (i) via dimerization and subsequent binding to specific DNA sequences so-called glucocorticoid response elements, (GREs), thereby positively affecting the expression of target genes (activated via classical GREs) or preventing transcription (via nGREs); (ii) by protein–protein interactions with other transcription factors (such as CREB, AP-1, Stat5), also modulating transcription positively or negatively, respectively. For the analysis of the part of GR dimers acting at GREs and nGREs, a pointmutation was introduced into the dimerization domain (exon 4) preventing dimerization and thus DNA binding. These so-called GR^{dim} mice survive to adulthood, thereby conquering one of the major caveats of classical GR mutants. GR^{dim} mice show increased plasma corticosterone levels, but normal ACTH release. Furthermore, an impairment in spatial memory was described (Oitzl et al. 2001). However, emotional behaviours have never been analysed in this strain (Reichardt et al. 2000).

GR^{NesCre} mice represent a model of Cushing's disease but display reduced anxiety

Since conventional GR knockout mice do not survive, nervous system specific knockout mice have been generated using the Cre/loxP recombination system under the control of the rat nestin promoter (Tronche et al. 1999). These so-called GR^{NesCre} mice are viable and lack the GR in neurons and glial cells throughout the CNS. As one might have expected, the HPA-system of these animals is severely disinhibited/over-activated due to the lack of the negative feedback normally exerted at the level of the hypothalamus via GR, with drastically elevated levels of CRH, ACTH, and corticosterone (Tronche et al. 1999). This results in a (neuro)endocrinological phenotype resembling Cushing's disease in man (a disease that is quite often associated with depression), with a redistribution of body fat, osteoporosis, and immunological abnormalities. This phenotype of GR^{NesCre} mice is not surprising, because GR signalling outside the nervous system is intact in this strain.

What was unexpected, however, was that GR^{NesCre} mice do not show a depression-like phenotype in respective behavioural paradigms. They do not exhibit increased despair-like behaviour in the forced swim test (FST) as it would be expected in depressive mice (Tronche et al. 1999). Moreover, applying standardized anxiety tests such as the dark-light box test and the elevated o-maze these animals display less anxiety-related behaviour than wild-type littermate controls (Tronche et al. 1999). This paradoxical finding can be explained by the fact that the neurons of GR^{NesCre} mice do not express the GR. As a result, the hypercortisolism cannot affect neurons and cause subsequent changes in behaviour. Thus, despite their hypercortisolism, these mice most likely represent a genetic model of resistance to depression. To test this hypothesis, they have to be subjected to stress-induced behavioural depression paradigms, such as the learned helplessness paradigm or a chronic stress model of depression.

GR-antisense mice exhibit some endocrinological but no behavioural features associated with depression

A different approach to interfere with GR functioning in the brain is the induction of GR-antisense sequences, generating mice with reduced expression of GR in the brain and some peripheral tissues as well (Pepin et al. 1992b). GR-antisense mice exhibit a reduced CRF expression in the hypothalamus, but no changes in ACTH and corticosterone levels at various timepoints of the circadian rhythm (Barden et al. 1997; Dijkstra et al. 1998; Karanth et al. 1997). The expected upregulation of the HPA-system in these mice only becomes apparent under stressful conditions (Pepin et al. 1992a, b) and is reversed by antidepressant treatment (Barden, 1996; Montkowski et al. 1995). Moreover, similar to depressed patients, GR-antisense mice are non-suppressors in the dexamethasone (DEX) suppression test (Barden et al. 1997).

Behaviourally – comparable to GR^{NesCre} mice – GR-antisense mice present reduced depression-like despair behaviour in the FST (Montkowski et al. 1995), and also demonstrate less anxiety in the elevated plus-maze as well as after predator stress (Montkowski et al. 1995; Rochford et al. 1997; Strohle et al. 1998). Furthermore, they display locomotor hyperactivity when exposed to a novel environment (Beaulieu et al. 1994) and exhibit enhanced responses to novelty with increased conditioned approach responses, altogether again in contrast to the predictions of the theory of a depression-like phenotype in these mice (Steckler and Holsboer, 1999). Taken together, GR-antisense mice display only some of the neuroendocrinological, but no behavioural features observed in depression. However, due to the possibility to reverse most of the observed alterations by pharmacological antidepressant treatment, this mouse strain might be a valid tool for the development of new antidepressive agents (Montkowski et al. 1995).

$GR^{+/-}$ mice represent a mouse model of depression with good construct and face validity

Glucocorticoid receptor heterozygous mice, in which one GR allele has been ablated, were recently designed by a conventional knockout strategy (Tronche et al. 1998). This leads to a reduction (about 50%) of GR expression on the protein level in the brain (Ridder et al. 2005). Such $GR^{+/-}$ mice do however not show a phenotype when compared to their wild-type littermates when they were analysed by a large well-established test battery for emotional behaviours including tests for depression-like signs such as despair (i.e. Porsolt FST and tail suspension test) (Ridder et al. 2005). Moreover, they reveal normal circadian levels of corticosterone (Ridder et al. 2005). When subjected to stress, though, $GR^{+/-}$ mice display a predisposition for depressive-like behaviours becoming obvious in the learned helplessness paradigm and they exhibit furthermore depression-like neuroendocrinological abnormalities.

In the learned helplessness procedure, a valid animal model in many species, mice are exposed to series of unpredictable, unavoidable, and uncontrollable footshocks on two consecutive days. On day three, about 30% of the animals demonstrate helplessness, that is, coping deficits in a test situation (within a shuttle box apparatus) where aversive stimuli (footshocks) would be avoidable, since they are announced by a light, signalling the mice to switch to the opposite compartment and thereby avoiding the shock (Chourbaji et al. 2005a). $GR^{+/-}$ mice demonstrate significantly increased helplessness compared to their wild-type littermates, measured by prolonged escape latencies and an increased number of failures in the shuttle box. The impaired coping of $GR^{+/-}$ mice represents a correlate of depression-like behaviour (Ridder et al. 2005).

An altered reaction to stress in this strain is also found on the neuroendocrinological level. Immobilization stress evokes a significant change in the response of the HPA-system in GR$^{+/-}$ animals. Since depression is a multigenetic/multifactorial disease, the dysregulation of a single system may not be sufficient to induce depression-like alterations in mice under basal conditions but render the affected individuals more sensitive to further environmental influences. In this context it is of interest that a selective impairment of GR function in hepatocytes does not affect gluconeogenesis under basal conditions, but evokes a gluconeogenesis deficit only under challenge conditions (by fasting the animals) (Opherk et al. 2004).

In accordance with an altered stress sensitivity of the HPA system, GR$^{+/-}$ mice exhibit a pathological DEX/CRH test, at present the most relevant biological indication for both, florid depression and the risk to develop a depressive episode. In several depressive patients, the alteration of the HPA system is also absent under baseline conditions (e.g. morning cortisol blood levels) but becomes evident under challenge conditions only, as it may be artificially modelled by the DEX/CRH test.

In GR$^{+/-}$ animals, external stressors provoke a behavioural as well as a neuroendocrinological phenotype resembling depression (Ridder et al. 2005). This can be regarded as strong point of the model since humans with a vulnerability to depression often manifest a depressive episode in response to external or internal stress factors only. One more environmental risk factor could be an early childhood trauma (e.g. maternal separation) that may significantly modify emotional behaviour in GR$^{+/-}$ mice. So far, however, respective experiments have not been performed with this strain.

YGR mice represent a model of resistance to depression

To verify the concept strengthened by the results obtained in GR$^{+/-}$ mice, the study by Ridder et al. (2005) implied another mouse strain that represents, from a molecular viewpoint, the opposite phenotype of GR$^{+/-}$ mice. In this approach, the so-called YGR mice overexpress GR by a yeast artefical chromosome, which results in a twofold increase of GR expression in the brain (Reichardt et al. 2000). One would assume that these animals show a phenotype opposite to the one described for GR$^{+/-}$ mice. In fact – opposite to the increased stress sensitivity of GR$^{+/-}$ mice – YGR mice exhibit a stress-resistant phenotype on behavioural and neuroendocrinological level. YGR mice demonstrated less helplessness, reduced stress-induced corticosterone levels, and oversuppression in the dexamethasone suppression test (Ridder et al. 2005). Thus, YGR mice substantiate the specificity of the findings in GR$^{+/-}$ mice. Generally speaking, their phenotype is also in good conformity with the 'Stress Hypothesis', predicting a protective effect by GR overexpression against stress.

Both, GR$^{+/-}$ and YGR mice confirm the predictions of the 'Neurotrophin Hypothesis of Depression'

An additional molecular theory of depression, the so-called 'Neurotrophin Hypothesis' postulates that a downregulation of the neurotrophin brain-derived neurotrophic factor (BDNF) is essential in the pathogenesis of depression in humans and rodents (Altar, 1999; Duman et al. 1997). In conjunction with the 'Stress Hypothesis', the 'Neurotrophin Hypothesis' predicts that stress characterized by high levels of circulating glucocorticoids leads, by activation of GRs, to a decrease of the neurotrophin brain-derived neurotrophic factor, to a subsequent underactivation of its tyrosine kinase receptor TrkB and possibly via the transcription factor CREB to molecular alterations that underlie depressive behaviours. In agreement with these hypotheses, GR$^{+/-}$ mice – which have a predisposition to stress-induced depression-like behaviour – show a significant downregulation of BDNF in the hippocampus, while YGR mice exhibit a significant BDNF upregulation (Schulte-Herbruggen et al. 2006a, b; 2007). Indeed, these findings have been the first experimental confirmation that an affected GR function concurrently evokes a BDNF dysregulation and a predisposition to depressive behaviour. However, there are also controversial findings with regard of the classical 'Neurotrophin Hypothesis'. Thus, the behavioural induction of a depression-like state in mice via the learned helplessness procedure or by olfactory bulbectomy does not result in alterations of hippocampal BDNF levels, and the latter model even resulted in a BDNF upregulation in the frontal cortex (Hellweg et al. 2007; Schulte-Herbruggen et al. 2006a; 2007) Moreover, a murine social defeat model that has some face value similarities with certain aspects of depression relies on intact (not compromised) BDNF levels in the mesolimbic dopamine system (Berton et al. 2006; Chen et al. 2006). In good agreement with the 'Neurotrophin Hypothesis', however, are recent findings in mice carrying a genetic variant BDNF, that is, in humans described as Val66Met-polymorphism, and show an increase in anxiety-like behaviour (Berton et al. 2006; Chen et al. 2006). The controversies around this area are also discussed in Chapter 11 of this book.

Forebrain-specific GR knockout (FBGRKO) mice represent a valid animal model of depression

Recently, a depressive-like phenotype has also been described in mice with a forebrain-specific complete GR knockout induced via the calcium-calmodulin-dependent protein kinase II (CamKII) promoter (Boyle et al. 2005). These animals exhibit an impaired negative feedback regulation of the HPA-axis, as well as increased depression-like behaviours, which have been demonstrated in the FST and tail suspension tests as well as in terms of anhedonic sucrose preference (Boyle et al. 2005). In contrast to $GR^{+/-}$ mice, the depression-like phenotype became apparent at four months of age already under basal (unstressed) conditions (Boyle et al. 2005). Additionally, forebrain-specific complete GR knockout mice also exhibit increased anxiety-like behaviours in the elevated plus-maze and the dark-light box (Boyle et al. 2006). While depression-like symptoms are reversable by chronic treatment with the tricyclic antidepressant imipramine, anxiety-related behaviours do not respond to treatment (Boyle et al. 2005; 2006). These findings nicely demonstrate that by the use of conditional gene-targeting strategies, alterations of GR expression or function in specific brain regions can be correlated with the occurrence of a depressive-like phenotype.

Mice overexpressing GR specifically in the forebrain (GRov) show increased emotional lability

Using a similar CamKII-promoter construct as Boyle et al ., Wei and colleagues generated a mouse strain overexpressing GR specifically in the forebrain (Wei et al. 2004). In contrast to the stress-resistent YGR mice with a general GR overexpression (see above), forebrain-specific overexpressing GR mice display increased immobility in the Porsolt FST and increased anxiety-like behaviour in the elevated plus-maze and in the dark-light box (Wei et al. 2004). These somewhat surprising results in light of similar findings obtained in forebrain-specific GR knockout mice have been interpreted by the authors as 'increased emotional lability' (Wei et al. 2004). In a recent study addressing the role of the MR, it was shown, that overexpression of this type of corticosteroidreceptor in the forebrain decreases anxiety-like behaviour and alters the stress response in mice, which point to the importance to consider also the ratio of MR and GR, which modulates emotional reactivity (Rozeboom et al. 2007).

Are the findings in GR mutant animals transferable to psychiatric conditions?

Translational approaches with regard to human diseases, that should be mimicked by animals require exact background knowledge of what is exactly investigated and has to consider both, inter-species similarities and differences to avoid artefacts due to misinterpretations. Therefore, a suitable election of solid parameters, which may be measured and replicated representatively, guarantees a valid illustration of a pathological state.

As it was stated at the beginning of the chapter, suitable animal models should implicate valid construct validity, that is, aetiology (which may be represented by a distinct genetic background), face validity, represented by respective symptomatolgy, and predictive validity, which demands that the symptoms are reversible by antidepressive treatment. Some of the listed mutants indeed unite these requirements reviewed.

Substantiating the concept that depression is a multi-aetiological disorder (Claes, 2004), GR mutant mice represent potentially adequate models for combined effects of genetic and environmental manipulations (Howell and Muglia, 2006). In particular $GR^{+/-}$ mice as characterized by Ridder et al. mimic the human condition in depressive disorders, since they resemble individuals, which are vulnerable to become depressive after stressful challenges (Ridder et al. 2005). In this respect, $GR^{+/-}$ mice are different from such mice with a forebrain-specific complete GR knockout (Boyle et al. 2005), which develop depression-like behavioural and neurochemical characteristics during adulthood already under baseline conditions. However, the findings in both strains prove that compromised GR function constitutes a crucial molecular risk factor in the pathophysiology of depression, indicating that both mouse lines are models with good face validity and may serve for future target-oriented physiological, biochemical, and pharmacological investigations of GR function in human depressive disorders. Besides such aspects relating to the serotonergic and noradrenergic systems (e.g. monoamine tissue levels, monoamine transporter expression and function, pre- and postsynaptic receptor expression) it seems of great interest to analyse the importance of critical periods, in which the effects of chronic stress are considered, like in a recent study of Sterlemann et al. (2008) where this type of 'representative' stress evoked persistent effects on physiological and behavioural parameters throughout life (Sterlemann et al. 2008). Recently conducted experiments in GR under- and overexpressing mice argue against a prominent role of the serotonin and norepinephrine metabolism in these models, since both monoamines and their metabolites show regular levels and normal diurnal variations in several forebrain and limbic system areas of these strains (Schulte-Herbruggen et al. 2006a, b; 2007). Thanks to the accessibility of brain tissue, neuroanatomical studies are also feasible, for example, relating to neurogenesis and dendritic spine plasticity. Furthermore, GR mutant mice may be good models to better characterize potential diagnostic tools for depressive patients, in whom different facets of depression may be treated systematically (Schatzberg and Lindley, 2008). Thus, GR deficient mice can be used to calibrate flow cytometry methods for analyses of GR expression of lymphocytes, or might be used to assess the quality of potential GR ligands for positron emission tomography (PET) investigations (Wüst et al. 2003). Furthermore they might be interesting models with regard to the investigation of drugs interfering with stress components like MR and/or GR mediators of the cell death cascade, thereby providing important targets for the modulation of mood and memory (Lucassen et al. 2006). With respect to effectiveness and potential mechanisms of pharmacotherapy, these models can be used to study which antidepressive substances, for example, GR antagonists, work in mouse models of depression based on GR deficiency, and which depressive features are reversed by these substances. Thus, chronic treatment with the tricyclic antidepressant imipramine reverses the behavioural despair phenotype and influences the HPA-axis abnormalities in forebrain specific GR knockout mice (Boyle et al. 2005). In contrast, the anxiety-related behavioural signs observed in this model are not attenuated by treatment with imipramine (Boyle et al. 2006). Consequently, the exact biological effects that underlie the potential clinical improvements need to be studied and optimal doses for long-term administration (with fewer side effects) to handle specific diseases have to be established efficiently.

Outlook

Different depression-related phenotypes, as they were presented here, support the assumption of varying types of depression that have to be approached accordingly. Therefore, the generation of diverse animal models, in which particular pathogenetic aspects may be focussed separately, seems to be a good strategy to improve a suitable prescription of antidepressants, which may be matched more precisely to the respective form of depression. The findings in some of the mouse strains presented in this chapter support the idea that compromised GR function constitutes a crucial molecular risk factor in the pathophysiology of depression-like behaviours. Accordingly, it would be of great interest to intensify the state of scientific knowledge by analysing the action of GR antagonists in some of the mice specified in this chapter (e.g. GR heterozygotes or forebrain-specific GR knockouts). GR antagonists may gain importance, since promising effects were observed in human patients. In this respect, GR knockout mice could represent valuable tools to determine molecular and biochemical downstream effects of these drugs, which should be missing in GR mutant mice but be present in wild-type controls. Furthermore, the mouse strains discussed here seem to be a good tool to further study molecular, pathophysiological, and cellular/structural alterations that underlie specific behavioural features such as despair or helplessness. By using brain region or neuronal cell type specific conditional transgenic strategies it should even be possible to attribute crucial GR functions to specific brain areas or neuronal networks, which may open new possibilities to investigate essential coherencies of different aspects which could influence the manifestation of depression, such as disturbances in sleep, cognition, mood, intermediary metabolism, maintenance of cardiovascular tone, inflammatory processes as well as growth and reproduction. Of course, other genes apart from the GR may participate in the development of the characteristic alterations observed in GR compromised animals and these genes should be considered in parallel. However, since clinical data indicate that impairment of GR function define a specific neuroendocrinological endophenotype of (severe) depression, GR mutant animals may represent a model with good construct and face validity for this subgroup of depressed patients. Some of the patients' symptomatology might be attributable to the same brain regions identified in GR mutant mice. On the therapeutic side it has been demonstrated that specific behavioural changes in GR mutant mice respond to specific drug treatments (e.g. imipramine), while other behavioural abnormalities remain unchanged (Boyle et al. 2005; 2006). A major challenge is to work out, which kind of symptomatic appearances in patients match to the animal despair, and helplessness constructs, and to elucidate, whether it is possible to gain insights from the animals' response to specific treatments for human therapy. This approach may be even supported by the extension of investigation of promising mutants in paradigms that include, for example, the examination of naturalistic stressors such as predator or environmental stress evoked by high density or poor environments. However, it could be an interesting point to address, in how far not only pharmacological intervention but also environmental factors (i.e. enriched environment, social support) modulate a stress-related disease such as depression – maybe in a beneficial way by alleviating the individual allostatic overlaod.

Acknowledgements

This work was supported by a grant from the Deutsche Forschungsgemeinschaft to P.G. (SFB636/B3). We thank Christiane Brandwein and Miriam A. Vogt for critically reading the manuscript.

References

Altar, C.A. (1999). Neurotrophins and depression. *Trends in Pharmacological Sciences*, **20**, 59–61.

Arborelius, L., Owens, M.J., Plotsky, P.M., and Nemeroff, C.B. (1999). The role of corticotropin-releasing factor in depression and anxiety disorders. *Journal of Endocrinology*, **160**, 1–12.

Barden, N. (1996). Modulation of glucocorticoid receptor gene expression by antidepressant drugs. *Pharmacopsychiatry*, **29**, 12–22.

Barden, N., Stec, I.S., Montkowski, A., Holsboer, F., and Reul, J.M. (1997). Endocrine profile and neuroendocrine challenge tests in transgenic mice expressing antisense RNA against the glucocorticoid receptor. *Neuroendocrinology*, **66**, 212–220.

Beato, M., Herrlich P., and Schütz G. (1995). Steroid hormone receptors: many actors in search of a plot: *Cell*, **83**, 851–857.

Beaulieu, S., Rousse, I., Gratton, A., Barden, N., and Rochford, J. (1994). Behavioral and endocrine impact of impaired type II glucocorticoid receptor function in a transgenic mouse model. *Annals of the New York Academy of Sciences*, **746**, 388–391.

Berton, O., McClung, C.A., Dileone, R. J. et al. (2006). Essential role of BDNF in the mesolimbic dopamine pathway in social defeat stress. *Science*, **311**, 864–368.

Biondi, M. and Picardi, A. (1999). Psychological stress and neuroendocrine function in humans: the last two decades of research. *Psychotherapy and Psychosomatics*, **68**, 114–150.

Boyle, M.P., Brewer, J.A., Funatsu, M. et al. (2005). Acquired deficit of forebrain glucocorticoid receptor produces depression-like changes in adrenal axis regulation and behavior. *Proceedings of the National Academy of Sciences USA*, **102**, 473–478.

Boyle, M.P., Kolber, B.J., Vogt, S.K., Wozniak, Muglia, L.J. (2006). Forebrain glucocorticoid receptors modulate anxiety-associated locomotor activation and adrenal responsiveness. *Journal of Neuroscience*, **26**, 71–78.

Brown, E.S., Rush, A.J., and McEwen, B.S. (1999). Hippocampal remodeling and damage by corticosteroids: implications for mood disorders. *Neuropsychopharmacology*, **21**, 474–484.

Chen, Z.Y., Jing, D., Bath, K.G. et al. (2006). Genetic variant BDNF (Val66Met) polymorphism alters anxiety-related behavior. *Science*, **314**, 140–143.

Chourbaji, S., Zacher, C., Sanchis-Segura, C., Dormann, C., Vollmayr, B., and Gass, P. (2005a). Learned helplessness: validity and reliability of depressive-like states in mice. *Brain Research Brain Research Protocols*, **16**, 70–78.

Chourbaji, S., Zacher, C., Sanchis-Segura, C., Spanagel, Gass, P. (2005b). Social and structural housing conditions influence the development of a depressive-like phenotype in the learned helplessness paradigm in male mice. *Behavioural Brain Research*, **164**, 100–106.

Claes, S.J. (2004). CRH, stress, and major depression: a psychobiological interplay. *Vitamins and Hormones*, **69**, 117–150.

Cole, T.J., Blendy, J.A., Monaghan, A.P. et al. (1995). Targeted disruption of the glucocorticoid receptor gene blocks adrenergic chromaffin cell development and severely retards lung maturation. *Genes & Development*, **9**, 1608–1621.

Cole, T.J., K. Myles, J.F. Purton, et al. (2001). GRKO mice express an aberrant dexamethasone-binding glucocorticoid receptor, but are profoundly glucocorticoid resistant. *Molecular Cell Endocrinology*, **173**, 193–202.

de Kloet, E.R., Vreugdenhil, E., Oitzl, M.S., and Joels, M. (1998). Brain corticosteroid receptor balance in health and disease. *Endocrine Reviews*, **19**, 269–301.

Dijkstra, I., Tilders, F.J., Aguilera, G. et al. (1998). Reduced activity of hypothalamic corticotropin-releasing hormone neurons in transgenic mice with impaired glucocorticoid receptor function. *Journal of Neuroscience*, **18**, 3909–3918.

Duman, R.S., Heninger, G.R., Nestler, E.J. (1997). A molecular and cellular theory of depression. *Archives of General Psychiatry*, **54**, 597–606.

Hellweg, R., Zueger, M., Fink, K., Hortnagl, H., and Gass P. (2007). Olfactory bulbectomy in mice leads to increased BDNF levels and decreased serotonin turnover in depression-related brain areas. *Neurobiology of Disease*, **25**, 1–7.

Heuser, I., Yassouridis, A., Holsboer, F. (1994). The combined dexamethasone/CRH test: a refined laboratory test for psychiatric disorders. *Journal of Psychiatry Research*, **28**, 341–356.

Heuser, I. J., Schweiger, U., Gotthardt, U. et al. (1996). Pituitary-adrenal-system regulation and psychopathology during amitriptyline treatment in elderly depressed patients and normal comparison subjects. *American Journal of Psychiatry*, **153**, 93–99.

Holsboer, F. and Barden, N. (1996). Antidepressants and hypothalamic-pituitary-adrenocortical regulation: *Endocrine Reviews*, **17**, 187–205.

Holsboer, F. (2000). The corticosteroid receptor hypothesis of depression. *Neuropsychopharmacology*, **23**, 477–501.

Howell, M.P. and Muglia, L.J. (2006). Effects of genetically altered brain glucocorticoid receptor action on behavior and adrenal axis regulation in mice. *Frontiers in Neuroendocrinol*, **27**, 275–284.

Karanth, S., Linthorst, A.C., Stalla, G.K., Barden, N., Holsboer, F., and Reul, J.M. (1997). Hypothalamic-pituitary-adrenocortical axis changes in a transgenic mouse with impaired glucocorticoid receptor function. *Endocrinology*, **138**, 3476–3485.

Lucassen, P.J., Heine, V.M., Muller, M.B. et al. (2006). Stress, depression and hippocampal apoptosis. *CNS & Neurological Disorders Drug Targets*, **5**, 531–546.

Montkowski, A., Barden, N., Wotjak, C. et al. (1995). Long-term antidepressant treatment reduces behavioural deficits in transgenic mice with impaired glucocorticoid receptor function. *Journal of Neuroendocrinology*, **7**, 841–845.

Oitzl, M.S., Reichardt, H.M., Joels, M., and de Kloet, E.R. (2001). Point mutation in the mouse glucocorticoid receptor preventing DNA binding impairs spatial memory. *Proceedings of the National Academy of Sciences USA*, **98**, 12790–12795.

Opherk, C., Tronche, F., Kellendonk et al. (2004). Inactivation of the glucocorticoid receptor in hepatocytes leads to fasting hypoglycemia and ameliorates hyperglycemia in streptozotocin-induced diabetes mellitus. *Molecular Endocrinology*, **18**, 1346–1353.

Pepin, M.C., Govindan, M.V., and Barden, N. (1992a). Increased glucocorticoid receptor gene promoter activity after antidepressant treatment. *Molecular Pharmacology*, **41**, 1016–1022.

Pepin, M.C., Pothier, F., and Barden, N. (1992b). Impaired type II glucocorticoid-receptor function in mice bearing antisense RNA transgene. *Nature*, **355**, 725–728.

Reichardt, H.M., Umland, T., Bauer, A., Kretz, O., and Schutz, G. (2000). Mice with an increased glucocorticoid receptor gene dosage show enhanced resistance to stress and endotoxic shock. *Molecular Cell Biology*, **20**, 9009–9017.

Reul, J.M., Gesing, A., Droste, S. et al. (2000). The brain mineralocorticoid receptor: greedy for ligand, mysterious in function. *European Journal of Pharmacology*, **405**, 235–249.

Ridder, S., Chourbaji, S., Hellweg, R. et al. (2005). Mice with genetically altered glucocorticoid receptor expression show altered sensitivity for stress-induced depressive reactions. *Journal of Neuroscience*, **25**, 6243–6250.

Rochford, J., Beaulieu, S., Rousse, I., Glowa, J.R., and Barden, N. (1997). Behavioral reactivity to aversive stimuli in a transgenic mouse model of impaired glucocorticoid (type II) receptor function effects of diazepam and FG-7142. *Psychopharmacology (Berl)*, **132**, 145–152.

Rozeboom, A.M., Akil, H., and Seasholtz, A.F. (2007). Mineralocorticoid receptor overexpression in forebrain decreases anxiety-like behavior and alters the stress response in mice. *Proceedings of the National Academy of Sciences USA*, **104**, 4688–4693.

Steckler, T. and Holsboer, F. (1999). Enhanced conditioned approach responses in transgenic mice with impaired glucocorticoid receptor function. *Behavioural Brain Research*, **102**, 151–163.

von Bardeleben, U. and Holsboer F. (1991). Effect of age on the cortisol response to human corticotropin-releasing hormone in depressed patients pretreated with dexamethasone. *Biological Psychiatry*, **29**, 1042–1050.

Schatzberg, A.F. and Lindley, S. (2008) Glucocorticoid antagonists in neuropsychotic disorders. *European Journal of Pharmacology*, **583**, 358–364.

Schulte-Herbruggen, O., Chourbaji, S., Muller, H. et al. (2006a). Differential regulation of nerve growth factor and brain-derived neurotrophic factor in a mouse model of learned helplessness. *Experimental Neurology*, **202**, 404–409.

Schulte-Herbruggen, O., Chourbaji, S., Ridder, S. et al. (2006b). Stress-resistant mice overexpressing glucocorticoid receptors display enhanced BDNF in the amygdala and hippocampus with unchanged NGF and serotonergic function. *Psychoneuroendocrinology*, **31**, 1266–1277.

Schulte-Herbruggen, O., Hellweg, R., Chourbaji, S. et al. (2007). Differential regulation of neurotrophins and serotonergic function in mice with genetically reduced glucocorticoid receptor expression. *Experimental Neurology*, **204**, 307–316.

Sterlemann, V., Ganea, K., Liebl, C. et al. (2008). Long-term behavioral and neuroendocrine alterations following chronic social stress in mice: implications for stress-related disorders. *Hormones & Behaviour*, **53**, 386–394.

Strohle, A., Poettig, M., Barden, N., Holsboer, F., and Montkowski, A. (1998). Age- and stimulus-dependent changes in anxiety-related behaviour of transgenic mice with GR dysfunction. *Neuroreport*, **9**, 2099–2102.

Tronche, F., Kellendonk, C., and Kretz, O. (1999). Disruption of the glucocorticoid receptor gene in the nervous system results in reduced anxiety. *Nature Genetics*, **23**, 99–103.

Tronche, F., Kellendonk, C., Reichardt, H.M., and Schutz, G. (1998). Genetic dissection of glucocorticoid receptor function in mice. *Current Opinion in Genetics and Development*, **8**, 532–538.

Urani, A., Chourbaji, S., Henn, F., and Gass, P. (2003). The Neurotrophin hypothesis of depression revistited by transgenic mice. *Clinical Neuroscience Research*, **3**, 263–269.

van Rossum, E.F., Binder, E.B., Majer, M. et al. (2006). Polymorphisms of the glucocorticoid receptor gene and major depression. *Biological Psychiatry*, **59**, 681–688.

Wei, Q., Lu, X.Y., Liu, L. et al. (2004). Glucocorticoid receptor overexpression in forebrain: a mouse model of increased emotional lability. *Proceedings of the National Academy of Sciences USA*, **101**, 11851–11856.

Wüst, F., Carlson, K.E., Katzenellenbogen J.A. (2003). Synthesis of novel arylpyrazolo corticosteroids as potential ligands for imaging brain glucocorticoid receptors. *Steroids*, **68**, 177–191.

Yehuda, R. (2001). Are glucocortoids responsible for putative hippocampal damage in PTSD? How and when to decide. *Hippocampus*, **11**, 85–89; discussion 82–84.

Zobel, A.W., Nickel, T., Sonntag, A., Uhr, M., Holsboer, F., and Ising, M. (2001). Cortisol response in the combined dexamethasone/CRH test as predictor of relapse in patients with remitted depression. a prospective study. *Journal of Psychiatry Research*, **35**, 83–94.

Chapter 10

Cytokines and depression: experimental evidence and intermediate mechanisms

Robert Dantzer, Jason C. O'Connor,
Nathalie Castanon, Jacques Lestage, and
Keith W. Kelley

From cytokine-induced sickness behaviour to depression

The innate immune system is activated by specific molecular motifs that are an intrinsic component of microbial pathogens and are called pathogen-associated molecular patterns. Cells of the innate immune system recognize these motifs via specialized receptors called toll-like receptors (TLRs). Activation of TLRs induces a cascade of intracellular events that ultimately lead to the synthesis and release of inflammatory mediators including chemokines and proinflammatory cytokines. Chemokines permit the local recruitment of phagocytic cells. The proinflammatory cytokines that are produced by these phagocytic cells include a wide variety of molecular factors of which the most intensely studied are interleukin (IL)-1β, tumour necrosis factor (TNF)-α, IL-6 and the interferons (IFN). They are the first molecular signals of inflammation. Their production is modulated by a number of molecules known as cryogens or anti-inflammatory cytokines that are either specific of a given cytokine (e.g. the antagonist of the type I IL-1 receptor, IL-1RA, or the soluble form of the type II IL-1 receptor) or exert their inhibitory activity on multiple cytokines (e.g. IL-10) at the level of intracellular signalling pathways.

Major advances made in the study of inflammation have now elucidated the principal molecular actors of the inflammatory response, their cellular targets and their role in mounting the innate and adaptive immune responses. Simultaneously, it has been possible to elucidate the pathophysiological role of these actors in various inflammatory conditions ranging from autoimmune diseases such as rheumatoid arthritis and multiple sclerosis (Andreakos et al. 2004) to functional disorders such as chronic fatigue (Bower, 2007). What has been certainly the least easily predicted result of this research is the discovery of the profound action of cytokines on brain functions and their involvement in many behavioural and mood disorders (Dantzer, 2007).

In physiological terms, the proinflammatory cytokines that are released at the site of infection by innate immune cells act not only locally to coordinate the local inflammatory response but also systemically. The systemic response is known as the acute phase reaction. It involves the production of acute phase proteins by the liver in response to IL-6 and the fever response. Since the fever response is mediated mainly by changes in neuronal activity in the anterior preoptic area of the hypothalamus, it has long been considered the prototypical example of the brain action of peripheral cytokines (Blatteis, 2007). These cytokines were initially termed pyrogens before they were cloned and produced as recombinant proteins. However, the fever response does not take place in a vacuum in the sense that a febrile organism needs to drastically alter its behavioural priorities in order to increase thermogenesis and reduce its thermolysis so as to elevate and maintain its temperature at a higher set point than normal. The adaptive nature of fever was recognized well before the discovery of cytokines (Kluger, 1978); whereas, the conceptualization of sickness behaviour as an adaptive response to immune activation has been slower to emerge (Dantzer and Kelley, 2007; Hart, 1988). Sickness behaviour refers to the collective set of behavioural changes that take place in an infected organism. It includes decreased motor activity, social withdrawal, reduction in food and water intake, pilo-erection and adoption of a hunched posture, and it is often accompanied by altered cognition and mood, fatigue, modified pain sensitivity and fragmented sleep with a general decrease in rapid eye movement sleep and an increase in slow wave sleep.

Like fever, sickness behaviour is normally a fully reversible response once microbial pathogens have been cleared and the innate immune system is no longer activated. However, in conditions of chronic inflammation or when the activation of the innate immune system remains unabated, sickness behaviour can persist much longer and become pathological disorders that affect functionality and manifest as symptoms of depression, fatigue, pain and altered cognition.

In terms of mechanisms, cytokine-induced sickness behaviour is now well-known to be due to the action of proinflammatory cytokines that are produced by macrophage-like cells in the brain in response to peripherally released proinflammatory cytokines. The objective of the present chapter is not to review the mechanisms of propagation of the peripheral immune message to the brain nor the mode of action of brain cytokines on behaviour. Several review articles are already available for this (Dantzer et al. 2007; 2008b; Dunn, 2002; Hayley and Anisman, 2005). We will instead concentrate on the evidence for a role of cytokines in the development of clinical signs of depression, and discuss possible mechanisms that are involved in these effects. In order to do so, we will first discuss whether it is really possible to study depression in laboratory animals before presenting the evidence in favour of a role of cytokines in the depressive-like behaviours that are displayed by immunochallenged animals. We will then examine the mechanisms that are potentially involved in the development of inflammation-associated depression at the light of the very recent experimental results obtained in the field. This is the first of four chapters in this book that specifically discuss the role of inflammation in affective disorders, together with Chapters 11, 16, and 17.

The limitations of animal models of depression

The mere possibility that major depressive disorders can be studied in animal models is often met with scepticism and incredulity. There is nothing there that is specific to depression, since the same issue plagues research on anxiety and other mental disorders including schizophrenia and autism. Ideally an animal model of a human disease is supposed to share with the disease under consideration similar pathogenic factors, symptoms, and treatment. Most psychiatric disorders are only described in terms of symptomatology because of the lack of knowledge concerning the causes of these disorders, which explains why treatments are de facto targeting symptoms and not causal factors. This accounts for why most animal models of depression are usually seen as nothing else as convenient bioassays for preclinical drug screening of potential antidepressant drugs. For instance, this applies to antagonism of reserpine-induced ptosis (Dhawan et al. 1970) or to normalization of behavioural abnormalities in olfactory bulbectomized rodents (Song and Leonard, 2005). A few animal models are assumed to feature some symptom homology with major depression, for instance the apparent resignation or 'helplessness' that is assumed to underlie the immobility that quickly replaces struggling in animals submitted to inescapable stressors in the form of painful electric shocks, forced swimming in small water tanks or tail suspension (Maier, 1984; Willner, 1984). The same applies to the decreased preference for a sweet solution that is interpreted to model anhedonia or decreased sensitivity to reward, a key symptom of depression in humans (Willner et al. 1992).

A few animal models of depression are claimed to be etiopathogenic because they involve exposure to some form of stress, and stress is well known to precipitate the occurrence of major depressive disorders in vulnerable individuals. The best known case is the model of chronic mild stress in which rats or mice are exposed to a series of mild stressors that occur daily in an unpredictable basis and are repeated over several weeks (Willner et al. 1992). Their home cage is tilted on one day; on the other day the litter is dampened; the next day they are deprived of food or the light–dark cycle is modified, and so on. Other more severe forms of stress involve exposure to an aggressive conspecific and social defeat either in an acute or in a chronic manner (Buwalda et al. 2005).

In all of these models, the gold standard is the reversal of the observed behavioural alterations by chronic antidepressant treatment. However, this inevitably leads to circularity. An animal model of depression is by definition a valid model if it is sensitive to already known antidepressant drugs. As a consequence the probability of finding a treatment of depression that is different from those that already exist is very low. In addition, the heuristic value of these models is very limited since a good animal model of depression needs to be sensitive to all classes of antidepressants whatever their mechanism of action. There is no simple explanation as to why antidepressants are able to treat depression, yet in some cases called treatment-resistant depression why they are actually unable to do so. Also, all this fails to take into account the controversy about antidepressant drugs not being better than placebos at least for non-severe forms of depression (Hansen et al. 2005; Schatzberg and Kraemer, 2000).

Within this context, it sounds like the recourse to animal models of depression to study the relationship between inflammation and depression is a dead end or nothing else than a series of variation on a familiar tune for which the issue is fully predictable. However, things are not that bad and actually the situation is a priori much more favourable than what the present status of the psychopharmacology of depression would imply. The reason for this relative optimism is that activation of the immune system has already been demonstrated in the clinics to be a causative factor for the occurrence of depression. Direct evidence is provided by the quasi-experimental model of cytokine-induced depression (Raison et al. 2006; and Chapter 17 in this book). In this model, one-third to half the cancer patients and hepatitis C patients who are treated with IFN-α develop major depressive disorders that regress upon discontinuation of immunotherapy and are sensitive to antidepressant treatment. Indirect evidence is the increased prevalence of major depressive disorders in physically ill patients with chronic inflammation. Since activation of the immune system is conducive to depression, it should be sufficient to activate the immune system of laboratory animals to have an etiopathogenic model of cytokine-induced depression. As we will see below, this is indeed the case but some precautions are necessary to dissociate cytokine-induced depression from cytokine-induced sickness behaviour.

Cytokines induce depressive-like behaviour

Raz Yirmiya was the first one to point to the similarity between signs of sickness behaviour in laboratory animals as defined empirically and signs of depression in humans as defined by the DSM-IV. This led him to assess the effects of a well-known activator of the innate immune system, lipopolysaccharide (LPS), on saccharin preference and to demonstrate that the reduced saccharin preference of LPS-treated rats could be alleviated by chronic but not acute pre-treatment with imipramine, a representative of tricyclic antidepressant drugs (Yirmiya, 1996). The problem with this study as well as with subsequent studies with fluoxetine, a representative of specific serotonin reuptake inhibitors (SSRIs) (Yirmiya et al. 1999), is that the behaviours under consideration, whether they were represented by decreased saccharin preference or by indices of sickness, were mostly measured at the peak of cytokine-induced sickness behaviour, that is, 4 hour after LPS administration. The issue under debate is whether cytokine-induced sickness can be equated with depression or if there is a difference. This is not a purely semantic issue since administration of IL-2 and/or IFN-α to patients very rapidly induces flu-like symptoms that are equivalent to the cytokine-induced sickness behaviour that develops in rats or mice treated with immune activators. However, depressive symptoms typically develop a few days to a few weeks later depending on the exact regimen of immunotherapy (Raison et al. 2006). Even if major depressive disorders caused by immune activation include sickness-like symptoms corresponding to the so-called neurovegetative symptoms of depression (e.g. fatigue, reduced appetite, psycho-motor retardation), they are not the only symptoms since true psychological symptoms of depression are observed simultaneously (Raison et al. 2005). They include in particular depressed mood, self-depreciation, and suicidal thoughts. The neurovegetative symptoms of depression are clearly different from the psychological symptoms since the last but not the first ones are sensitive to pre-treatment with paroxetine, another SSRI. In this context, it is not indifferent to note that SSRIs are in general less active on cytokine-induced sickness in rodent models of depression than imipramine.

A solution to this dilemma is to measure behavioural changes induced by activation of the innate immune system only when sickness has dissipated. The conceptual limitation of this approach is that cytokine-induced depression develops on a background of sickness and, as noted before, this form of depression includes some signs of sickness, so that the separation cannot be absolute but only relative. It is still the case that in conditions of acute as well as chronic immune activation it is possible to observe the development of depressive-like behaviour in animals at a time at which locomotor activity and food intake have returned to normal (Fig. 10.1). Using this approach, Frenois et al. showed that LPS-treated mice displayed an increased immobility in the

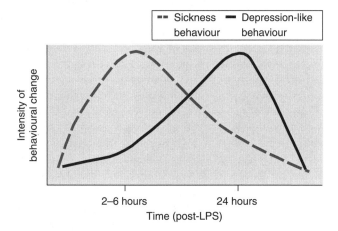

Fig. 10.1 LPS-induced depression-like behaviour develops on a background of sickness behaviour that peaks 2–6 hours post-injection. Recent experimental approaches have studied depression-like behaviours, including increased duration of immobility in the forced swim or tail suspension tests and reduced preference for a sweetened solution as they emerge following recovery from acute sickness behaviours. Reprinted by permission from Macmillan Publishers Ltd *Nature Reviews Neuroscience* Jan; 9(1):46-56 2008.

forced swim and tail suspension tests and decreased sucrose consumption at 24 hour post-LPS, a time at which sickness behaviour, as measured by decreased locomotor activity and reduced food intake, had disappeared (Frenois et al. 2007). In the same manner, Moreau et al. showed that chronic activation of the immune system in mice by inoculation of an attenuated form of Mycobacterium bovis, Bacillus Calmette-Guerin (BCG), increased the duration of immobility in the forced swim and tail suspension test, reduced voluntary wheel running and decreased preference for sucrose (Moreau et al. 2008). All these behavioural changes were observed between 7 and 21 days after BCG inoculation, when the infection was still active but the short-term signs of sickness had dissipated.

Aging is associated with a chronic state of inflammation that is not only present at the periphery but also in the central nervous system, as demonstrated for instance by the enhanced expression of IL-6 and the reduced expression of IL-10 in aged mice. In accordance with this low level of chronic inflammation, aged mice were shown to be not only more sensitive to LPS-induced sickness but also to LPS-induced depressive-like behaviour. In both cases, aged mice did not differ from young adults by their peak response to LPS but by the duration of the effect. In particular, the LPS-induced depressive-like behaviour that was observable at 24 hour post-LPS in young adult mice was of the same intensity in aged mice. However, it was still apparent at 72 hour post-LPS in aged but not in young adult mice (Godbout et al. 2007).

If these behavioural changes that are supposed to be indicative of depression based on the previously delineated animal models of depression have anything to do with depression, they should be reversed by antidepressant pre-treatment. This has been tested in the case of LPS-induced depressive-like behaviour (Yirmiya et al. 1999) but not yet for BCG-induced-depressive-like behaviour.

Is there an involvement of cytokines in depression independently of any immune activation?

So far the discussion on cytokines and depression has been limited to those cases in which cytokines are induced by pathogen-associated molecular patterns. To put this in perspective, it is important to keep in mind that proinflammatory cytokines are not supposed to be produced in baseline conditions, in the absence of any activation of the innate immune system. However, this applies only to phagocytic cells at the periphery and glial cells in the central nervous system, whereas other cells such as neurons can express relatively low levels of proinflammatory cytokines at baseline. In a very schematic manner it is possible to contrast an inducible compartment of cytokines that would be mainly glial with a constitutive compartment of cytokines that would be mainly neuronal (Dantzer, 2007). Constitutively expressed cytokines are supposed to play a key role in neuronal plasticity. Although it involves constitutive glial TNFα instead of neuronal TNFα, a good example of this is provided by the phenomenon of synaptic scaling (Stellwagen and Malenka, 2006). Inhibition of neuronal activity by tetrodotoxin in rat hippocampal slices leads to a compensatory increase in the number of a-amino-3-hydroxy-5-methyl-4-isoxazole propionic acid (AMPA) receptors on the membrane of neurons that is mediated by the release of TNFα by adjoining glial cells. A similar phenomenon involving the nuclear factor-kappa B signalling pathway has been evidenced in the glutamatergic neuromuscular junction of the drosophila (Heckscher et al. 2007), indicating that this role of cytokines is probably phylogenetically ancient.

In general, the constitutive and the inducible compartments of proinflammatory cytokines exert opposite roles. For instance, in the case of learning and memory, constitutive IL-1β promotes hippocampal-dependent memory whereas inducible IL-1β impairs it (Goshen et al. 2007).

In the case of depression, however, the available evidence indicates that if constitutively expressed cytokines play any role, this role is identical to that of inducible cytokines, that is, both forms of cytokines promote the development of depressive-like behaviour.

Neuronal expression of the proinflammatory cytokine TNFα has been proposed to play a pivotal role in the mechanism of the antidepressant efficacy of desipramine, which is usually attributed to its ability to increase synaptic concentrations of norepinephrine. According to Spengler and colleagues, the increased noradrenergic neurotransmission induced by desipramine would be secondary to what they originally presented as an increased expression of neuronal TNFα based on Northern blot analysis (Ignatowski and Spengler, 1994) before re-qualifying it as a decreased expression of this cytokine in neurons based on immunohistochemistry (Ignatowski et al. 1997) and in situ hybridization data (Nickola et al. 2001; Reynolds et al. 2005). The proposed mechanism for this effect is that desipramine would block the physiological inhibition exerted by neuronal TNFα on the release of norepinephrine (Reynolds et al. 2004; 2005).

In a series of elegant experiments conducted with IL-1-deficient mice that were chosen either for their lack of the type I IL-1 receptor or for their excessive production of IL-1RA, Yirmiya and colleagues showed that chronic mild stress was no longer able to induce depressive-like behaviours, including decreased sucrose preference, reduced social exploration, and increased adrenocortical activation (Goshen et al. 2008). Chronic administration of IL-1β in wild-type mice was used in these experiments to control for the depressogenic-like effects of immune activation. In a different series of experiments built along the same line of reasoning, Koo and Duman (Koo and Duman, 2008) observed that blocking the type I IL-1 receptor by administration of IL-1RA or use of type I IL-1 receptor-deficient mice blocked the anhedonic effects of chronic mild stress. It could be argued that there is nothing exceptional there since stressors are known to activate proinflammatory cytokine production although the exact conditions under which this can happen especially when the stress is chronic are still unclear. Although an obvious candidate is increased permeability of the gut mucosal barrier leading to bacterial translocation, this possibility remains to be tested.

A role for constitutive TNFα in depression has been proposed using relatively rudimentary behavioural phenotyping approaches of TNFα receptor knockout mice. Deletion of TNFR1 that is necessary for TNFα-induced sickness behaviour (Palin et al. 2007) leads to an antidepressant phenotype in the forced swim test and to decreased fear conditioning (Simen et al. 2006). TNFR2 deficiency that does not impact on TNFa-induced sickness behaviour had similar consequences in the forced swim test and increased appetence for sucrose.

IL-6 has also been reported to be upregulated in the brains, plasma and cerebrospinal fluid of depressed patients (Maes et al. 1995), while antidepressant treatment normalized IL-6 expression (Benedetti et al. 2002; Frommberger et al. 1997). Using a similar behavioural phenotyping approach as the one described above (Simen et al. 2006), Chourbaji and colleagues demonstrated that IL-6-deficient mice exhibit an antidepressant phenotype characterized by reduced behavioural despair during the forced swim and tail suspension tests. These mice also display reduced fear conditioning and heightened hedonic behaviour as measured by a two-bottle sucrose preference paradigm (Chourbaji et al. 2006). The potential importance of IL-6 in depression is likely context specific, however, because acute induction of depressive-like behaviours by restraint stress or direct administration of IL-1β, IL-6, or LPS results in a similar induction of depressive-like behaviours in both WT and IL-6-deficient mice (Swiergiel and Dunn, 2006). Although, this particular study tested the mice within the first 2 hours after stress or immune activation, so a role for IL-6-inducing depressive behaviours at a later time or following chronic treatments remains possible.

Mechanisms of the depression-inducing effects of cytokines and the role of tryptophan metabolites

The observation that major depression or depressive symptoms are often accompanied by changes in the proinflammatory cytokine profile has become fairly well accepted. Numerous clinical and experimental studies have reported observations linking proinflammatory processes to depression and depressive symptoms. However, for a number of reasons, the molecular mechanisms by which cytokines may causally contribute to or precipitate depression in patients remain poorly understood. Given current technology and ethical limitations, analysis of samples from depressed patients is limited to those that can be obtained either relatively non-invasively, including blood or in some cases cerebrospinal fluid or postmortem. The utilization of animal (mostly rodent) models of depression has recently provided a great deal of insight into the potential molecular actions of cytokines in depression.

One currently favoured hypothesis of how proinflammatory cytokines can induce depression is by disrupting synaptic plasticity and neurogenesis. Imaging studies and postmortem brain analysis have revealed atrophy of the prefrontal cortex and reduced hippocampal volume in depressed patients (Sheline et al. 1996), some of which are reversed by antidepressant treatment (Czeh et al. 2001). In the Koo and Duman study cited above, the anhedonic behaviour induced by acute foot shock stress or intracerebroventricular administration of IL-1β was accompanied by a reduction in hippocampal cell proliferation (neurogenesis). Moreover, inhibition of IL-1 receptor activation not only prevented the anhedonia but also restored hippocampal neurogenesis (Koo and Duman, 2008). While this recent finding supports a potential role for IL-1β in mediating both hippocampal neurogenesis and the onset of anhedonic behaviour, it is not clear at present what the true role is, if there is one, of adult neurogenesis in the development of depression.

Postulates claiming an essential role of neurogenesis in depressive pathophysiology have largely been based on studies showing that neurogenesis and the induction of brain neurotrophins, such as brain-derived neurotrophic factor (BDNF), VGF nerve growth factor, vascular endothelial growth factor (VEGF), and insulin-like growth factor (IGF)-I are consistently associated with antidepressant effects. In fact, focal X-ray irradiation of the hippocampus in mice prevented both the neurogenic and behavioural antidepressant effects of fluoxetine and imipramine indicating a necessary role of neurogenesis (Santarelli et al. 2003). The antidepressant effects of exercise have also been shown to be dependent on the upregulation of VGF nerve growth factor (Hunsberger et al. 2007) and BDNF (Duman et al. 2008). Direct administration of VGF nerve growth factor (Hunsberger et al. 2007), IGF-I or BDNF (Hoshaw et al. 2005) elicits behavioural changes in rodents that are reminiscent of antidepressant activity. While the vast majority of these studies have been conducted in laboratory animals, a recent meta-analysis confirmed the observation of abnormally low serum BDNF levels in patients suffering from major depressive disorder and the normalization of these levels following antidepressant treatment (Sen et al. 2008).

Interestingly, the antagonism between proinflammatory cytokines and growth factors has been recognized for some years now, but this has been done outside the context of depression. Proinflammatory cytokines, including IL-1β and TNFα antagonize the cell survival and proliferative properties of growth factors (Broussard et al. 2004; Shen et al. 2004; Strle et al. 2004). Induction of these cytokines either by immune activation, or direct administration of the cytokines themselves, precipitates depressive-like behaviour in rodents (Dantzer et al. 2008b). Conversely, administration of exogenous growth factors overcomes cytokine-induced sickness behaviour and altered spatial memory in a Y maze (Bluthe et al. 2005; 2006). A potential mechanism by which proinflammatory cytokines may impair growth factor function is by inducing a state of 'resistance' that probably occurs at the level of cellular signalling pathways (O'Connor et al. 2008b). While these molecular interactions are very well characterized in diseases like type 2 diabetes, our understanding of the signalling pathways that underlie these cytokine-growth factor interactions in depression remain in its infancy, even if there is some evidence to point to the mitogen-activated protein kinase (MAPK) and stress-activated protein kinase (SAPK) pathways as likely targets (Malemud and Miller, 2008; Palin et al. 2008). The controversies around this area are discussed in Chapter 11 of this book.

Upregulation of the tryptophan degrading enzyme indoleamine 2,3-dioxygenase (IDO) is another molecular mechanism that has been postulated to mediate depression precipitated by proinflammatory cytokines (Fig. 10.2). Clinical observations made over the past 25 years within a wide range of contexts (e.g. major depressive disorders [Maes et al. 1995], HIV comorbid depression [Fuchs et al. 1990], and depression precipitated by cytokine immunotherapy [Capuron et al. 2002; Wichers et al. 2005; and Chapter 17 in this book]) have found an association between reduced circulating tryptophan levels and major depressive disorders. The reduced levels of tryptophan are often accompanied by an increase in kynurenine that is the main metabolite of tryptophan. Furthermore depression scores correlated in some instances with increases in serum kynurenine/tryptophan ratio (Capuron et al. 2002; Wichers et al. 2005). IDO is well known to be inducible by proinflammatory cytokines, like IFNγ and TNFα, and evidence of IDO activation can be found in a number of neuroinflammatory and neurodegenerative diseases. The problem with all these data is that they are only suggestive but not demonstrative of a possible role of IDO in mediating cytokine-induced depression.

Although IDO has been mainly studied for its role in immune tolerance there is a wealth of research on the consequences of IDO activation on brain functions. IDO is the first and rate-limiting enzyme that degrades tryptophan along the kynurenine pathway. IDO is ubiquitously expressed in extrahepatic tissues including the brain. This enzyme is activated during pathological conditions by proinflammatory cytokines. Because of its situation within the metabolic pathway of tryptophan, increased IDO activity has the capacity to influence a number of neuroactive pathways that may contribute to the development of depression. Tryptophan is the biosynthetic precursor for the synthesis of serotonin (5-HT), and increased degradation of tryptophan along

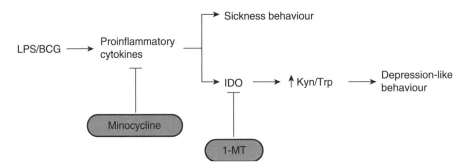

Fig. 10.2 Immune activation induces the production of proinflammatory cytokines responsible for inducing both sickness behaviours and the tryptophan degrading enzyme indoleamine 2,3 dioxygenase (IDO). Activation of IDO results in an increase in the kynurenine/tryptophan ratio. Indirect inhibition of IDO with the anti-inflammatory tetracycline antibiotic, minocycline, or directly with the competitive inhibitor, 1-methyltryptophan normalizes the kynurenine/tryptophan ratio and prevents the development of depression-like behaviours. Reprinted by permission from Macmillan Publishers Ltd *Nature Reviews Neuroscience* Jan; 9(1):46-56 2008.

the alternative kynurenine pathway has been postulated to reduce the availability of this ami-noacid for serotonin synthesis. Additionally, the kynurenine pathway generates several other neuroactive tryptophan metabolites that can act outside of the serotoninergic system. Most notably, kynurenine is further metabolized into 3-hydroxykynurenine (3HK) en route to the formation of quinolinic acid (QA) and NAD+. Kynurenine can also be metabolized along a second route that ends with the formation of kynurenic acid (KA). Increased levels of QA can be excitotoxic via activation of NMDA receptors and the generation of free radicals. Conversely, KA at high concentrations antagonizes both ionotropic NMDA and α7 nicotinic acetylcholine receptors. 3-HK does not appear to interact with a specific receptor; rather, its neural-damaging properties are via free radical generation (Schwarcz and Pellicciari, 2002).

The role of increased kynurenine pathway metabolism has been most heavily studied in the context of neuronal death and neurodegenerative diseases. However, recent experimental studies have begun to substantiate a pivotal role of increased IDO metabolism in the pathogenesis of cytokine-induced depression. As discussed previously, models of acute (LPS) (Frenois et al. 2007; O'Connor et al. 2008) or chronic (BCG) (Moreau et al. 2008) immune activation have now been used to dissociate early sickness behaviours from depressive-like behaviours that develop later and can persist for several weeks. In both cases, the occurrence of depressive-like behaviours occurs simultaneously with a profound increase in proinflammatory cytokine and IDO expression. This increase in IDO expression translates into heightened IDO enzymatic activ-ity and elevated kynurenine/tryptophan ratios similar to those observed in depressed patients. Moreover, when aged rodents were challenged with LPS, not only was the resultant depressive-like behavioural response more persistent than in LPS-treated young mice, but also upregulation of proinflammatory cytokines and IDO activity was markedly higher in the aged mice (Godbout et al. 2007). These experimental data strongly implicated IDO upregulation in the development of depressive-like behaviours.

Not until more recent experiments, however, where either the IDO inducing cytokines or IDO itself have been targeted was a causal effect for IDO established. Two independent labo-ratories have conduced experimental studies targeting IDO upregulation indirectly using the anti-inflammatory tetracycline, minocycline. Minocycline is particularly well suited for use in these studies as it readily enters the brain and potently suppresses production of IDO-inducing proinflammatory cytokines. Indeed, minocycline pre-treatment of mice prior to acute periph-eral immune activation with LPS attenuated the upregulation of IDO, normalized the increased kynurenine/tryptophan ratio, and prevented the development of depressive-like behaviours (increased immobility during the forced swim and tail suspension tests or anhedonia) (Henry et al. 2008; O'Connor et al. 2008). In a similar set of studies, the BCG model of chronic inflam-mation induced depressive-like behaviour developed by Moreau and colleagues (Moreau et al. 2008) was employed in either WT control mice, mice pre-treated with the TNFα-binding protein, etanercept, and mice lacking functional type 1 IFNγ receptors. As expected BCG precipitated the development of depressive-like behaviours in mice; however, specifically targeting the IDO-inducing proinflammatory cytokine TNFα attenuated both the IDO and behavioural responses (O'Connor et al. 2009a). IFNγ receptor deficient mice altogether failed to develop BCG-induced upregulation of IDO and depressive-like behaviours (O'Connor et al. 2009a).

Indoleamine 2,3-dioxygenase can be directly inhibited in vivo using a competitive inhibi-tor, 1-methyltryptophan (1-MT). This inhibitor was chronically administered in the form of a subcutaneously implanted pellet prior to LPS challenge (O'Connor et al. 2008). Mice with the 1-MT pellet displayed a normal acute sickness response, yet they failed to develop depressive-like behaviours. In a similar series of studies in BCG inoculated mice, 1-MT pre-treatment or genetic deletion of IDO both normalized the kynurenine/tryptophan ratio and prevented the

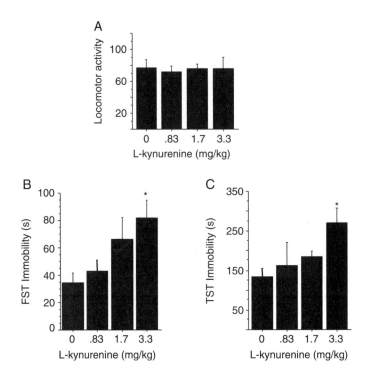

Fig. 10.3 The IDO generated tryptophan metabolite, L-kynurenine, dose-dependently induces depression-like behaviour without affecting general locomotor activity in the absence of peripheral immune activation. Mice were injected intraperitoneally with increasing doses of L-kynurenine, and behavioural testing was carried out 2 hours later. Reprinted by permission from Macmillan Publishers Ltd *Molecular Psychiatry* Jan 15 2008.

development of depressive-like behaviours (O'Connor et al. 2008). Of note, while both acute and chronic peripheral immune activation reduced circulating tryptophan no evidence was found to suggest that brain 5-HT levels were subsequently affected (O'Connor et al. 2009b; O'Connor et al. 2008). Rather, direct peripheral administration of L-kynurenine, without immune activation, dose-dependently induced depressive-like behaviours, supporting a direct role for tryptophan metabolites in the development of depressive behaviours (O'Connor et al. 2008) (Fig. 10.3). These results do not exclude the possible role of other factors such as the activating effects of proinflammatory cytokines on the serotonin transporter (Zhu et al. 2006). However, they clearly point to a pivotal role of IDO activation in mediating cytokine-induced depression probably via the production of neuroactive kynurenine metabolites (Schwarcz and Pellicciari, 2002).

Conclusion

Enough evidence has accumulated during the last ten years or so to accept the fact that proinflammatory cytokines play a pathogenic role in the development of major depressive disorders associated with inflammation and that the degradation of tryptophan along the kynurenine pathway is certainly a pivotal contributing factor to this phenomenon. Several issues are still at stake, from the role of these mechanisms in non-immune-mediated depressive disorders to the respective importance of peripheral versus the central production of tryptophan metabolites.

At the conceptual level, it is obvious that there is no single theory to account for the many facets of the biological psychiatry of major depressive disorders and the (relative) efficacy of antidepressant treatments. Impaired neurogenesis and its consequences on hippocampal volume is the latest a-la-mode theory. Its unrestricted diffusion and popularization has led to the point that some researchers and professionals are tempted to see depression as the result of a shrinkage of the hippocampus in the same way as Parkinson's disease is caused by a gradual disappearance of the dopaminergic cell bodies in the substantia nigra. Scientific research cannot ignore popular representations. Any new molecular factor is immediately gauged with reference to fashionable theories. As we have discussed above, this applies to growth factors that promote neurogenesis and therefore mediate antidepressant activity as well as to cytokines that inhibit neurogenesis and therefore promote depression. A spoon of cortisol resistance on top of this makes the plate even more palatable especially since chronic inflammation can induce glucocorticoid resistance (Miller et al. 2005; Pace et al. 2007). However, since old recipes have not provided anything revolutionary in the field of depression, it is important to question whether reviving them via the consequences of cytokine expression and action in the brain is a worthwhile enterprise. A paradigmatic shift would certainly be more appropriate and at least there is nothing much there to lose.

Concerning the role of immune versus non-immune processes at the origin of a role of cytokines in depression, we have made clear in the present chapter that the evidence in favour of a causal relationship between inflammation and depression is mainly based on studies assessing the functional consequences of immune activation. The evidence for a possible role of non-immune factors is still very limited and non-conclusive. It would be therefore very premature to make the cytokine signalling theory a universal theory of depression. It is important to note en passant that this issue applies as well to the role of cytokines in other symptoms associated with inflammation, from fatigue to pain and sleep disorders (Dantzer et al. 2008a; Speciale et al. 1989).

Al contrario, the above cautionary note should not act as a deterrent for this type of research but rather favour the consideration of a possible involvement of immune factors in conditions that apparently lack any obvious immune component. To take just one example, there is no obvious reason why the increased prevalence of depression that is observed in adults having a history of childhood maltreatment should be associated with a pattern of elevated inflammatory biomarkers (Danese et al. 2007; 2008). However, there is an increasing body of literature showing that maternal deprivation in rats induces gut permeability (Barreau et al. 2007). In addition, this effect as well as some of the pathophysiological consequences of maternal separation can be alleviated by probiotic treatment of rat pups (Eutamene et al. 2007; Garcia-Rodenas et al. 2006; Gareau et al. 2007). Bacterial translocation plays certainly a crucial role in this phenomenon (Caso et al. 2008). Together with the observation that immune stimulation at an early age can alter programming of the neuroendocrine and immune systems (Karrow, 2006), this is certainly sufficient to call for a re-examination of the gut-brain axis in the pathophysiology of major depressive disorders (Maes et al. 2008).

The demonstration of the causative role of immune factors in the pathophysiology of depression calls for a re-examination of the temptation of locating the putative mechanisms of depression exclusively in the brain. If it is clear that the ultimate target is the brain it does not mean that the causal mechanisms originate in the brain. Besides the gut-brain axis mentioned in the previous paragraph, the generation of tryptophan metabolites by IDO activation is much more abundant at the periphery than in the brain so that the molecular factors that are ultimately causing depression can actually be generated at the periphery and enter the brain by diffusion or active transport. The avidity with which glial cells uptake kynurenine (Speciale et al. 1989) is certainly an important factor to be considered in respect to this possibility and further studies are clearly needed to clarify these aspects.

Acknowledgements

Supported by NIH grants to KWK (R01 MH 051569 and R01 AG 029573) and RD (R01 MH 071349 and R01 MH 079829).

References

Andreakos, E., Foxwell, B. and Feldmann, M. (2004). Is targeting Toll-like receptors and their signaling pathway a useful therapeutic approach to modulating cytokine-driven inflammation? *Immunol Rev.*, **202**, 250–265.

Barreau, F., Cartier, C., Leveque, M. et al. (2007). Pathways involved in gut mucosal barrier dysfunction induced in adult rats by maternal deprivation: corticotrophin-releasing factor and nerve growth factor interplay. *J Physiol.*, **580**, 347–356.

Benedetti, F., Lucca, A., Brambilla, F., Colombo, C., and Smeraldi, E. (2002). Interleukine-6 serum levels correlate with response to antidepressant sleep deprivation and sleep phase advance. *Prog Neuropsychopharmacol Biol Psychiatry*, **26**, 1167–1170.

Blatteis, C.M. (2007). The onset of fever: new insights into its mechanism. *Prog Brain Res.*, **162**, 3–14.

Bluthe, R.M., Frenois, F., Kelley, K.W., and Dantzer, R. (2005). Pentoxifylline and insulin-like growth factor-I (IGF-I) abrogate kainic acid-induced cognitive impairment in mice. *J Neuroimmunol.*, **169**, 50–58.

Bluthe, R.M., Kelley, K.W., and Dantzer, R. (2006). Effects of insulin-like growth factor-I on cytokine-induced sickness behavior in mice. *Brain Behav Immun.*, **20**, 57–63.

Bower, J.E. (2007). Cancer-related fatigue: links with inflammation in cancer patients and survivors. *Brain Behav Immun.*, **21**, 863–871.

Broussard, S.R., Mccusker, R.H., Novakofski, J.E. et al. (2004). IL-1beta impairs insulin-like growth factor i-induced differentiation and downstream activation signals of the insulin-like growth factor i receptor in myoblasts. *J Immunol.*, **172**, 7713–7720.

Buwalda, B., Kole, M.H., Veenema, A.H. et al. (2005). Long-term effects of social stress on brain and behavior: a focus on hippocampal functioning. *Neurosci Biobehav Rev.*, **29**, 83–97.

Capuron, L., Ravaud, A., Neveu, P. J., Miller, A.H., Maes, M., and Dantzer, R. (2002). Association between decreased serum tryptophan concentrations and depressive symptoms in cancer patients undergoing cytokine therapy. *Mol Psychiatry*, **7**, 468–473.

Caso, J.R., Leza, J.C. and Menchen, L. (2008). The effects of physical and psychological stress on the gastro-intestinal tract: lessons from animal models. *Curr Mol Med*, **8**, 299–312.

Chourbaji, S., Urani, A., Inta, I. et al. (2006). IL-6 knockout mice exhibit resistance to stress-induced development of depression-like behaviors. *Neurobiol Dis.*, **23**, 587–594.

Czeh, B., Michaelis, T., Watanabe, T. et al. (2001). Stress-induced changes in cerebral metabolites, hippocampal volume, and cell proliferation are prevented by antidepressant treatment with tianeptine. *Proc Natl Acad Sci USA*, **98**, 12796–12801.

Danese, A., Pariante, C.M., Caspi, A., Taylor, A., and Poulton, R. (2007). Childhood maltreatment predicts adult inflammation in a life-course study. *Proc Natl Acad Sci USA*, **104**, 1319–1324.

Danese, A., Moffitt, T.E., Pariante, C.M., Ambler, A., Poulton, R., and Caspi, A. (2008). Elevated inflammation levels in depressed adults with a history of childhood maltreatment. *Arch Gen Psychiatry*, **65**, 409–415.

Dantzer, R. (2007). Expression and action of cytokines in the brain: Mechanisms and pathophysiological implications. In Ader, R. (Ed.) *Psychoneuroimmunology 4th Edition.* Amsterdam, Elsevier.

Dantzer, R. and Kelley, K.W. (2007). Twenty years of research on cytokine-induced sickness behavior. *Brain Behav Immun.*, **21**, 153–160.

Dantzer, R., Bluthe, R., Castanon, N. (2007). Cytokines, sickness behavior, and depression. In Ader, R. (ed.) *Psychoneuroimmunology 4th Edition.* Amsterdam, Elsevier.

Dantzer, R., Capuron, L., Irwin, M.R. et al. (2008a). Identification and treatment of symptoms associated with inflammation in medically ill patients. *Psychoneuroendocrinology, 33,* 18–29.

Dantzer, R., O'Connor, J.C., Freund, G.G., Johnson, R.W., and Kelley, K.W. (2008b). From inflammation to sickness and depression: when the immune system subjugates the brain. *Nat Rev Neurosci., 9,* 46–56.

Dhawan, K.N., Jaju, B.P., and Gupta, G.P. (1970). Validity of antagonism of different effects of reserpine as test for anti-depressant activity. *Psychopharmacologia., 18,* 94–98.

Duman, C.H., Schlesinger, L., Russell, D.S., and Duman, R.S. (2008). Voluntary exercise produces antidepressant and anxiolytic behavioral effects in mice. *Brain Res., 1199,* 148–158.

Dunn, A. J. (2002). Mechanisms by which cytokines signal the brain. *Int Rev Neurobiol., 52,* 43–65.

Eutamene, H., Lamine, F., Chabo, C. et al. (2007). Synergy between Lactobacillus paracasei and its bacterial products to counteract stress-induced gut permeability and sensitivity increase in rats. *J Nutr., 137,* 1901–1907.

Frenois, F., Moreau, M., O'Connor, J. et al. (2007). Lipopolysaccharide induces delayed FosB/DeltaFosB immunostaining within the mouse extended amygdala, hippocampus and hypothalamus, that parallel the expression of depressive-like behavior. *Psychoneuroendocrinology, 32,* 516–531.

Frommberger, U.H., Bauer, J., Haselbauer, P., Fraulin, A., Riemann, D., and Berger, M. (1997). Interleukin-6-(IL-6) plasma levels in depression and schizophrenia: comparison between the acute state and after remission. *Eur Arch Psychiatry Clin Neurosci., 247,* 228–233.

Fuchs, D., Moller, A.A., Reibnegger, G., Stockle, E., Werner, E.R., and Wachter, H. (1990). Decreased serum tryptophan in patients with HIV-1 infection correlates with increased serum neopterin and with neurologic/psychiatric symptoms. *J Acquir Immune Defic Syndr., 3,* 873–876.

Garcia-Rodenas, C.L., Bergonzelli, G.E., Nutten, S. et al. (2006). Nutritional approach to restore impaired intestinal barrier function and growth after neonatal stress in rats. *J Pediatr Gastroenterol Nutr., 43,* 16–24.

Gareau, M.G., Jury, J., Macqueen, G., Sherman, P.M., and Perdue, M.H. (2007). Probiotic treatment of rat pups normalises corticosterone release and ameliorates colonic dysfunction induced by maternal separation. *Gut, 56,* 1522–1528.

Godbout, J.P., Moreau, M., Lestage, J. et al. (2007). Aging exacerbates depressive-like behavior in mice in response to activation of the peripheral innate immune system. *Neuropsychopharmacology 33,* 2341–2351.

Goshen, I., Kreisel, T., Ounallah-Saad, H. et al. (2007). A dual role for interleukin-1 in hippocampal-dependent memory processes. *Psychoneuroendocrinology, 32,* 1106–1115.

Goshen, I., Kreisel, T., Ben-Menachem-Zidon, O. et al. (2008). Brain interleukin-1 mediates chronic stress-induced depression in mice via adrenocortical activation and hippocampal neurogenesis suppression. *Mol Psychiatry, 13,* 717–728.

Hansen, R.A., Gartlehner, G., Lohr, K.N., Gaynes, B.N., and Carey, T.S. (2005). Efficacy and safety of second-generation antidepressants in the treatment of major depressive disorder. *Ann Intern Med.,* s143, 415–426.

Hart, B.L. (1988). Biological basis of the behavior of sick animals. *Neurosci Biobehav Rev., 12,* 123–137.

Hayley, S. and Anisman, H. (2005). Multiple mechanisms of cytokine action in neurodegenerative and psychiatric states: neurochemical and molecular substrates. *Curr Pharm Des., 11,* 947–962.

Heckscher, E.S., Fetter, R.D., Marek, K.W., Albin, S.D., and Davis, G.W. (2007). NF-kappaB, IkappaB, and IRAK control glutamate receptor density at the Drosophila NMJ. *Neuron., 55,* 859–873.

Henry, C.J., Huang, Y., Wynne, A. et al. (2008). Minocycline attenuates lipopolysaccharide (LPS)-induced neuroinflammation, sickness behavior, and anhedonia. *J Neuroinflammation, 5,* 15.

Hoshaw, B.A., Malberg, J.E., and Lucki, I. (2005). Central administration of IGF-I and BDNF leads to long-lasting antidepressant-like effects. *Brain Res., 1037,* 204–208.

Hunsberger, J.G., Newton, S.S., Bennett, A.H. et al. (2007). Antidepressant actions of the exercise-regulated gene VGF. *Nat Med.*, **13**, 1476–1482.

Ignatowski, T.A. and Spengler, R.N. (1994). Tumor necrosis factor-alpha: presynaptic sensitivity is modified after antidepressant drug administration. *Brain Res.*, **665**, 293–299.

Ignatowski, T.A., Noble, B.K., Wright, J.R., Gorfien, J.L., Heffner, R.R., and Spengler, R.N. (1997). Neuronal-associated tumor necrosis factor (TNF alpha): its role in noradrenergic functioning and modification of its expression following antidepressant drug administration. *J Neuroimmunol.*, **79**, 84–90.

Karrow, N.A. (2006). Activation of the hypothalamic-pituitary-adrenal axis and autonomic nervous system during inflammation and altered programming of the neuroendocrine-immune axis during fetal and neonatal development: lessons learned from the model inflammagen, lipopolysaccharide. *Brain Behav Immun.*, **20**, 144–158.

Kluger, M.J. (1978). The evolution and adaptive value of fever. *Am Sci*, **66**, 38–43.

Koo, J.W. and Duman, R.S. (2008). IL-1beta is an essential mediator of the antineurogenic and anhedonic effects of stress. *Proc Natl Acad Sci USA*, **105**, 751–756.

Maes, M., Smith, R., and Scharpe, S. (1995). The monocyte-T-lymphocyte hypothesis of major depression. *Psychoneuroendocrinology*, **20**, 111–116.

Maes, M., Kubera, M., and Leunis, J.C. (2008). The gut-brain barrier in major depression: intestinal mucosal dysfunction with an increased translocation of LPS from gram negative enterobacteria (leaky gut) plays a role in the inflammatory pathophysiology of depression. *Neuro Endocrinol Lett.*, **29**, 117–124.

Maier, S. F. (1984). Learned helplessness and animal models of depression. *Prog Neuropsychopharmacol Biol Psychiatry*, **8**, 435–446.

Malemud, C.J. and Miller, A.H. (2008). Pro-inflammatory cytokine-induced SAPK/MAPK and JAK/STAT in rheumatoid arthritis and the new anti-depression drugs. *Expert Opin Ther Targets*, **12**, 171–183.

Miller, G.E., Rohleder, N., Stetler, C., and Kirschbaum, C. (2005). Clinical depression and regulation of the inflammatory response during acute stress. *Psychosom Med.*, **67**, 679–687.

Moreau, M., Andre, C., O'Connor, J.C. et al. (2008). Inoculation of Bacillus Calmette-Guerin to mice induces an acute episode of sickness behavior followed by chronic depressive-like behavior. *Brain Behav Immun.*, **22**, 1087–1095.

Nickola, T.J., Ignatowski, T.A., Reynolds, J.L., and Spengler, R.N. (2001). Antidepressant drug-induced alterations in neuron-localized tumor necrosis factor-alpha mRNA and alpha(2)-adrenergic receptor sensitivity. *J Pharmacol Exp Ther.*, **297**, 680–687.

O'Connor, J.C., Lawson, M.A., Andre, C. et al. (2008). Lipopolysaccharide-induced depressive-like behavior is mediated by indoleamine 2,3-dioxygenase activation in mice. *Mol Psychiatry, doi*: 10.1038/sj.mp.4002148.

O'Connor, J.C., André, C., Wang, Y. et al. (2009a). Interferon-γ and tumor necrosis factor-α mediate the upregulation of indoleamine 2,3- dioxygenase and the induction of depressive-like behaviour in mice in response to Bacillus Calmette-Guérin. *J Neurosci*, Accepted for Publication.

O'Connor, J.C., Lawson, M.A., André, C. et al. (2009b). Induction of IDO by bacille Calmete-Guérin is responsible for development of murine depressive-like behaviour. *J Immunol*, **182**, 3202–3212.

Pace, T. W., Hu, F., and Miller, A.H. (2007). Cytokine-effects on glucocorticoid receptor function: relevance to glucocorticoid resistance and the pathophysiology and treatment of major depression. *Brain Behav Immun.*, **21**, 9–19.

Palin, K., Bluthe, R.M., McCusker, R.H., Moos. F., Dantzer, R., and Kelley, K.W. (2007). TNF alpha-induced sickness behaviour in mice with functional 55 kD TNF receptors is blocked by central IGF-1 *J Neuroimmunol*, **187**, 55–60.

Palin, K., Mccusker, R.H., Strle, K., Moos, F., Dantzer, R., and Kelley, K.W. (2008). Tumor necrosis factor-alpha-induced sickness behavior is impaired by central administration of an inhibitor of c-jun N-terminal kinase. *Psychopharmacology (Berl)*, **197**, 629–635.

Raison, C.L., Capuron, L., and Miller, A.H. (2006). Cytokines sing the blues: inflammation and the pathogenesis of depression. *Trends Immunol., 27,* 24–31.

Raison, C.L., Demetrashvili, M., Capuron, L., and Miller, A.H. (2005). Neuropsychiatric adverse effects of interferon-alpha: recognition and management. *CNS Drugs, 19,* 105–123.

Reynolds, J.L., Ignatowski, T.A., Sud, R., and Spengler, R.N. (2004). Brain-derived tumor necrosis factor-alpha and its involvement in noradrenergic neuron functioning involved in the mechanism of action of an antidepressant. *J Pharmacol Exp Ther., 310,* 1216–1225.

Reynolds, J.L., Ignatowski, T.A., Sud, R., and Spengler, R.N. (2005). An antidepressant mechanism of desipramine is to decrease tumor necrosis factor-alpha production culminating in increases in noradrenergic neurotransmission. *Neuroscience, 133,* 519–531.

Santarelli, L., Saxe, M., Gross, C. et al. (2003). Requirement of hippocampal neurogenesis for the behavioral effects of antidepressants. *Science, 301,* 805–809.

Schatzberg, A.F. and Kraemer, H.C. (2000). Use of placebo control groups in evaluating efficacy of treatment of unipolar major depression. *Biol Psychiatry, 47,* 736–744.

Schwarcz, R. and Pellicciari, R. (2002). Manipulation of brain kynurenines: glial targets, neuronal effects, and clinical opportunities. *J Pharmacol Exp Ther., 303,* 1–10.

Sen, S., Duman, R., and Sanacora, G. (2008). Serum brain-derived neurotrophic factor, depression, and antidepressant medications: meta-analyses and implications. *Biol Psychiatry, 64,* 527–532.

Sheline, Y.I., Wang, P.W., Gado, M.H., Csernansky, J.G., and Vannier, M.W. (1996). Hippocampal atrophy in recurrent major depression. *Proc Natl Acad Sci USA, 93,* 3908–3913.

Shen, W.H., Zhou, J.H., Broussard, S.R., Johnson, R.W., Dantzer, R., and Kelley, K.W. (2004). Tumor necrosis factor alpha inhibits insulin-like growth factor I-induced hematopoietic cell survival and proliferation. *Endocrinology, 145,* 3101–3105.

Simen, B.B., Duman, C.H., Simen, A.A., and Duman, R.S. (2006). TNFalpha signaling in depression and anxiety: behavioral consequences of individual receptor targeting. *Biol Psychiatry., 59,* 775–785.

Song, C. and Leonard, B.E. (2005). The olfactory bulbectomised rat as a model of depression. *Neurosci Biobehav Rev., 29,* 627–647.

Speciale, C., Hares, K., Schwarcz, R., and Brookes, N. (1989). High-affinity uptake of L-kynurenine by a Na+-independent transporter of neutral amino acids in astrocytes. *J Neurosci., 9,* 2066–2072.

Stellwagen, D. and Malenka, R.C. (2006). Synaptic scaling mediated by glial TNF-alpha. *Nature, 440,* 1054–1059.

Strle, K., Broussard, S.R., Mccusker, R.H. et al. (2004). Proinflammatory cytokine impairment of insulin-like growth factor I-induced protein synthesis in skeletal muscle myoblasts requires ceramide. *Endocrinology, 145,* 4592–4602.

Swiergiel, A.H. and Dunn, A.J. (2006). Feeding, exploratory, anxiety- and depression-related behaviors are not altered in interleukin-6-deficient male mice. *Behav Brain Res., 171,* 94–108.

Wichers, M.C., Koek, G.H., Robaeys, G., Verkerk, R., Scharpe, S., and Maes, M. (2005). IDO and interferon-alpha-induced depressive symptoms: a shift in hypothesis from tryptophan depletion to neurotoxicity. *Mol Psychiatry, 10,* 538–544.

Willner, P. (1984). The validity of animal models of depression. *Psychopharmacology (Berl), 83,* 1–16.

Willner, P., Muscat, R., and Papp, M. (1992). Chronic mild stress-induced anhedonia: a realistic animal model of depression. *Neurosci Biobehav Rev., 16,* 525–534.

Yirmiya, R. (1996). Endotoxin produces a depressive-like episode in rats. *Brain Res., 711,* 163–174.

Yirmiya, R., Weidenfeld, J., Pollak, Y. et al. (1999). Cytokines, 'depression due to a general medical condition', and antidepressant drugs. *Adv Exp Med Biol., 461,* 283–316.

Zhu, C.B., Blakely, R.D., and Hewlett, W.A. (2006). The proinflammatory cytokines interleukin-1beta and tumor necrosis factor-alpha activate serotonin transporters. *Neuropsychopharmacology, 31,* 2121–2131.

Chapter 11

Do depression, stress, sleep disruption, and inflammation alter hippocampal apoptosis and neurogenesis?

Paul J. Lucassen, P. Meerlo, A.S. Naylor, A.M. van Dam, A.G. Dayer, B. Czeh, and Charlotte A. Oomen

We discuss the regulation of cellular plasticity, focusing on neurogenesis and apoptosis in the adult hippocampus, by stress, sleep, inflammation, and depression. This is the fourth of five chapters in this book that present not only clinical data but also experimental evidence from animal models relevant to the role of the hypothalamo-pituitary-adrenal (HPA) in affective disorders, together with Chapters 7, 8, 9, and 26. Moreover, this is the second of four chapters in this book that discuss the role of inflammation in affective disorders, together with Chapters 10, 16, and 17.

Stress

Stress represents an essential alarm system that is activated whenever a discrepancy occurs between an organism's expectation and the reality it encounters. Lack of information, loss of control, unpredictability, or psychosocial demands can all produce stress. The same holds for perturbations of a more biological nature, like blood loss, metabolic crises, or inflammation. Various sensory and cognitive signals then converge to activate a stress response that triggers several adaptive processes in the body and brain aimed at restoring homeostasis.

In mammals, the stress response develops through a rapid release of epinephrine and norepinephrine from the adrenal. These hormones elevate metabolic rate and redirect blood flow to vital organs like the heart and muscles. Shortly after, the limbic HPA system is activated, a classic neuroendocrine circuit in which limbic and hypothalamic brain structures integrate cognitive, neuroendocrine, and autonomic inputs and together determine the magnitude and duration of the organism's response to stress.

Stress-induced activation of the HPA axis involves the production of corticotropin-releasing hormone (CRH) in the hypothalamic paraventricular nucleus (PVN), which induces adrenocorticotropin hormone (ACTH) release from the anterior pituitary gland, which causes the release of glucocorticoids (GC) (cortisol in primates, corticosterone in rodents) from the adrenal cortex. When stress is prolonged, the stimulatory effect on ACTH release is potentiated through co-expression of vasopressin (AVP) by parvocellular CRH neurons.

Upon their release, GC mobilize energy and affect carbohydrate, lipid and mineral metabolism in the periphery. If stress becomes chronic, an imbalance may occur that can exert deleterious effects and induce, for example, muscle wasting and suppression of the immune system. Although fast effects have also been described (de Kloet et al. 2008), traditional GC effects involve slow genomic actions following activation of mineralocorticoid (MR) and glucocorticoid receptors (GR).

The MR has a high affinity for corticosterone and is highly expressed in the hippocampus, lateral septum, and amygdala. The GR has a tenfold lower affinity and is ubiquitously distributed, with enrichments in the hippocampus, PVN and pituitary, that is, the main feedback sites through which GCs regulate their own release. Also the amygdala and prefrontal cortex, a.o., modulate HPA feedback (de Kloet et al. 2005; Joels et al. 2007).

The degree of MR and GR occupation depends on circulating GC levels, that fluctuate over the day. During rest, GC levels are low and mainly activate MRs. After stress, GRs become activated as well. Given its high MR and GR levels, the hippocampus, at least in rat, is very sensitive to stress. It is also involved in emotional processing and cognition. Differences in MR/GR ratio influence gene expression and may alter electrophysiological properties of the hippocampus. While short-term exposure induces behavioural adaptation, prolonged stress exposure can alter HPA feedback responsivity, overexposing brain and body to aberrant GC levels. Such conditions represent risk factors for depression in susceptible individuals (de Kloet et al. 2005). Even though feedback is largely GR-mediated, chronic stress may also alter MR function that has been implicated in HPA axis inhibition and neurogenesis (Fischer et al. 2002; Gesing et al. 2001).

Major depression is presumed to result from an interaction between environmental stressors and genetic/developmental predispositions. Long-lasting hyper(re)activity of the CRH neurons, accompanied by an increased stress responsiveness and a glucocorticoid resistant state, is indeed common in depression (de Kloet et al. 2005; Swaab et al. 2005).

Stress effects on hippocampal function and structure

Although depressive disorders are traditionally considered to have a neurochemical basis, impairments of structural plasticity are likely involved as well (Fuchs et al. 2004; 2006). Hence, various studies have addressed the consequences of stress for hippocampal function as well as structure. Chronic stress is generally associated with reductions in hippocampal excitability, long-term potentiation, and hippocampal memory, but positive effects of stress on these parameters have also been described, that depend on the timing and type of stressor (Kim and Diamond, 2002; Joels et al. 2007).

After chronic stress, reductions in neuropil and hippocampal volume occur. Chronic psychosocial stress, for example, reduces hippocampal volume of tree shrews by approximately 10% (Czeh et al. 2001; Fuchs et al. 2004). Also in depression, numerous in vivo imaging studies report structural changes in the human prefrontal cortex and hippocampus. Moreover, duration of the depressive episode is closely paralleled by volumetric changes, with longer periods of depression generally corresponding to smaller hippocampi (Bremner, 2002; Campbell et al. 2004; Drevets, 2000; Drevets et al. 2003; MacQueen et al. 2003; Sheline, 2000, 2003).

Although chronic stress was previously reported to induce hippocampal neuronal loss particularly in the CA3 subregion (Sapolsky et al. 1990), more recent studies could not find massive loss of the principal hippocampal cells after chronic stress or chronic corticosteroid application in animals, nor in the hippocampus of depressed individuals (Lucassen et al. 2001; 2006; Lucassen and de Kloet, 2001; Muller et al. 2001; O'Brien et al. 2001; Sousa et al. 1998).

Major neuronal loss or massive apoptosis is thus not responsible for hippocampal volume changes after stress, consistent with observations that many of the stress-induced structural changes are reversible after appropriate recovery periods (Heine et al. 2004c). Therefore, volume changes must be derived from other factors. Candidate factors include: somatodendritic components, that will be discussed below, neurogenesis, an event that is sensitive to stress but likely occurs at very low rates in adult or elderly subjects (Boekhoorn et al. 2006; Eriksson et al. 1998; Manganas et al. 2007), and glial changes that may contribute to hippocampal shrinkage in stress-related disorders like depression (Czeh et al. 2006), while shifts in fluid balance cannot be excluded either, as discussed in detail elsewhere (Czeh and Lucassen, 2007).

Structural plasticity: stress effects on dendrites and synapes

The structural substrates for stress-induced functional alterations generally involve axonal changes, synaptic loss, alterations in postsynaptic densities, and dendritic reorganization. Chronic stress, or increased corticosterone levels, initially induce atrophy of the apical dendrites of the CA3 and to a lesser extent of CA1 cells and DG granule cells (Fuchs et al. 2006). Furthermore, (transient) alterations in CA3 synapses and mossy fibre terminals have been described (Sandi, 2004). This synaptic remodelling may also involve cortical areas, where changes in cell adhesion molecule expression, memory and fear conditioning often occur in parallel. Dendritic changes appear to occur early and are generally lasting (Sandi, 2004) but can grow or shrink depending on the brain region involved, even after a single or acute stressor (Alfarez et al. 2008; Mitra and Sapolsky, 2008). Concluding, effects of stress on hippocampal structure are relatively mild and subregion-specific and appear to occur already shortly after the onset of stress, but prior to cognitive disturbances.

Structural plasticity: stress and adult neurogenesis

Adult neurogenesis (AN) refers to the generation of new neurons in an adult brain. This special form of adult neuroplasticity occurs in the dentate gyrus (DG) of the hippocampal formation (Fig. 11.1) in many mammalian species (Zhao et al. 2008), including humans (Eriksson et al. 1998). In young adult rats thousands of new DG neurons are born every day (Oomen et al. 2007), but no quantitative data are yet available in humans. AN declines with age (Heine, 2004a; Manganas et al. 2007) and is dynamically regulated by numerous environmental factors. (Lucassen et al. 2008)

Neurogenesis also occurs in the subventricular zone (SVZ) of ventricle wall in many mammals but conflicting results are reported in humans (Curtis et al. 2007; Sanai et al. 2007). In this system, newborn neurons originating from the SVZ migrate long distances in the rostral migratory stream before reaching the olfactory bulb where they differentiate into functional neurons (Lledo and Saghatelyan, 2005).

In other brain structures such as the amygdala, striatum, and neocortex several independent groups have observed low levels of neurogenesis but negative results exist as well (Cameron and Dayer, 2008; Gould, 2007; Rakic, 2002). Part of the difficulty in studying AN in regions such as the neocortex could reside in the fact that new cortical neurons probably belong to small subclasses of interneurons dispersed in large neocortical volumes (Cameron and Dayer, 2008). Only new labelling methodologies will help resolve this ongoing controversy.

Adult neurogenesis is potently stimulated by exercise and enriched environment but inhibited by stress and GC exposure (Van Praag et al. 1999; Brown et al. 2003; Naylor et al. 2005; Oomen et al. 2007). Both psychosocial (Dong et al. 2004; Gould et al. 1997; Tanapat et al. 2001) and physical stressors (Heine et al. 2004c; Malberg and Duman, 2003; Pham et al. 2003; Veenema et al. 2007; Vollmayr et al. 2003) all inhibit one or more phases of the neurogenesis process.

After birth, newly generated neurons undergo a process of competitive selection that will determine their successful integration in the existing hippocampal network. Although AN is extensive in the adult rat, about half of the newborn cells die within one month under normal laboratory conditions (Dayer et al. 2003). The surviving new neurons integrate in the existing hippocampal circuitry and two months after birth they continue to modify their synaptic connectivity.

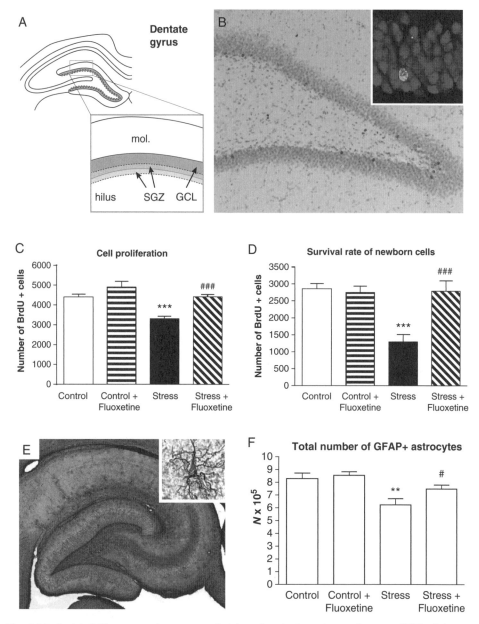

Fig. 11.1 A: Adult hippocampal neurogenesis takes place in the subgranular zone (SGZ) of the DG adjacent to the granule cell layer (GCL). B: Newborn granule cells (brown) in the rat DG. Insert in B shows a confocal image of a double labelled cell: red reflects mature neurons (NeuN), green-yellow is the proliferative marker BrdU labelling a newly generated neuron. C–D: Chronic social stress inhibits both the cell proliferation rate and survival rate of the newly generated cells, whereas concomitant fluoxetine treatment can counteract this effect of stress. E: A representative image of GFAP-staining in the DG. GFAP labels astroglia, insert shows an individual GFAP+ astrocyte. F: Chronic stress results in reduced numbers of astroglia in the hippocampus, whereas fluoxetine blocked this effect of stress. $P < 0.05$ compared to Control; # $P < 0.05$ compared to stress. See colour plate section for colour version.

The survival rate of newly generated neurons can be modified by hippocampus-dependent forms of learning (Aimone et al. 2006; Dupret et al. 2007; 2008; Gould et al. 1999). The effects of learning on cell survival are complex and depend on the age of the newborn neurons (Dupret, 2007) and on the type of learning (Dalla et al. 2007; Leuner et al. 2006). Specific phases of spatial learning can induce apoptosis only in a targeted population of young newborn neurons within a specific time window (Dupret, 2007) and learning can increase or decrease the survival of newborn neurons depending on training intensity and duration and cognitive status (Döbrössy et al. 2003; Drapeau et al. 2007; Olariu et al. 2005). Factors like stress and antidepressants (AD) (Lucassen et al. 2004; 2006) also modify DG apoptosis and survival of newborn neurons. The close correlation between cell birth and death in the adult DG implies a continuous turnover of a pool of granule cells, and a very heterogeneous composition of the DG. Importantly, although a stress-induced change in DG turnover rate may not directly influence total DG cell number, it will change the overall composition, average age of the DG cells, and thereby properties of the hippocampal network (Joels et al. 2007).

Methodological considerations

When studying effects of stress on changes in structural plasticity, like neurogenesis, many variables influence these effects, including inter-individual and gender differences in stress coping. In a laboratory setting, also handling, time of day at sacrifice and previous exposure to stressful learning tasks, for example, (Holmes et al. 2004; Kochman et al. 2006; Lu et al. 2003) can all be of influence (Namestkova et al. 2005; Ehninger and Kempermann, 2006). Furthermore, inter-individual differences in HPA reactivity and neurogenesis can be influenced by early life stressors (Caldji et al. 2000; Seckl, 2001; Lucassen et al. 2009; Oomen et al. 2009).

Many studies on AN have employed stressors that are both uncontrollable and unpredictable (Malberg and Duman, 2003; Shors et al. 2007). An uncontrollable stressor generally induces stronger HPA-axis activation than controllable stressors. Chronic restraint is an uncontrollable and strong, but very predictable stressor, that causes adaptation of the stress response when applied for prolonged periods (Pham et al. 2003). Active avoidance learning in contrast, is stressful but controllable and does not affect DG proliferation (van der Borght et al. 2005). Housing and stress can differently impact male vs. female animals (Lagace et al. 2007; Ormerod et al. 2004).

Stress effects on neurogenesis

As reviewed recently (Lucassen et al. 2008a), some exceptions exist (Pham et al. 2003; Thomas et al. 2006), but most studies in rats, mice, tree shrews, and monkeys report (transient) reductions in the proliferation of adult-generated cells after acute stress (Alonso et al. 2004; Gould et al. 1997; Heine et al. 2004c; Malberg and Duman, 2003; Veenema et al. 2007). Cell proliferation and neurogenesis is also decreased following chronic stress, without affecting DG-GCL cell number and volume (Fig. 11.1) (Alonso et al. 2004; Czeh et al. 2001; Heine et al. 2004c; Lee et al. 2006; Malberg and Duman, 2003; Vollmayr et al. 2003) although exceptions exist (Jayatissa et al. 2008; Pham et al. 2003).

Effects of stress on AN are largely mediated by GC but also by other steroids (Ambrogini et al. 2005; Galea et al. 2006; Karishma and Herbert, 2002). Steroid removal by adrenalectomy increases proliferation and neurogenesis (Cameron and McKay, 1999; Krugers et al. 2007) whereas increased GC levels inhibit proliferation and neurogenesis (Fig. 11.2) (Ambrogini et al. 2002; Mayer et al. 2006; Wong and Herbert, 2006). Also, manipulations interfering with HPA axis activity such as

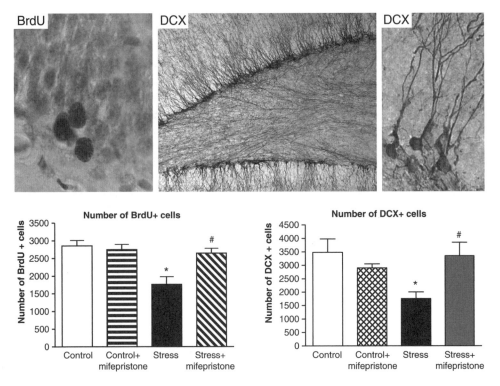

Fig. 11.2 Top panels show examples of BrdU+ and Doublecortin (DCX)+ immunostained cells in the DG. DCX+ somata are located in the SGZ with extensions passing through the GCL. Lower panels display BrdU- and DCX-positive cell numbers in rats subjected to 21 days of chronic unpredictable stress. The significant reduction in both BrdU- (21-day-old cells) and DCX-positive cell numbers after chronic stress, or corticosteroid treatment is normalized by four days of high-dose treatment with the GR antagonist mifepristone, whereas the drug alone has no effect (see Mayer et al. 2006; Oomen et al. 2007 for details). See colour plate section for colour version.

pharmacological blockade of CRF-1, V1b, or GR (Fig. 11.2), normalize stress or corticosterone-induced reductions in adult neurogenesis (Alonso et al. 2004; Mayer et al. 2006; Oomen et al. 2007; Wong and Herbert, 2006). The normalizing effect of the GR blocker mifepristone occurs only in a 'high corticoid' or 'high stress' environment and mifepristone, unlike classic antidepressant drugs (Malberg et al. 2000), does not stimulate neurogenesis in control animals (Mayer et al. 2006; Oomen et al. 2007). Of interest, treatment with mifepristone was recently reported to ameliorate symptoms of psychotic depression already after a few days of treatment (Belanoff et al. 2001; 2002; Flores et al. 2006).

Perinatal stress

The set point of HPA-axis activity is programmed by genotype, but can be changed by early development. In humans, early life stressors are among the strongest predisposing factors for major depression in later life. Aversive experiences, both in utero or neonatally, like early maternal separation or abuse, can result in sustained HPA-axis activation and lasting alterations in the stress response that may predispose individuals to adult onset depression, anxiety disorder, or both (de Kloet et al. 2005).

The juvenile and early perinatal phase offers a time window in which maternal factors and corticosterone can induce lasting programming effects on AN, stress reactivity, hippocampal function, and behaviour in the offspring (Caldji et al. 2000; Fenoglio et al. 2006; Seckl, 2001). For rat pups, an important environmental factor during development is the mother. Variations in maternal care determine HPA-axis properties through epigenetic modulation (Liu et al. 2000). Pups that receive more maternal care are less anxious later in life and show enhanced cell survival in the DG (Bredy et al. 2003).

Also, subjecting pregnant rats or macaques to stress, for example, induces lifelong reductions in adult DG proliferation in the offspring (Bosch et al. 2006; Coe et al. 2003; Lemaire et al. 2000; Lucassen et al. 2008b), parallel to hippocampal learning impairments, that can be normalized by handling (Lemaire et al. 2006). Chronic stress in pregnant mice induces increased anxiety-related behaviour, prolonged HPA axis dysfunction and sleep disturbances in the adult offspring. Also, changes in AN and cell death occur following early maternal separation, notably in a sex-dependent manner (Mirescu et al. 2004; Oomen et al. 2008; Zhang et al. 2002) that could be normalized by fluoxetine (Lee et al. 2001). Chapter 8 of this book describes specifically the concept of in utero 'programming'.

Sleep disruption as a stressor

In addition to stress, sleep disruption can modulate neurogenesis. Increasing evidence suggests that disturbed sleep may not only be a symptom of depression but may also sensitize individuals to the development of mood disorders. In agreement, primary insomnia often precedes and predicts a depressive episode (Riemann and Voderholzer, 2003). Also, experimental studies in rodents show that chronic sleep curtailment gradually leads to neurobiological changes similar to those found in depression (Novati et al. 2008; Roman et al. 2005a). Several rodent studies have shown that chronically disrupted and restricted sleep can reduce hippocampal proliferation and neurogenesis (Guzman-Marin et al. 2007; Mirescu et al. 2006; Mueller et al. 2008; Roman et al. 2005b; for review see Meerlo et al. 2008b). On the basis of these findings it has been hypothesized that chronically disrupted sleep, by inhibiting neurogenesis, might be one of the factors contributing to depression aetiology.

Especially chronic sleep disruption or restriction may have cumulative effects that cause decreases in proliferation and neurogenesis (Meerlo et al. 2008b). Yet, although sleep disruption for a period shorter than one day has little effect on basal rates of cell proliferation and neurogenesis (Guzman-Marin et al. 2007; Roman et al. 2005b), one study in rodents showed that even mild restriction of sleep may prevent the increase in neurogenesis that occurs with hippocampus-dependent learning (Hairston et al. 2005). Since sleep deprivation also disturbs hippocampus-dependent memory formation (Stickgold and Walker, 2005), these data suggest that sleep loss may interfere with cognition by affecting stages of hippocampal neurogenesis.

The mechanisms by which sleep disruption affects hippocampal neurogenesis are not fully understood. It has been proposed that effects of prolonged sleep deprivation might be an indirect result of stress (Mirescu et al. 2006). Indeed, sleep loss could be considered as stressful and is sometimes associated with mildly elevated GC levels. Also, prolonged sleep disruption gradually causes alterations in HPA-axis regulation similar to those in depression (Meerlo et al. 2002; Novati et al. 2008). One study has suggested that lowering GC levels may prevent sleep deprivation-induced suppression of hippocampal neurogenesis (Mirescu et al. 2006). However, a number of studies with adrenalectomized rats have clearly shown that prolonged sleep loss

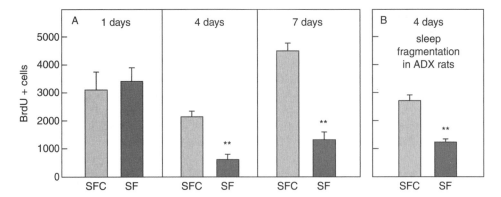

Fig. 11.3 A: Hippocampal cell proliferation in rats subjected to sleep fragmentation (SF) by forced treadmill walking and in control animals that were subjected to forced walking but had sufficient time to sleep (SFC). Whereas 1 day of SF had no effect on cell proliferation, the numbers of BrdU-positive cells in the dorsal DG was significantly reduced after four or seven days of SF. B: Effects of four days SF on cell proliferation in adrenalectomized (ADX) rats that received basal corticosterone in their drinking water. Independent of changes in corticosterone, a 55% reduction in the number of BrdU positive cells was found after SF compared with ADX SF controls. *P* < 0.01 compared to controls. Reprinted from *Neuroscience* 148,1 Hippocampal neurogenesis is reduced by sleep fragmentation in the adult rat Guzman-Marin, R. et al p9 2007, with permission from Elsevier.

can inhibit neurogenesis by ways that are independent of adrenal stress hormones (Fig. 11.3) (Guzman-Marin et al. 2007; Mueller et al. 2008).

Besides GC, many other systems are affected by sleep deprivation or disruption that may provide a link between insufficient sleep and reductions in AN. Serotonin, for example, promotes hippocampal cell proliferation and neurogenesis, in part via the serotonin-1A receptor (Banasr et al. 2004). Recent studies in rats show that chronic sleep restriction reduces the sensitivity of the serotonin-1A receptor system (Roman et al. 2005a). This reduction develops during the course of prolonged sleep restriction, consistent with the finding that suppression of AN generally occurs only after a prolonged period of sleep disturbance. A reduction in neurogenesis following sleep deprivation might also be related to increased levels of pro-inflammatory cytokines (see next paragraph). Both interleukin (IL) 6 and tumour necrosis factor (TNF)-α are increased after sleep restriction (Haack et al. 2007; Irwin et al. 2006). Also, plasma IL-6 levels are, for example, increased in patients with primary insomnia (Burgos et al. 2006). Exposure to both IL-6 and TNF-α decrease neurogenesis in vitro suggesting these cytokines may mediate detrimental effects of neuroinflammation on hippocampal neurogenesis in vivo (Monje et al. 2003). Clearly, the mechanisms by which prolonged sleep disturbance affects AN involve several complex factors, with some being relevant for depression aetiology.

Inflammation as a stressor: microglia

Effects of both stress and sleep disruption on hippocampal neurogenesis may in part be mediated by pro-inflamatory cytokines. The HPA-axis is not only activated by stress, but also during disease processes and by pro-inflammatory cytokines such as interleukin-6 or exogenous interferon gamma (Cassidy and O'Keane, 2000). During inflammation, cells of the immune system produce pro-inflammatory cytokines. Interleukin-1β (IL-1β) and interleukin-6 (IL-6) then elicit various (patho)physiological reactions that together coordinate the 'nonspecific symptoms of sickness' and activate the HPA-axis; elevated GC levels are immunosuppressive and prevent the immune system from overshooting. Thus, a clear bi-directional communication exists between the immune and neuroendocrine system.

Interleukins are also produced within the brain during ischemia, dementia, multiple sclerosis, and epilepsy. In most of these conditions, microglial cells produce interleukins that are generally considered detrimental for neuronal viability. However, interleukins have also been implicated in processes like brain plasticity. Hence, neuroinflammation, defined by microglia activation and the presence of pro-inflammatory mediators, represents a stressor that may affect AN. Moreover, synthetic GCs such as prednisone and dexamethasone are often prescribed for the treatment of inflammatory disorders, that also inhibit AN, thus suggesting an indirect, GC-mediated, inhibitory effect of neuroinflammation on neurogenesis.

Inflammation and cytokine expression can affect AN directly (Monje et al. 2003; Vallieres et al. 2002) while immune modulators like transforming growth factor (TGF)-β (Wachs et al. 2006) have a (concentration-dependent) neurogenic potential in the adult brain (Battista et al. 2006). Other pro-inflammatory cytokines such as tumour necrosis factor-alpha (TNF-α) (Iosif et al. 2006) or interferon-α decrease AN through modulation of IL-1 (Kaneko et al. 2006). In addition, impairment of IL-1β action prevents the attenuated rate of AN in response to stress, supporting the idea that pro-inflammatory mediators and local cues in the brain play a role in restricting AN.

Conversely, factors capable of affecting cell genesis can also influence microglial activation. As part of the neuroinflammatory response, activated microglia modulate the neurogenic niche and, dependent on whether they are activated by IL-4 or by IFN-γ, microglia cells can differentially induce oligodendrogenesis and neurogenesis, respectively (Butovsky et al. 2006).

Reducing neuroinflammation by specific drugs can further restore or increase AN in different pathological models (Ekdahl et al. 2003; Monje et al. 2003) while T-cells even seem to underlie hippocampal plasticity and function through an effect on progenitor cells (Ziv et al. 2006).

The general picture emerging from these studies is that inflammatory responses in the brain influence AN, which may be mediated through elevated GC levels. Of interest, inflammatory mediators have also been implicated in the pathophysiology of depression (Dantzer et al. 2008; and Chapter 10 of this book).

Remaining issues and mechanistic remarks

Stress-induced reductions in proliferation could result from apoptosis of progenitor cells, or from cell cycle arrest. After acute stress, a reduction in proliferation was found that was paralleled by increased numbers of apoptotic cells, yet no distinction was made between apoptosis of new-born or mature cells. Following chronic stress, both proliferation and apoptosis were reduced, parallel to increases in the cell cycle inhibitor p27Kip1, indicating that more cells had entered cell cycle arrest and that DG turnover had slowed down (Heine et al. 2004b, c).

The suppressing effects of GCs or stress on individual precursor cells are most likely mediated either directly through specific GR or NMDA receptors on the precursor cells themselves (Garcia et al. 2004; Nacher et al. 2007), indirectly through growth factor release from neighbouring cells, or through the local environment. Important mediators include; insulin-like growth factor-1 (IGF-1), brain-derived neurotrophic factor (BDNF), epidermal growth factor (EGF) (Aberg et al. 2000; Kuhn et al. 1997) and VEGF (Heine et al. 2005). The proximity of the precursors to blood vessels suggests a strong interaction with the vasculature. Also, astrocytes are important as they support the survival of developing neurons, possess GRs and are significantly affected by some but not all types of stress (Fig. 11.1)(Czeh et al. 2006; Oomen et al. 2009).

Several examples of a persistent inhibition of AN exist, despite normalized GC levels. Early life stressors, for example, decrease neurogenesis, an effect that can last into adulthood (Lemaire et al. 2000; Lucassen et al. 2009; Mirescu et al. 2004). Similar findings were shown in the 'learned helplessness' paradigm where reductions in proliferation are induced, that last up to ages where no corticosterone differences are present anymore (Malberg and Duman, 2003). These findings suggest that while GC may be involved in the initial suppression of cell proliferation, particularly in early life, they are not always necessary for the maintenance of this effect. Alternatively, dynamic GC changes may have been replaced by alterations in mediators of steroid action like CBG or 11BOHSD (Lucassen et al. 2009).

An interesting contradiction also exists in the direction of the generally positive effect of exercise on AN. Exercise is generally associated with beneficial changes, also in its effects on depression (Brené et al. 2007; Ernst et al. 2006). In rats, short-term voluntary running for nine days potently stimulated neurogenesis whereas long-term running for 24 days induced a strong downregulation of progenitor proliferation rate to 50% of non-running controls (Fig. 11.4). This finding was paralleled by a strong activation of the HPA axis and opioid system (Droste et al. 2003; Naylor et al. 2005). Furthermore, by decreasing the daily running distance of long-term running animals, the HPA-axis was not stimulated and a return to normal proliferation levels was found (Naylor et al. 2005). Hence, prolonged running can develop into a stressor, overruling its positive effects on AN, and may even induce dependency-like behaviour (Droste et al. 2003), suggesting that positive stimuli for AN can only be effective when HPA axis activation is minimal.

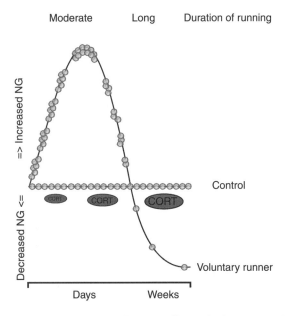

Fig. 11.4 Schematic representation of the differential effects of voluntary running on adult hippocampal neurogenesis. Whereas short-term running for nine days potently increases neurogenesis levels (>400%), prolonged running for 24 days induces a strong reduction in neurogenesis to approximately 50% of control levels. These changes are paralleled by the development of an activated HPA axis and a gradual rise in corticosterone levels, as represented by the size of the red ovals (see Naylor et al. 2005; Droste et al. 2003).

Stress induced changes in adult neurogenesis: relevant for depression?

Stress and GCs play important roles in various clinical disorders and alterations of HPA axis (re) activity are common in major depression. Also, in many animal models of stress, symptoms of depression can be reproduced (de Kloet et al. 2005; Swaab et al. 2005). The set point of HPA-axis activity appears to be programmed by genotype but can be altered by development or by stress (Kendler et al. 1999; Seckl, 2001). Although initial studies implicated AN in depression, current evidence indicates that AN most likely does not contribute to depression per se, but may be involved in the action of antidepressant drugs. Of note, ADs exert very diverse actions not only on AN but also on apoptosis, glia, dendritic complexity, spine density, and hippocampal volume (Czeh and Lucassen, 2007; Lucassen et al. 2004; Norrholm and Ouimet, 2001; Sairanen et al. 2007). Furthermore, reduced AN is not specific for depression as it has been additionally implicated in various other psychiatric disorders (e.g. schizophrenia, dementia, addiction) suggesting an involvement in the cognitive impairments common in these illnesses (Kempermann et al. 2008; Sahay and Hen, 2007).

The demonstration that chronic AD treatment can stimulate AN (Malberg and Duman, 2003) has been followed quickly by compelling experimental evidence (generated exclusively from preclinical studies) that stress-induced reductions of adult DG neurogenesis can be reversed by various AD treatments including selective serotonin reuptake inhibitors (SSRIs), tricyclic ADs (TCAs), ECT and atypical antipsychotics and GR antagonists (Oomen et al. 2007; Sahay and Hen, 2007; Warner-Schmidt and Duman, 2006).

Together with the demonstration that the behavioural effects of ADs require neurogenesis (Airan et al. 2007; Santarelli et al. 2003), these findings have strengthened the concept that lasting reductions in AN after stress could be implicated in AD action (Jacobs et al. 2000; Sahay and Hen, 2007). Hence, promotion of neurogenesis has been regarded as a promising strategy for identifying new AD targets. Accordingly, when tested in chronic stress paradigms, several potential antidepressant compounds, like selective neurokinin-1 (NK1) receptor antagonists (Czeh et al. 2005), corticotrophin-releasing factor (CRF1) and vasopressin (V1b) or GR antagonist (Alonso et al. 2004; Oomen et al. 2007) could indeed normalize inhibitory effects of stress on proliferation or neurogenesis.

It should be emphasized that the functional significance of the newly generated neurons in the aetiology of depression, or in hippocampal volume changes, is still subject to debate. Depletion of neurogenesis by means other than stress for example, fails to produce a 'depressive-like' state in animals (Czeh and Lucassen, 2007; Sahay and Hen, 2007). Also, AN is difficult to study in human brain. So far, one study (Reif et al. 2006) examined cell proliferation in depressed subjects and, while confirming its rare occurrence (Boekhoorn et al. 2006; Eriksson et al. 1998; Manganas et al. 2007), no changes were found in depression. However many patients were, or had been, on antidepressant medication.

Concluding remarks

Stress, GC, inflammation and sleep deprivation modulate different phases of AN that can normalize again, for example, after exercise, recovery periods, or AD treatment. Although neurogenesis has been implicated in learning and is stimulated by many ADs, its functional impact and contribution to depression aetiology remains unclear. A lasting reduction in neurogenesis may be indicative of impaired hippocampal plasticity but is, by itself, unlikely to produce depression.

Lasting reductions in DG turnover rate will, however, affect average age and overall composition of the DG, and thereby influence properties of the hippocampal memory circuit and thereby cognitive function. Whether stress-induced reductions in AN occur in humans, awaits further investigation.

Acknowledgements

PJL is supported by the VolkswagenStiftung Germany, the University of Amsterdam, the European Union (MCTS NEURAD), Corcept Inc. and the Nederlandse HersenStichting. We are grateful to J. Muller-Keuker (GPZ) for her help in the preparation of the figures.

References

Aberg, M.A., Aberg, N.D., Hedbacker, H., Oscarsson, J., and Eriksson P.S. (2000). Peripheral infusion of IGF-I selectively induces neurogenesis in the adult rat hippocampus. *J Neurosci.*, **20**, 289–903.

Aimone, J.B., Wiles, J., and Gage, F.H. (2006). Potential role for adult neurogenesis in the encoding of time in new memories. *Nat Neurosci.*, **9**, 723–727.

Alfarez, D.N., Karst, H., Velzing, E.H., Joëls, M., and Krugers, H.J. (2008). Opposite effects of glucocorticoid receptor activation on hippocampal CA1 dendritic complexity in chronically stressed and handled animals. *Hippocampus*, **18**, 20–28.

Alonso, R., Griebel, G., Pavone, G., Stemmelin, J., Le Fur, G., and Soubrie, P. (2004). Blockade of CRF(1) or V(1b) receptors reverses stress-induced suppression of neurogenesis in a mouse model of depression. *Mol Psychiatry*, **9**, 278–286.

Ambrogini, P., Orsini, L., Mancini, C., Ferri, P., Barbanti, I., and Cuppini, R. (2002). Persistently high corticosterone levels but not normal circadian fluctuations of the hormone affect cell proliferation in the adult rat dentate gyrus. *Neuroendocrinology*, **76**, 366–372.

Ambrogini, P., Cuppini, R., Ferri, P. et al. (2005). Thyroid hormones affect neurogenesis in the dentate gyrus of adult rat. *Neuroendocrinology*, **81**(4), 244–253.

Banasr, M., Hery, M., Printemps, R., and Daszuta, A. (2004). Serotonin induced increases in adult cell proliferation and neurogenesis are mediated through different and common 5-HT receptor subtypes in the dentate gyrus and the subventricular zone. *Neuropsychopharmacology*, **29**, 450–460.

Belanoff, J.K., Flores, B.H., Kalezhan, M., Sund, B., and Schatzberg, A.F. (2001). Rapid reversal of psychotic depression using mifepristone. *J Clin Psycho-pharmacol.*, **21**, 516–521.

Belanoff, J.K., Rothschild, A.J., Cassidy, F. et al. (2002). An open label trial of C-1073 (mifepristone) for psychotic major depression. *Biol Psychiatry*, **52**, 386–392.

Boekhoorn, K., Joels, M., and Lucassen, P.J. (2006). Increased proliferation reflects glial and vascular-associated changes, but not neurogenesis in the presenile Alzheimer hippocampus. *Neurobiol Dis.*, **24**, 1–14.

Bredy, T.W., Grant, R.J., Champagne, D.L., and Meaney, M.J. (2003). Maternal care influences neuronal survival in the hippocampus of the rat. *Eur J Neurosci.*, **18**, 2903–2909.

Bremner, J.D. (2002). Structural changes in the brain in depression and relationship to symptom recurrence. *CNS Spectr.*, **7**, 129–130, 135–139.

Brené, S., Bjørnebekk, A., Aberg, E., Mathé, A.A., Olson, L., and Werme, M. (2007). Running is rewarding and antidepressive. *Physiol Behav.*, **92**, 136–140.

Brown, J., Cooper-Kuhn, C.M., Kempermann, G. et al. (2003). Enriched environment and physical activity stimulate hippocampal but not olfactory bulb neurogenesis. *Eur J Neurosci.*, **17**, 2042–2046.

Burgos, I., Richter, L., Klein, T. et al. (2006). Increased nocturnal interleukin-6 excretion in patients with primary insomnia: a pilot study. *Brain Behav Immun.*, **20**, 246–253.

Butovsky, O., Ziv, Y., Schwartz, A. et al. (2006). Microglia activated by IL-4 or IFN-gamma differentially induce neurogenesis and oligodendrogenesis from adult stem/progenitor cells. *Mol Cell Neurosci.*, **31**, 149–160.

Caldji, C., Diorio, J., and Meaney, M.J. (2000). Variations in maternal care in infancy regulate the development of stress reactivity. *Biol Psychiatry,* **48**, 1164–1174.

Cameron, H.A. and Dayer, A.G. (2008). New interneurons in the adult neocortex: small, sparse, but significant? *Biol Psychiatry,* **63**, 650–655.

Cameron, H.A. and McKay, R.D. (1999). Restoring production of hippocampal neurons in old age. *Nat Neurosci.,* **2**, 894–897.

Campbell, S., Marriott, M., Nahmias, C., and MacQueen, G.M. (2004). Lower hippocampal volume in patients suffering from depression: a meta-analysis. *Am J Psychiatry,* **161**, 598–607.

Coe, C.L., Kramer, M., Czeh, B. et al. (2003). Prenatal stress diminishes neurogenesis in the dentate gyrus of juvenile rhesus monkeys. *Biol Psychiatry,* **54**, 1025–1034.

Curtis, M.A., Kam, M., Nannmark, U. et al. (2007). Human neuroblasts migrate to the olfactory bulb via a lateral ventricular extension. *Science,* **315**, 1243–1249.

Czeh, B., Michaelis, T., Watanabe, T. et al. (2001). Stress-induced changes in cerebral metabolites, hippocampal volume, and cell proliferation are prevented by antidepressant treatment with tianeptine. *Proc Natl Acad Sci USA,* **98**, 12796–12801.

Czeh, B., Pudovkina, O., van der Hart, M.G. et al. (2005). Examining SLV-323, a novel NK1 receptor antagonist, in a chronic psychosocial stress model for depression. *Psychopharmacology(Berl),* **180**, 548–557.

Czeh, B., Simon, M., Schmelting, B., Hiemke, C., and Fuchs, E. (2006). Astroglial plasticity in the hippocampus is affected by chronic psychosocial stress and concomitant fluoxetine treatment. *Neuropsychopharmacology,* **31**, 1616–1626.

Czeh, B. and Lucassen, P.J. (2007). Hippocampal volume changes in depression: are neurogenesis, gliogenesis and apoptosis causally involved? *Eur Arch Gen Psy and Clin Med.,* **257**, 250–260.

Dalla, C., Bangasser, D.A., Edgecomb, C., and Shors, T.J. (2007). Neurogenesis and learning: acquisition and asymptotic performance predict how many new cells survive in the hippocampus. *Neurobiol Learn Mem.,* **88**, 143–148.

Dantzer, R., O'Connor, J.C., Freund, G.G., Johnson, R.W., and Kelley, K.W. (2008). From inflammation to sickness and depression: when the immune system subjugates the brain. *Nat Rev Neurosci.,* **9**, 46–56.

Dayer, A.G., Ford, A.A., Cleaver, K.M., Yassaee, M., and Cameron, H.A. (2003). Short-term and long-term survival of new neurons in the rat dentate gyrus. *J Comp Neurol.,* **460**, 563–572.

de Kloet, E.R., Joels, M., and Holsboer, F. (2005). Stress and the brain: from adaptation to disease. *Nat Rev Neurosci.,* **6**, 463–475.

de Kloet, E.R., Karst, H., and Joëls, M. (2008). Corticosteroid hormones in the central stress response: quick-and-slow. *Front Neuroendocrinol.,* **29**, 268–272.

Döbrössy, M.D., Drapeau, E., Aurousseau, C., Le Moal, M., Piazza, P.V., and Abrous, D.N. (2003). Differential effects of learning on neurogenesis: learning increases or decreases the number of newly born cells depending on their birth date. *Mol Psychiatry,* **8**, 974–982.

Drevets, W.C. (2000). Functional anatomical abnormalities in limbic and prefrontal cortical structures in major depression. *Prog Brain Res.,* **126**, 413–431.

Droste, S.K., Gesing, A., Ulbricht, S., Muller, M.B., Linthorst, A.C., and Reul, J.M. (2003). Effects of long-term voluntary exercise on the mouse hypothalamic-pituitary-adrenocortical axis. *Endocrinology,* **144**, 3012–3023.

Ehninger, D. and Kempermann, G. (2006). Paradoxical effects of learning the Morris water maze on adult hippocampal neurogenesis in mice may be explained by a combination of stress and physical activity. *Genes Brain Behav.,* **5**, 29–39.

Ekdahl, C.T., Claasen, J.H., Bonde, S., Kokaia, Z., and Lindvall, O. (2003). Inflammation is detrimental for neurogenesis in adult brain. *Proc Natl Acad Sci USA,* **100**, 13632–13637.

Eriksson, P.S., Perfilieva, E., Bjork-Eriksson, T. et al. (1998). Neurogenesis in the adult human hippocampus. *Nat Med.,* **4**, 1313–1317.

Ernst, C., Olson, A.K., Pinel, J.P., Lam, R.W., and Christie, B.R. (2006). Antidepressant effects of exercise: evidence for an adult-neurogenesis hypothesis? *J Psychiatry Neurosci.*, **31**, 84–92.

Fenoglio, K.A., Brunson, K.L., and Baram, T.Z. (2006). Hippocampal neuroplasticity induced by early-life stress: functional and molecular aspects. *Front Neuroendocrinol.*, **27**, 180–192.

Fischer, A.K., von Rosenstiel, P., Fuchs, E., Goula, D., Almeida, O.F., and Czeh, B. (2002). The prototypic mineralocorticoid receptor agonist aldosterone influences neurogenesis in the dentate gyrus of the adrenalectomized rat. *Brain Res.*, **947**, 290–293.

Fuchs, E., Czeh, B., Kole, M.H., Michaelis, T., and Lucassen, P.J. (2004). Alterations of neuroplasticity in depression: the hippocampus and beyond. *Eur Neuropsychopharmacol.*, **14** Suppl 5, S481–S490.

Fuchs, E., Flugge, G., and Czeh, B. (2006). Remodeling of neuronal networks by stress. *Front Biosci.*, **11**, 2746–2758.

Galea, L.A., Spritzer, M.D., Barker, J.M., Pawluski, J.L. (2006). Gonadal hormone modulation of hippocampal neurogenesis in the adult. *Hippocampus*, **16**, 225–232.

Garcia, A., Steiner, B., Kronenberg, G., Bick-Sander, A., and Kempermann, G. (2004). Age-dependent expression of glucocorticoid- and mineralocorticoid receptors on neural precursor cell populations in the adult murine hippocampus. *Aging Cell*, **3**, 363–371.

Gesing, A., Bilang-Bleuel, A., Droste, S.K., Linthorst, A.C., Holsboer, F., and Reul, J.M. (2001). Psychological stress increases hippocampal mineralocorticoid receptor levels: involvement of corticotropin-releasing hormone. *J Neurosci.*, **21**, 4822–4829.

Gould, E., McEwen, B.S., Tanapat, P., Galea, L.A., and Fuchs, E. (1997). Neurogenesis in the dentate gyrus of the adult tree shrew is regulated by psychosocial stress and NMDA receptor activation. *J Neurosci.*, **17**, 2492–2498.

Gould, E., Beylin, A., Tanapat, P., Reeves, A., and Shors, T.J. (1999). Learning enhances adult neurogenesis in the hippocampal formation. *Nat Neurosci.*, **2**, 260–5.

Gould, E. (2007). How widespread is adult neurogenesis in mammals? *Nat Rev Neurosci.*, **8**, 481–488.

Guzman-Marin, R., Bashir, T., Suntsova, N., Szymusiak, R., and McGinty, D. (2007). Hippocampal neurogenesis is reduced by sleep fragmentation in the adult rat. *Neuroscience.*, **148**, 325–333.

Haack, M., Sanchez, E., and Mullington, J.M. (2007). Elevated inflammatory markers in response to prolonged sleep restriction are associated with increased pain experience in healthy volunteers. *Sleep.*, **30**, 1145–1152.

Hairston, I.S., Little, M.T., Scanlon, M.D. et al. (2005). Sleep restriction suppresses neurogenesis induced by hippocampus-dependent learning. *J Neurophysiol.*, **94**, 4224–4233.

Heine, V.M., Maslam, S., Joels, M., and Lucassen, P.J. (2004a). Prominent decline of newborn cell proliferation, differentiation, and apoptosis in the aging dentate gyrus, in absence of an age-related hypothalamus–pituitary–adrenal axis activation. *Neurobiol Aging*, **25**, 361–375.

Heine, V.M., Maslam, S., Joels, M., and Lucassen, P.J. (2004b). Increased P27KIP1 protein expression in the dentate gyrus of chronically stressed rats indicates G1 arrest involvement. *Neuroscience*, **129**, 593–601.

Heine, V.M., Maslam, S., Zareno, J., Joels M., and Lucassen, P.J. (2004c). Suppressed proliferation and apoptotic changes in the rat dentate gyrus after acute and chronic stress are reversible. *Eur J Neurosci.*, **19**, 131–144.

Heine, V.M., Zareno, J., Maslam, S., Joels, M., and Lucassen, P.J. (2005). Chronic stress in the adult dentate gyrus reduces cell proliferation near the vasculature and VEGF and Flk-1 protein expression. *Eur J Neurosci.*, **21**, 1304–1314.

Holmes, M.M., Galea, L.A., Mistlberger, R.E., and Kempermann, G. (2004). Adult hippocampal neurogenesis and voluntary running activity: circadian and dose-dependent effects. *J Neurosci Res.*, **76**, 216–222.

Iosif, R.E., Ekdahl, C.T., Ahlenius, H. et al. (2006). Tumor necrosis factor receptor 1 is a negative regulator of progenitor proliferation in adult hippocampal neurogenesis. *J Neurosci.*, **26**, 9703–12.

Irwin, M.R., Wang, M., Campomayor, C.O., Collado-Hidalgo, A., and Cole, S. (2006). Sleep deprivation and activation of morning levels of cellular and genomic markers of inflammation. *Arch Intern Med.,* **166**, 1756–1762.

Jacobs, B.L., van Praag, H., and Gage, F.H. (2000). Adult brain neurogenesis and psychiatry: a novel theory of depression. *Mol Psychiatry,* **5**, 262–9.

Jayatissa, M.N., Bisgaard, C.F., West, M.J., and Wiborg, O. (2008). The number of granule cells in rat hippocampus is reduced after chronic mild stress and re-established after chronic escitalopram treatment. *Neuropharmacology,* **54**, 530–541.

Joels, M., Karst, H., Krugers, H.J., and Lucassen, P.J. (2007). Chronic stress; implications for neuron morphology, function and neurogenesis. *Frontiers in Neuroendocrinology,* **28**, 72–96.

Kaneko, N., Kudo, K., Mabuchi, T. et al. (2006). Suppression of cell proliferation by interferon-alpha through interleukin-1 production in adult rat dentate gyrus. *Neuropsychopharmacology,* **31**, 2619–2626.

Karishma, K.K., and Herbert, J. (2002). Dehydroepiandrosterone (DHEA) stimulates neurogenesis in the hippocampus of the rat, promotes survival of newly formed neurons and prevents corticosterone-induced suppression. *Eur J Neurosci.,* **16**, 445–453.

Kempermann, G., Krebs, J., and Fabel, K. (2008). The contribution of failing adult hippocampal neurogenesis to psychiatric disorders. *Curr Opin Psychiatry,* **21**, 290–295.

Kendler, K.S., Karkowski, L.M., and Prescott, C.A. (1999). Causal relationship between stressful life events and the onset of major depression. *Am J Psychiatry,* **156**, 837–841.

Kim, J.J., and Diamond, D.M. (2002). The stressed hippocampus, synaptic plasticity and lost memories. *Nat Rev Neurosci.,* **3**, 453–462.

Krugers, H.J., van der Linden, S., van Olst, E. et al. (2007). Dissociation between apoptosis, neurogenesis, and synaptic potentiation in the dentate gyrus of adrenalectomized rats. *Synapse,* **61**, 221–230.

Kuhn, H.G., Winkler, J., Kempermann, G., Thal, L.J., and Gage, F.H. (1997). Epidermal growth factor and fibroblast growth factor-2 have different effects on neural progenitors in the adult rat brain. *J Neurosci.,* **17**, 5820–5829.

Lagace, D.C., Fischer, S.J., and Eisch, A.J. (2007). Gender and endogenous levels of estradiol do not influence adult hippocampal neurogenesis in mice. *Hippocampus,* **17**, 175–180.

Lee, H.J., Kim, J.W., Yim, S.V. et al. (2001). Fluoxetine enhances cell proliferation and prevents apoptosis in dentate gyrus of maternally separated rats. *Mol Psychiatry,* **6**, 610, 725–8.

Lee, K.J., Kim,S.J., Kim, S.W. et al. (2006). Chronic mild stress decreases survival, but not proliferation, of new-born cells in adult rat hippocampus. *Exp Mol Med.,* **38**, 44–54.

Lemaire, V., Koehl, M., Le Moal, M., and Abrous, D.N. (2000). Prenatal stress produces learning deficits associated with an inhibition of neurogenesis in the hippocampus. *Proc Natl Acad Sci USA.,* **97**, 11032–11037.

Lemaire, V., Lamarque, S., Le Moal, M., Piazza, P.V., and Abrous, D.N. (2006). Postnatal stimulation of the pups counteracts prenatal stress-induced deficits in hippocampal neurogenesis. *Biol Psychiatry,* **59**, 786–792.

Leuner, B., Gould, E., and Shors, T.J. (2006). Is there a link between adult neurogenesis and learning? *Hippocampus,* **16**, 216–24.

Liu, D., Diorio, J., Day, J.C., Francis, D.D., and Meaney, M.J. (2000). Maternal care, hippocampal synaptogenesis and cognitive development in rats. *Nat Neurosci.,* **3**, 799–806.

Lledo, P.M., and Saghatelyan, A. (2005). Integrating new neurons into the adult olfactory bulb: joining the network, life-death decisions, and the effects of sensory experience.*Trends Neurosci.,* **28**, 248–254.

Lucassen, P.J. and De Kloet, E.R. (2001). Glucocorticoids and the aging brain; cause or consequence? In P. Hof, C. Mobbs (ed.) *Functional Neurobiology of Aging,* pp. 883–905. New York, Academic Press.

Lucassen, P.J., Muller, M.B., Holsboer, F. et al. (2001). Hippocampal apoptosis in major depression is a minor event and absent from subareas at risk for glucocorticoid overexposure. *Am J Pathol.,* **158,** 453–468.

Lucassen, P.J., Fuchs, E., and Czeh, B. (2004). Antidepressant treatment with tianeptine reduces apoptosis in the hippocampal dentate gyrus and temporal cortex. *Biol Psychiatry,* **55,** 789–796.

Lucassen, P.J., Heine, V.M., Muller, M.B. et al. (2006). Stress, depression and hippocampal apoptosis. *CNS Neurol Disord Drug Targets,* **5,** 531–546.

Lucassen, P.J., Oomen, C.A., van Dam, A.-M., and Czéh, B. (2008). Regulation of hippocampal neurogenesis by systemic factors including stress, glucocorticoids, sleep, and inflammation. In (eds. F.H. Gage, G. Kempermann, and H. Song) pp. 363–395. *Adult Neurogenesis,* Cold Spring Harbor, New York, Cold Spring Harbor Laboratory Press.

Lucassen, P.J., Bosch, O., Jousma, E. et al. (2008b). Prenatal stress reduces postnatal neurogenesis in rats selectively bred for high, but not low anxiety: possible key role of lack of induction of placental 11B-hydroxysteroid dehydrogenase type 2. *Eur. J. Neurosci.,* **29,** 97–103.

MacQueen, G.M., Campbell, S., McEwen, B.S. et al. (2003). Course of illness, hippocampal function, and hippocampal volume in major depression. *Proc Natl Acad Sci USA,* **100,** 1387–1392.

Malberg, J.E., Eisch, A.J., Nestler, E.J., and Duman, R.S. (2000). Chronic antidepressant treatment increases neurogenesis in adult rat hippocampus. *J Neurosci.,* **20,** 9104–9110.

Malberg, J.E., and Duman, R.S. (2003). Cell proliferation in adult hippocampus is decreased by inescapable stress: reversal by fluoxetine treatment. *Neuropsychopharmacology,* **28,** 1562–1571.

Manganas, LN, Zhang, X, Li, Y et al. (2007). Magnetic resonance spectroscopy identifies neural progenitor cells in the live human brain. *Science,* **9,** 318(5852), 980–985.

Mayer, J.L., Klumpers, L., Maslam, S., de Kloet, E.R., Joels, M., and Lucassen, P.J. (2006). Brief treatment with the glucocorticoid receptor antagonist mifepristone normalises the corticosterone-induced reduction of adult hippocampal neurogenesis. *J Neuroendocrinol.,* **18,** 629–631.

Mayo, W., Lemaire, V., Malaterre, J. et al. (2005). Pregnenolone sulfate enhances neurogenesis and PSA-NCAM in young and aged hippocampus. *Neurobiol Aging,* **26,** 103–114.

Meerlo, P., Koehl,M., Van der Borght, K., and Turek, F.W. (2002). Sleep restriction alters the hypothalamic–pituitary–adrenal response to stress. *J Neuroendocrinol.,* **14,** 397–402.

Meerlo, P., Sgoifo, A., and Suchecki, D. (2008a). Restricted and disrupted sleep: Effects on autonomic function, neuroendocrine stress systems and stress responsivity. *Sleep Med Rev.,* **12,** 197–210.

Meerlo, P., Mistlberger, R.E., Jacobs, B.L., Heller, H.C., and McGinty, D. (2008b). New neurons in the adult brain: the role of sleep and consequences of sleep loss. *Sleep Med Rev.,* Epub ahead of print.

Mirescu, C., Peters, J.D., and Gould, E. (2004). Early life experience alters response of adult neurogenesis to stress. *Nat Neurosci.,* **7,** 841–846.

Mirescu, C., Peters, J.D., Noiman, L., and Gould, E. (2006). Sleep deprivation inhibits adult neurogenesis in the hippocampus by elevating glucocorticoids. *Proc Natl Acad Sci USA,* **103,** 19170–5.

Mitra, R., and Sapolsky, R.M. (2008). Acute corticosterone treatment is sufficient to induce anxiety and amygdaloid dendritic hypertrophy. *Proc Natl Acad Sci USA,* **105,** 5573–5578.

Monje, M.L., Toda, H., and Palmer, T.D. (2003). Inflammatory blockade restores adult hippocampal neurogenesis. *Science,* **302,** 1760–1765.

Montero-Pedrazuela, A., Venero, C., Lavado-Autric, R. et al. (2006). Modulation of adult hippocampal neurogenesis by thyroid hormones: implications in depressive-like behavior. *Mol Psychiatry,* **11,** 361–371.

Mueller, A., Pollock, M.S., Lieblich, S.E., Epp, J., Galea, L.A.M., and Mistlberger R.E. (2008). REM sleep deprivation can inhibit adult hippocampal neurogenesis independent of adrenal stress hormones. *Am J Physiol.,* **294,** R1693–1703.

Muller, M.B., Lucassen, P.J., Yassouridis, A., Hoogendijk, W.J., Holsboer, F., and Swaab, D.F. (2001). Neither major depression nor glucocorticoid treatment affects the cellular integrity of the human hippocampus. *Eur J Neurosci.,* **14,** 1603–1612.

Nacher, J., Varea, E., Miguel Blasco-Ibanez, J. et al. (2007). N-methyl-d-aspartate receptor expression during adult neurogenesis in the rat dentate gyrus. *Neuroscience, ***144**, 855–864.

Naylor, A.S., Persson, A.I., Eriksson, P.S., Jonsdottir, I.H., and Thorlin, T. (2005). Extended voluntary running inhibits exercise-induced adult hippocampal progenitor proliferation in the spontaneously hypertensive rat. *J Neurophysiol., ***93**, 2406–2414.

Novati, A., Roman, V., Cetin, T. et al. (2008). Chronically restricted sleep leads to depression-like changes in neurotransmitter receptor sensitivity and neuroendocrine stress reactivity in rats. *Sleep, ***31**, 1579–1585.

O'Brien, J., Thomas, A., Ballard, C. et al. (2001). Cognitive impairment in depression is not associated with neuropathologic evidence of increased vascular or Alzheimer-type pathology. *Biol Psychiatry, ***49**, 130–136.

Olariu, A., Cleaver, K.M., Shore, L.E., Brewer, M.D., and Cameron, H.A. (2005). A natural form of learning can increase and decrease the survival of new neurons in the dentate gyrus. *Hippocampus, ***15**, 750–762.

Oomen, C.A., Mayer, J.L., Joels, M., de Kloet, E.R., and Lucassen P.J. (2007). Brief treatment with the GR antagonist mifepristone normalizes the reduction in neurogenesis after chronic stress. *Eur.J. Neurosci., ***26**, 3395–3401.

Oomen, C.A., Girardi, C.E.N., Cahyadi, R. et al. (2009). Opposite effects of early maternal deprivation on neurogenesis in male versus female rats. *PLOS One, ***3**, e3675–3688.

Ormerod, B.K., Lee, T., and Galea, L.A. (2004). Estradiol enhances neurogenesis in the dentate gyri of adult male meadow voles by increasing the survival of young granule neurons. *Neuroscience, ***128**, 645–654.

Pham, K., Nacher, J., Hof, P.R., and McEwen, B.S. (2003). Repeated restraint stress suppresses neurogenesis and induces biphasic PSA-NCAM expression in the adult rat dentate gyrus. *Eur J Neurosci., ***17**, 879–886.

Rakic, P. (2002). Neurogenesis in adult primate neocortex: an evaluation of the evidence. *Nat Rev Neurosci., ***3**, 65–71.

Riemann, D. and Voderholzer, U. (2003). Primary insomnia: a risk factor to develop depression? *J Aff Disord, ***76**, 255–259.

Reif, A., Fritzen, S., Finger, M. et al. (2006). Neural stem cell proliferation is decreased in schizophrenia, but not in depression. *Mol Psychiatry, ***11**, 514–522.

Roman, V., Walstra, I., Luiten, P.G., and Meerlo, P. (2005a). Too little sleep gradually desensitizes the serotonin 1A receptor system. *Sleep, ***28**, 1505–1510.

Roman, V., Van der Borght, K., Leembur S.A., Van der Zee, E.A., and Meerlo, P. (2005b). Sleep restriction by forced activity reduces hippocampal cell proliferation. *Brain Res., ***1065**, 53–59.

Sahay, A., and Hen, R. (2007). Adult hippocampal neurogenesis in depression. *Nat Neurosci., ***10**, 1110–1115.

Sairanen, M., O'Leary, O.F., Knuuttila, J.E., and Castren, E. (2007). Chronic antidepressant treatment selectively increases expression of plasticity-related proteins in the hippocampus and medial prefrontal cortex of the rat. *Neuroscience, ***144**, 368–374.

Sanai, N., Berger, M.S., Garcia-Verdugo, J.M., and Alvarez-Buylla, A. (2007). Comment on 'Human neuroblasts migrate to the olfactory bulb via a lateral ventricular extension.' *Science, ***318**, 393.

Sandi, C. (2004). Stress, cognitive impairment and cell adhesion molecules. *Nat Rev Neurosci., ***5**, 917–930.

Santarelli, L., Saxe, M., Gross, C. et al. (2003). Requirement of hippocampal neurogenesis for the behavioral effects of antidepressants. *Science, ***301**, 805–809.

Seckl, J.R. (2001). Glucocorticoid programming of the fetus; adult phenotypes and molecular mechanisms. *Mol Cell Endocrinol., ***185**, 61–71.

Sheline, Y.I. (2000). 3D MRI studies of neuroanatomic changes in unipolar major depression: the role of stress and medical comorbidity. *Biol Psychiatry., ***48**, 791–800.

Sheline, Y.I. (2003). Neuroimaging studies of mood disorder effects on the brain. *Biol Psychiatry., ***54**, 338–352.

Shors, T.J., Mathew, J., Sisti, H.M., Edgecomb, C., Beckoff, S., and Dalla, C. (2007). Neurogenesis and helplessness are mediated by controllability in males but not in females. *Biol Psychiatry.*, **62**, 487–495.

Sousa, N., Almeida, O.F., Holsboer, F., Paula-Barbosa, M.M., and Madeira, M.D. (1998). Maintenance of hippocampal cell numbers in young and aged rats submitted to chronic unpredictable stress. Comparison with the effects of corticosterone treatment. *Stress*, **2**, 237–249.

Stickgold, R., and Walker, M.P. (2005). Memory consolidation and reconsolidation: what is the role of sleep? *Trends Neurosci.*, **28**, 408–415.

Swaab, D.F., Bao, A.M., and Lucassen, P.J. (2005). The stress system in the human brain in depression and neurodegeneration. *Ageing Res Rev.*, **4**, 141–194.

Tanapat, P., Hastings, N.B., Rydel, T.A., Galea, L.A., and Gould, E. (2001). Exposure to fox odor inhibits cell proliferation in the hippocampus of adult rats via an adrenal hormone-dependent mechanism. *J Comp Neurol.*, **437**, 496–504.

Thomas, R.M., Urban, J.H., and Peterson, D.A. (2006). Acute exposure to predator odor elicits a robust increase in corticosterone and a decrease in activity without altering proliferation in the adult rat hippocampus. *Exp Neurol.*, **201**, 308–315.

Vallieres, L., Campbell, I.L., Gage, F.H., and Sawchenko, P.E. (2002). Reduced hippocampal neurogenesis in adult transgenic mice with chronic astrocytic production of interleukin-6. *J Neurosci.*, **22**, 486–492.

van der Borght, K., Meerlo, P., Luiten, P.G., Eggen, B.J., and Van der Zee, E.A. (2005). Effects of active shock avoidance learning on hippocampal neurogenesis and plasma levels of corticosterone. *Behav Brain Res.*, **157**, 23–30.

van Praag, H., Christie, B.R., Sejnowski, T.J., and Gage, F.H. (1999). Running enhances neurogenesis, learning, and long-term potentiation in mice. *Proc Natl Acad Sci USA*, **96**, 13427–13431.

Veenema, A.H., De Kloet, E.R., De Wilde, M.C. et al. (2007). Differential effects of stress on adult hippocampal cell proliferation in low and high aggressive mice. *J.Neuroendocrinol.*, **19**, 489–498.

Vollmayr, B., Simonis, C., Weber, S., Gass, P., and Henn, F. (2003). Reduced cell proliferation in the dentate gyrus is not correlated with the development of learned helplessness. *Biol Psychiatry*, **54**, 1035–1040.

Wachs, F.P., Winner, B., Couillard-Despres, S. et al. (2006). Transforming growth factor-beta1 is a negative modulator of adult neurogenesis. *J Neuropathol Exp Neurol.*, **65**, 358–370.

Warner-Schmidt, J.L., and Duman, R.S. (2006). Hippocampal neurogenesis: opposing effects of stress and antidepressant treatment. *Hippocampus*, **16**, 239–49.

Wong, E.Y., and Herbert, J. (2006). Raised circulating corticosterone inhibits neuronal differentiation of progenitor cells in the adult hippocampus. *Neuroscience*, **137**, 83–92.

Zhang, L.X., Levine, S., Dent, G. et al. (2002). Maternal deprivation increases cell death in the infant rat brain. *Dev Brain Res.*, **133**, 1–11.

Zhao, C., Deng, W., and Gage, F.H. (2008). Mechanisms and functional implications of adult neurogenesis. *Cell*, **132**, 645–660.

Ziv, Y., Ron, N., Butovsky, O. et al. (2006). Immune cells contribute to the maintenance of neurogenesis and spatial learning abilities in adulthood. *Nat Neurosci.*, **9**, 268–275.

Chapter 12

The role of the medial prefrontal cortex in mediating resistance and vulnerability to the impact of adverse events

Steven F. Maier, Jose Amat, Michael V. Baratta,
Sondra T. Bland, John C. Christianson,
Brittany Thompson, Robert R. Rozeske, and
Linda R. Watkins

The aetiology of many psychological/psychiatric disorders involves a complex interplay between genetic predispositions and the experience of traumatic, adverse, or stressful events. The prevailing evidence suggests that trauma can dysregulate stress-responsive brainstem and limbic circuits, the proximate cause of some aspects of anxiety and depression (Charney, 2004). However, the exact circuits that are dysregulated and the manner in which this dysregulation occurs are not well understood. In addition, the consequences of exposure to aversive events is not determined solely by the physical nature of the event, but rather by complex cognitive factors relating to the individuals appraisal of the event and perceived ability to cope (Chorpita and Barlow, 1998). How such factors regulate the impact of the event on stress-responsive neural circuits is largely unknown. Moreover, individuals differ in their susceptibility and resilience to adverse events, and the experiential factors that determine vulnerability and resistance are only poorly understood. The present chapter will summarize the implications of the research that has been conducted with a particular animal paradigm for these issues. Clinical data relevant to the conceptualization of vulnerability and resilience are discussed in Chapter 14 of this book.

Serotonin and the dorsal raphe nucleus

Basic organization. A large number of structures and transmitters/modulators are responsive to environmental challenges and play roles in mediating the behavioural sequelae of exposure to such challenges. Recent evidence suggests that among these regions and transmitters, serotonergic (5-HT) neurons projecting from the dorsal (DRN) and median (MRN) raphe nuclei appear to have pivotal functions. There has been considerable controversy concerning whether 5-HT neurons are selectively or dedicatedly 'stress-responsive' (Rueter et al. 1997). This is in part due to the seemingly diffuse anatomical organization of 5-HT projections. Virtually all 5-HT cell bodies are located within the 9 raphe nuclei located in the brainstem. The DRN and MRN provide virtually all of the 5-HT innervation of forebrain and limbic structures, yet are themselves small brainstem regions that contain very few neurons. The rat DRN, for example, contains only 20 000–30 000 neurons, with perhaps 2/3 being 5-HT neurons. This organization means that a small number of cells innervate large areas of the brain, with this being possible because projecting 5-HT neurons arborize quite widely. At first glance, an arrangement in which a small number of neurons project from a discrete structure and connect with widespread regions would be well suited to regulate and be responsive to very general features of functioning such as arousal and generalized motor activity (Jacobs and Fornal, 1999), and indeed many 5-HT neurons do have this property of covarying with 'behavioral state' (Rueter et al. 1997). Moreover, 5-HT often acts in a modulatory fashion, with a significant portion of 5-HT transmission occurring via volume, rather than tight synaptic transmission (Ridet and Privat, 2000).

However, recent evidence suggests that there is some topographical organization to 5-HT systems (Lowry, 2002) and that there is a subpopulation of 5-HT neurons that may be selectively 'stress-responsive' and that play an important role in mediating aspects of anxiety and/or depression. Exposure to a variety of stressors has been shown to increase 5-HT metabolism or release in the medial prefrontal cortex (Kawahara et al. 1993), hippocampus (Amat et al. 1998b), amygdala (Adell et al. 1997), and nucleus accumbens (Inoue et al. 1994). Interestingly, these structures do not receive innervation from all raphe nuclei, or even all parts of the MRN and DRN. Rather, they receive 5-HT projections from only a part of the MRN and the caudal parts of the DRN, particularly the intrafascicular part. This anatomy, as well as other considerations, has led Lowry and colleagues (Lowry et al. 2005) to argue that there exists a discrete mesolimbocortical 5-HT system projecting from the caudal DRN and a closely related part of the MRN that is critical to the mediation of stress-related behavioural change (also see below). In support of this proposal, a variety of anxiogenic pharmacological agents have been shown to selectively increase the activity of 5-HT neurons in this subregion as assessed by Fos expression (Abrams et al. 2005; Singewald and Sharp, 2000) (also see below). Furthermore, pharmacological blockade of 5-HT receptors (Campbell and Merchant, 2003) and genetically reduced 5-HT release (Jennings et al. 2006) in projection regions of the caudal DRN, such as the basolateral amygdala, has been reported to decrease anxiety-related behaviours.

Relationship between corticotrophin releasing hormone (CRH) and 5-HT. An enormous body of evidence indicates that brain CRH systems serve a critical role in mediating the behavioural effects of stressor exposure (Smagin et al. 2001) and are involved in mediating anxiety and depression (Southwick et al. 2005). Obviously, the DRN does not operate in isolation, and so it is natural to inquire into possible relationships between non-hypothalamic CRH neurons and DRN 5-HT neurons in mediating the impact of adverse events. There are two major types of CRH receptors (CRHR1 and CRHR2). CRHR1 is widely distributed throughout the brain, but CRHR2 has a much more restricted distribution. Interestingly, the DRN is unusual in expressing a high density of CRHR2 (Chalmers et al. 1995).

There are data suggesting that CRH both excites (Lowry et al. 2000) and inhibits (Price et al. 1998) DRN 5-HT neurons. It is possible that this apparent discrepancy is produced by the presence of both CRHR1 and CRHR2 within the DRN. Ligands with high affinity for CRHR2, such as urocortin 2 (UcnII), have been shown to activate discrete populations of DRN neurons that are the same as or similar to those activated by stressors and anxiogenic drugs (Staub et al. 2005). With regard to CRH, there are data to suggest that low doses inhibit DRN 5-HT neurons, while higher doses are excitatory. Since CRH has a relatively low affinity for CRHR2 relative to CRHR1, the overall pattern of the results would follow if CRHR2 were differentially expressed on 5-HT neurons, whereas CRHR1 are also expressed on GABAergic inhibitory interneurons. There is some anatomical evidence that this distribution does indeed occur (Day et al. 2004).

Stressor controllability

Basic paradigm. Complex cognitive factors that in humans mediate the impact of stressors are difficult to study in animals, where the underlying neurochemistry can be explored. The stressor controllability/learned helplessness paradigm is an exception. Actual or perceived behavioural control (ability to alter the onset, termination, intensity, or pattern of an aversive event by behavioural responses) is a key element of coping processes, and can be studied in animals. In our laboratory rats are placed in small boxes with a small wheel mounted on the front wall that the rat can turn with its paws. The rat's tail extends from the rear of the chamber and electric shock can be delivered to the tail. Rats are run in triplets and two of the rats receive periodic tailshock. If one of the rats, designated 'Escape', turns the wheel during a tailshock then that tailshock terminates immediately. If the Escape rat does not turn the wheel, the shock remains present until a cut-off is reached. Thus, this rat has behavioural control over the termination of each of the tailshocks. The other rat, designated Yoked is paired with the Escape subject. For this rat each tailshock begins at the same time as it does for the Escape subject, but terminates when the Escape subject turns the wheel – for the Yoked rat turning the wheel has no consequence. Thus, the Escape and Yoked subjects receive *physically identical* stressors, but one has behavioural control (escapable shock – ES) and the other does not (IS). The third rat is a control that is either restrained in the apparatus or left in the home cage. With this design it is possible to determine whether any behavioural or physiological outcome of exposure to the stressor is caused by exposure to the stressor per se, the physical aspect, or to the psychological dimension of control.

Behavioural outcomes. Numerous studies have examined the behavioural outcomes that follow exposure to escapable (ES) and yoked inescapable (IS) shock. The earliest reported study (Seligman and Maier, 1967) found that subjects given IS later failed to learn to escape footshock in a shuttlebox, while subjects that had received equivalent ES learned normally. This phenomenon was called the 'learned helplessness effect', and has been often used as a behavioural endpoint in explorations of the neurobiology of stressor control. Failure to escape in a shuttlebox after IS but not ES was followed by reports indicating that a variety of behavioural changes (see Table 12.1) follow IS, but that ES leaves these behaviours unchanged. Some of the behavioural sequelae of IS appear to be 'depression-like', and some 'anxiety-like'.

Three points are worth making concerning these behavioural outcomes. The first is that not all of the behavioural changes that follow exposure to this stressor are modulated by controllability (e.g. Woodmansee et al. 1993), that is, there are a number of changes that follow ES as well as IS (e.g. reduced activity in a running wheel). Second, most of the behaviours that have been shown to be sensitive to stressor controllability have a finite time-course after IS. The impact of IS persists for 2–4 days, depending on the behavioural measure, and then dissipates (e.g. Maier et al. 1979). However, the behavioural effects of IS can be maintained for long periods of time if the subject (typically rats) is periodically made to 're-experience' the IS episode by being re-exposed to the

Table 12.1 Behavioural changes that follow exposure to inescapable, but not equal escapable stressor exposure

Depression-like Consequences	Anxiety-like Consequences
♦ Reduced aggressive, social, and sexual behavior	♦ Exaggerated fear conditioning
♦ Reduced food and water intake	♦ Exaggerated fear to ambiguous cues
♦ Reduced responding for Reduced motor activity in response to aversive events	♦ Neophobia
♦ Reduced escape behavior	♦ Anxious behavior in "tests" of anxiety (social interaction, elevated plus mtaze, zero maze)
♦ Reduced exploration brain stimulation reward	♦ Exaggerated attention to external cues
♦ Sensitivity to antidepressant drugs	♦ Timecourse
	♦ Sensitivity to blockade by anxiolytic drugs
	♦ Induction by anxiogenic drugs

environment in which IS had occurred (Maier, 2001). Third, because the pattern of findings was typically one in which IS produced an outcome, but ES failed to do so and appeared to produce a subject no different than non-shocked controls, it was natural to assume that it is the lack of control that is the active ingredient that is learned about and that initiates a neural cascade of events that produce the behavioural outcomes such as failure to learn in a shuttlebox. Controllable stressors were assumed to merely lack that key ingredient and to simply not produce the critical neurochemical alterations produced by the uncontrollable stressor. That is, the experience of controllable stressor was assumed to leave the organism relatively unchanged.

Uncontrollable stressors and the DRN

Given the assumption that it is uncontrollability that is the active ingredient that produces behavioural change, it was only natural to focus on determining the neurochemical changes that are produced by IS, and how these neurochemical changes mediate subsequent behaviours, such as poor escape learning. Indeed, many investigators did not even include ES groups in their studies, and simply compared IS to non-shocked subjects. Because the behavioural changes that follow IS are broad and mediated by a diverse array of neural structures (e.g. escape by the dorsal periaqueductal grey (dPAG), fear by the amygdala, etc.), it was logical to begin by determining whether structures that project widely, including to regions that are proximate mediators of behaviours that are altered by IS, might be key nodes. The locus coeruleus (LC) and the DRN were obvious possibilities. The LC sends noradrenergic projections to much of the forebrain, and its involvement in stressor controllability phenomena has been studied by Jay Weiss and his colleagues (Weiss et al., 1981). The DRN sends 5-HT projections widely, including to the dPAG and amygdala. Indeed, 5-HT released in the dPAG inhibits escape, while 5-HT released in the amygdala potentiates fear (Graeff et al. 1997), the exact pattern produced by IS.

Our laboratory has focused on the role of the DRN, and it is indeed a critical structure in the mediation of the behavioural sequelae of uncontrollable stressors. The most important findings have been the following:

(1) IS produces a much greater activation of DRN 5-HT neurons than does exactly equal amounts of ES (Grahn et al. 1999), leading to greater release of 5-HT in projection regions of the DRN such as the amygdala (Amat et al. 1998a). Interestingly, this differential activation is restricted to the same caudal part of the DRN that has been reported to be activated by anxiogenics (see above).

(2) The intense activation of the DRN produced by IS leads to the sensitization of DRN 5-HT neurons for a period of a number of days, at least in part because inhibitory somatodendritic 5-HT1A autoreceptors on DRN 5-HT neurons are desensitized/downregulated (Greenwood et al. 2003). This 5-HT1A downregulation likely occurs because IS produces an accumulation of high levels of extracellular 5-HT within the DRN (Maswood et al. 1998) from release by axon collaterals within the DRN.

(3) This sensitization leads to the release of exaggerated levels of 5-HT in projection regions of the DRN in response to input to the DRN. For example, two footshocks are not sufficient to increase 5-HT efflux within the basolateral amygdala under normal conditions, but produces large increases in rats that had experienced IS, but not ES, 24 hour earlier (Amat et al. 1998a);

(4) The excessive release of 5-HT from these sensitized DRN 5-HT neurons appears to be both necessary and sufficient to produce the typical behavioural consequences of IS. It is necessary because either lesion of the DRN (Maier et al. 1993) or selective inhibition of DRN 5-HT

activity, either at the time of IS or later behavioural testing, prevents the behavioural effects of IS (e.g. shuttlebox escape learning deficits now do not occur) from occurring (Maier et al. 1994). DRN 5-HT activation is sufficient because the intense activation of DRN 5-HT activation via the microinjection of pharmacological activating agents, in the absence of any shock stressor at all, produces later behavioural changes that mimic those produced by IS (Maier et al. 1995).

Although the DRN is a key node in the mediation of the behavioural consequences of IS, it does not receive direct somatosensory projections and so must receive input from other structures that leads to IS-induced activation. Given the topic of this book, it should be noted that CRH or some other ligand for the CRH receptor plays an important role in activating the DRN during IS. Thus, microinjection of a CRH antagonist into the caudal (but not rostral) DRN blocks the behavioural effects of IS (Hammack et al. 2002), and microinjection of UcnII without any shock produces them (Hammack et al. 2003). These data suggest that there is a critical CRH or other CRH-like ligand input to the DRN during IS, possibly from the bed nucleus of the stria terminalis (Hammack et al. 2004) and that the DRN is a target of CRH action. CRH input is not only signalling to the DRN that is critical in the mediation of IS behavioural effects (Amat et al. 2001; Grahn et al. 2002), but a discussion of this issue is beyond the scope of this chapter.

The ventral medial prefrontal cortex

The research alluded to above uncovered a number of critical inputs to the DRN that are required for activation during IS, but none discriminated between IS and ES (Amat et al. 2001). That is, they provided excitatory input whether the stressor was uncontrollable or controllable. Given that ES produces a much smaller activation of DRN 5-HT neurons than does IS, this pattern of data implies that the presence of behavioural control leads to an active suppression of DRN 5-HT activation. This could occur because the DRN itself detects the presence of behavioural control, or because some other structure detects control and then sends input to the DRN that inhibits 5-HT activity. Obviously, what defines control here is that a motor response (turning the wheel) reliably precedes the termination of each of the tailshocks. A structure that detects the presence of control must be able to compute that the conditional probability of shock termination given that the wheel has been turned is greater than the conditional probability of shock termination given that the wheel has not been turned. Thus, in order to detect or compute whether behavioural control is present a brain region would need somatomotor input that provides information regarding whether motor responses have or have not occurred, and somatosensory information indicating whether tailshock is or is not present. The DRN does not receive such input.

In general terms it is the cortex that receives sensory and feedback motor input and performs sensory-motor integration. Interestingly, the DRN receives virtually all of its cortical input from prelimbic (PL) and infralimbic (IL) regions of the ventral medial prefrontal cortex (vmPFC) (Gabbott et al. 2005). Glutamatergic afferents from the vmPFC synapse preferentially on GABAergic interneurons within the DRN (Jankowski and Sesack, 2004). Thus, activation of vmPFC output would be expected to inhibit DRN 5-HT neuronal activity, a finding that has been reported by several groups (Celada et al. 2001; Hajos et al. 1998). If some aspect of behavioural control is processed by the vmPFC with consequent input to the DRN via direct projections, then the regulation of DRN 5-HT activity would have to be inhibitory. This suggests that perhaps it is control, not the lack of control that is the active ingredient producing controllability differences. In this scheme the DRN is driven from brain regions that respond to aversive stimulation per se, whether it is controllable or uncontrollable. The presence of control would be detected by the vmPFC, with vmPFC output to the DRN inhibiting the activation produced by the stressor (see Fig. 12.1).

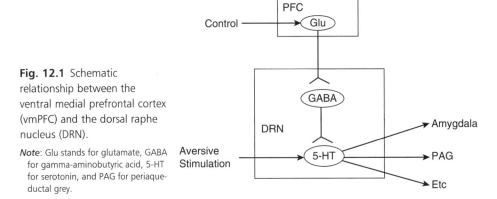

Fig. 12.1 Schematic relationship between the ventral medial prefrontal cortex (vmPFC) and the dorsal raphe nucleus (DRN).

Note: Glu stands for glutamate, GABA for gamma-aminobutyric acid, 5-HT for serotonin, and PAG for periaqueductal grey.

Control, the vmPFC, the DRN, and learned helplessness. The most obvious implications of the model shown in Fig. 12.1 are that the differential DRN 5-HT activation and DRN-dependent behavioural outcomes produced by IS and ES are dependent on vmPFC activation during ES. Clearly, if vmPFC output to the DRN is prevented during the ES and IS experiences, now ES should produce the same high level of DRN 5-HT activation and behavioural consequences typical of IS. Amat et al. (2005) examined just these possibilities by inactivating the vmPFC by microinjection of the GABAa agonist muscimol during ES and yoked IS. DRN activation was assessed by measuring the expression of Fos in 5-HT labelled neurons within the DRN and extracellular levels of 5-HT within the DRN. The latter is a measure of DRN 5-HT activation because activated DRN 5-HT neurons release 5-HT within the DRN from axon collaterals, as well as in projection regions. Inhibition of the vmPFC during the stressor did not alter the intense activation of the DRN produced by IS, but it radically altered the outcome of ES – now ES produced an intense activation of DRN 5-HT neurons equal to that produced by IS. Consistent with this effect on the DRN, inactivation of the vmPFC led ES to produce the same behavioural consequence (deficits in shuttlebox escape learning–the learned helplessness effect) as are normally produced only by IS.

It is important to note that vmPFC inactivation during ES did not interfere with the rats learning to turn the wheel to escape during ES. That is, the rat acquired the wheel turn escape response normally, but when the vmPFC was inactivated the DRN responded as if the rat was not performing wheel turn escape responses. Furthermore, subsequent behaviour was as if the rat had not actually been able to escape, even though escape behaviour was performed perfectly. This pattern becomes sensible when it is recognized that the vmPFC is not involved in habit learning (Dalley et al. 2004). Instead, what the vmPFC appears to be doing is to use the presence or absence of the stressor controlling escape response to regulate the DRN response to the stressor.

If the difference in consequences between uncontrollable and controllable stressors occurs because the ability to exert behavioural control activates vmPFC output to the DRN, then simple pharmacological activation of the vmPFC during stressor exposure should prevent DRN activation and later failure to learn to escape, even if the stressor were uncontrollable. To test this idea Amat et al. (2008) microinjected picrotoxin, a GABA-A antagonist, during exposure to ES and yoked IS. Since the pyramidal output neurons from the vmPFC are under GABAergic inhibition, picrotoxin activates vmPFC output (Berretta, 2005). vmPFC activation during the stressors led IS to appear as if it was ES – DRN 5-HT activity was reduced to the usual level produced by ES and later escape learning deficits did not occur. Thus, vmPFC inactivation led ES to function as if it was IS, and vmPFC activation led IS to function as if it was ES. Clearly, what is critical is whether vmPFC output is activated or not, not whether the stressor is actually under behavioural control.

Control, the vmPFC, the DRN, and immunization. Exposure to a stressor often alters the organism's responses to a subsequent stressor. Interestingly, the controllability of the initial stress experience determines the nature of this proactive effect. Several studies have reported that an initial experience with ES blocks the usual behavioural consequences of later IS, while an initial exposure to IS either has no effect on, or potentiates the impact of later IS (Moye et al. 1983; Williams and Maier, 1977). Is the vmPFC critical to the immunizing effects of ES? To answer this question Amat et al. (2006) exposed rats to either ES, yoked IS, or control treatment, with separate groups receiving vmPFC microinjection of muscimol during this Day 1 treatment. Seven days later the rats all received IS and DRN activation during the IS and later behaviour was measured. The initial exposure to ES prevented the normal high level of DRN activation during the later IS – that is, the DRN acted as if the IS was actually escapable. Subsequent behaviour followed suit and now IS did not produce later escape learning deficits. Importantly, prior IS did not reduce the IS-induced DRN activation or the effects of IS on later behaviour. Thus, the protective effects were specific to ES. vmPFC inactivation during ES eliminated the immunizing effects of ES – now ES did not reduce the DRN activation produced by subsequent IS nor did it reduce the behavioural impact of IS.

One way to explain these proactive effects of ES is to imagine that there is plasticity in the vmPFC so that activation by ES alters it in such a fashion that it is now later activated by IS, thereby inhibiting the DRN and blocking behavioural outcomes. If this were so, then ES-induced immunization would require vmPFC activation at the time of the later IS, as well as during the initial ES. To test this possibility Amat et al. (2006) inactivated the vmPFC during the second IS experience, rather than during the initial ES, and this eliminated the reduction in DRN activation and the protection against the behavioural effects of IS afforded by the initial ES experience. Thus, the vmPFC is needed to allow the organism to utilize the prior exposure to ES in regulating the DRN and behaviours that are a consequence of DRN 5-HT sensitization. Again, the subjects will have learned about control during the Day 1 treatment, but the later use of this information requires the vmPFC. The data would suggest that perhaps the experience of ES 'ties' or associates the activation of the vmPFC to the tailshock stimulus or to some aspect of the cascade of neural and endocrine changes induced by the shock so that the later occurrence of even IS will now activate the vmPFC output to the DRN. If this is so, then there would have to be long-term plasticity in the vmPFC, and it can be noted that the intra-vmPFC microinjection of the protein synthesis inhibitor anisomycin after ES blocked the immunizing effects of ES (Amat et al. 2006). This is noteworthy because persistent plasticity requires the synthesis of new proteins (Gold, 2008).

The implication of the data reviewed above is that activation of the vmPFC during a stressor alters vmPFC function in such a way that it is later activated by stimuli that share some aspect in common with the initial stressor. If this is so, then pharmacological activation of vmPFC should produce immunization against later IS, but only if is paired with exposure to the stressor. Amat et al. (2008) microinjected picrotoxin in the vmPFC before either ES, IS, or no shock control treatment. IS followed seven days later. Mere exposure to picrotoxin did not block the later effects of IS. However, picrotoxin given during the initial IS experience blocked the DRN activation during later IS, as well as the behavioural effects of the IS. That is, the simple activation of the vmPFC during the stressor was protective. Clearly, the non-specific activation of the vmPFC with picrotoxin duplicates the effects of having behavioural control.

Control, the vmPFC, the amygdala, and fear conditioning. The research described above focused on vmPFC regulation of the DRN and behaviours that result from DRN activation. However, the vmPFC projects to other stress-responsive structures, with the amygdala being notable in this regard (Vertes, 2004). The amygdala serves a variety of functions, but plays a clear role in fear conditioning. In fear conditioning an association is formed between external stimuli such as tones or lights (the CS) and an aversive stimulus, typically a footshock (the UCS). Neurons encoding the CS and UCS project to the basolateral region of the amygdala (BLA), and here the association between them is formed. The BLA then sends input to the CeA, with the CeA sending projections to the regions of the brain that produce the individual responses that constitute fear. For example, the CeA projects to the periaqueductal grey, with the periaqueductal grey producing the freezing that is characteristic of fear in rodents. Thus, the BLA is where the conditioning occurs and the CeA produces the fear response output (see Fanselow and Poulos, 2005; Kim and Jung, 2006; Walker and Davis, 2002, for reviews).

The data from the vmPFC inactivation and activation studies above suggests that the experience of ES alters the vmPFC in such a way that it is later activated by shocks that are uncontrollable as well as shocks that are controllable. What if after experience with ES fear would activate the vmPFC? If this were to occur, then prior exposure to ES might be expected to retard fear conditioning. Baratta et al. (2007) exposed rats to ES, yoked IS, or control treatment. Fear conditioning in which a tone was paired with footshock occurred seven days later, with testing for the amount of fear conditioned to the tone and to the shock context occurring 24 hour later. As might be expected (Rau et al. 2005), prior IS facilitated fear conditioning, that is, more fear was conditioned to the tone and to the shock context than in non-shocked controls. However, prior ES actually retarded fear conditioning. This result is quite striking as ES is not negatively fearful or stressful, it is quite aversive (Maier et al. 1986), but it reduced the fear conditioned to the tone and context.

The role of IL and PL cortices in fear processes: control alters the expression but not the learning of conditioned fear. There has been a great deal of recent interest in the role of the vmPFC in fear conditioning and extinction, and a consideration of this literature suggests an interpretation of the impact of control on later fear acquisition. The literature on the function of the vmPFC in fear is inconsistent. The inconsistencies are likely in part due to the use of lesions versus chemical inactivation and failures to distinguish the PL and IL regions of the vmPFC. The IL and PL regions have different projections to the amygdala. The PL projects primarily to the basal nucleus (McDonald et al. 1996) and appears to be excitatory in nature (Likhtik et al. 2005). As noted above, the basal nucleus projects to the CeA and the connection is excitatory (Quirk et al. 2003), leading to output from the CeA to the proximate mediators of fear responses. In contrast, the IL sends glutamatergic projections to GABAergic cells in the lateral subdivision of the central nucleus and the intercalated cell mass (ITC) (Sesack et al. 1989). These GABAergic cells inhibit the CeA output neurons (Royer et al. 1999). Vidal-Gonzalez et al. (2006) have summarized this anatomy in the schematic shown in Fig. 12.2.

This anatomy would suggest that PL and IL manipulation might exert opposite effects on fear responses. Clearly, PL stimulation should increase the *expression* of conditioned fear responses, while IL stimulation should reduce the expression of fear. Milad et al. (2004) conditioned fear responses to a tone and then added IL microstimulation to the presentation of the tone. This decreased fear on the very first trail, demonstrating that the effect was on expression rather than learning. Conversely, PL microstimulation proved to increase fear responses when added to the CS (Vidal-Gonzalez et al. 2006). In addition to regulating the expression of fear via its connections to the amygdala, the vmPFC may also be a site of plasticity in the formation of fear conditioning or in fear extinction (Quirk and Mueller, 2008), but this is not an issue here. The clinical evidence supporting a role for PFC and emotional processing in affective disorders is also discussed in Chapters 13 and 22 of this book.

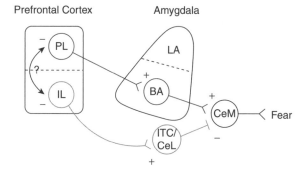

Prefrontal Cortex   Amygdala

Fig. 12.2 Relationship between the ventral medial prefrontal cortex and amygdala (from Vidal-Gonzalez et al. 2006). See colour plate section for colour version.

Note: PL stands for prelimbic, IL for infralimbic, LA for lateral amygdala, BL for absl amygdala, ITC for interca-lated region, CeL for lateral division of the central nucleus, and CeMfor the mdiql division of the central nucleus.

The foregoing suggests that perhaps the experience of ES did not facilitate the fear conditioning process itself, that is, the formation of the association between CS and UCS. Rather, it might have increased the amount of fear expressed to a CS without altering its level of association with the UCS, and it might have done so while altering the vmPFC in such a way that IL input to the amygdala was enhanced during the testing for fear. To examine these possibilities Baratta et al. (2008) conducted the same three-stage experiment as above – exposure to ES, fear conditioning, and then fear testing. The critical new finding was that intra-IL microinjection of muscimol before testing restored the level of fear in the ES subjects to control levels. That is, ES reduced the measured fear response following conditioning as before, but the impact of the ES was eliminated by inhibition of the IL during the testing. Thus, the association of CS and UCS had clearly been formed in an intact manner, but prior ES simply reduced the expression of that association in fear behaviour.

Summary

It has been clear for many years that the degree of behavioural control that the organism has over adverse events is a potent modulator of the behavioural and physiological impact of that event. The earliest thinking was that the differential effects of inescapable and escapable stressors occurred because the organism learns about the uncontrollability of the inescapable stressor, with this learning of uncontrollability then initiating a cascade of events that produces the behavioural consequences of IS (Maier et al. 1969). The presence of control was not viewed as inducing active processes of its own, but rather as simply lacking the active uncontrollability ingredient. This thinking is evident in the terms that were given for the initial phenomenon –'learned helplessness' and 'behavioural depression'. The recent research reviewed above suggests a quite different interpretation. At least as far as the vmPFC is concerned, the data imply that it is the presence of control that initiates vmPFC action. When the vmPFC was inhibited during ES and IS regions of the brain innervated by the vmPFC and behaviour acted as if both ES and IS were uncontrollable. Conversely, when the vmPFC was activated during ES and IS both the brain and behaviour responded as if the stressor were controllable.

The foregoing suggests that the 'default option' for subcortical brain structures is that a stressor cannot be controlled by behavioural responses. That is, it would appear that regions such as the DRN are activated by both uncontrollable and controllable stress, but are actively inhibited by the vmPFC if the stressor is controllable (Fig. 12.1). This would seem to be a sensible arrangement from an evolutionary perspective. The vmPFC is a relatively recently evolved structure, and more primitive organisms can be argued to have little reason for great sensitivity to the dimension of behavioural control. Many primitive organisms do not have extensive behavioural repertoires that can be used to deal with threatening stimuli, and many of the adjustments that occur to such stimuli are physiological in nature. Thus, it would be sensible for phylogenetically old stress-responsive brain structures to be activated by stressors per se without regard to complex factors such as behavioural control. These physiological adjustments often involve the sensitization of defensive reflexes and the production of energy (Clatworthy et al. 1994). The processes involved (e.g. glucocorticoid secretion) can be costly and catabolic in nature (e.g. breakdown of muscle), and so it would be useful to keep them in check under circumstances where they are not needed. If behavioural coping is possible it might be better to deal with a threat behaviourally than to allow persistent activation of metabolically demanding and potentially injurious processes. Thus, as the evolving organism's behavioural repertoire became more complex it would be sensible that 'higher' brain structures inhibit the activation of 'lower' stress-responsive structures if behavioural coping is possible.

Emotional regulation

The data and perspective presented here are consistent with recent human research that is described as concerning 'emotion regulation'. A variety of human research has focused on the 'top-down' regulation of emotion (e.g. Phan et al. 2005) and has suggested that this regulation may be compromised in a variety of psychological disorders (Taylor and Liberzon, 2007). Neuroimaging studies of emotional reappraisal have implicated precisely the neural interactions suggested by our animal data reviewed above. In these studies subjects are shown pictures that either arouse negative affect or are neutral and asked either to (a) simply attend to the pictures, (b) reduce the affect produced by the picture by viewing the situation depicted as being fake or as having an outcome different from the one shown (e.g. victims of a car accident were not really hurt badly and survived well), or (c) increase the affect by imagining themselves as experiencing the situation depicted or imagining a more extreme outcome than the one shown (e.g. in response to a picture of a ferocious dog the subject might imagine that the leash broke and that they were attacked). The first studies using this type of paradigm (e.g. Oschner et al. 2002) found that when subjects were asked to decrease their negative affect there was decreased amygdala activity, as would be expected, and an increase in activity in lateral and dorsal regions of PFC. However, it is difficult for the lateral PFC and amygdala changes to be directly related since there are no direct connections between lateral and dorsal parts of the PFC and the amygdala. However, the vmPFC does project to the amygdala in humans (Ongur and Price, 2000) and so Urry et al. (2006) examined whether there is an inverse relationship between vmPFC and amygdala activity during negative emotional regulation. Indeed, the more successful the subject was at reducing the affective impact of the pictures the less the amygdala activity and the greater vmPFC activity. There was a strong negative correlation between vmPFC and amygdala activity, and further analysis has indicated that the vmPFC–amygdala relationship fully accounts for the dorsal/lateral PFC-amygdala correlation. Interestingly, this vmPFC-amygdala inverse relationship during negative emotion regulation is lost in depressed individuals (Johnstone et al. 2007).

This top-down regulation of amygdala activity by the vmPFC during the voluntary reduction of negative emotion is exactly what our experiments have uncovered in a different domain, the effects of behavioural control over stressors in animals. Thus, it may be useful to view behavioural control within the broader context of emotion regulation, with the presence of control blunting emotional responsivity to adverse events. Deficient regulation would allow brainstem and limbic stress-responsive structures to be activated in an unrestrained fashion, which is precisely the pattern when control is absent. Perhaps a loss of top-down vmPFC inhibitory control is a key element in the aetiology of affective disorders.

References

Abrams, J.K., Johnson, P.L., Hay-Schmidt, A., Mikkelsen, J.D., Shekhar, A., and Lowry, C.A. (2005). Serotonergic systems associated with arousal and vigilance behaviors following administration of anxiogenic drugs. *Neuroscience, 133*, 983–997.

Adell, A., Casanovas, J.M., and Artigas, F. (1997). Comparative study in the rat of the actions of different types of stress on the release of 5-HT in raphe nuclei and forebrain areas. *Neuropharmacology, 36*, 735–741.

Amat, J., Matus-Amat, P., Watkins, L.R., and Maier, S.F. (1998a). Escapable and inescapable stress differentially alter extracellular levels of 5-HT in the basolateral amygdala of the rat. *Brain Res., 812*, 113–120.

Amat, J., Matus-Amat, P., Watkins, L.R., and Maier, S.F. (1998b). Escapable and inescapable stress differentially and selectively alter extracellular levels of 5-HT in the ventral hippocampus and dorsal periaqueductal gray of the rat. *Brain Res., 797*, 12–22.

Amat, J., Sparks, P.D., Matus-Amat, P., Griggs, J., Watkins, L. R., and Maier, S.F. (2001). The role of the habenular complex in the elevation of dorsal raphe nucleus serotonin and the changes in the behavioral responses produced by uncontrollable stress. *Brain Res., 917*, 118–126.

Amat, J., Baratta, M.V., Paul, E., Bland, S.T., Watkins, L.R., and Maier, S.F. (2005). Medial prefrontal cortex determines how stressor controllability affects behavior and dorsal raphe nucleus. *Nat Neurosci., 8*, 365–371.

Amat, J., Paul, E., Zarza, C., Watkins, L.R., and Maier, S.F. (2006). Previous experience with behavioral control over stress blocks the behavioral and dorsal raphe nucleus activating effects of later uncontrollable stress: role of the ventral medial prefrontal cortex. *J Neurosci., 26*, 13264–13272.

Amat, J., Paul, E., Watkins, L.R., and Maier, S.F. (2008). Activation of the ventral medial prefrontal cortex during an uncontrollable stressor reproduces both the immediate and long-term protective effects of behavioral control. *Neuroscience, in press.*

Baratta, M.V., Christianson, J.P., Gomez, D.M. et al. (2007). Controllable versus uncontrollable stressors bi-directionally modulate conditioned but not innate fear. *Neuroscience, 146*, 1495–1503.

Baratta, M.V., Lucero, T.R., Amat, J., Watkins, L.R., and Maier, S.F. (2008). Role of the ventral medial prefrontal cortex in mediating behavioral control-induced reduction of later conditioned fear. *Learn Mem., 15*, 84–87.

Berretta, S., Pantazopoulos, H., Caldera, M., Pantazopoulos, P., and Pare, D. (2005). Infralimbic cortex activation increases c-Fos expression in intercalated neurons of the amygdala. *Neuroscience, 132*, 943–953.

Campbell, B.M. and Merchant, K.M. (2003). Serotonin 2C receptors within the basolateral amygdala induce acute fear-like responses in an open-field environment. *Brain Res., 993*, 1–9.

Celada, P., Puig, M.V., Casanovas, J.M., Guillazo, G., and Artigas, F. (2001). Control of dorsal raphe serotonergic neurons by the medial prefrontal cortex: Involvement of serotonin-1A, GABA(A), and glutamate receptors. *J Neurosci., 21*, 9917–9929.

Chalmers, D.T., Lovenberg, T.W., and De Souza, E.B. (1995). Localization of novel corticotropin-releasing factor receptor (CRF2) mRNA expression to specific subcortical nuclei in rat brain: comparison with CRF1 receptor mRNA expression. *J Neurosci., 15*, 6340–6350.

Charney, D.S. (2004). Psychobiological mechanisms of resilience and vulnerability: implications for successful adaptation to extreme stress. *Am J Psychiatry., 161*, 195–216.

Chorpita, B.F. and Barlow, D.H. (1998). The development of anxiety: the role of control in the early environment. *Psychol Bull., 124*, 3–21.

Clatworthy, A.L., Castro, G.A., and Walters, E.T. (1994). Induction of a cellular defense reaction is accompanied by an increase in sensory neuron excitability in Aplysia. *Ann N Y Acad Sci., 712*, 335–337.

Dalley, J.W., Cardinal, R.N., and Robbins, T.W. (2004). Prefrontal executive and cognitive functions in rodents: neural and neurochemical substrates. *Neurosci Biobehav Rev.*, **28**, 771–784.

Day, H.E., Greenwood, B.N., Hammack, S.E. et al. (2004). Differential expression of 5HT-1A, alpha 1b adrenergic, CRF-R1, and CRF-R2 receptor mRNA in serotonergic, gamma-aminobutyric acidergic, and catecholaminergic cells of the rat dorsal raphe nucleus. *J Comp Neurol.*, **474**, 364–378.

Fanselow, M.S., and Poulos, A.M. (2005). The neuroscience of mammalian associative learning. *Annu Rev Psychol.*, **56**, 207–234.

Gabbott, P.L., Warner, T.A., Jays, P.R., Salway, P., and Busby, S.J. (2005). Prefrontal cortex in the rat: projections to subcortical autonomic, motor, and limbic centers. *J Comp Neurol.*, **492**, 145–177.

Gold, P. E. (2008). Protein synthesis inhibition and memory: formation vs amnesia. *Neurobiol Learn Mem.*, **89**, 201–211.

Graeff, F.G., Viana, M.B., and Mora, P.O. (1997). Dual role of 5-HT in defense and anxiety. *Neurosci Biobehav Rev.*, **21**, 791–799.

Grahn, R.E., Will, M.J., Hammack, S.E. et al. (1999). Activation of serotonin-immunoreactive cells in the dorsal raphe nucleus in rats exposed to an uncontrollable stressor. *Brain Res.*, **826**, 35–43.

Grahn, R.E., Hammack, S.E., Will, M.J. et al. (2002). Blockade of alpha1 adrenoreceptors in the dorsal raphe nucleus prevents enhanced conditioned fear and impaired escape performance following uncontrollable stressor exposure in rats. *Behav Brain Res.*, **134**, 387–392.

Greenwood, B.N., Foley, T.E., Day, H.E. et al. (2003). Freewheel running prevents learned helplessness/ behavioral depression: role of dorsal raphe serotonergic neurons. *J Neurosci.*, **23**, 2889–2898.

Hajos, M., Richards, C.D., Szekely, A.D., and Sharp, T. (1998). An electrophysiological and neuroanatomical study of the medial prefrontal cortical projection to the midbrain raphe nuclei in the rat. *Neuroscience*, **87**, 95–108.

Hammack, S.E., Richey, K.J., Schmid, M.J., LoPresti, M.L., Watkins, L.R., and Maier, S. F. (2002). The role of corticotropin-releasing hormone in the dorsal raphe nucleus in mediating the behavioral consequences of uncontrollable stress. *J Neurosci.*, **22**, 1020–1026.

Hammack, S.E., Schmid, M.J., LoPresti, M.L. et al. (2003). Corticotropin releasing hormone type 2 receptors in the dorsal raphe nucleus mediate the behavioral consequences of uncontrollable stress. *J Neurosci.*, **23**, 1019–1025.

Hammack, S.E., Richey, K.J., Watkins, L.R., and Maier, S.F. (2004). Chemical lesion of the bed nucleus of the stria terminalis blocks the behavioral consequences of uncontrollable stress. *Behav Neurosci.*, **118**, 443–448.

Inoue, T., Tsuchiya, K., and Koyama, T. (1994). Regional changes in dopamine and serotonin activation with various intensity of physical and psychological stress in the rat brain. *Pharmacol Biochem Behav.*, **49**, 911–920.

Jacobs, B.L., and Fornal, C.A. (1999). Activity of serotonergic neurons in behaving animals. *Neuropsychopharmacology*, **21**, 9S–15S.

Jankowski, M.P. and Sesack, S.R. (2004). Prefrontal cortical projections to the rat dorsal raphe nucleus: ultrastructural features and associations with serotonin and gamma-aminobutyric acid neurons. *J Comp Neurol.*, **468**, 518–529.

Jennings, K.A., Loder, M.K., Sheward, W.J. et al. (2006). Increased expression of the 5-HT transporter confers a low-anxiety phenotype linked to decreased 5-HT transmission. *J Neurosci.*, **26**, 8955–8964.

Johnstone, T., van Reekum, C.M., Urry, H.L., Kalin, N.H., and Davidson, R.J. (2007). Failure to regulate: counterproductive recruitment of top-down prefrontal-subcortical circuitry in major depression. *J Neurosci.*, **27**, 8877–8884.

Kawahara, H., Yoshida, M., Yokoo, H., Nishi, M., and Tanaka, M. (1993). Psychological stress increases serotonin release in the rat amygdala and prefrontal cortex assessed by in vivo microdialysis. *Neurosci Lett.*, **162**, 81–84.

Kim, J.J., and Jung, M.W. (2006). Neural circuits and mechanisms involved in Pavlovian fear conditioning: a critical review. *Neurosci Biobehav Rev.*, **30**, 188–202.

Likhtik, E., Pelletier, J.G., Paz, R., and Pare, D. (2005). Prefrontal control of the amygdala. *J Neurosci.*, **25**, 7429–7437.

Lowry, C.A., Rodda, J.E., Lightman, S.L., and Ingram, C.D. (2000). Corticotropin-releasing factor increases in vitro firing rates of serotonergic neurons in the rat dorsal raphe nucleus: evidence for activation of a topographically organized mesolimbocortical serotonergic system. *J Neurosci.*, **20**, 7728–7736.

Lowry, C.A. (2002). Functional subsets of serotonergic neurones: implications for control of the hypothalamic-pituitary-adrenal axis. *J Neuroendocrinol.*, **14**, 911–923.

Lowry, C.A., Johnson, P.L., Hay-Schmidt, A., Mikkelsen, J., and Shekhar, A. (2005). Modulation of anxiety circuits by serotonergic systems. *Stress*, **8**, 233–246.

Maier, S.F., Seligman, M.E.P., and Solomon, R.L. (1969). Pavlovian fear conditioning and learned helplessness: effects on escape and avoidance behavior of (a) the CS-US contingency, and (b) the independence of the US and voluntary responding. In B. A. Campbell and R. M. Church (Eds.), *Punishment*, pp. 110–145. New York, Appleton-Century-Crofts.

Maier, S.F., Coon, D.J., McDaniel, M., and Jackson, R.L. (1979). The time course of learned helplessness, inactivity, and nociceptive deficits in rats. *Learning And Motivation*, **10**, 467–488.

Maier, S.F., Ryan, S.M., Barksdale, C.M., and Kalin, N.H. (1986). Stressor controllability and the pituitary-adrenal system. *Behav Neurosci.*, **100**, 669–674.

Maier, S.F., Grahn, R.E., Kalman, B.A., Sutton, L.C., Wiertelak, E.P., and Watkins, L.R. (1993). The role of the amygdala and dorsal raphe nucleus in mediating the behavioral consequences of inescapable shock. *Behav Neurosci.*, **107**, 377–388.

Maier, S.F., Kalman, B.A., and Grahn, R.E. (1994). Chlordiazepoxide microinjected into the region of the dorsal raphe nucleus eliminates the interference with escape responding produced by inescapable shock whether administered before inescapable shock or escape testing. *Behav Neurosci.*, **108**, 121–130.

Maier, S.F., Busch, C.R., Maswood, S., Grahn, R.E., and Watkins, L.R. (1995). The dorsal raphe nucleus is a site of action mediating the behavioral effects of the benzodiazepine receptor inverse agonist DMCM. *Behav Neurosci.*, **109**, 759–766.

Maier, S.F. (2001). Exposure to the stressor environment prevents the temporal dissipation of behavioral depression/learned helplessness. *Biol Psychiatry*, **49**, 763–773.

Maswood, S., Barter, J.E., Watkins, L.R., and Maier, S.F. (1998). Exposure to inescapable but not escapable shock increases extracellular levels of 5-HT in the dorsal raphe nucleus of the rat. *Brain Res.*, **783**, 115–120.

McDonald, A.J., Mascagni, F., and Guo, L. (1996). Projections of the medial and lateral prefrontal cortices to the amygdala: a Phaseolus vulgaris leucoagglutinin study in the rat. *Neuroscience*, **71**, 55–75.

Milad, M.R., Vidal-Gonzalez, I., and Quirk, G. J. (2004). Electrical stimulation of medial prefrontal cortex reduces conditioned fear in a temporally specific manner. *Behav Neurosci.*, **118**, 389–394.

Moye, T.B., Hyson, R.L., Grau, J.V., and Maier, S.F. (1983). Immunization of opioid analgesia: effects of prior escapable shock on subsequent shock-induced and morphine-induced antinociception. *Learning and Motivation*, **14**, 238–251.

Ochsner, K.N., Bunge, S.A., Gross, J.J., and Gabrieli, J.D. (2002). Rethinking feelings: an FMRI study of the cognitive regulation of emotion. *J Cogn Neurosci.*, **14**, 1215–1229.

Ongur, D., and Price, J.L. (2000). The organization of networks within the orbital and medial prefrontal cortex of rats, monkeys and humans. *Cereb Cortex*, **10**, 206–219.

Phan, K.L., Fitzgerald, D.A., Nathan, P.J., Moore, G.J., Uhde, T.W., and Tancer, M.E. (2005). Neural substrates for voluntary suppression of negative affect: a functional magnetic resonance imaging study. *Biol Psychiatry*, **57**, 210–219.

Price, M.L., Curtis, A.L., Kirby, L.G., Valentino, R.J., and Lucki, I. (1998). Effects of corticotropin-releasing factor on brain serotonergic activity. *Neuropsychopharmacology*, **18**, 492–502.

Quirk, G.J., Likhtik, E., Pelletier, J.G., and Pare, D. (2003). Stimulation of medial prefrontal cortex decreases the responsiveness of central amygdala output neurons. *J Neurosci., 23*, 8800–8807.

Quirk, G.J., and Mueller, D. (2008). Neural mechanisms of extinction learning and retrieval. *Neuropsychopharmacology, 33*, 56–72.

Rau, V., DeCola, J.P., and Fanselow, M.S. (2005). Stress-induced enhancement of fear learning: an animal model of posttraumatic stress disorder. *Neurosci Biobehav Rev., 29*, 1207–1223.

Ridet, J. and Privat, A. (2000). Voliume transmission. *Treends in Neuroscience, 23*, 58–59.

Royer, S., Martina, M., and Pare, D. (1999). An inhibitory interface gates impulse traffic between the input and output stations of the amygdala. *J Neurosci., 19*, 10575–10583.

Rueter, L.E., Fornal, C.A., and Jacobs, B.L. (1997). A critical review of 5-HT brain microdialysis and behavior. *Rev Neurosci., 8*, 117–137.

Seligman, M.E.P. and Maier, S.F. (1967). Failure to escape traumatic shock. *Journal of Experimnetal Psychology, 74*, 1–9.

Sesack, S.R., Deutch, A.Y., Roth, R.H., and Bunney, B.S. (1989). Topographical organization of the efferent projections of the medial prefrontal cortex in the rat: an anterograde tract-tracing study with Phaseolus vulgaris leucoagglutinin. *J Comp Neurol., 290*, 213–242.

Singewald, N. and Sharp, T. (2000). Neuroanatomical targets of anxiogenic drugs in the hindbrain as revealed by Fos immunocytochemistry. *Neuroscience, 98*, 759–770.

Smagin, G.N., Heinrichs, S.C., and Dunn, A.J. (2001). The role of CRH in behavioral responses to stress. *Peptides, 22*, 713–724.

Southwick, S.M., Vythilingam, M., and Charney, D.S. (2005). The psychobiology of depression and resilience to stress: implications for prevention and treatment. *Annu Rev Clin Psychol., 1*, 255–291.

Staub, D.R., Spiga, F., and Lowry, C.A. (2005). Urocortin 2 increases c-Fos expression in topographically organized subpopulations of serotonergic neurons in the rat dorsal raphe nucleus. *Brain Res., 1044*, 176–189.

Taylor, S.F. and Liberzon, I. (2007). Neural correlates of emotion regulation in psychopathology. *Trends Cogn Sci., 11*, 413–418.

Urry, H.L., van Reekum, C.M., Johnstone, T. et al. (2006). Amygdala and ventromedial prefrontal cortex are inversely coupled during regulation of negative affect and predict the diurnal pattern of cortisol secretion among older adults. *J Neurosci., 26*, 4415–4425.

Vertes, R.P. (2004). Differential projections of the infralimbic and prelimbic cortex in the rat. *Synapse., 51*, 32–58.

Vidal-Gonzalez, I., Vidal-Gonzalez, B., Rauch, S.L., and Quirk, G.J. (2006). Microstimulation reveals opposing influences of prelimbic and infralimbic cortex on the expression of conditioned fear. *Learn Mem., 13*, 728–733.

Walker, D.L. and Davis, M. (2002). The role of amygdala glutamate receptors in fear learning, fear-potentiated startle, and extinction. *Pharmacol Biochem Behav., 71*, 379–392.

Weiss, J.M., Goodman, P.A., Losita, B.A., Corrigan, S., Charry., and Bailey, W.H. (1981). Behavioral depression produced by an uncontrollable stressor: relationship to norepinephrine, dopamine, and serotonin levels in various regions of rat brain. *Brain Research Reviews, 3*, 36–97.

Williams, J.L. and Maier, S.F. (1977). Transituational imunization and thereapy of learned helplessness in the rat. *Journal of Experimental Psychology: Animal Behavior Processes, 3*, 240–253.

Woodmansee, W.W., Silbert, L.H., and Maier, S.F. (1993). Factors that modulate inescapable shock-induced reductions in daily activity in the rat. *Pharmacol Biochem Behav., 45*, 553–559.

Chapter 13

Is it all monoamines?

Philip J. Cowen and Catherine J. Harmer

Monoamines and depression

There are two monoamine theories of depression. The first suggests that depression is caused by a central deficiency of catecholamines, principally noradrenaline (NA) while the other implicates deficient serotonin (5-HT) activity. Of course these theories are not mutually exclusive though some authors have suggested that there might be different 'kinds' of depression relating to NA and serotonin deficiency, respectively. There is, however, little empirical evidence for this interesting idea (Nelson et al. 2005). Some of the experimental evidence underlying these ideas is presented in Chapter 12 of this book, while other biological observations in clinical samples that are relevant to these ideas are discussed in Chapters 22, 24, and 25.

The origin of the monoamine hypothesis lay in the astute clinical observations that the monoamine oxidase inhibitor (MAOI) isoniazid, and the tricyclic antidepressant (TCA), imipramine were useful in treating clinical depression (Healy, 2002). Prior to this there were no effective medications for the treatment of depression so these discoveries transformed the field. Subsequent work in animals showed that both MAOIs and TCAs potentiated the function of monoamines, MAOIs by preventing their metabolism and TCAs by blocking the re-uptake of NA and 5-HT into the pre-synaptic nerve ending (Healy, 2002). This naturally led to the idea that perhaps depression itself might be caused by a monoamine deficiency. At a time when there was no good neurobiological understanding of depression this notion was intriguing and, equally important, potentially testable. This is why the monoamine theory of depression has had such a big impact on psychopharmacology.

In this review we shall cover the evidence for the presence of monoamine abnormalities in depressed patients and also discuss the psychological effects of monoamine depletion, which may provide the best evidence for a role of monoamines in acute depressive states. Finally we will outline recent studies on the effects of monoamine manipulation on the processing of emotional information. This work allows an insight into the way in which monoamine manipulation can alter the way the brain processes emotional data and thereby influence mood.

Evidence for 5-HT abnormalities in depression

At the time Alec Coppen proposed the 5-HT hypothesis of depression (Coppen, 1967), direct investigation of the living human brain was not possible and a variety of indirect biochemical measures were employed to support the notion that depressed patients had abnormalities in brain 5-HT function (Table 13.1). From this early stage it was apparent that assessing 5-HT abnormalities in depressed patients was a challenging task for several reasons, particularly the inconsistency of findings from different laboratories as well as the problem of taking into account biochemical effects of current and previous antidepressant treatment. The most reliable evidence for 5-HT abnormalities from this era in depressed patients were diminished uptake of 5-HT by

Table 13.1 Abnormalities in 5-HT mechanisms in depressed patients

5-HT measure	Abnormality reported in depression	Reliability of finding
Platelet 5-HT uptake	Diminished	High
Platelet imipramine binding	Low	Modest
Platelet 5-HT$_{2A}$ receptor binding	Increased	Poor
Plasma tryptophan	Low	High
CSF-HIAA	Low	Weak, may be stronger in suicidal subgroup
Prolactin response to 5-HT re-uptake blockers	Diminished	High (also diminished in recovered patients)
Brain 5-HT$_{2A}$ receptor binding (postmortem)	Increased	Modest (in subgroup of suicides who employed violent methods)
Brain 5-HT$_{1A}$ receptor binding (PET)	Low	High (also diminished in recovered patients)
Brain 5-HT$_{2A}$ receptor binding (PET/SPET)	Low/increased/normal	Poor
Brain 5-HT transporter binding (PET/SPET)	Low/increased/normal	Poor

platelets (Coppen et al. 1978) and lowered levels in plasma of the amino acid precursor of 5-HT, tryptophan (Cowen et al. 1990).

The platelet 5-HT transporter can also be investigated using ligand-binding techniques and labelled imipramine has been a widely used ligand for this purpose. Consistent with the 5-HT uptake data, generally platelet imipramine binding is lower in depressed patients; however, this abnormality is less reliable than the decrease in platelet 5-HT uptake (Mössner et al. 2007). Platelets also have membrane receptor for 5-HT$_{2A}$ receptors but there is no consistent evidence for any particular alteration in this measure in depressed patients (Mendelson, 2000).

Measurements of 5-HT and its major metabolite in postmortem studies of depressed patients, usually dying by suicide, produced inconsistent findings; however, it is possible that people who die using more violent means have increased 5-HT$_{2A}$ receptor binding in frontal cortex (Horton, 1992). The same is true of measurement of the 5-HT metabolite, 5-hydroxyindoleacetic acid (5-HIAA) in lumbar cerebrospinal fluid (CSF), in that while findings in depressed patients in general are inconclusive, there is better evidence that depressed patients who have made impulsive and more dangerous suicide attempts have low CSF 5-HIAA level. This finding is not restricted to patients with depression. It has also been reported in, for example, patients with schizophrenia and personality disorder who have histories of aggressive behaviour directed towards themselves or other people. It has been proposed that low levels of CSF 5-HIAA, while not related specifically to depression, may be associated with a tendency of individuals to respond in an impulsive and hostile way to life difficulties (Placidi et al. 2001).

The development of neuroendocrine challenge techniques-enabled assessments of brain 5-HT function to be carried out in unmedicated depressed patients. These investigations yielded more reliable evidence of abnormalities in brain 5-HT function, albeit in hypothalamic regions. The most consistent changes were found using 5-HT re-uptake inhibitors where acute drug challenge is reliably associated with diminished prolactin release in unmedicated depressed patients (Cowen, 2001), suggesting lowered 5-HT-mediated neuroendocrine responses. This could be due to decreased levels of synaptic 5-HT or reduced responsivity of post-synaptic 5-HT receptors in hypothalamic areas.

It is not clear, however, whether this abnormality in 5-HT-mediated neuroendocrine response is specific for depression, as opposed, for example, to anxiety disorders. In addition the prolactin response to intravenous citalopram remains blunted even when patients have recovered and withdrawn from drug treatment (Bhagwagar et al. 2002). This suggests that impaired 5-HT-mediated prolactin release may be associated with vulnerability to depression but is not necessarily associated with the symptomatic state of depression.

More modern investigations have employed brain-imaging techniques, in particular ligand-imaging in conjunction with positron emission tomography (PET) and single photon emission tomography (SPET). This enables more direct investigation of 5-HT receptors in the living human brain (Grasby, 2002). These data have provided consistent and convincing evidence that the binding density of $5-H_{1A}$ receptors shows a widespread decrease in depressed patients (Drevets et al. 2007; Sargent et al. 2000). However, as with the prolactin response to citalopram, the binding appears to remain low in recovered depressed patients suggesting that it is not a marker of the acute depressive state (Bhagwagar et al. 2004). In addition, $5-HT_{1A}$ receptor binding is also lowered in patients with panic disorder; however, these patients usually have high rates of co-morbid depression (Neumeister et al. 2004a).

Other 5-HT receptors, for example, the $5-HT_{2A}$ receptor and the 5-HT transporter, have also been widely studied in imaging investigations in depressed patients. However, the data from this work are contradictory showing that even using state-of-the-art imaging to measure 5-HT receptors in unmedicated patients, classified with reliable diagnostic systems, is insufficient to overcome clinical heterogeneity or technical variability between different laboratories (see Bhagwagar et al. 2006; 2007). In schizophrenia the ability to use PET and SPET to measure in vivo dopamine release has produced important advances in understanding pathophysiology (Laruelle and Abi-Dargham, 1999). It has been difficult to apply the same methodology to measure 5-HT release in vivo but a recent study shows that it may be possible to use $5-HT_{1A}$ ligand PET to measure the release of 5-HT onto $5-HT_{1A}$ autoreceptors in the raphe nuclei (Sibon et al. 2008). This could be an important methodological development.

Tryptophan depletion, 5-HT and depression

Another approach to elucidating the role of 5-HT in depression is to assess the effect of lowering brain 5-HT function and examining its clinical and neuropsychological effects. The technique employed 'tryptophan depletion' (TRD) takes advantage of the fact that is possible to ower plasma and brain tryptophan by administering an amino-acid mixture free of the 5-HT precursor, tryptophan. Because the conversion of tryptophan to 5-hydroxytryptophan by tryptophan hydroxylase is the rate-limiting step in 5-HT synthesis, TRD is able to produce a transient lowering of brain 5-HT activity (see Young et al. 1985).

In healthy volunteers with no vulnerability factors for the development of depression, TRD does not produce consistent changes in mood (see Ruhe et al. 2007). This suggests that lowering brain 5-HT is not of itself sufficient to cause clinical depressive symptomatology. However, in recovered depressed patients withdrawn from medication, TRD causes, in a high proportion of participants, a transient but striking return of depressive symptomatology (Ruhe et al. 2007; Smith et al. 1997). This suggests that in those with risk factors for depression, lowering brain 5-HT function can indeed cause clinical depressive symptomatology.

Why should recovered depressed patients show a depressive response to TRD when healthy controls do not? It is worth noting at this point that people at high genetic risk of depression who have not suffered a personal episode of illness do not experience clinical symptomatology after TRD though they may be more likely than controls to experience transient dysphoria, measurable on adjective check lists (see Ruhe et al. 2007). This suggests that most of the overt clinical relapse experienced by recovered depressed patients following TRD is related to the experience of having been depressed before. This could be a consequence of previous treatment, for example, with SSRIs, but in our own TRD study we also saw clinical relapses following TRD in patients who had recovered spontaneously or after psychotherapy (Smith et al. 2007). Therefore it seems more likely that depression itself may cause persistent neurobiological changes that produce a depressogenic response when affected individuals are exposed to low brain 5-HT activity.

Some workers have combined TRD with functional brain imaging to identify the brain circuitry involved in TRD-induced relapse. For example, Neumeister et al. (2004b) reported changes in activity in orbitofrontal cortex, anterior cingulate cortex, and ventral striatum and similar findings were obtained by Smith et al. (1999). These brain regions have been implicated in the processing of emotional information (Phillips et al. 2003a) and it may be that in patients who have experienced depression, the circuitry involved in emotional expression and regulation are particularly susceptible to the effects of diminished 5-HT activity.

Evidence for catecholamine abnormalities in depression

The catecholamine theory of depression was proposed by Joseph Schildkraut (Schildkraut, 1965) (Table 13.2). As with abnormalities of 5-HT the data for changes in NA and dopamine in unmedicated depressed patients are rather inconsistent. In addition there is a dearth of suitable NA ligands for PET and SPET imaging so this aspect of brain NA activity has not been explored in depression.

Blood platelets have membrane receptors for α_2-adrenoceptors and there are some evidence, albeit inconsistent, that the number of platelet α_2-adrenoceptors is increased in depressed patients (Leonard, 2000). Postmortem studies of NA and its metabolites have been unrevealing (Horton, 1992). There is some postmortem evidence for increased binding of α_2-adrenoceptor in certain brain regions in depressed suicide victims (Escriba et al. 2004). One of the more consistent findings for an NA abnormality in depression comes from neuroendocrine challenge studies where the growth hormone response to the noradrenergic TCA, desipramine, as well as the α_2-adrenoceptor agonist, clonidine, is decreased in unmedicated depressed patients (Cowen, 2001). This again suggests an abnormality in post-synaptic α_2-adrenoceptor function

Table 13.2 Abnormalities in catecholamine mechanisms in depressed patients

Measure	Abnormality reported in depression	Reliability of finding
Platelet α_2-adrenoceptor binding	Increased	Modest
Brain α_2-adrenoceptor binding	Increased	Modest
Growth hormone response to clonidine and desipramine	Diminished	High
CSF-HVA	Low	High
Dopamine D_2 brain receptor binding	Low/increased/high	Poor

in depression but the blunted endocrine response to clonidine would not be consistent with the increase in brain α_2-adrenoceptor expression noted in the postmortem studies.

Dopamine has been less studied than NA in depression, but there is reliable evidence for a decrease in CSF of its main metabolite, homovanillic acid (Reddy et al. 1992). This has been linked inconsistently to particular clinical features of depression, for example, motor retardation or melancholia (Roy et al. 1985). There have been several PET and SPET studies of dopamine D_2 receptor binding in depression but the data are inconsistent (see Hirvonen et al. 2008). A SPET study that employed [^{123}I]IBZM displacement in conjunction with amphetamine challenge found no change in dopamine release in acutely depressed patients (Parsey et al. 2001).

Catecholamine depletion, noradrenaline, dopamine, and depression

It is possible to lower the synthesis of catecholamines by inhibiting the enzyme tyrosine hydroxylase, which catalyses the conversion of the amino acid, tyrosine to L-DOPA, a precursor of both NA and dopamine. The drug used to achieve this effect is α-methyl-para-tyrosine (AMPT). In healthy subjects, AMPT produces sedation but not significant depressive symptoms (see Ruhe et al. 2007). As with TRD, however, when administered to recovered depressed patients off drug treatment, it causes a striking clinical relapse in depressive symptomatology (Berman et al. 1999). This could be mediated either by diminished dopamine or NA function, or by combined inhibition of both these neurotransmitters.

It is possible to lower plasma tyrosine levels using a similar technique to that employed in TRD but omitting tyrosine and its precursor, phenylalanine, from the mixture. This manoeuvre lowers plasma tyrosine and impairs brain dopamine release. However, NA activity appears to be relatively unaffected (McTavish et al. 1999). McTavish et al. (2005) found that tyrosine depletion did not produce depressive symptoms in recovered depressed patients. This suggests that the mood-lowering effect of AMPT is presumably mediated via depletion of NA rather than dopamine or perhaps by NA and dopamine acting together. Bremner et al. (2003) used PET to study the neural circuitry involved in the depressive relapse caused by AMPT. Interestingly, similar regions were identified as during TRD, including orbitofrontal cortex, dorsolateral prefrontal cortex, and thalamus.

Emotional processing, monoamines, and depression

Negative biases in depressed patients

It is very well recognized that depressed patients have negative cognitive biases in the way they view themselves and the world. Such biases are most obvious at a conscious level, where negative interpretations of neutral or ambiguous events and experience almost defines the state of depression. However, the underlying neuropsychological mechanisms can also be demonstrated in laboratory studies of how emotional material is perceived, remembered, and evaluated. For example, depressed patients show increased attention to sad and fearful facial expressions and in memory tasks recall a higher proportion of negative self-descriptor words and fewer positive words (see Leppänen, 2006).

Neuroimaging studies using functional magnetic resonance (fMRI) are able to illustrate the neural basis of these emotional biases and, more generally, to define the circuitry involved in emotional regulation. Relevant brain regions include orbitofrontal cortex, dorsolateral prefrontal cortex, amygdala, ventral striatum, and thalamus (Phillips et al. 2003a, b). As noted above these areas receive a prominent innervation from monoaminergic neurones. Therefore it seems plausible that one of the ways that monoamine function might impact on mood is through alteration of emotional biases and thereby in the processing of emotional information.

Effects of short-term antidepressant treatment

We have explored this idea by studying the effect of short-term monoamine manipulation on emotional processing in healthy volunteers using selective 5-HT and NA promoting agents, specifically the SSRI citalopram and the selective NA re-uptake inhibitor, reboxetine, both of which are licensed antidepressants. Short-term antidepressant treatment does not affect the mood of non-depressed individuals; hence any changes in emotional processing are likely to be due to a direct effect of the antidepressant rather than due to a primary effect on mood.

We found in healthy subjects that a weeks' treatment with citalopram and reboxetine, produce biases in emotional processing that are generally the opposite of those seen in depression. For example, both drugs decreased the recognition of fearful facial expressions, and people treated with citalopram were more likely to classify equivocal facial expression of negative emotions as happy. In addition, both reboxetine and citalopram significantly increased the number of positive words recalled in a self-descriptor memory task. These changes occurred in the absence of any subjective alteration in mood (Harmer et al. 2004).

These positive biases in emotional processing were apparent after one week of treatment, rather earlier than the therapeutic effects of antidepressants are generally thought to occur. However, we have seen also positive biases in emotional processing after single doses of reboxetine and citalopram, both of which increased the recognition of happy facial expressions (Harmer et al. 2003a, b). This suggests that the ability of antidepressants to elicit positive biases might occur very early in treatment.

In subsequent work we used fMRI to determine the effect of antidepressant administration on the neural response to facial expressions. We found that a week of treatment with both reboxetine and citalopram attenuated the amygdala response to masked fearful faces while reboxetine also increased the activity of the fusiform gyrus to presentation of happy faces (Harmer et al. 2006; Norbury et al. 2007; 2008). Thus antidepressants are able to modify the neural circuitry involved in emotional processing without any change in subjective mood. Moreover, the changes in emotional processing extend to stimuli presented outside conscious awareness.

Implications for how monoamines modify mood

Our findings in healthy subjects suggest that antidepressants produce very early changes in the processing of emotional information. Both NA and 5-HT potentiation lead to positive biases in emotional perception and memory, that is, the opposite effects to those seen in the depressed state. We also have preliminary data that a single dose of reboxetine normalizes the decreased recognition of happy facial expressions and impaired memory for positive emotional information seen in depressed patients, again prior to any changes in mood (Harmer in preparation). We therefore propose that the primary neuropsychological action of antidepressants is exerted on emotional processing and the improvement in mood occurs as a secondary consequence of this. These data are consistent with the notion that the effect of monoamines such as 5-HT and NA on mood is not exerted directly but rather via altered biases in the way that emotional experience is appraised and interpreted.

It is also possible that the ability of low 5-HT and NA states to induce depressed mood is exerted through effects on emotional processing. We have some evidence for the latter possibility in that TRD, given in a dose insufficient to produce subjective mood change, caused negative biases in the recognition of facial expressions in recovered depressed patients but not in healthy controls (Hayward et al. 2005). This supports the PET imaging data referred to above, suggesting that the circuitry involved in emotional processing is particularly susceptible to monoamine depletion in recovered depressed patients.

Conclusions

Unmedicated depressed patients have abnormalities in both NA and 5-HT mechanisms; the evidence for abnormalities in 5-HT is currently rather stronger. However, many of these changes, particularly in 5-HT, apparently persist into clinical recovery, suggesting that that they may represent vulnerability factors or 'scars' of previous illness. The best evidence for a role of 5-HT and NA in acute depression is the ability of TRD and AMPT to produce transient depressive relapse in unmedicated recovered depressed patients.

Positron emission tomography studies show that depression caused by TRD and AMPT is associated with changes in activity of the neural circuitry that underpins the processing of emotional information. This suggests that the impact of monoamine depletion on mood could be mediated by changes in the appraisal of emotional data. In support of this hypothesis, studies in healthy participants with 5-HT and NA re-uptake inhibitors show that monoamine potentiation produces positive changes in emotional biases which could plausibly lead in time to a clinical antidepressant effect.

At the moment, the treatment of depression really is 'all monoamines'. The moderate efficacy of current antidepressants, though welcome, implies that other biochemical mechanisms will need to be recruited to improve clinical efficacy. The effects of TRD and AMPT suggest that monoamines are involved in vulnerability to depression and its clinical symptomatology. However, monoamines are but one element in the chemically and anatomically addressed neural circuitry responsible for emotional expression and regulation. Progress in understanding the neurobiology of emotion will help us improve our insight into the aetiology of clinical depression and the options for treatment.

Acknowledgement

The studies of the authors were supported by the Medical Research Council.

References

Berman, R.M., Narasimhan, M., Miller, H.L. et al. (1999). Transient depressive relapse induced by catecholamine depletion: potential phenotypic vulnerability marker? *Archives of General Psychiatry*, **56**, 395–403.

Bhagwagar, Z., Whale, R., and Cowen, P.J. (2002). State and trait abnormalities in serotonin function in major depression. *British Journal of Psychiatry*, **180**, 24–28.

Bhagwagar, Z., Rabiner, E.A., Sargent, P.A., Grasby, P.M., and Cowen, P.J. (2004). Persistent reduction in brain serotonin1A receptor binding in recovered depressed men measured by positron emission tomography with [11C]WAY-100635. *Molecular Psychiatry*, **9**, 386–392.

Bhagwagar, Z., Hinz, R., Taylor, M., Fancy, S.L., Cowen, P.J., and Grasby P.M. (2006). Increased 5-HT(2A) receptor binding in euthymic, medication-free patients recovered from depression: a positron emission study with [(11)C]MDL 100,907. *American Journal of Psychiatry*, **163**, 1580–1587.

Bhagwagar Z., Murthy, N., Selvaraj, S. et al. (2007). 5-HTT binding in recovered depressed patients and healthy volunteers: a positron emission tomography study with [11C]DASB. *American Journal of Psychiatry*, **164**, 1858–1865.

Bremner, J.D., Vythilingam, M., Vermetten, E. et al. (2003). Regional brain metabolic correlates of a-methylparatyrosine-induced depressive symptoms: implications for the neural circuitry of depression. *Journal of the American Medical Association*, **289**, 3125–3134.

Coppen, A. (1967). The biochemistry of affective disorders. *British Journal of Psychiatry*, **113**, 1237–1264.

Coppen, A., Swade, C., and Wood, K. (1978). Platelet 5-hydroxytryptamine accumulation in depressive illness. *Clinica Chimica Acta*, **87**,165–168.

Cowen, P.J., Parry-Billings, M., and Newsholme, E.A. (1989). Decreased plasma tryptophan levels in major depression. *Journal of Affective Disorders*, **16**, 27–31.

Cowen, P.J. (2001). Neuroendocrine markers of depression and antidepressant drug action. In B.E Leonard (ed.). *Antidepressants*, pp. 95–107. Switzerland, Birkhauser.

Drevets, W.C., Thase, M.E., Moses-Kolko, E.L. et al. (2007). Serotonin-1A receptor imaging in recurrent depression: replication and literature review. *Nuclear Medicine and Biology*, **34**, 865–877.

Escriba, P.V., Ozaita, A., and Garcia-Sevilla, J.A. (2004). Increased mRNA expression of α2A-adrenoceptors, serotonin receptors and mu-opioid receptors in the brains of suicide victims. *Neuropsychopharmacology*, **29**, 1512.

Grasby, P.M. (2002). Imaging the neurochemical brain in health and disease. *Clinical Medicine*, **2**, 67–73.

Harmer, C.J., Bhagwagar, Z., Perrett, D.I., Vollm, B.A., Cowen, P.J., and Goodwin, G.M. (2003a). Acute SSRI administration affects the processing of social cues in healthy volunteers. *Neuropsychopharmacology*, **28**,148–152.

Harmer, C.J., Hill, S.A, Taylor, M.J., Cowen, P.J., and Goodwin, G.M. (2003b). Toward a neuropsychological theory of antidepressant drug action: increase in positive emotional bias after potentiation of norepinephrine activity. *American Journal of Psychiatry*, **160**, 990–992.

Harmer, C.J., Shelley, N.C. Cowen, P.J., and Goodwin, G.M. (2004). Increased positive versus negative affective perception and memory in healthy volunteers following selective serotonin and norepinephrine reuptake inhibition. *American Journal of Psychiatry*, **161**, 256–1263.

Harmer, C.J., Mackay, C.E, Reid, C.B, Cowen, P.J., and Goodwin G.M. (2006). Antidepressant drug treatment modifies the neural processing of nonconscious threat cues. *Biological Psychiatry*, **59**, 816–820.

Hayward, G., Goodwin, G.M., Cowen, P.J., and Harmer, C.J. (2005). Low-dose tryptophan depletion in recovered depressed patients induces changes in cognitive processing without depressive symptoms. *Biological Psychiatry*, **57**, 517–524.

Healy, D., Carney, P.A., O'Halloran, A., and Leonard, B.E. (1985). Peripheral adrenoceptors and serotonin receptors in depression: changes associated with response to treatment with trazodone or amitriptyline. *Journal of Affective Disorders*, **9**, 285–296.

Healy, D. (2002). *The Creation of Psychopharmacology*. Cambridge, Massachusetts, Harvard University Press.

Hirvonen, J., Karlsson, H., Kajander, J. et al (2008). Striatal dopamine D_2 receptors in medication-naive patients with major depressive disorder as assessed with [^{11}C]raclopride PET. *Psychopharmacology*, **197**, 581–590.

Horton, R. W. (1992). The neurochemistry of depression: evidence derived from studies of post-mortem brain tissue. *Molecular Aspects of Medicine*, **13**, 191–203.

Laruelle, M. and Abi-Dargham, A. (1999). Dopamine as the wind of the psychotic fire: new evidence from brain imaging studies. *Journal of Psychopharmacology*, **13**, 358–371.

Leonard, B.E. (2000). Peripheral markers of depression. *Current Opinion in Psychiatry*, **13**, 61–68.

Leppanen, J.M. (2006). Emotional processing in mood disorders: a review of behavioral and neuroimaging findings. *Current Opinion in Psychiatry*, **19**, 34–39.

McTavish, S.F.B, Cowen, P.J., and Sharp, T. (1999). Effect of a tyrosine-free amino acid mixture on regional brain catecholamine synthesis and release. *Psychopharmacology*, **141**, 182–188.

McTavish, S.F.B., Mannie, Z.N., Harmer, C.J., and Cowen, P.J. (2005). Lack of effect of tyrosine depletion on mood in recovered depressed women. *Neuropsychopharmacology*, **30**, 786–911.

Mendelson, S.D. (2000). The current status of the platelet 5-HT(2A) receptor in depression. *Journal of Affective Disorders*, **57**, 13–24.

Mössner, R., Mikova, O., Koutsilieri, E. et al. (2007). Consensus paper of the WFSBP task force on biological markers: biological markers in depression. *World Journal of Biological Psychiatry*, **8**, 141–174.

Nelson, J.C, Portera. L., and Leon, A.C. (2005). Are there differences in the symptoms that respond to a selective serotonin or norepinephrine reuptake inhibitor. *Biological Psychiatry*, **57**, 1535–1542.

Neumeister, A., Bain, E., Nugent, A.C. et al. (2004a). Reduced serotonin type 1A receptor binding in panic disorder. *Journal of Neuroscience*, **24**, 589–591.

Neumeister, A., Nugent. A.C., Waldeck, T. et al. (2004b). Neural and behavioral responses to tryptophan depletion in unmedicated patients with remitted major depressive disorder and controls. *Archives of General Psychiatry*, **61**, 765–773.

Norbury, R., Mackay, C.E, Cowen, P.J., Goodwin, G.M., and Harmer, C.J. (2007). Short-term antidepressant treatment and facial processing. *British Journal of Psychiatry*, **190**, 531–532.

Norbury, R., Mackay, C.E., Cowen, P.J., Goodwin, G.M., and Harmer, C.J. (2008). The effects of reboxetine on emotional processing in healthy volunteers: an fMRI study. *Molecular Psychiatry* (in press).

Parsey, R.V., Oquendo, M.A., Zea-Ponce, Y. et al. (2001). Dopamine D_2 receptor availability and amphetamine-induced dopamine release in unipolar depression. *Biological Psychiatry*, **50**, 313–322.

Philips, M.L., Drevets, W.C., Rausch, S.L., and Lane, R. (2003a). Neurobiology of emotion perception I: implications for major psychiatric disorders. *Biological Psychiatry*, **54**, 504–514.

Phillips, M.L., Drevets, W.C, Rauch, S.L., and Lane, R. (2003b). Neurobiology of emotion perception II: implications for major psychiatric disorders. *Biological Psychiatry*, **54**, 515–528.

Placidi, G.P, Oquendo, M.A., Malone, K.M., Huang, Y.Y, Ellis, P., and Mann, J.J. (2001). Aggressivity, suicide attempts and depression: relationship to cerebrospinal fluid monoamine metabolite levels. *Biological Psychiatry*, **50**, 783–791.

Reddy, P.L., Khanna, S. Subhash, M.N., Channabasavanna, S.M., Sridhara Rama, and Rao, B.S. (1992). CSF amine metabolites in depression. *Biological Psychiatry*, **31**, 112–118.

Roy, A., Pickar, D., Linnoila, M. et al. (1985). Cerebrospinal fluid monoamine and monoamine metabolite concentrations in melancholia. *Psychiatry Research*, **15**, 281–292.

Ruhe, H.G., Mason, N.S., and Schene, A.H. (2007). Mood is indirectly related to serotonin, norepinephrine and dopamine levels in humans: a meta-analysis of monoamine depletion studies. *Molecular Psychiatry*, **12**, 331–359.

Sargent, P.A., Kjaer, K.H., Bench, C.J. et al. (2000). Brain serotonin1A receptor binding measured by positron emission tomography with [11C]WAY-100635: effects of depression and antidepressant treatment. *Archives of General Psychiatry*, **57**, 174–180.

Schildkraut, J.J. (1965). The catecholamine hypothesis of affective disorders: a review of supporting evidence. *Journal of Neuropsychiatry and Clinical Neuroscience*, **7**, 524–533.

Sibon, I., Benkelfat, C., Gravel, P. et al. (2008). Decreased [(18)F]MPPF binding potential in the dorsal raphe nucleus after a single oral dose of fluoxetine: a positron-emission tomography study in healthy volunteers. *Biological Psychiatry* (in press).

Smith, K.A., Fairburn, C.G., and Cowen, P.J. (1997). Relapse of depression after rapid depletion of tryptophan. *Lancet*, **349**, 915–919.

Smith, K.A, Morris, J.S., Friston, K.J., Cowen, P.J., and Dolan, R.J. (1999). Brain mechanisms associated with depressive relapse and associated cognitive impairment following acute tryptophan depletion. *British Journal of Psychiatry*, **174**, 525–529.

Young, S.N., Smith, S.E., Pihl, R.O., and Ervin, F.R. (1985). Tryptophan depletion causes a rapid lowering of mood in normal males. *Psychopharmacology*, **87**, 73–177.

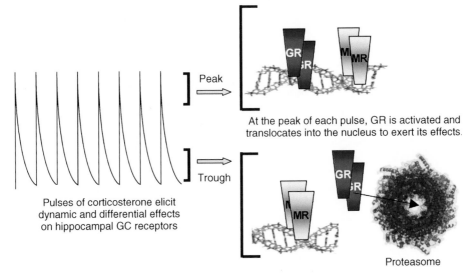

Pulses of corticosterone elicit
dynamic and differential effects
on hippocampal GC receptors

Peak

At the peak of each pulse, GR is activated and
translocates into the nucleus to exert its effects.

Trough

Proteasome

At the trough of each pulse, GR is cleared from the
nucleus by a proteasome-dependent mechanism,
leaving activated MR in the nucleus.

Fig. 7.7 Proposed model of pulsatile corticosterone regulation of glucocorticoid receptors in the hippocampus. Reprinted with permission from Endocrinology, Proteasome-dependent down-regulation of activated nuclear hippocampal glucocorticoid receptors determines dynamic responses to corticosterone, B L Conway-Campbell. 148, 5470-7. © 2007 The Endocrine Society. See p. 86.

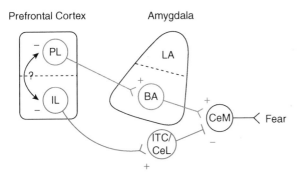

Prefrontal Cortex

Amygdala

Fig. 12.2 Relationship between the ventral medial prefrontal cortex and amygdala (from Vidal-Gonzalez et al. 2006). See p.165.

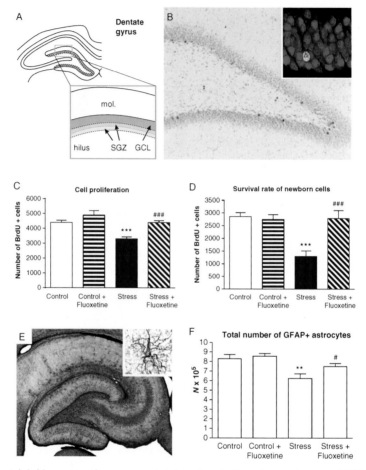

Fig. 11.1 A: Adult hippocampal neurogenesis takes place in the subgranular zone (SGZ) of the DG adjacent to the granule cell layer (GCL). B: Newborn granule cells (brown) in the rat DG. Insert in B shows a confocal image of a double labelled cells: red reflects mature neurons (NeuN), green-yellow is the proliferative marker BrdU labelling a newly generated neuron. C–D: Chronic social stress inhibits both the cell proliferation rate and survival rate of the newly generated cells, whereas concomitant fluoxetine treatment can counteract this effect of stress. E: A representative image of GFAP-staining in the DG. GFAP labels astroglia, insert shows an individual GFAP+ astrocyte. F: Chronic stress results in reduced numbers of astroglia in the hippocampus, whereas fluoxetine blocked this effect of stress. $P < 0.05$ compared to Control; # $P < 0.05$ compared to stress. See p. 142.

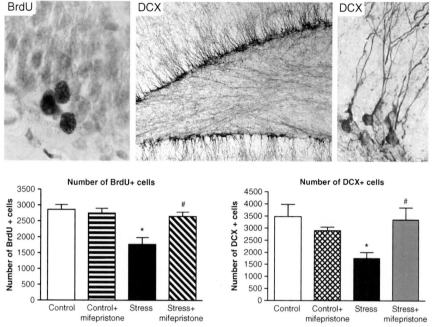

Fig. 11.2 Top panels show examples of BrdU+ and Doublecortin (DCX)+ immunostained cells in the DG. DCX+ somata are located in the SGZ with extensions (arrowheads) passing through the GCL. Lower panels display BrdU- and DCX-positive cell numbers in rats subjected to 21 days of chronic unpredictable stress. The significant reduction in both BrdU- (21-day-old cells) and DCX-positive cell numbers after chronic stress or corticosterone treatment is normalized by four days of high-dose treatment with the GR antagonist mifepristone, whereas the drug alone has no effect (see Mayer et al. 2006; Oomen et al. 2007 for details). See p. 144.

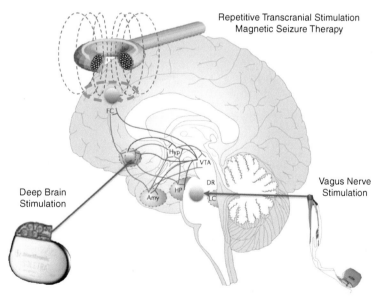

Fig. 25.1 The figure shows schematically that the described targeted neuromodulatory interventions might act on a network that processes affective stimuli at different sites. This network has been identified and described using functional neuroimaging methods in depressed patients. See p. 338.

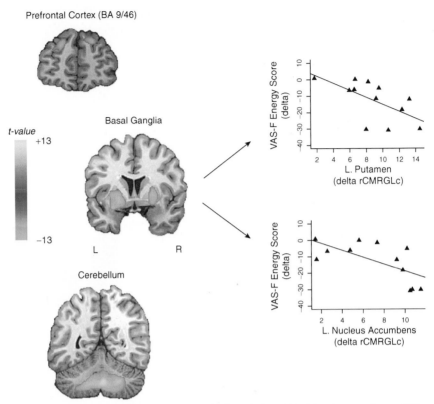

Fig. 17.2 Changes in regional brain glucose metabolism during IFN–alpha therapy. See p. 228.

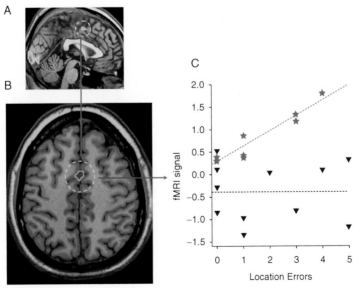

Fig. 17.3 Increased activation in the dACC of IFN-alpha-treated subjects. Reprinted by permission of Elsevier from Anterior cingulate activation and error processing during interferon-alpha treatment by Capuron, L et al *Biological Psychiatry*, 58, 190-6 2005. See p. 231.

Chapter 14

The role of affective processing in vulnerability to and resilience against depression

Nicole Geschwind, Jim van Os, Frenk Peeters, and Marieke Wichers

Introduction: depression as a complex disorder

Unlike Mendelian diseases, depression is not caused by a single gene alteration but is the product of multiple interacting causes (Cannon and Keller, 2005; van Praag et al. 2004). Recent findings underscore just how complex these interactions can be. Genes may interact with the environment (e.g. the serotonin transporter polymorphism has been found to interact with stress) (Caspi et al. 2003) or increase the risk of exposure to certain environments (e.g. through mediation of such personality traits as neuroticism or sensation-seeking) (van Praag et al. 2004). Environmental risk factors may interact or correlate with each other (e.g. childhood adversity was found to be associated with a higher occurrence of life events) (Wichers et al. 2008d). Gene x gene x environment interactions have also been reported. For example, regarding risk for depression, the serotonin transporter polymorphism and a gene coding for brain-derived neurotrophic factor (BDNF) were shown to interact with each other as well as with childhood maltreatment and social support (Kaufman et al. 2006). Furthermore, new insights demonstrate that genetic regulation is more complex than previously thought (Pearson, 2006). Genes can be functionally altered by insertions, deletions, or duplications. Furthermore, as has been demonstrated in the rapidly developing field of epigenetics, a gene can be silenced through the addition of a methyl group to the gene. Methylation of genes is reversible and can be influenced by environmental factors as well as be inherited (Mill and Petronis, 2007; Pearson, 2006). In a study on rat pups, for example, it was found that the degree of maternal care influenced gene methylation, which in turn was associated with altered HPA axis functioning (Fish et al. 2004).

Given this challengingly complex situation, there is an urgent need for multidisciplinary studies involving epidemiology, psychology, genetics, psychiatry, pharmacology, and neuroscience (The European Network of Schizophrenia Networks for the Study of Gene-Environment Interactions (EU-GEI) in press, Moffitt et al. 2005). Where possible, such studies should focus on endophenotypes rather than on disorder outcomes (Caspi and Moffitt, 2006). Endophenotypes are intermediate phenotypes (expressions of genes) that lie somewhere on the pathway between disease-promoting genetic variation, biological vulnerability, and disorder (Cannon and Keller, 2005). They are assumed to be more biologically homogeneous than the current nosological categories of disorders. Examining endophenotypes may facilitate the identification of susceptibility genes and gene-environment interactions (Bearden and Freimer, 2006). The nature of endophenotypes may be biological (e.g. HPA axis functioning) or psychological (e.g. sensitivity to stress).

Several assessment issues are important especially when studying psychological endopheno-types. Assessment should be (i) repeated (rather than cross-sectional / one-time assessment), because repeated measurements increase reliability and sensitivity; (ii) prospective (rather than retrospective); and (iii) based on a short and recent time span (rather than covering longer periods of time), thereby decreasing memory bias (Delespaul, 1995). In contrast to clinical interviews and standardized questionnaires, the experience sampling method (ESM) meets all these require-ments (see Fig. 14.1). In ESM research, participants' reactions to random real-life situations are recorded in a booklet at multiple times a day for several days, assessing context, emotions, and cognitions as they occur. This repeated measurement of daily life situations endows ESM with particularly high ecological validity and reliability (de Vries, 1992; Eck et al. 1998). ESM thus makes it possible to study disorder-relevant endophenotypes in daily life, that is, in the context in which they take place. Examples of ESM endophenotypes are stress sensitivity (often defined as negative affect reactivity to daily life stressors) or reward experience (often defined as positive affect reactivity to pleasant daily life events) (e.g. Wichers et al. 2009). The measurement of ESM endophenotypes can of course be combined with genetic information or biological measurements (e.g. cortisol, see Wichers et al. 2008c). The above-mentioned features make ESM an ideal instrument for the study of gene-environment interaction research.

In the past, research has largely focused on what makes us vulnerable to psychopathology (Seligman and Csikszentmihalyi, 2000). With the advent of the positive psychology movement, researchers have started to show more interest in protective influences (Gable and Haidt, 2005). While some people are particularly vulnerable to becoming depressive, others show remarkable resilience. Studying both vulnerability and resilience will enable us to get a more complete pic-ture of how to best prevent and treat depression. This chapter therefore deals with research into both vulnerability to and resilience against depression with the complexity of co-occurring and

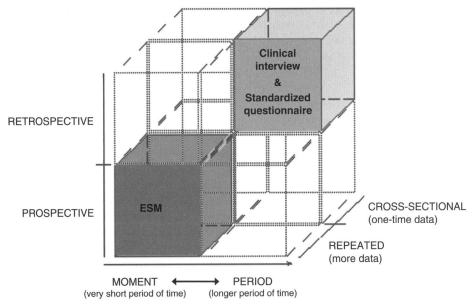

Fig. 14.1 Comparison of the experience sampling method (ESM) and conventional measures. ESM is prospective, repeated, and concerned with very short moments of time, compared to conventional methods such as clinical interviews and standardized questionnaires. (Figure reproduced with permission from Delespaul, 1995.)

interacting genetic and environmental processes in mind. The discussion focuses on the latest findings concerning the role of affective processing in relation to vulnerability and resilience, with special attention to gene-environment research using ESM.

Vulnerability to and resilience against depression

Depression is a multifaceted disorder: emotion, perception, cognition, self-esteem, personality, social support, and coping are only some of the many factors involved in its aetiology and maintenance. However, the scope of this chapter is limited to affective processing. Investigations into the factor structure of emotion have converged on two-factor models, commonly labelled positive and negative affect (PA and NA, respectively) (Almagor and Ben-Porath, 1989; Watson and Tellegen, 1985). PA is associated with behavioural approach and characterized by such feelings as enthusiasm, interest, and happiness. NA is associated with behavioural withdrawal and includes such feelings as distress, sadness, and hostility. Evidence suggests that PA and NA are related yet independent systems (Watson et al. 1999).

In depression, the processing of both NA and PA appears to be altered (Leppänen, 2006). Increased NA as well as a reduced capacity to experience PA (anhedonia) are core symptoms of depression (American Psychiatric Association, 2000). Much if not most of people's emotional experience is influenced by events in their daily lives. A genuine smile can make someone feel happy and elated, whereas a careless word can make someone feel upset or angry. Tendencies to react to daily life events in a certain way not only have short-term effects (in terms of e.g. altered mood) but also appear to have long-term consequences. For example, the tendency to react to daily life stressors with a large increase in NA appears to be a risk indicator for depression (Jacobs et al. 2006; Wichers et al. 2007b). On the other hand, a tendency to experience more positive emotions has been found to have several protective effects (e.g. Danner et al. 2001; Fredrickson 2001). Experimental evidence relevant to our understanding of vulnerability and resilience is presented in Chapter 12 of this book.

Vulnerability to depression: negative affect and stress sensitivity

Increased NA and withdrawn behaviour are core symptoms of depression. As argued above, stress sensitivity is likely a main contributor to daily life NA. Stress sensitivity also has biological plausibility as an endophenotype, given that depressed individuals frequently display excessive HPA axis activation and that HPA axis functioning has been linked to stress responses (e.g. see Hasler et al. 2004). An ESM twin study showed that participants with a co-twin with lifetime depression have a different diurnal cortisol profile than those without, suggesting that altered HPA axis functioning is an indicator of depression liability, and not just a consequence of being depressed (Wichers et al. 2008c).

It has been shown that both genetic and environmental risk factors can produce long-term increases in sensitivity to stressful events. For example, women with a history of childhood abuse displayed an augmented ACTH and cortisol response as well as elevated heart rate in a laboratory public-speaking psychosocial stress task of public speaking (Heim et al. 2000). A history of childhood abuse has also been found to make women more sensitive to the depressogenic effects of stressful life events (SLEs) (Kendler et al. 2004). In a study by van Os and Jones (1999), higher maternal neuroticism was associated with higher sensitivity to SLEs, indicating familial transmission of vulnerability factors. Momentary assessment technology using ESM is particularly well suited to provide ecological validation of the notion of sensitivity to stress as embodied in, for example, the personality trait neuroticism. Recent ESM data indicate that neuroticism expresses itself in daily life through lower PA and increased NA instability (Jacobs et al. submitted). Poorer childhood mental health and higher levels of childhood neuroticism were associated with higher sensitivity to SLEs, too, suggesting that altered stress sensitivity may be one of the mechanisms linking poorer childhood mental health to enduring affective psychopathology in adulthood (van Os and Jones, 1999). Taken together, these studies suggest that heightened stress sensitivity is a risk factor and endophenotype for depression.

A recent ESM study confirmed that daily life stress sensitivity (operationalized as NA reactivity to daily life stressors) is an important endophenotype for depression. Study participants with the highest genetic risk of depression (measured by co-twin lifetime depression status) reacted to daily life stressors with more NA than did participants with low genetic risk (Wichers et al. 2007b). Prospective follow-up measurements showed that daily life stress sensitivity indeed predicts future depression (Wichers et al. submitted). As a whole, these studies show that depression is associated with higher stress sensitivity and suggest that heightened stress sensitivity represents a vulnerability to depression rather than a consequence of being depressed.

Sensitization and stress sensitivity

Knowing that stress sensitivity plays an important role in depression, it is important to examine the mechanisms through which people become more sensitive to stress. A likely mechanism contributing to the development of stress sensitivity is 'sensitization'.

In order to explain the long-term effects of early stress on later adult vulnerability, Post (1992) suggested (on the basis of animal laboratory studies) that, in some individuals, a process of 'sensitization' to stressors occurs over the course of development. Early stress may trigger structural changes due to the induction of gene-transcription factors. These structural changes likely result in long-term changes in the expression of neurotransmitters, receptors, and neuropeptides. These changes are assumed to induce progressively lower thresholds to stress, so that with each further exposure less stress is required for similar behavioural (and biological) responses (Monroe and Harkness, 2005; Post, 1992). Findings concerning stress and depression in the literature – for example, the fact that recurrent episodes of depression become more and more independent of major life stressors and can eventually be triggered even by minor events – support the notion that a process of sensitization may be involved (Kendler et al. 2001; Monroe and Harkness, 2005).

A recent ESM study that tested the hypothesis that sensitization processes underlie the development of stress sensitivity, found that previously experienced stress exposures – such as childhood adversity and SLEs in adulthood – increased adult stress sensitivity to small stressors in the flow of daily life in a dose-response relationship: the greater the number of adversities people had faced, the higher their stress sensitivity. Furthermore, genes appeared to potentiate this effect: participants with a high genetic risk for depression developed higher levels of daily life stress sensitivity in response to pre-natal and postnatal adversities than did those with a low genetic risk (see Fig. 14.2). Childhood adversity seemed to play the most important role in the vicious circle of increased stress sensitivity in those at high genetic risk for depression, because it was associated with both increased stress sensitivity and a higher occurrence of SLEs. In fact, the effect of adult SLEs on stress sensitivity disappeared when controlled for childhood adversity (Wichers et al. 2008d). An effect of childhood adversity on stress sensitivity was also found in another ESM study on frequent attendees of general practitioners (Glaser et al. 2006), as well as in laboratory and naturalistic studies (e.g. Heim et al. 2000; Kendler et al. 2004). The genetic regulation of the stress response is also discussed in Chapter 5 of this book.

Taken together, these studies show that adverse events render especially the genetically vulnerable more sensitive to stress, and support the hypothesis that genes contribute to vulnerability partly by facilitating the process of sensitization after stress exposure. However, many questions remain. For example, it is unknown what the exact mechanisms of stress sensitization are or how epigenetic changes influence stress sensitization.

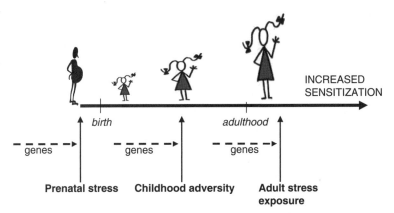

Fig. 14.2 It is hypothesized that stress exposures during the course of development increase future stress sensitization. Genetic factors may impact on sensitization by increasing the effects of stressors on the sensitization process. Thus, genes interact with environmental stressors at different stages of development.

Resilience against depression: the role of positive emotions

Along with the frequent experience of negative emotions, the diminished experience of positive emotions lies at the heart of depressive symptomatology. Anhedonia is a core symptom of major depressive disorder, and experimental studies showed that depressed individuals generated less positive affect from pleasant stimuli than did non-depressed individuals (Dunn et al. 2004; Sloan et al. 1997). However, compared to the extensive literature on negative emotions, relatively little attention has been paid to the role of positive emotions in depression. Some studies, though, have been performed in this area.

Positive emotions and having a positive attitude seem to have beneficial effects on mental and physical health (Seligman et al. 2005). For example, positive emotions speed up cardiovascular recovery from stress and improve immune system functioning, and are associated with increased longevity (Fredrickson 2001; Tugade and Fredrickson 2004; Tugade et al. 2004). In Danner and colleagues' well-known nun study (2001), positive emotional content in early-life autobiographies was strongly associated with longevity 60 years later, with a 2.5-fold difference in risk for mortality between nuns in the lowest and those in the highest quartile of positive emotion expression. A meta-analysis of cross-sectional, longitudinal, and experimental studies demonstrated that happiness was associated with and preceded success, indicating that happiness facilitates accomplishment (Lyubomirsky et al. 2005). In a study in which women with chronic pain were interviewed weekly, higher levels of overall PA predicted lower levels of pain in subsequent weeks, demonstrating that positive affect can be a source of resilience in chronic pain. Higher weekly PA also resulted in lower negative affect both directly and in interaction with stress and pain (Zautra et al. 2005).

The latest ESM studies that additionally examined gene-environment interactions confirm the protective function of positive emotions. An ESM twin study showed that the experience of positive emotions during moments of daily life stress protects against stress sensitivity by buffering negative reactivity to stressful events (Wichers et al. 2007a). Moreover, the experience of positive emotions also attenuated the expression of genetic vulnerability on negative mood bias in the flow of daily life (Wichers et al. 2007a). On average, having a twin (especially a monozygotic twin) with a lifetime history of depression is associated with increased NA in response to stressful situations (Wichers et al. 2007b). However, this effect of genetic vulnerability is weakened during the co-experience of positive emotions (Wichers et al. 2007a).

The protective effect of positive emotions on genetic vulnerability was also found in ESM studies that examined specific genes, for example, the gene encoding for brain-derived neurotrophic factor (BDNF). BDNF is important for neuronal survival and synaptic plasticity (Nair and Vaidya, 2006). Stress has been found to decrease BDNF expression in the hippocampus (Duman and Monteggia, 2006), and there is evidence that BDNF plays a role in such stress-related disorders as depression (Chen et al. 2006; Hashimoto, 2007; Hashimoto et al. 2004; Lang et al. 2005; Nair and Vaidya, 2006). The gene coding for BDNF contains a functional polymorphism (Val66Met). Of the two genetic versions, Valine (Val) is the more active variant and is therefore associated with higher BDNF secretion than is Methionine (Met). A recent ESM study found that carriers of the BDNF Val/Met combination displayed a significantly larger NA response to social stress than did carriers of the Val/Val combination (Wichers et al. 2008b). Interestingly, this gene-environment interaction was moderated by the experience of positive emotions. The experience of positive emotions during social stress decreased BDNF genetic moderation of the NA response. When Val/Met carriers experienced high levels of positive emotion at times of social stress, their NA levels were comparable to those of BDNF Val/Val carriers (see Fig. 14.3).

The studies described above suggest that genetic effects do not influence stress sensitivity in a deterministic manner and may be modified by targeting the ability to generate positive emotions in daily life. Furthermore, a decreased ability to generate positive emotions may contribute to a loss of resilience against stressful events in daily life. Therefore, since daily life stress sensitivity is likely on the causal pathway to depression, an increased ability to generate positive emotions may contribute to resilience against the development of depression. This hypothesis is confirmed by a randomized controlled trial that compared the antidepressant imipramine with placebo. A six-week treatment with imipramine decreased daily life stress sensitivity (measured with ESM) and increased the amount of positive emotion generated from daily life activities (Wichers et al. 2009). Importantly, only increases in the ability to experience positive emotion discriminated between treatment responders and non-responders. This implies that the restoration of the ability to experience positive affect is required for response to treatment in depression, and further underlines the value of targeting positive emotions in particular.

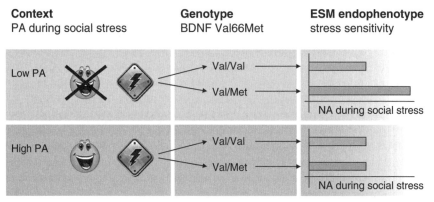

Fig. 14.3 The experience of positive emotions at times of social stress decreases the genetic moderation of the BDNF Val66Met polymorphism on the NA response to social stress. When PA is low, Val/Met carriers experience significantly more NA than do Val/Val carriers during social stress. When PA is high, however, this difference in sensitivity to social stress diminishes (graphic summary of data from Wichers et al. 2009).

To conclude, the existing literature on positive emotions demonstrates that positive emotions have important protective functions and that mechanisms of resilience related to the experience of positive emotions clearly deserve further attention in future research and therapy efforts. The potential of positive emotions to diminish the expression of genetic vulnerability suggests that focusing on positive emotions may be especially beneficial in certain subgroups. This possibility is discussed in the following paragraph.

Targeting positive emotions: personalized medicine?

The above-mentioned finding that BDNF Val/Met carriers in particular benefit from experiencing positive emotion at times of social stress (Wichers et al. in 2008b) suggests possible advantages of 'personalized medicine' (targeting treatment to an individual's needs on the basis of personal characteristics). Targeting the ability to experience positive emotions appears to be especially relevant in individuals who have at least one copy of the Met variant, because teaching them to experience more positive emotions may have a protective influence on their genetic predisposition to experience more social stress.

Other studies suggest that variations in the catechol-O-methyl transferase (COMT) Val158Met polymorphism may be associated with the ability to experience positive emotions. COMT is an enzyme that breaks down dopamine, and dopamine has been found to be associated with positive affect (Burgdorf and Panksepp, 2006). Met is less active than Val, leading to lower levels of COMT and, as a result, higher prefrontal levels of dopamine (Egan et al. 2002). In a recent ESM study on the COMT Val158Met polymorphism, it was found that the ability to generate positive emotions from daily life events increased with an increase in the number of the subject's Met alleles (Wichers et al. 2008) (see Fig. 14.4). This raises the question whether targeting the ability to experience positive emotions may be especially useful in Val/Val carriers – because they seem to be less efficient in experiencing PA – or in Met/Met carriers, because they may have a greater capacity for experiencing PA. Two recent studies show that having at least one Met allele is associated with a faster (Yoshida et al. 2008) and a better (Baune et al. 2008) response to antidepressant medication (although see also Szegedi et al. 2005). This may suggest that Met/Met carriers have a higher natural capacity to recover from depression, possibly via PA, and that especially carriers of Val/Val may benefit from additional treatment that targets positive emotions. However, such suggestions are highly speculative at this point.

To conclude, while the notion of 'personalized medicine' is certainly attractive, much more research is needed in order to determine what the optimal individual treatment strategies may be.

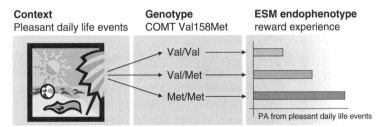

Fig. 14.4 Genetic moderation by the COMT Val158Met polymorphism on the PA response to pleasant daily life events (here called 'reward experience'). In a recent ESM study, the ability to generate positive emotions from daily life events was found to increase with the number of Met alleles of the subject (graphic summary of data from Wichers et al. 2008).

Targeting positive emotions: how?

Increasing the ability to experience positive emotions could play an important role in making people less stress sensitive and more resilient against depression. Furthermore, response to treatment of depression may be conditional on restoration of the ability to experience PA (Wichers et al. 2009). The question arises how PA may be best targeted, either as prevention strategy to make people more resilient against depression, or in combination with pharmacological treatment in order to obtain an optimal treatment response.

Meditation-based techniques, such as mindfulness-based cognitive therapy (MBCT), may offer a way to modify the experience of PA. More advanced meditators have been found to possess greater self-awareness and to experience more positive emotions (Easterlin and Cardena, 1998–99), and people have been found to report more positive emotions when in a mindful compared to a non-mindful state (Brown and Ryan, 2003). During mindfulness training sessions, people are trained towards increased moment-to-moment awareness of experience, resulting in increased openness or receptiveness (Baer, 2003). Although studies have shown that mindfulness training is effective in reducing depressive symptoms and relapse probability (Baer 2003; Coelho et al. 2007; Teasdale et al. 2000), the mechanism remains unknown. It can be hypothesized that mindfulness training is a tool that increases the ability to make use of natural, moment-to-moment rewards in the environment, thereby increasing positive affect. Whether this is indeed the case should be evaluated in future research.

Conclusion/future directions

Sensitive and ecologically valid gene-environment interaction research focusing on daily life (ESM) endophenotypes is badly needed in order to further unravel the very complex gene-environment interactions associated with depression. Recent ESM studies have shown that heightened stress sensitivity is both a risk factor and an endophenotype of depression, and suggest that PA plays a role in making people more resilient to stress. Focusing treatment and prevention efforts on heightening positive affect therefore appears to be a promising venue to reduce stress sensitivity. Further research is necessary in order to answer such questions as how the ability to experience positive emotions is best modified, and who will benefit most from a treatment aimed at increasing PA.

Acknowledgement

Marieke Wichers was supported by the Dutch Medical Council (VENI grant nr 916.76.147).

References

Almagor, M. and Ben-Porath, Y.S. (1989). The two-factor model of self-reported mood: a cross-cultural replication. *Journal of Personality Assessment*, **53**, 10–21.

American Psychiatric Association. (2000). *Diagnostic and Statistical Manual of Mental Disorders*. Washington, DC.

Baer, R.A. (2003). Mindfulness training as a clinical intervention: a conceptual and empirical review. *Clinical Psychology: Science and Practice*, **10**, 125–143.

Baune, B.T., Hohoff, C., Berger, K. et al. (2008). Association of the COMT Val158Met variant with antidepressant treatment response in major depression. *Neuropsychopharmacology*, **33**, 924–932.

Bearden, C.E. and Freimer, N.B. (2006). Endophenotypes for psychiatric disorders: ready for primetime? *Trends in Genetics*, **22**, 306–313.

Brown, K.W. and Ryan, R.M. (2003). The benefits of being present: mindfulness and its role in psychological well-being. *Journal of Personality and Social Psychology*, **84**, 822–48.

Burgdorf, J. and Panksepp, J. (2006). The neurobiology of positive emotions. *Neuroscience and Biobehavioral Reviews*, **30**, 173–187.

Cannon, T. and Keller, M.C. (2005). Endophenotypes in the genetic analyses of mental disorders. *Annual Review of Clinical Psychology*, **2**, 267–290.

Caspi, A., Sugden, K., Moffitt, T.E. et al. (2003). Influence of life stress on depression: moderation by a polymorphism in the 5-HTT gene. *Science*, **301**, 386–389.

Caspi, A. and Moffitt, T.E. (2006). Gene-environment interactions in psychiatry: joining forces with neuroscience. *Neuroscience*, **7**, 583–590.

Chen, Z.-Y., Jing, D., Bath, K.G. et al. (2006). Genetic variant BDNF (Val66Met) polymorphism alters anxiety-related behavior. *Science*, **314**, 140–143.

Coelho, H.F., Canter, P.H., and Ernst, E. (2007). Mindfulness-based cognitive therapy: evaluating current evidence and informing future research. *Journal of Consulting and Clinical Psychology*, **75**, 1000–1005.

Danner, D.D., Snowdon, D.A., and Friesen, W.V. (2001). Positive emotions in early life and longevity: findings from the nun study. *Journal of Personality and Social Psychology*, **80**, 804–813.

De Vries, M. (ed.) (1992). *The Experience of Psychopathology: Investigating Mental Disorders in Their Natural Settings*. Cambridge, Cambridge University Press.

Delespaul, P.A.E.G. (1995). *Assessing Schizophrenia in Daily Life. The Experience Sampling Method*. Maastricht, Maastricht University Press.

Duman, R.S. and Monteggia, L.M. (2006). A neurotrophic model for stress-related mood disorders. *Biological Psychiatry*, **59**, 1116–1127.

Dunn, B.D., Dalgleish, T., Lawrence, A.D., Cusack, R., and Ogilvie, A.D. (2004). Categorical and dimensional reports of experienced affect to emotion-inducing pictures in depression. *Journal of Abnormal Psychology*, **113**, 654–666.

Easterlin, B. and Cardena, E. (1998–1999). Cognitive and emotional differences between short and long term Vipassana meditators. *Imagination, Cognition, & Personality*, **18**, 69–81.

Eck, M.V., Nicolson, N.A., and Berkhof, J. (1998). Effects of stressful daily events on mood states: relationship to global perceived stress. *Journal of Personality and Social Psychology*, **75**, 1572–1585.

Egan, M., Goldman, D., and Weinberger, D. (2002). The human genome. *American Journal of Psychiatry*, **159**, 12.

Fish, E.W., Shahrokh, D., Bagot, R. et al. (2004). Epigenetic programming of stress responses through variations in maternal care. *Annals of the New York Academy of Science*, **1036**, 167–180.

Fredrickson, B.L. (2001). The role of positive emotions in positive psychology: the broaden-and-build theory of positive emotions. *American Psychologist*, **56**, 218–226.

Gable, S.L. and Haidt, J. (2005). What (and why) is positive psychology? *Review of General Psychology*, **9**, 103–110.

Glaser, J.-P., Van Os, J., Portegijs, P.J.M., and Myin-Germeys, I. (2006). Childhood trauma and emotional reactivity to daily life stress in adult frequent attenders of general practitioners. *Journal of Psychosomatic Research*, **61**, 229–236.

Hashimoto, K., Shimizu, E., and Iyo, M. (2004). Critical role of brain-derived neurotrophic factor in mood disorders. *Brain Research Reviews*, **45**, 104–114.

Hashimoto, K. (2007). BDNF variant linked to anxiety-related behaviors. *BioEssays*, **29**, 116–119.

Hasler, G., Drevets, W.C., Manji, H.K., and Charney, D.S. (2004). Discovering endophenotypes for major depression. *Neuropsychopharmacology*, **29**, 1765–1781.

Heim, C., Newport, D.J., Heit, S. et al. (2000). Pituitary-adrenal and autonomic responses to stress in women after sexual and physical abuse in childhood. *JAMA*, **284**, 592–597.

Jacobs, N., Kenis, G., Peeters, F., Derom, C., Vlietinck, R., and Van Os, J. (2006). Stress-related negative affectivity and genetically altered serotonin transporter function: evidence of synergism in shaping risk of depression. *Archives of General Psychiatry*, **63**, 989–996.

Jacobs, N., Van Os, J., Mengelers, R., Thiery, E., Delespaul, P., and Wichers, M. (submitted). Neuroticism explained: from a non-informative vulnerability maker to informative person-context interactions in the realm of daily life.

Kaufman, J., Yang, B.-Z., Douglas-Palumberi, H. et al. (2006). Brain-derived neurotrophic factor-5-HTTLPR gene interactions and environmental modifiers of depression in children. *Biological Psychiatry*, **59**, 673–680.

Kendler, K.S., Thornton, L.M., and Gardner, C.O. (2001). Genetic risk, number of previous depressive episodes, and stressful life events in predicting onset of major depression. *American Journal of Psychiatry*, **158**, 582–586.

Kendler, K.S., Kuhn, J.W., and Prescott, C.A. (2004). Childhood sexual abuse, stressful life events and risk for major depression in women. *Psychological Medicine*, **34**, 1475–1482.

Lang, U.E., Hellweg, R., Kalus, P. et al. (2005). Association of a functional BDNF polymorphism and anxiety-related personality traits. *Psychopharmacology*, **180**, 95–99.

Leppänen, J.M. (2006). Emotional information processing in mood disorders: a review of behavioral and neuroimaging findings. *Current Opinion in Psychiatry*, **19**, 34–39.

Lyubomirsky, S., King, L., and Diener, E. (2005). The benefits of frequent positive affect: does happiness lead to success? *Psychological Bulletin*, **131**, 803–855.

Mill, J. and Petronis, A. (2007). Molecular studies of major depressive disorder: the epigenetic perspective. *Molecular Psychiatry*, **12**, 799–814.

Moffitt, T.E., Caspi, A., and Rutter, M. (2005). Strategy for investigating interactions between measured genes and measured environments. *Arch Gen Psychiatry*, **62**, 473–481.

Monroe, S.M. and Harkness, K.L. (2005). Life stress, the 'kindling'hypothesis, and the recurrence of depression: considerations from a life stress perspective. *Psychological Review*, **112**, 417–445.

Nair, A. and Vaidya, V.A. (2006). Cyclic AMP response element binding protein and brain-derived neurotrophic factor: molecules that modulate our mood? *Journal of Bioscience*, **31**, 423–434.

Pearson, H. (2006). What is a gene? *Nature*, **441**, 399–401.

Post, R.M. (1992). Transduction of psychosocial stress into the neurobiology of recurrent affective disorder. *American Journal of Psychiatry*, **149**, 999–1010.

Seligman, M.E.P. and Csikszentmihalyi, M. (2000). Positive psychology: an introduction. *American Psychologist*, **55**, 5–14.

Seligman, M.E.P., Steen, T.A., and Peterson, C. (2005). Positive psychology progress: empirical validation of interventions. *American Psychologist*, **60**(5), 410–421.

Sloan, D.M., Strauss, M.E., Quirk, S.W., and Sajatovic, M. (1997). Subjective and expressive emotional responses in depression. *Journal of Affective Disorders*, **46**, 135–141.

Szegedi, A., Rujescu, D., Tadic, A. et al. (2005). The catechol-o-methyltransferase val108/158met polymorphism affects short-term treatment response to mirtazapine, but not to paroxetine in major depression. *The Pharmacogenomics Journal*, **5**, 49–53.

Teasdale, J.D., Segal, Z.V., Williams, J.M.G., Ridgeway, V.A., Soulsby, J.M., and Lau, M.A. (2000). Prevention of relapse/recurrence in major depression by mindfulness-based cognitive therapy. *Journal of Consulting and Clinical Psychology*, **68**, 615–623.

The European Network of Schizophrenia Networks for the Study of Gene-Environment Interactions (Eu-Gei) (2008). Schizophrenia aetiology: do gene-environment interactions hold the key? Comment on Tandon et al. *Schizophrenia Research*, **102**, 21–26.

Tugade, M.M. and Fredrickson, B.L. (2004). Resilient individuals use positive emotions to bounce back from negative emotional experiences. *Journal of Personality and Social Psychology*, **86**, 320–333.

Tugade, M.M., Fredrickson, B.L., and Barrett, L. F. (2004). Psychological resilience and positive emotional granularity: examining the benefits of positive emotions on coping and health. *Journal of Personality*, **72**, 1161–1190.

Van Os, J. and Jones, P. B. (1999). Early risk factors and adult person-environment relationships in affective disorder. *Psychological Medicine*, **29**, 1055–1067.

Van Praag, H.M., De Kloet, R., and Van Os, J. (2004). *Stress, the Brain, and Depression.* Cambridge, Cambridge University Press.

Watson, D. and Tellegen, A. (1985). Toward a consensual structure of mood. *Psychological Bulletin*, **98**, 219–235.

Watson, D., Wiese, D., Vaidya, J., and Tellegen, A. (1999). The two general activation systems of affect: structural findings, evolutionary considerations, and psychobiological evidence. *Journal of Personality and Social Psychology*, **76**, 820–838.

Wichers, M., Aguilera, M., Kenis, G. et al. (2008a). The catechol-O-methyl transferase (COMT) Val(158) Met polymorphism and experience of reward in the flow of daily life. *Neuropsychopharmacology*, **33**, 3030–3036.

Wichers, M., Barge-Schaapveld, D.Q.C.M., Mengelers, R., Nicolson, N.A., Peeters, F., and Os, J. V. (2009). Reduced stress-sensitivity or increased reward experience: the psychological mechanism of response to antidepressant medication. *Neuropsychopharmacology,* **34**, 923–931.

Wichers, M., Geschwind, N., Jacobs, N. et al. (submitted-a). The transition from stress-sensitivity to depressive state: a longitudinal twin study.

Wichers, M., Kenis, G., Jacobs, N. et al. (2008b). The psychology of psychiatric genetics: evidence that positive emotions moderate genetic stress sensitivity to social stress associated with the BDNF Val66Met polymorphism. *Journal of Abnormal Psychology*, **117**, 699–704.

Wichers, M., Myin-Germeys, I., Jacobs, N. et al. (2008c). Susceptibility to depression expressed as alterations in cortisol day curve: a cross-twin, cross-trait study. *Psychosomatic Medicine*, **70**, 314–318.

Wichers, M., Myin-Germeys, I., Jacobs, N. et al. (2007a). Evidence that moment-to-moment variation in positive emotions buffers genetic risk for depression: a momentary assessment twin study. *Acta Psychiatrica Scandinavia*, **115**, 451–457.

Wichers, M., Myin-Germeys, I., Jacobs, N. et al. (2007b). Genetic risk of depression and stress-induced negative affect in the flow of daily life. *British Journal of Psychiatry*, **191**, 218–223..

Wichers, M., Schrijvers, D., Geschwind, N. et al. (2008d). The mechanism of gene-environment interactions in depression: evidence that genes potentiate multiple sources of adversity. *Psychological Medicine*, **6**, 1–10.

Yoshida, K., Higuchi, H., Takahashi, H. et al. (2008). Influence of the tyrosine hydroxylase Val81Met polymorphism and catechol-O-Methyltransferase Val158Met polymorphism on the antidepressant effect of milnacipran. *Human Psychopharmacology: Clinical and Experimental*, **23**, 121–128.

Zautra, A.J., Johnson, L.M., and Davis, M.C. (2005). Positive affect as a source of resilience for women in chronic pain. *Journal of Consulting and Clinical Psychology*, **73**, 212–220.

Chapter 15

PTSD and HPA axis: same hormones, different disorders

Elizabeth A. Young

Major life stressors have been strongly associated with psychiatric disorders, particularly major depression. However, with the arrival of post-traumatic stress disorder in the 1980s, stressors were subdivided into stressors and traumas. While major life stressors were associated with the onset of major depression, trauma was associated with post-traumatic stress disorder (PTSD). By DSM-IV definition, traumas are not associated with depression and other stressors are not associated with PTSD. The hypothalamic-pituitary-adrenal (HPA) axis pattern was proposed to show the biological validation of the distinction between depression and trauma, since opposite patterns of HPA axis activation were found in these disorders. And since the HPA axis is the main hormonal stress system it is a logical place to examine the relationship between stress, trauma, depression, and PTSD. The role of the HPA axis in affective disorders and other stress-related conditions is discussed in several other Chapters of this book (Chapters 5, 7–9, 11, 16, 19, 21, and 26).

HPA axis regulation

The hypothalamic-pituitary-adrenal (HPA) axis transforms stressful input into hormonal messages that enable the organism to adapt to the stressful stimulus. Neurons in the paraventricular nucleus (PVN) of the hypothalamus synthesize CRH which is secreted into the hypophyseal portal system via the median eminence (Swanson et al. 1983). In humans, CRH is believed to be the primary secretagogue driving pituitary corticotropes to release ACTH. The stimulus for CRH secretion can be either 'physical', for example, hypotension or exercise, or 'psychological', for example,, perceived danger or stressful events. Brainstem catecholamine systems are critical circuits involved in the 'activation' pathways for CRH release (Herman et al. 1990; Plotsky, 1987; Plotsky et al. 1989). CRH release stimulates the secretion of ACTH from pituitary corticotropes which, in turn, stimulates the secretion of cortisol from the adrenal cortex in a feed-forward cascade. Glucocorticoid secretion is tightly controlled and limited by negative feedback effects of glucocorticoids at both pituitary and brain sites. Negative feedback on secretion can occur very rapidly, within 5–10 minutes, and provides real-time inhibition to limit the stress response and prevents oversecretion of glucocorticoids (Keller-Wood and Dallman, 1985). In addition to rapid effects on secretion, glucocorticoids exert negative feedback effects on messenger ribonucleic acid (mRNA) and subsequent protein stores for both CRH and the ACTH precursor, proopiomelanocortin (POMC) (Roberts et al. 1979). Regulation of gene transcription can occur directly via glucocorticoid responsive elements, as has been shown for POMC. Glucocorticoid negative feedback may also involve trans-synaptic influences and 'inhibition' circuits within the brain. In the case of glucocorticoid regulation of the CRH gene, strong data suggest that these trans-synaptic inhibition circuits are critical in regulating CRH mRNA levels in the PVN (Herman et al. 1989).

Negative feedback regulation of the HPA axis occurs through a dual receptor system, mineralocorticoid receptors (MR) and glucocorticoid receptors (GR) (de Kloet et al. 1985; McEwen et al. 1968; Reul and de Kloet, 1985; Spencer et al. 1990). These two receptors differ in their affinity for glucocorticoids, with MR demonstrating the highest affinity for cortisol while GR demonstrates lower affinity for cortisol (de Kloet et al. 1985; McEwen et al. 1968; Reul and de Kloet, 1985; Spencer et al. 1990). In addition, their distribution in rodent brain differs with MR predominantly in limbic areas particularly hippocampus while GR is more widely distributed across all brain regions (Herman et al. 1989; McEwen et al. 1968); in primates, MR is also found in cortex and subcortical structures (Patel et al. 2000). Thus MR is a high-affinity, low-capacity receptor while GR is the low-affinity, high-capacity receptor. Because of the low levels of circulating cortisol in the nadir, MR is believed to be more important in the regulation of HPA axis drive in the evening, the time when depressed patients are most likely to demonstrate increased central drive (de Kloet et al. 1998; Dallman et al. 1989; Reul and de Kloet, 1985; Sapolsky et al. 1990; Spencer et al. 1990; Young et al. 1997).

Mineralocorticoid receptors and GR can form heterodimers and thus cooperate in the regulation of genes, and these heterodimers have been demonstrated to be more active than either MR–MR or GR–GR homodimers in some systems (Bradbury et al. 1994). While MR and GR are synergistic in their effects on HPA axis inhibition, this not the case in all systems (de Kloet and Reul, 1987; Joels and de Kloet, 1994; Kuroda et al. 1994; Lopez et al. 1997; Meijer and de Kloet, 1994; Trapp and Holsboer, 1996). In fact, the effects of MR and GR can be antagonistic as has been demonstrated for neuronal excitability in the hippocampus (Joels and de Kloet, 1994). Furthermore, other studies have demonstrated that acute activation of MR lowers 5HT release and turnover and reduces 5HT-mediated responses in the hippocampus (Joels and de Kloet, 1994). In contrast, high levels of glucocorticoids trigger GR-stimulated serotonin transmission and lead to increased 5HT responses (Joels and de Kloet, 1994). These at times opposing activities of MR and GR have led to the proposal of an MR:GR balance that is necessary for proper regulation of a number of physiological systems (de Kloet and Reul, 1987).

The hippocampus is believed to be an important site of negative feedback regulation. The hippocampus is a site that is richly endowed with both GR and MR. As such, prior work in animals focused on the hippocampus and its role in both basal and stress induced glucocorticoid secretion. Lesions of the hippocampus increase basal glucocorticoid secretion and CRH mRNA in PVN (Herman et al. 1992). Lesions also prolong stress-induced glucocorticoid secretion (Herman et al. 2003). Stimulation of the hippocampus in humans reduces cortisol (Rubin et al. 1966), consistent with the animal literature. Following adrenalectomy, implantation of corticosterone directly in the hypothalamus is ineffective in reducing basal ACTH secretion, while local implantation of corticosterone in the hippocampus reduces ACTH (Kovacs and Makara, 1988). The hippocampus provides no direct input to the PVN but rather inhibitory output flows through the bed nucleus of the stria terminalis (Herman et al. 2003). The medial prefrontal cortex also provides indirect feedback signals to the PVN. It should be noted that the standard experimental animal used to study the HPA axis, the rat, is not the best model for defining these circuits in humans. Furthermore, the distribution of GR and MR in the hippocampus and cortex is somewhat different in non-human primates than rats (Patel et al. 2000; Sanchez et al. 2000). Studies in rats have focused on the negative feedback effects of the hippocampus because of the predominance of MR in the hippocampus which shows little distribution of MR outside of the hippocampus. In the squirrel monkey MR is found in the outer five layers of the anterior cingulate cortex and the dorsolateral prefrontal cortex contains abundant MR (Patel et al. 2000). In rhesus monkeys, Sanchez et al. (2000) reported that GR was less abundant in the hippocampus but dense labelling for GR mRNA occurred in cingulate and prefrontal cortex. This suggests that these frontal cortical regions may be even more important in regulating negative feedback in primate brains than data suggests for rodent brains. Furthermore, the data suggest that MR's role in HPA axis regulation in primates has been underestimated. Bilateral lesions of anterior cingulate or medial prefrontal cortex (in rats) enhance corticosterone response to stress as well as activation within the PVN (Brake et al. 2000; Diorio et al. 1993). Evidence suggests lateralization of this function with only bilateral or right prefrontal lesions associated with negative feedback (Sullivan and Gralton, 1997). There are no direct inputs from cortex to the PVN and thus multisynaptic inputs may flow through the BNST, or may flow through and modulate amygdala activation, or may involve the PVN of the thalamus, which has been associated with chronic stress-induced changes in stress reactivity (Bhatnagar et al. 1998).

In addition to stress as an activator of the HPA axis, intrinsic rhythmic elements in the suprachiasmatic nucleus (SCN) also drive secretion from the HPA axis in a circadian pattern (Krieger, 1979). ACTH secretion is pulsatile in nature with the trough of integrated secretion occurring in the evening and early night and the peak of secretion occurring just before awakening. Active secretion continues through the morning and early afternoon. Even in the absence of corticosteroid feedback (adrenalectomy), ACTH continues to demonstrate a circadian rhythm (Jacobson et al. 1989). The circadian rhythm of ACTH is believed to be secondary to a circadian rhythm in CRH secretion, although it is difficult to assess this since cannulation of the hypophyseal portal system in anesthetized rats causes near maximal CRH secretion. An alternative is to examine CRH mRNA levels in the PVN, to determine if circadian-driven CRH secretion causes changes in mRNA levels. CRH mRNA does indeed demonstrate a circadian rhythm that is independent of glucocorticoid secretion, but is synchronized with and phase-advanced to the plasma ACTH and cortisol rhythm, suggesting that circadian neural inputs are turning on CRH transcription in advance of the anticipated period of active CRH secretion (Kwak et al. 1993). These data suggest that there are intrinsic neural elements responsible for both the initiation and inhibition of the CRH/ACTH/cortisol circadian rhythm and that glucocorticoids act to dampen the overall amount of secretion, that is, absolute values of the hormones, as well as the amplitude of the rhythm. Furthermore, from studies examining the circadian rhythm of ACTH under metyrapone blockade, it appears that glucocorticoids alter the timing of the circadian peak and nadir (Veldhuis et al. 2001; Young and Ribiero, 2006), although they are not themselves directly responsible for the inhibition of PVN CRH secretion during the quiescent phase. As elaborated in the following section, existing data suggest differences in the roles of MR and GR in feedback inhibition across the circadian rhythm.

HPA axis abnormalities in depression

Stress plays a critical role in the precipitation of major depression and numerous studies have shown the importance of life stressors in depression. The link between stress and depression is further validated by the overactivity of the HPA axis as manifested by an increase in cortisol secretion, a well-established phenomenon in depression (Carroll et al. 1976; Sachar et al. 1973). The original studies of Sachar et al. (1973) suggested that depressed patients demonstrate increased cortisol secretory activity as measured by mean plasma cortisol concentration, the number of cortisol secretory episodes and the number of minutes of active secretion. Later studies have continued to validate this hypercortisolemia in depression (Carroll et al. 1973; Rubin et al. 1987; Halbreich et al. 1985; Pfohl et al. 1985). As many as two-thirds of endogenously depressed patients fail to suppress cortisol, or show an early escape of cortisol, following overnight administration of 1 mg of dexamethasone (dex), using a cortisol cut-off of 5 µg/dl to define 'escape' (Carroll et al. 1981). While non-suppression of cortisol to dexamethasone is strongly associated with endogenous depression, this finding is less robust in outpatients with depression. Although both hypercortisolemia and feedback abnormalities to dexamethasone are present in depressed patients, they do not necessarily occur in the same individuals (Carroll et al. 1981; Halbreich et al. 1985). Nor is non-suppression of ACTH/ß-endorphin to dexamethasone at the pituitary closely associated with the classic DST non-suppression. In our studies of 73 patients with major depression using a within-subject design to classify suppressor and non-suppressor at the pituitary using ß-endorphin-IR as a measure of corticotroph secretion, we found that 53% of patients showed non-suppression at the pituitary while only 11% of these same patients were DST non-suppressors using the 5 µg/dl cut-off. Using a multiple regression model, the strongest predictor of feedback resistance to dexamethasone as measured by pituitary suppression to dex was basal cortisol and aging with a combined correlation coefficient $r = 0.8$. We have also examined glucocorticoid fast feedback (Young et al. 1991) and found this to be abnormal in major depression. A blunted ACTH response to oCRF has also been reported in depressed patients (Gold et al. 1986; Holsbeoer et al. 1984; Young et al. 1990). The blunted response to oCRF appears to be dependent upon increased baseline cortisol, since blockade of cortisol production with metyrapone normalizes the ACTH response (von Bardeleben et al. 1988; Young et al. 1995). More recently, the combination of dexamethasone with administration of CRH has been used as a challenge (Heuser et al. 1994). While Holsboer has argued that the abnormal response to the dex/CRH test reflects elevated AVP tone, there is little human data to support this. Most studies have found that dexamethasone acts predominantly at the level of the pituitary, since the P-glycoprotein transporter excludes dexamethsone from the brain (Karssen et al. 2005). Furthermore, CRH is considered a challenge of the sensitivity of CRH receptors on the pituitary. Thus the combination acts predominantly at the pituitary. While the classical DST relies on endogenous drive to provide activation of the HPA axis, the dex/CRH test provides both the negative feedback stimulus (dex) and the 'drive' by administering CRH. By now a large number of studies have confirmed that both the ACTH and cortisol response to the dex/CRH test are increased in depressed patients compared to controls (Ising et al. 2005). Furthermore, studies have found 'normalization' with antidepressant treatment and that failure to normalize predicts relapse (Hatzinger et al. 2000; Zobel et al. 2001). All of these studies parallel the findings with the older DST literature (Arana et al. 1985). In an interesting report, Stuart Watson (Watson et al. 2006) compared the dex/CRH test to the DST in 82 patients and 28 controls and found that there was a close correlation between the cortisol responses on the two tests ($r = 0.73$, $p < 0.0005$) and that the DST showed slightly better sensitivity (66%) versus sensitivity of 61.9% for dex/CRH test. Overall, the two tests are closely related and they both evaluate the sensitivity of predominantly GR to suppression.

Given that basal cortisol is elevated in major depression, it was expected that increased cortisol would be accompanied by an increased level of ACTH in plasma. Two studies, as well as data from our group (Pfohl et al. 1985; Linkowski et al. 1985; Young et al. 2001) have been able to demonstrate small differences between normal controls and depressed subjects in their mean 24-hour plasma ACTH levels. The demonstration of enhanced sensitivity to ACTH 1-24 in depressed patients suggests that increased ACTH secretion is not necessarily the cause of increased cortisol secretion (Amsterdam et al. 1983). However, other studies using very low 'threshold' doses of ACTH 1-24 have not been able to demonstrate an increased sensitivity to ACTH in depressed patients (Krishnan et al. 1990), which suggests that increased cortisol secretion is secondary to increased ACTH secretion. Our 24 -hour studies of ACTH and cortisol secretion demonstrated that subjects with increased mean cortisol also demonstrated increased mean ACTH, supporting a central origin of the HPA axis overactivity. (Young et al. 2001). In summary, regarding the HPA axis profile in depression, it appears likely that there is increased CRF/ACTH secretion, which is then likely amplified at the adrenal to lead to increased cortisol. These changes in cortisol secretion are commonly considered to be 'state' changes and resolve when the depression resolves. However, almost all studies examining the HPA axis in major depression in euthymic subjects have examined patients on antidepressants, which exert direct effects on the HPA axis.

When stress response was examined in major depression, we found that patients with depression continued to respond to stress with increased cortisol despite elevated resting cortisol levels, which should inhibit the stress response (Young et al. 2000). In fact, given their resting cortisol levels, depressed patients clearly hyper-responded compared to normal subjects with similar cortisol levels. The AUC cortisol response to the Trier Social Stress Test (TSST) for high cortisol controls (with mean basal cortisol of 13 μg/dl) was 8.7 ± 30, while depressed patients (mean basal cortisol of 15 μg/dl), showed AUC cortisol response of 139 ± 39. The correlation between pre-stress cortisol and AUC ACTH was $r = 0.65$ in the normal subjects, demonstrating an important role of basal cortisol on stress responsiveness. We found an exaggerated ACTH response to the TSST in depressed patients with comorbid social phobia, while the response in social phobia alone was normal (Young et al. 2004). Likewise Heim et al. (2000) found that the response to the TSST was greatly exaggerated in women with child abuse plus depression, an extremely common occurrence in patients with major depression. In our study of child abuse in UM psychiatry clinics, we found that 37.5% of depressed patients had a history of childhood emotional, physical, or sexual abuse (Young et al. 1997).

The HPA axis in trauma and post-traumatic stress disorder

Basal studies

The majority of studies examining trauma have focused upon PTSD. Given that PTSD is stress-related in aetiology, it was expected that PTSD patients would show HPA axis abnormalities similar to that seen in depressed patients or chronically stressed animals. However, that is not clearly the case. An initial report by Mason et al. (1986) found that urinary free cortisol (UFC) excretion was *lower* in PTSD than MDD. But, Pittman and Orr (1990) found *increased* UFC excretion in outpatient PTSD veterans compared to combat controls without PTSD. Yehuda and colleagues have reported data consistent with Mason's, showing decreased UFC excretion in PTSD *male* veterans compared to normal controls in a number of studies (Yehuda et al. 1991). However, later reports from Mason (Mason et al. 2002), in male combat veterans, suggest that these findings are less certain. The most comprehensive studies of PTSD by Yehuda and colleagues (see Yehuda, 2002 for review) continue to show low cortisol and enhanced suppression to dexamethasone (dex) in combat veterans with PTSD. Furthermore, the presence of comorbid MDD does not change the neuroendocrine picture. A recent study (de Kloet et al. 2007) in Dutch veterans found a blunted saliva cortisol awakening response and enhanced suppression to dex in both PTSD and combat exposed controls. Plasma cortisol and ACTH pre- and post-dex was not different between PTSD and combat exposed controls. Yehuda's group (Golier et al. 2006) examined veterans from the first Gulf war and found normal basal saliva cortisol and GR number but enhanced cortisol suppression to dex in both combat-exposed veterans and those with PTSD only, compared to non-combat-exposed controls. Those with comorbid MDD and PTSD did not show enhanced suppression to dex. Since women are most likely to experience PTSD in the community, male combat veterans are not representative of the community where this psychiatric disease is most likely to occur (Breslau et al. 1991; 1995; Kessler et al. 1995). Furthermore significant confounds with current and past alcohol and substance abuse occur in the Vietnam veteran population.

A number of studies have sought to address this problem by using non-veteran subjects recruited from clinics and the community. The majority of these studies have examined women with childhood sexual abuse. While some studies have demonstrated increased UFC (Lemieux and Coe, 1995), others have demonstrated similar plasma cortisol (Rassmussen et al. 2001) and still others have found lower cortisol and enhanced suppression to dex (Stein et al. 1997). Yehuda examined Holocaust survivors, who also were predominantly exposed early in life, and observed lower UFC and enhanced suppression to dexamethasone in this population (Yehuda, 2000). A recent Dutch study of chronic PTSD in civilian trauma found lower 9AM plasma cortisol in PTSD subjects (Olff et al. 2006). A comprehensive study examining cortisol production rate over 24 hours in 10 subjects with PTSD and 10 age, sex-matched controls found normal production rate, normal 24 -hour plasma cortisol, and normal saliva cortisol and normal lymphocyte GR receptor number and affinity (Wheler et al. 2006). However, UFC was lower in PTSD subjects, but this was not confirmed by GC/mass spec analysis of the urine. Studies examining motor vehicle accident survivors (Hawk et al. 2000) found no difference in cortisol between those with and without PTSD six months later. Studies of male and female adults with exposure to mixed traumas have found either no effect of PTSD on basal cortisol (Kellner et al. 2002; 2003) or elevated basal cortisol (Atmaca et al. 2002; Lindley et al. 2004).

Epidemiological-based samples in adults have focused upon natural disasters and have generally examined exposure with high- and low-PTSD symptoms (Anisman et al. 2001; Davidson and Baum 1986; Fukuda et al. 2000), but without diagnostic information. One exception was the study of Maes et al. (1998) which looked at PTSD subjects recruited from community disasters and demonstrated increased UFC in PTSD. However, this study was small and there is no evidence that the subjects recruited into the biological study were representative of the subjects exposed to disasters. In general, community-based studies suggest that exposure to disaster increases plasma (Fukuda et al. 2000) and saliva cortisol (Anisman et al. 2001) and UFC (Davidson and Baum, 1986). To add further complexity, the majority of studies of trauma and PTSD included subjects with comorbid depression and commonly subjects have both disorders.

In addition to the issue of exposure to trauma, the persistence of the neuroendocrine changes following recovery from PTSD is unclear. In an early study Yehuda et al. (1995) reported that Holocaust survivors with past but not current PTSD demonstrated normal UFC, while later studies of offspring of Holocaust survivors (Yehuda, 2000; Yehuda et al. 2002) suggested that changes in cortisol may persist beyond the duration of the symptoms, and thus may be a marker of underlying vulnerability to PTSD. The large analysis by Boscarino (1996) of cortisol data from several thousand combat veterans showed a very small effect of current PTSD on basal cortisol, but a very clear effect of combat exposure with increasing levels of severity of combat exposure associated with increasingly lower cortisol. In this study lifetime PTSD was not associated with lower cortisol. But another recent study found elevated cortisol in women with partner violence related lifetime PTSD (Inslicht et al. 2006).

Response to HPA axis challenges

Studies examining the response to low dose dex in PTSD veterans, combat-exposed veterans without PTSD, and normal controls found enhanced feedback to dex in veterans with PTSD, whether or not co-morbid MDD was present; combat-exposed controls demonstrated normal suppression compared to non-combat normal subjects (Yehuda, 2000). Similar enhanced suppression to dex has been found in Holocaust survivors with PTSD and their offspring (Yehuda, 2000; Yehuda et al. 2007). This enhanced suppression to dex has been found in studies looking at either plasma or saliva cortisol (Yehuda, 2000). In Yehuda's studies (2000), as well as the report by Stein et al. (1997) the enhanced suppression is also paired with low baseline cortisol. Lindley et al. (2004) examined a treatment seeking non-veteran PTSD population and found elevated basal cortisol and normal suppression to dex in subjects with PTSD. Kellner examined response to low dose dex in anxiety disorders and found a *normal* response in both PTSD and patients with panic disorders (Kellner et al. 2004). Few other groups have utilized the low dose dex suppression test, to determine whether this is a replicable finding in PTSD and whether it is present in other anxiety disorders. More recent studies continue to show variable results (Golier et al. 2006; Inslicht et al. 2006; Kellner et al. 2004; Olff et al. 2006)

Activational challenges have generally used CRF challenge. An initial CRF challenge study in combat-related PTSD showed normal to increased plasma cortisol at time of challenge (Smith et al. 1989) and a decreased ACTH response in subjects with high baseline cortisol. A study by Rasmussen et al. (2001) examined women with history of childhood abuse who met criteria for PTSD. Women with PTSD showed enhanced cortisol response to CRF and to exogenous ACTH infusion, as well as a trend towards higher 24-hour UFC. Interestingly, all the women with PTSD had either past or current major depression, so comorbidity was the rule. In the study by Heim et al. (2001) examining response to CRF in women with major depression, with and without childhood abuse, 14 of 15 childhood abuse MDD patients also met criteria for PTSD. This group, with comorbid MDD and PTSD, demonstrated a blunted ACTH response to CRF challenge, similar to that observed in MDD alone without PTSD. The abused groups also demonstrated lower baseline and stimulated cortisol in response to CRF challenge as well as following ACTH infusion. These same groups of women showed a significantly *greater* HPA response to the TSST, despite *smaller* responses to CRF (Heim et al. 2001).

Several additional studies have evaluated response to stressors. An early study by Liberzon et al. (1999) using combat noise versus white noise in male veterans with PTSD showed elevated basal and post-provocation cortisol compared to combat controls, but no evidence of a difference between the combat and white noise days. A study by Bremner et al. (2003) of PTSD subjects of both sexes used a stressful cognitive challenge and found elevated basal saliva cortisol and continuing higher cortisol for 60 minutes post challenge. Eventually the saliva cortisol of the PTSD group returned to the same level as controls, raising the issue of whether the 'basal' samples were truly basal or were influenced by the anticipation of the challenge. Similar data were found in the study of Elzinga et al. (2003) using trauma scripts in women with childhood abuse and PTSD versus abused-no PTSD. In that study saliva cortisol was again significantly elevated at baseline, increased in response to the challenge (while controls showed no response) and then greatly decreased following the stressor, compatible with the idea that 'basal' levels already reflected exaggerated stress sensitivity in this group. Using a one-minute cold pressor test, a very recent report (Santa Ana et al. 2006) compared the plasma ACTH and cortisol response in PTSD subjects with either childhood trauma or adult trauma to controls and saw lower basal cortisol in the childhood abuse group. However, their data do not support an actual change in ACTH or cortisol in response to the stressor in any group so it is difficult to take their findings as reflecting differences in the stress response in subjects with PTSD. Together the existing stress data suggest an exaggerated stress response in PTSD.

Other challenges include metyrapone. One study by Yehuda (2000) of combat veterans with PTSD demonstrated greater rebound ACTH secretion compared to controls following administration of metyrapone in the morning, indicating that increased CRF drive is present in the morning and normally restrained by cortisol feedback. The other three studies examining metyrapone challenge in PTSD found a normal ACTH response to afternoon or overnight metyrapone as well as a normal response to cortisol infusion in PTSD subjects and panic disorder subjects (Kanter et al. 2001; Kellner et al. 2004a, b). However, two studies examining overnight metyrapone showed a blunted response in male and female PTSD subjects (Neylan et al. 2003; Otte et al. 2007). Of note, our studies in major depression show the overnight response to be normal while the evening response is increased (Young and Ribiero, 2006). Finally one study of serial CSF sampling of CRH has demonstrated increased CSF CRH in PTSD despite normal 24-hour UFC in the PTSD group (Baker et al. 1999).

The role of comorbidity

The issue of comorbid depression in the PTSD population is not clear, with most studies including comorbid individuals and few analysing the data by the absence or presence of comorbid depression. The original studies by Yehuda et al. (2000) found that comorbidity with major depression had no effect on the HPA axis findings in PTSD, and that despite the general picture of decreased sensitivity to dex found in subjects with major depression, that subjects with PTSD and major depression showed enhanced negative feedback to dexamethasone. The studies of Heim et al. (2001; 2001) focusing upon childhood abuse and MDD examined multiple HPA axis challenges in the same subjects and included many subjects with both PTSD and MDD. Their studies found an effect of early abuse (with comorbid PTSD in 11/13 subjects) and MDD on stress reactivity, with both an increased ACTH and cortisol response to the stressor compared to either controls or depressed patients without childhood abuse. In the same subjects, they found a blunted response to CRH challenge in MDD patients with or without childhood abuse, but an increased response to CRH in abused without MDD. The abused subjects also showed a blunted cortisol response to ACTH 1-24. Furthermore, they found lower cortisol and enhanced feedback to low dose dex in the same subjects (Newport et al. 2004). Thus childhood abuse produced 'enhanced pituitary response with counter-regulatory adrenal adaptations', a change compatible with low or normal basal cortisol. The dexamethasone challenge data were analysed by the presence or absence of PTSD as the primary diagnosis and again found enhanced feedback in PTSD.

To date, the challenge studies suggest that the picture is complicated in PTSD with comorbid depression; the findings of some studies look like depression while others look quite different, for example, showing a smaller response to ACTH infusion when MDD patients show an augmented response. This confusion led us to conduct two epidemiological-based studies on PTSD in the community.

Our studies of PTSD in representative community samples

These three studies (Young and Breslau, 2004a, b; Young et al. 2004) used community based samples with biological samples representative of both those exposed to trauma and those with PTSD. The first study involved the Detroit area study (Breslau et al. 2000; 2003). Subjects were selected by the following criteria: (1) all new exposures since previous wave; (2) all subjects ever diagnosed with PTSD; and (3) a random selection of the remainder of subjects. Subjects were excluded if they were on psychotropic medications, had recent substance abuse or could not abstain from smoking overnight. However, no eligible subjects were excluded on the basis of these criteria. Subjects came into Henry Ford sleep laboratory and urine was collected in 3 eight-hour collections and then assayed for cortisol. For analysis, both current and past PTSD were collapsed although data with current PTSD did not show any different conclusion than those analyses with lifetime PTSD. The data for 24-hour UFC for exposed/No PTSD versus PTSD versus non-exposed is shown in Fig. 15.1. As can be observed, we found no evidence of any change in UFC in subjects with PTSD. We also examined the data by comorbidity resulting in a four group analysis: neither PTSD nor MDD, PTSD alone, MDD alone, nor both disorders. Because we found sex-specific differences, the data for each sex are shown in Figs 15.2 and 15.3. In these analyses we found a significant effect of time and a significant group by sex interaction as well as a significant sex difference. Post-hoc analyses found the following: in men an elevation with MDD compared to the no-disorder group and to the MDD + PTSD group; in women, a significant elevation in the MDD+PTSD group compared to each of the other three groups. Additional analyses found an effect of recent exposure on UFC in men and *no significant effect* of childhood abuse on UFC.

Study 2 involved the same original cohort but recruited 516 of the 913 subjects still in follow-up to participate in at-home saliva cortisol collection; in the morning at awakening and around 7.00 p.m. in the evening. In this study we used no exclusions but examined the effects of potential

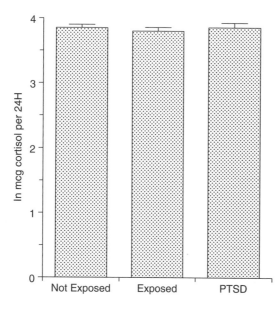

Fig. 15.1 24-hour cortisol in urine in persons with no exposure to trauma, exposure to trauma without PTSD and exposed to trauma with PTSD. There was no difference in 24-hour cortisol among groups or in any pair-wise comparison.

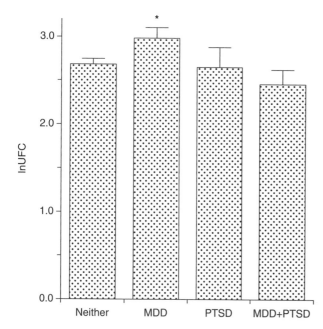

Fig. 15.2 8-HR UFC (Corrected for Diurnal Variation) in Men.

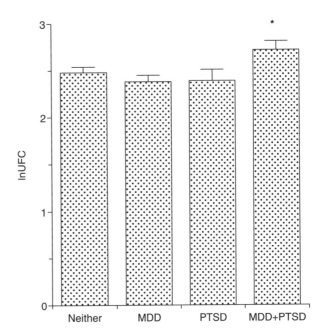

Fig. 15.3 8-Hour UFC (Corrected for Diurnal Variation) in Women

confounds. We found no effect of smoking status on saliva cortisol. We also found no effect of oral contraceptives or hormone replacement on saliva (free) cortisol. Finally, we found no effect of antidepressants or other psychotropics on saliva cortisol. Thus the analysis did not exclude any subjects based upon these potential confounds. Furthermore, for saliva cortisol we found no sex differences in patterns. Thus Fig. 15.4 presents the data for both sexes for PTSD, exposed to trauma and non-exposed groups. As can be seen in Fig. 15.4, we found a significant increase in saliva cortisol overall, with post-hoc testing demonstrating that the increase was significant in the evening in the PTSD group compared to the exposed/no PTSD group. We also conducted a four-group analysis looking at the effect of comorbidity. In the analysis, shown in Fig. 15.5, we found that PTSD with comorbid MDD showed significantly increased PM saliva cortisol compared to the No PTSD/No MDD (Neither) group. No other groups differed from each other by post-hoc testing. Paired with the previous analysis, the overall conclusions were that PTSD alone had no effect on saliva cortisol but if comorbid MDD was present, then the HPA axis profile resembled the classic profile for MDD.

Study number three involved the Women's Employment Sample (WES), a low-income community-based welfare to work transition sample. Subjects were recruited in Flint area. This group had a large number of subjects with current or past PTSD, thus allowing a reliable comparison of these groups. However, it had almost no subjects who were unexposed to trauma. The comparison of past versus current (chronic) PTSD to not-exposed is shown if Fig. 15.6. As can be seen, there were no differences and no evidence that PTSD demonstrated *lower* cortisol. Furthermore, PTSD with comorbid MDD showed a similar pattern to that shown in the Detroit Area Study (Fig. 15.5). Furthermore, as a group the MDD subjects showed significantly increased evening cortisol (Fig. 15.7). Finally, we found an effect of recent (past year, $n = 70$) exposure to trauma causing increased saliva cortisol in those recently exposed (Fig. 15.8). Similar to analyses in the Detroit Area study, we found no significant effect of exposure to childhood abuse/trauma ($n = 89$) compared to those not exposed ($n = 98$).

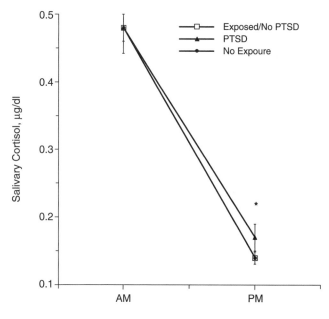

Fig. 15.4 Salivary Cortisol in Detroit Area Study (n=516)

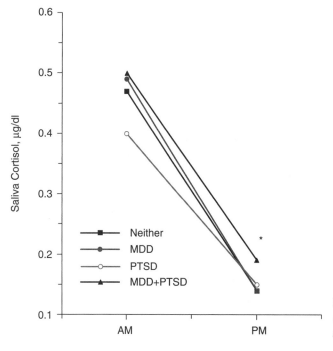

Fig. 15.5 Analysis of Saliva Cortisol in PTSD By Presence and Absence of MDD

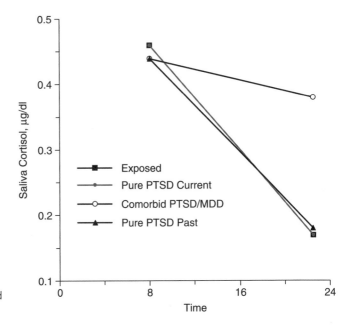

Fig. 15.6 Comparison of Past and Current PTSD vs Comorbid MDD +PTSD

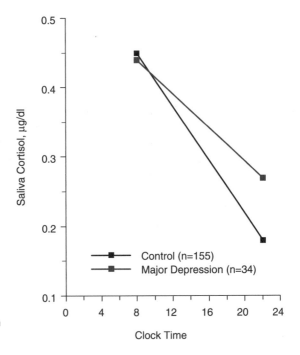

Fig. 15.7 Effect of Recent Major Depression (past year) in WES study

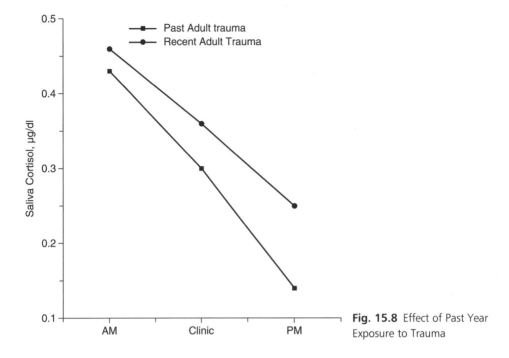

Fig. 15.8 Effect of Past Year Exposure to Trauma

Overall conclusions

From the reviewed studies of convenience populations with PTSD, it is clear that there are no consistent findings with regards to the effects of PTSD on basal cortisol. Early studies of combat veterans showed an effect but later studies have not. It may be that chronicity of the disorder or other factors such as age of trauma exposure have affected the results. Our studies of two epidemiological-based samples examining persons who represented the population at large with PTSD have shown no effect of PTSD on basal cortisol. However, unlike the studies of Yehuda (2000), we did find an effect of comorbid depression on the basal cortisol profile in PTSD, with those who were comorbid showing a pattern characteristic of major depression. Thus our findings do not support that comorbid PTSD affects depression to result in lower basal cortisol. It should be noted that our two studies, while complementary, still may suffer from too few men since women predominate with PTSD in community-based samples. However, the very large studies of Boscarino, on male Vietnam veterans only demonstrated an extremely small effect of current PTSD on plasma cortisol and no effect of past PTSD. Using a sample of 293 veterans with current PTSD versus 2197 veterans without current PTSD, he found an effect size of 0.12, a small-effect size. Furthermore, this study found a stronger effect of combat exposure on cortisol with an effect size of 0.22 between no exposure and the highest level of combat. Since PTSD diagnosis is confounded with severity of combat exposure, it is difficult to conclude that the effect of current PTSD is that of PTSD per se rather than combat exposure. Thus, little data support low basal cortisol in PTSD, in contrast to MDD, where increased cortisol has been a consistent finding.

References

Amsterdam, J.C., Winokur, A., Abelman, E., Lucki, I., and Richels, K. (1983). Co-syntropin (ACTH a[1–24]) stimulation test in depressed patients and healthy subjects. *American Journal of Psychiatry*, **140**, 907–909.

Anisman, H., Griffiths, J., Matheson, K., Ravindran, A.V., and Merali, Z. (2001). Posttraumatic stress symptoms and salivary cortisol levels. *American Journal of Psychiatry*, **158**, 1509–1511.

Arana, G.W., Baldessarini, R.J., and Ornsteen, M. (1985) The dexamethasone suppression test for diagnosis and prognosis in psychiatry. *Commentary and Review. Archives of General Psychiatry*, **42**, 1193–1204.

Atmaca, M., Kuloglu, M., Tezcan, E., Onal, S., Ustundag, B. (2002). Neopterin levels and dexamethasone suppression test in posttraumatic stress disorder. *European Archives of Psychiatry Clinical Neuroscience*, **252**, 161–165.

Baker, D.G., West, S.A., Nicholson, W.E. et al. (1999) Serial CSF corticotropin-releasing hormone levels and adrenocortical activity in combat veterans with posttraumatic stress disorder. *American Journal of Psychiatry*, 156, 585–588.

Bhatnagar, S., Dallman, M.F., Roderick, R.E., Basbaum, A.I., and Taylor, B.K. (1998) The effects of prior chronic stress on cardiovascular responses to acute restraint and formalin injection. *Brain Research*, **797**, 313–320.

Boscarino, J.A. (1996). Posttraumatic stress disorder, exposure to combat, and lower plasma cortisol among Vietnam veterans: findings and clinical implications. *Journal of Consulting and Clinical Psychology*, **64**, 191–201.

Bradbury, M.J., Akana, S.F., and Dallman, M.F. (1994). Roles of type I and II corticosteroid receptors in regulation of basal activity in the hypothalamo-pituitary-adrenal axis during the diurnal trough and the peak: evidence for a nonadditive effect of combined receptor occupation. *Endocrinology*, **34**, 1286–1296.

Brake, W.G., Flores, G., Francis, D., Meaney, M.J., Srivastava, L.K., and Gratton,A. (2000). Enhanced nucleus accumbens dopamine and plasma corticosterone stress responses in adult rats with neonatal excitotoxic lesions to the medial prefrontal cortex. *Neuroscience*, **96**, 687–695.

Bremner, J.D., Vythilingam, M., Vermetten, E. et al. (2003). Cortisol response to a cognitive stress challenge in posttraumatic stress disorder (PTSD) related to childhood abuse. *Psychoneuroendocrinology*, **28**, 733–735.

Breslau, N., Davis, G.C., Andreski, P., and Peterson, E. (1991). Traumatic events and posttraumatic stress disorder in an urban population of young adults. *Archives of General Psychiatry*, **48**, 216–222.

Breslau, N., Davis, G.C., and Andreski, P. (1995). Risk factors for PTSD-related traumatic events: a prospective analysis. *American Journal of Psychiatry*, **152**, 529–535.

Breslau, N., Davis, G.C., Peterson, E.L., and Schultz, L.R. (2000). A second look at comorbidity in victims of trauma: the post-traumatic stress disorder-major depression connection. *Biological Psychiatry*, **48**, 902–909.

Breslau, N., Davis, G.C., and Schultz, L. (2003). PTSD and the incidence of nicotine, alcohol and drug disorders in victims of trauma. *Archives of General Psychiatry*, **60**, 289–229.

Carroll, B.J., Curtis, G.C., and Mendels, J. (1976). Neuroendocrine regulation in depression I. Limbic system-adrenocortical dysfunction. *Archives of General Psychiatry*, **33**, 1039–1044.

Carroll, B.J., Feinberg, M., Greden, J.F. et al. (1981). A specific laboratory test for the diagnosis of melancholia. *Archives of General Psychiatry*, **38**, 15–22.

Dallman, M.F., Levin, N., Cascio, C.S., Akana, S.F., Jacobsen, L., and Kuhn, R.W. (1989). Pharmacological evidence that the inhibition of diurnal adrenocorticotropin secretion by corticosteroids is mediated via type I corticosterone-preferring receptors. *Endocrinology*, **124**, 2844–2850.

Davidson, L.M. and Baum, A. (1986). Chronic stress and posttraumatic stress disorders. *Journal of Consulting and Clincal Psychology*, **54**, 303–308.

de Kloet, C.S., Vermetten, E., Heijnen, C.J., Geuze, E., Lentjes, E,G., and Westenberg, H.G. (2007). Enhanced cortisol suppression in response to dexamethasone administration in traumatized veterans with and without posttraumatic stress disorder. *Psychoneuroendocrinology*, **32**, 215–226.

de Kloet, E.R. and Reul, J.M. (1987). Feedback action and tonic influence of corticosteroids on brain function: a concept arising from the heterogeneity of brain receptor systems. *Psychoneuroendocrinology*, **12**, 83–105.

de Kloet, E.R., Vreugdenhil, E., Oitzl, M.S., and Joels, M. (1998) Brain corticosteroid receptor balance in health and disease. *Endocrinology Review*, **19**, 269–230.

deKloet, E.R., Wallach, G., and McEwen, B.S. (1975). Differences in corticosterone and dexamethasone binding to rat brain and pituitary. *Endocrinology*, **96**, 598–605.

Diorio, D., Viau, V., and Meaney, M.J. (1993). The role of the medial prefrontal cortex (cingulate gyrus) in the regulation of hypothalamic-pituitary-adrenal responses to stress. *Journal of Neuroscience*, **13**, 3839–3847.

Elzinga, B.M., Schmahl, C.G., Vermetten, E., van Dyck, R., and Bremner, J.D. (2003). Higher cortisol levels following exposure to traumatic reminders in abuse-related PTSD. *Neuropsychopharmacology*, **28**, 1656–1665.

Fukuda, S., Morimota, K., Kanae, M., and Maruyama, S. (2000). Effect of the Hanshin-Awaji earthquake on posttraumatic stress, lifestyle changes, and cortisol levels of victims. *Archives of Environmental Health*, **55**, 121–125.

Gold, P.W., Loriaux, D.L., and Roy, A. (1986). Response to corticotropin-releasing hormone in the hypercortisolism of depression and Cushing's disease. *New England Journal of Medicine*, **314**, 1329–1335.

Golier, J.A., Schmeidler, J., Legge, J., and Yehuda, R. (2006). Enhanced cortisol suppression to dexamethasone associated with Gulf War deployment. *Psychoneuroendocrinology*, **31**, 1181–1189.

Halbreich, U., Asnis, G.M., Schindledecker, R., Zurnoff, B., and Nathan, R.S. (1985). Cortisol secretion in endogenous depression I. Basal plasma levels. *Archives of General Psychiatry*, **42**, 909–914

Hatzinger, M., Hemmeter, U.M., Baumann, K., Brand, S., Holsboer-Trachsler, E. (2002). The combined DEX-CRH test in treatment course and long-term outcome of major depression. *Journal of Psychiatric Research*, **36**, 287–297.

Hawk, L.W., Dougall, A.L., Ursano, and R.J., Baum, A. (2000). Urinary catecholamines and cortisol in recent-onset posttraumatic stress disorder after motor vehicle accidents. *Psychosomatic Medicine*, **62**, 423–434.

Heim, C., Newport, D.J., Heit, S. et al. (2000). Pituitary-adrenal and autonomic responses to stress in women after sexual and physical abuse in childhood. *JAMA*, **284**, 592–597.

Heim, C., Newport, D.J., Bonsall, R., Miller, A.H., and Nemeroff, C.B. (2001). Altered pituitary-adrenal axis responses to provocative challenge tests in adult survivors of childhood abuse. *American Journal of Psychiatry*, **158**, 575–581.

Herman, J.P., Patel, P.D., Akil, H., and Watson, S. (1989). Localization and regulation of glucocorticoid and mineralocorticoid receptor messenger RNAs in the hippocampal formation of the rat. *Molecular Endocrinology*, **3**, 1886–1894.

Herman, J.P., Schafer, M.K.-H., Young, E.A. et al. (1989). Hippocampal regulation of the hypothalamo-pituitary-adrenocortical axis: in situ hybridization analysis of CRF and vasopressin messenger RNA expression in the hypothalamic paraventricular nucleus following hippocampectomy. *Journal of Neuroscience*, **9**, 3072–3082.

Herman, J.P., Wiegand, S., and Watson, S.J. (1990). Regulation of basal corticotropin releasing hormone and arginine vasopressin mRNA expression in the paraventricular nucleus: effects of selective hypothalamic deafferentation. *Endocrinology*, **127**, 2408–2417.

Herman, J.P., Cullinan, W.E., Young, E.A., Akil, H., and Watson, S.J. (1992). Selective forebrain fiber tract lesions implicate ventral hippocampal structures in tonic regulation of paraventricular nucleus corticotropin-releasing hormone (CRH) and arginine vasopressin (AVP) mRNA expression. *Brain Research*, **592**, 228–238.

Herman, J.P., Figueiredo, H., Mueller, N.K. et al. (2003). Central mechanisms of stress integration: hiearchical circuitry controlling hypothalamo-pituitary-adrenocortical responsiveness. *Frontiers in Neuroendocrinology*, **24**, 151–180.

Heuser, I., Yassouridis, A., and Holsboer F. (1994). The combined dexamethasone/CRH test: a refined laboratory test for psychiatric disorders. *Journal of Psychiatric Research*, **28**, 341–356.

Holsboer, F., Bardeleden, U., Gerken, A., Stalla, G., and Muller, O. (1984). Blunted corticotropin and normal cortisol response to human corticotropin-releasing factor in depression. *New England Journal of Medicine*, **311**, 1127.

Inslicht, S.S., Marmar, C.R., Neylan, T.C. et al. (2006). Increased cortisol in women with intimate partner violence-related posttraumatic stress disorder. *Annals of New York Academic Science*, **1071**, 428–429.

Ising, M., Kunzel, H.E., Binder, E.B., Nickel, T., Modell, S., and Holsboer, F. (2005). The combined dexamethasone/CRH test as a potential surrogate marker in depression. *Progress in Neuropsychopharmacology Biological Psychiatry*, **29**, 1085–1093.

Jacobson, L., Akana, S.F., Cascio, C.S., Scribner, K., Shinsako, J., and Dallman, M.F. (1989). The adrenocortical system responds slowly to removal of corticosterone in the absence of concurrent stress. *Endocrinology*, **124**, 2144–2152.

Joels, M. and de Kloet, E.R. (1994). Mineralocorticoid and glucocorticoid receptors in the brain. Implications for ion permeability and transmitter systems. *Progress in Neurobiology*, **43**, 1–36.

Kanter, E.D., Wilkinson, C.W., Radant, A.D. et al. (2001). Glucocorticoid feedback sensitivity and adrenocortical responsiveness in posttraumatic stress disorder. *Biological Psychiatry*, **50**, 238–245.

Karssen, A.M., Meijer, O.C., Berry, A., Sanjuan Pinol, R., and de Kloet, E.R. (2005). Low doses of dexamethasone can produce a hypocorticosteroid state in the brain. *Endocrinology*, **146**, 5587–5595.

Keller-Wood, M.E., and Dallman, M.F. (1985). Corticosteroid inhibition of ACTH secretion. *Endocrine Reviews*, **5**, 1–24.

Kellner, M., Baker, D.G., Yassouridis, A. et al. (2002). Mineralocorticoid receptor function in patients with posttraumatic stress disorder. *American Journal of Psychiatry*, **159**, 1938–1940.

Kellner, M., Yassouridis, A., Hubner, R., Baker, D.G., and Wiedemann, K. (2003). Endocrine and cardiovascular responses to corticotropin-releasing hormone in patients with posttraumatic stress disorder: a role for atrial natriuretic peptide? *Neuropsychobiology*, **47**, 102–108.

Kellner, M., Otte, C., Yassouridis, A., Schick, M., Jahn, H., and Wiedemann, K. (2004a). Overnight metyrapone and combined dexamethasone/metyrapone tests in post-traumatic stress disorder: preliminary findings. *European Neuropsychopharmacology*, **14**, 337–339.

Kellner, M., Schick, M., Yassouridis, A., Struttmann, T., Wiedemann, K., and Alm, B. (2004). Metyrapone tests in patients with panic disorder. *Biological Psychiatry*, **56**, 898–900.

Kessler, R.C., Sonnega, A., Bromet, E., Hughes, M., and Nelson, C.B. (1995). Posttraumatic stress disorder in the National Comorbidity Survey. *Archives of General Psychiatry*, **52**, 1048–1060.

Kovacs,K.J. and Makara,G.B. (1988). Corticosterone and dexamethasone act at different brain sites to inhibit adrenalectomy-induced adrenocorticotropin hypersecretion. *Brain Research*, **474**, 205–210.

Krieger, D.T. (1979). Rhythms in CRH, ACTH and corticosteroids. *Endocrine Reviews*, **1**, 123.

Krishnan, K.R.R., Ritchie, J.C., Saunders, W.B., Nemeroff, C.B., and Carroll, B.J. (1990). Adrenocortical sensitivity to low-dose ACTH administration in depressed patients. *Biological Psychiatry*, **27**, 930–933.

Kuroda, Y., Watanabe, Y., Albeck, D.S., Hastings, N.B., and McEwen, B.S. (1994). Effects of adrenalectomy and type I or type II glucocorticoid receptor activation on 5-HT1A and 5-HT2 receptor binding and 5-HT transporter mRNA expression in rat brain. *Brain Research*, **648**, 157–161.

Kwak, S.P., Morano, I.M., Young, E.A., Watson, S.J., and Akil, H. (1993). The diurnal CRH mRNA rhythm in the hypothalamus: decreased expression in the evening is not dependent on endogenous glucocorticoids. *Neuroendocrinology*, **57**, 96–105.

Lemieux, A.M. and Coe, C.L. (1995). Abuse-related posttraumatic stress disorder: evidence for chronic neuroendocrine activation in women. *Psychosomatic Medicine*, **57**, 105–115.

Liberzon, I., Abelson, J.L., Flagel, S.B., and Raz, J. (1999). Neuroendocrine and psychophysiological responses in PTSD: a symptom provocation study. *Neuropsychopharmacology*, **21**, 40–50.

Lindley, S.E., Carlson, E.B., and Benoit, M. (2004). Basal and dexamethasone suppressed salivary cortisol concentrations in a community sample of patients with posttraumatic stress disorder. *Biological Psychiatry*, **55**, 940–945.

Linkowski, P., Mendelwicz, J., LeClercq, R. et al. (1985). The 24 hour profile of ACTH and cortisol in major depressive illness. *Journal of Clinical Endocrinology and Metabolism*, **61**, 429–438.

López, J.F., Vázquez, D.M., Chalmers, D.T., Akil, H., and Watson, S.J. (1997). Regulation of 5-HT receptors and the Hypothalamic-Pituitary-Adrenal axis: implications for the neurobiology of suicide. *Annals of New York Academy of Sciences*, **836**, 106–134.

Maes, M., Lin, A., Bonaccorso, S., et al. (1998). Increased 24-hour urinary cortisol excretion in patients with post-traumatic stress disorder and patients with major depression, but not in patients with fibromyalgia. *Acta Psychiatria Scandinavia*, **98**, 328–335.

Mason, J.W., Giller, E.L., Kosten, T.R., Ostroff, R.B., and Podd, L. (1986). Urinary-free cortisol levels in posttraumatic stress disorder patients. *Journal of Nervous Mental Disorders*, **174**, 145–159.

Mason, J.W., Wang, S., Yehuda, R. et al. (2002). Marked lability in urinary cortisol levels in subgroups of combat veterans with posttraumatic stress disorder during an intensive exposure treatment program. *Psychosomatic Medicine*, **64**, 238–246.

McEwen, B.S., Weiss, J.M., and Schwartz, L.S. (1968). Selective retention of corticosterone by limbic structures in the rat brain. *Nature*, **220**, 911–913.

Meijer, O.C. and de Kloet, E.R. (1994). Corticosterone suppresses the expression of 5-HT1A receptor mRNA in rat dentate gyrus. *European Journal of Pharmacology*, **266**, 255–261.

Newport, D.J., Heim, C., Bonsall, R., Miller, A.H., and Nemeroff, C.B. (2004). Pituitary-adrenal responses to standard and low-dose dexamethasone suppression tests in adult survivors of child abuse. *Biological Psychiatry*, **55**, 10–20.

Neylan, T.C., Lenoci, M., Maglione, M.L. et al. (2003) Delta sleep response to metyrapone in post-traumatic stress disorder. *Neuropsychopharmacology*, **28**, 1666–1676.

Olff, M., Guzelcan, Y., de Vries, G.J., Assies, J., and Gersons, B.P. (2006). HPA- and HPT-axis alterations in chronic posttraumatic stress disorder. *Psychoneuroendocrinology*, **31**, 1220–1230.

Otte, C., Lenoci, M., Metzler, T., Yehuda, R., Marmar, C.R., and Neylan, T.C. (2007). Effects of metyrapone on hypothalamic-pituitary-adrenal axis and sleep in women with post-traumatic stress disorder. *Biological Psychiatry*, **61**, 952–956.

Patel, P.D., López, J.F., Lyons, D.M., Burke, S., Wallace, M., and Schatzberg, A.F. (2000). Glucocorticoid and mineralocorticoid receptor mRNA expression in squirrel monkey brain. *Journal of Psychiatric Research*, **34**, 383–392.

Paykel, E.S. (1994). Life events, social support and depression. *Acta Psychiatrica Scandinavia*, **377**, 50–58.

Pfohl, B., Sherman, B., Schlecte, J., and Stone, R. (1985). Pituitary/adrenal axis rhythm disturbances in psychiatric patients. *Archives of General Psychiatry*, **42**, 897–903.

Pittman, R.G. and Orr, S.P. (1990). Twenty-four hour urinary cortisol and catecholamine excretion in combat-related posttraumatic stress disorder. *Bioogical Psychiatry*, **27**, 245–247.

Plotsky, P.M. (1987). Facilitation of immunoreactive corticotropin-releasing factor secretion into the hypophyseal-portal circulation after activation of catechoaminergic pathways or central norepinepherine injection. *Endocrinology*, **121**, 924–930.

Plotsky, P.M., Cunningham, E.T., and Widmaier, E.P. (1989). Catecholaminergic modulation of corticotropin-releasing factor and adrenocorticotropin secretion. *Endocrine Reviews*, **10**, 437–458.

Rasmusson, A.M., Lipschitz, D.S., Wang, S. et al. (2001) Increased pituitary and adrenal reactivity in premenopausal women with posttraumatic stress disorder. *Biological Psychiatry*, **50**, 965–977.

Reul, J.M.H. and deKloet, E.R. (1985). Two receptor systems for corticosterone in rat brain: microdistribution and differential occupation. *Endocrinology*, **117**, 2505–2511.

Roberts, J.L., Budarf, M.L., Baxter, J.D., and Herbert, E. (1979). *Biochemistry*, **22**, 4907–4915.

Rubin, R., Mandell, A., and Crandall, P.H. (1966), Corticosteroid responses to limbic stimulation in man: localization of stimulus sites. *Science*, **153**, 767–768.

Rubin, R.T., Poland, R.E., Lesser, I.M., Winston, R.A., and Blodgett, N. (1987). Neuroendocrine aspects of primary endogenous depression I: Cortisol secretory dynamics in patients and matched controls. *Archives of General Psychiatry*, **44**, 328–336.

Sachar, E.J., Hellman, L., Roffwarg, H.P., Halpern, F.S., Fukush, D.K., and Gallagher, T.F. (1973). Disrupted 24 hour patterns of cortisol secretion in psychotic depressives. *Archives of General Psychiatry*, **28**, 19–24.

Sanchez, M.M., Young,.L.J., LPlotsky, P.M., and Insel, T.R. (2000). Distribution of corticosteroid receptors in the rhesus brain: relative absence of glucocorticoid receptors in the hippocampal formation. *Journal of Neuroscience*, **20**, 4657–4668.

Santa Ana, E.J., Saladin, M.E., Back, S.E. et al. (2006). PTSD and the HPA axis: differences in response to the cold pressor task among individuals with child vs. adult trauma. *Psychoneuroendocrinology*, **31**, 501–509.

Sapolsky, R.M., Armanini, M.P., Packan, D.R., Sutton, S.W., and Plotsky, P.M. (1990). Glucocorticoid feedback inhibition of adrenocorticotropic hormone secretagogue release: relationship to corticosteroid receptor occupancy in various limbic sites. *Neuroendocrinology*, **51**, 328–336.

Smith, M.A., Davidson, J., Ritchie, J.C. et al. (1989). The corticotropin-releasing hormone test in patients with posttraumatic stress disorder. *Biological Psychiatry*, **26**, 349–355.

Spencer, R.L., Young, E.A., Choo, P.H, and McEwen, B.S. (1990). Glucocorticoid Type I and Type II receptor binding: estimates of in vivo receptor number, occupancy and activation with varying levels of steroid. *Brain Research*, **514**, 37–48.

Stein, M.B., Yehuda, R., Koverola, C., and Hanna, C. (1997). Enhanced dexamethasone suppression of plasma cortisol in adult women traumatized by childhood sexual abuse. *Biological Psychiatry*, **42**, 680–686.

Sullivan, R.M. and Gratton, A. (1997). Relationships between stress-induced increases in medial prefrontal cortical dopamine and plasma corticosterone levels in rats: role of cerebral laterality. *Neuroscience*, **83**, 81–91.

Swanson, L.W., Sawchenko, P.E., Rivier, J., and Vale, W.W. (1983). Organization of ovine corticotropin-releasing factor immunoreactive cells and fibers in the rat brain: an immunohistochemical study. *Neuroendocrinology*, **36**, 165–186.

Trapp, T. and Holsboer, F. (1996). Heterodimerization between mineralocorticoid and glucocorticoid receptors increases the functional diversity of corticosteroid action. *Trends Pharmacological Sciences*, **17**, 145–149.

Veldhuis, J.D., Iranmanesh, A., Naftolowitz, D., Tatham, N., Cassidy, F., and Carroll, B.J. (2001). Corticotropin secretory dynamics in humans under low glucocorticoid feedback. *Journal of Clinical Endocrinology and Metabolism*, **86**, 5554–5563.

von Bardeleben, U., Stalla, G.K., Mueller, O.A., and Holsboer, F. (1988). Blunting of ACTH response to CRH in depressed patients is avoided by metyrapone pretreatment. *Biological Psychiatry*, **24**, 782–786.

Watson, S., Gallagher, P., Smith, M.S., Ferrier, I.N., and Young, A.H. (2006). The dex/CRH test–is it better than the DST? *Psychoneuroendocrinology*, **31**, 889–894.

Wheler, G.H., Brandon, D., Clemons, A. et al. (2006). Cortisol production rate in posttraumatic stress disorder. *Journal of Clinical Endocrinology and Metabolism*, **91**, 3486–3489.

Yehuda, R., Giller, E.L., Southwick, S.M., Lowy, M.T. and Mason J.W. (1991). Hypothalamic-pituitary-adrenal dysfunction in posttraumatic stress disorder. *Biological Psychiatry*, **30**, 1031–1048.

Yehuda, R., Kahana, B., Schmeidler, J., Southwick, S.M., Wilson, S., and Giller, E.L. (1995). Impact of cumulative lifetime trauma and recent stress on current posttraumatic stress disorder symptoms in holocaust survivors. *American Journal of Psychiatry*, **152**, 1815–1818.

Yehuda, R. (2002). Current status of cortisol findings in post-traumatic stress disorder. *Psychiatric Clinics of North America*, **25**, 341–368.

Yehuda, R., Halligan, S.L., Grossman, R., Golier, J.A., and Wong, C. (2002). The cortisol and glucocorticoid receptor response to low dose dexamethasone administration in aging combat veterans and holocaust survivors with and without posttraumatic stress disorder. *Biological Psychiatry*, **52**, 393–403.

Yehuda, R., Blair, W., Labinsky, E., and Bierer, L.M. (2007). Effects of parental PTSD on the cortisol response to dexamethasone administration in their adult offspring. *American Journal of Psychiatry*, **164**, 163–166.

Young, E.A., Watson, S.J., Kotun, J. et al. (1990) Response to low dose oCRH in endogenous depression: role of cortisol feedback. *Archives of General Psychiatry*, **47**, 449–457

Young, E.A., Haskett, R.F., Watson, S.J., and Akil, H. (1991). Loss of glucocorticoid fast feedback in depression. *Archives of General Psychiatry*, **48**, 693–699.

Young, E.A., Haskett, R.F., Grunhaus L. et al. (1994). Increased circadian activation of the hypothalamic pituitary adrenal axis in depressed patients in the evening. *Archives of General Psychiatry*, **51**, 701–707.

Young, E.A., Akil, H., Haskett, R.F., and Watson, S.J. (1995). Evidence against changes in corticotroph CRF receptors in depressed patients. *Biological Psychiatry*, **37**, 355–363.

Young, E.A., Abelson, J.L., Curtis, G.C., and Nesse, R.M. (1997). Childhood adversity and vulnerability to mood and anxiety disorders. *Depression and Anxiety*, **5**, 66–72.

Young, E.A., Lopez, J.F., Murphy-Weinberg, V., Watson, S.J., and Akil, H. (1997). Normal pituitary response to metyrapone in the morning in depressed patients: implications for circadian regulation of crh secretion. *Biological Psychiatry*, **41**, 1149–1155.

Young, E.A., Lopez, J.F., Murphy-Weinberg, V., Watson, S.J., and Akil, H. (2000). Hormonal evidence for altered responsiveness to social stress in major depression. *Neuropsychopharmacology*, **23**, 411–418.

Young, E.A., Carlson, N.E., and Brown, M.B. (2001). 24 hour ACTH and cortisol pulsatility in depressed women. *Neuropsychpoharmacology*, **25**, 267–276.

Young, E.A., Abelson, J.L., and Cameron, O.G. (2004). Effect of comorbid anxiety disorders on the hpa axis response to a social stressor in major depression, *Biological Psychiatry*, **56**, 113–120.

Young, E.A. and Breslau, N. (2004). Cortisol and Catecholamines in posttraumatic stress disorder: a community study. *Archives of General Psychiatry*, **61**, 394–401.

Young, E.A. and Breslau, N. (2004). Saliva cortisol in a community sample with posttraumatic stress disorder. *Biological Psychiatry*, **56**, 205–209.

Young, E.A., Tolman, R., Witkowski, K., and Kaplan, G. (2004). Salivary cortisol and ptsd in a low income community sample of women. *Biological Psychiatry*, **55**, 621–626.

Young, E.A. and Ribiero, S.C. (2006). Sex differences in the ACTH response to 24H metyrapone in depression. *Brain Research*, **1126**, 148–155.

Zobel, A.W., Nickel, T., Sonntag, A., Uhr, M., Holsboer, F., and Ising, M. (2001). Cortisol response in the combined dexamethasone/CRH test as predictor of relapse in patients with remitted depression: a prospective study. *Journal of Psychiatric Research*, **35**, 83–94.

Chapter 16

Neuroendocrine and immune crosstalk in major depression

Timothy G. Dinan and Peter Fitzgerald

There is overwhelming evidence to indicate that adaptation to chronic stress involves response from both the neuroendocrine and immune systems. While acute stress activates the sympathoad-renal medullary system (SAM) resulting in the components of the 'fight or flight' response with a release of catecholamines, chronic stress results in alterations of the hypothalamic-pituitary-adrenal axis (HPA) with changes in the release of cortisol (Rubin et al. 2001). At the same time chronic stress can result in alterations in both innate and adaptive immunity (Maes, 2001). There is a complex interplay between the HPA and the immune system as the body adapts to a stressor (Fig. 16.1). Major depression has long been recognized as a disorder, frequently driven by psychosocial stress and associated with changes in both immunity and the HPA. While knowl-edge of the biology of these complex systems is rapidly increasing, the reasons for the altered function in major depression are far less well understood. Here we examine the changes observed in HPA activity and in immunity in patients with major depression and examine possible links between both systems. This is the third of four chapters in this book that specifically discuss the role of inflammation in affective disorders, together with Chapters 10, 11, and 17. The role of the HPA axis in affective disorders and other stress-related conditions is discussed in several other Chapters of this book (Chapters 5, 7–9, 11, 15, 19, 21, and 26).

HPA

A wide variety of neurotransmitters influence the hypothalamic paraventricular nucleus regula-tion of the HPA. These transmitters include 5HT, noradrenaline, acetylcholine, and the opioids. Under basal conditions corticotrophin-releasing hormone (CRH) produced by the parvicellular neurones is the dominant regulator of the axis (Vale et al. 1981). In situations of chronic stress many parvicellar neurones co-express vasopressin (AVP), which plays an important role in sustaining HPA activation (Dinan and Scott, 2006). CRH and AVP act synergistically on the ante-rior pituitary corticotropes to bring about the release of ACTH (Aguilera et al. 2000). This in turn stimulates the release of cortisol for the adrenal cortex, which feeds back to suppress the axis. Negative feedback is defined in terms of speed of response into immediate, intermediate, and delayed (Tilbrook and Clarke, 2006). Much of the research in psychiatry has focused on delayed feedback While high cortisol provides a break on HPA activity it simultaneously has potent immuno-suppressive actions (Turnbull and Rivier, 1999).

Innate and acquired immunity

Immune defence mechanisms originated as a protection against microbial invasion and consist of both an innate and adaptive arm. The components of innate immunity are capable of recognizing

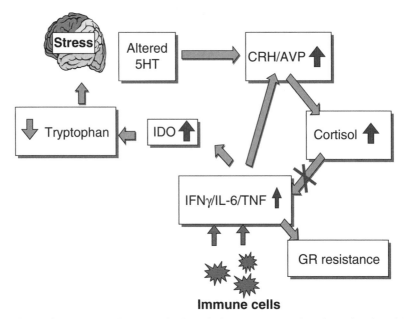

Fig. 16.1 shows the interaction between the hypothalamic-pituitary-adrenal axis (HPA) and the immune system. Chronic stress leads to activation of the HPA with increased release of cortisol via ACTH, which is stimulated by corticotrophin-releasing hormone (CRH) and vasopressin (AVP). Immune activation is reflected in an increase in pro-inflammatory cytokines which help sustain HPA activation and alter tryptophan metabolism by enhancing indoleamine 2, 3-dioxygenase (IDO). TNFα elevation may induce glucocorticoid receptor (GR) resistance which prevents the higher level of cortisol from suppressing immune activity and enhancing negative feedback in the HPA.

structures that are shared by various microbes but are not present on host cells. The major players in the detection of pathogens are the toll-like receptors (TLRs) which are pattern recognition receptors (Hawlisch and Kohl, 2006; Palsson-McDermott and O'Neill, 2007). Ten transmembrane TLRs have been identified in man. Of these TLR4 is the best characterized as the lipopolysaccharide recognition site for gram negative bacteria (McCoy and O'Neill, 2008). Expression of inflammatory cytokines subsequent to stimulation of TLR4 is dependent on the transcription factor NF-κB (Goldman, 2007). TLR2 detects components of gram-positive bacteria while TLR3 recognizes double-stranded RNA produced by many viruses. TLR5 recognizes bacterial flagella from both gram positive and negative bacteria. TLR7 and 8 recognize single-stranded RNA and TLR9 recognizes unmethylated CpG DNA. All ten TLRs are expressed on macrophages and phagocytosis is a major function of these cells. As well as recognizing foreign structures they also play a role in removing both apoptotic and necrotic cells. In contrast to innate immunity, the adaptive immune system is antigen-specific and operates through T and B cells (Harrington and Hall, 2008). Cytokines produced by the innate response determine the type of adaptive response. Naïve T cells activate to either a Th1 or Th2 phenotype (Schwarz et al. 2001). Th1 cells primarily produce IFN-γ, IL-2, IL-12, IL-18, and TNF-β. Th2 cells secrete IL-4, IL-5, IL-6, IL-10, IL-13, and TGF-β. These cytokines are large polypeptide mediators (8-60Kda) that regulate growth, differentiation, and function of many cell types (Turnbull and Rivier, 1999). Several cytokines are available in more than one form, as they are a product of more than one gene. These are distinguished using a suffix from the Greek alphabet, for example, α, β, or γ (Thompson, 1998). Most commonly cytokines have been classified into families of interleukins, tumour necrosis factors (TNF), interferons (INF), chemokines, haematopoietins, and colony-stimulating factors (CSF). As many cytokines exert a number of different actions, they may in fact belong to more than one cytokine family.

In the broadest terms the cytokines can be classed as pro-inflammatory or anti-inflammatory. Interleukin-1 (IL-1), interleukin-6 (IL-6), and TNF act as pro-inflammatory cytokines. Their actions include stimulating immune cells to exert their effects locally or through a remote site usually of cell injury. Anti-inflammatory cytokines include interleukin-4 (IL-4), interleukin-10 (IL-10), and interleukin-13 (IL-13). Anti-inflammatory cytokines serve to dampen the immune response and to hinder the production of further cytokines (Kiecolt-Glaser and Glaser, 2002).

The Th1 system produces cell-mediated immunity against intracellular pathogens while the Th2 system helps B-cell maturation and humoral immune responses against extracellular pathogens. Th3 cells secrete TGF-β while TH17 cells were characterized as a novel CD4(+) subset that preferentially produces IL-17, IL-17F, and IL-22 as the primary cytokines (Carrier et al. 2006). Th17 cells appear to play a major role in sustaining the inflammatory response and their presence is associated with autoimmune disease (Weber et al. 2008). They are induced by a combination of TGF-β and IL-6, while they are maintained by IL-23. Induction is dependent on the orphan nuclear receptor RORγt, which is expressed in response to either TGF-β or IL-6.

In contrast, Tregs are cells which suppress immune responses of other cells and express CD4, CD25, and Foxp3 (Coleman et al. 2007). These cells are involved in closing down immune responses after an invading organism has been eliminated and also in preventing autoimmune responses.

HPA in major depression

Multiple disturbances at different levels of the HPA have been described in patients with major depression. Linkowski et al. (1987) reported increased 24-hour mean plasma cortisol secretion, a decreased amplitude in the cortisol rhythm and shorter nocturnal quiescence of cortisol secretion in male patients with major depression. In a similar study Rubin et al. (1987) also reported hypercortisolism. This increase in plasma cortisol has been explained both by increased forward drive in the axis and decreased negative feedback. Nemeroff and colleagues (1984) reported increased levels of CRH-like immunoreactivity in the CSF of depressives while numerous studies report a failure to suppress cortisol in response to dexamethasone challenge (Carroll et al. 1981; Rubin and Poland, 1984). Using the low dose dexametasone challenge of 1 mg, patients with melancholic features have non-suppression rates of 40–70%.

ACTH responses to exogeneous CRH administration are often blunted in major depression (Gold et al. 1984; Holsboer et al. 1984). When this test is conducted following the administration of dexamethasone a paradoxical enhancement of response is observed in depressives relative to controls (von Bardeleben and Holsboer, 1989). Our recent studies have focused on the role of VAP in the increased HPA forward drive seen in depression. We examined a cohort of depressed subjects on two separate occasions, with CRH alone, and with the combination of CRH and ddAVP (desmopressin an analogue of AVP) (Dinan et al. 1999). A significant blunting of ACTH output to CRH alone was noted. Following the combination of CRH and ddAVP, the release of ACTH in depressives and healthy volunteers was indistinguishable. We concluded that while the CRH1 receptor is downregulated in depression, that a concomitant upregulation of the V3 (or V1b) receptor takes place. This is consistent with the animal models of chronic stress, described above, in which a switching from CRH to AVP regulation is observed. It is interesting that in CRH1 receptor-deficient mice, basal plasma AVP levels are significantly elevated, AVP mRNA is increased in the PVN and there is increased AVP-like immunoreactivity in the median eminence (Muller et al. 2000).

In a further study we have provided evidence for the upregulation of the anterior pituitary V3 receptor (Dinan et al. 2004). Fourteen patients with major depression and 14 age- and sex-matched healthy comparison subjects were recruited. ddAVP 10 µg was given intravenously and ACTH and cortisol release was monitored for 120 min. Both ACTH and cortisol responses were raised in the depressives relative to the controls. This suggests that patients with major depression have augmented ACTH and cortisol responses to desmopressin indicating enhanced V_3 responsivity.

Immune markers in depression

The majority of patients with major depression develop the syndrome within the context of chronic psychosocial stress. Such stress causes an increase in the number of circulating white blood cells, and decreases the number of NK cells, together with T and B cells. Unlike acute stress, chronic stress increases the CD4 to CD8 ratio (Herbert and Cohen, 1993; Raison et al. 2002). A study which looked at stress in caregivers to Alzheimer's patients and its relationship to rate of wound healing found that healing took significantly longer in caregivers compared to controls. This may have implications, for example, in recovery from surgery (Mercado and Glaser, 1995). A further study looked at the effect surgical stress had on immune function. Cell-mediated and antibody-mediated immunity as illustrated by type 1/type 2 T-helper cell balance were examined. The study concluded that there was a shift in type 1/ type 2 T-helper cell balance indicating a switch towards antibody-mediated immunity following surgery (Decker et al. 1996). Major depression has been shown to be associated with activation of the inflammatory response. These changes include increased numbers of peripheral leucocytes including monocytes and neutrophils (Herbert and Cohen, 1993; Maes, 1999). Positive acute phase proteins including C-reactive protein are increased (Maes, 1997; 1999; 2001; Song et al. 1994) while negative acute phase proteins are decreased, for example, albumin (Maes, 1997; 1999). We examined C-reactive protein (CRP) levels before and after a course of SSRI therapy (O'Brien et al. 2006). Antidepressant treatment resulted in a significant drop in CRP levels irrespective of whether or not patients showed a clinical improvement. Normalization of this aspect of immune function can therefore take place in the absence of a clinical response, just as patients with normal HPA function can be clinically depressed. Overall, the acute phase response is an integral part of the inflammatory response and its purpose is to enable protein mobilization, which serves to limit tissue damage and stimulate repair (Kushner, 1982). Elevations in CRP levels are reported as predictive of cardiovascular events (Haverkate et al. 1997).

Smith (1991) put forward the 'macrophage theory of depression' where he proposed that excessive secretion of macrophage cytokines such as IL-1, TNFα, and INFα were associated with major depression. Maes and his colleagues (1997) provided support for this theory, showing that there is increased production of IL-1, IL-2, IL-6, and IFNγ in depressive illness. In a study of CSF cytokine levels in patients with depression Levine et al. (1999) found that the depressed group had higher CSF IL-1β, lower IL-6, and no change in TNFα compared to the control group.

We examined pro- and anti-inflammatory cytokine levels in patients who were SSRI resistant (O'Brien et al. 2007). Patients with SSRI-resistant depression had significantly higher production of the pro-inflammatory cytokines IL-6 and TNF-a compared to normal controls. Euthymic patients who were formerly SSRI resistant had pro-inflammatory cytokine levels which were similar to the healthy subject group. Anti-inflammatory cytokine levels did not differ across the three groups. The suppression of pro-inflammatory cytokines does not occur in depressed patients who fail to respond to SSRIs and is necessary for clinical recovery.

Cytokines and HPA axis activity in depression

The pro-inflammatory cytokines TNF-α, IL-1, and IL-6 are primary HPA-stimulating cytokines acting directly on the hypothalamic paraventricular neurones. TNF appears first, followed by IL-1 and subsequently IL-6 (van Deventer et al. 1990). Both TNF and IL-1 stimulate further production of IL-6 but IL-6 then in turn inhibits production of both these cytokines. IL-6 acts synergically with glucocorticoids to stimulate acute phase proteins such as CRP initiating the acute phase response (Boumpas et al. 1993; Hirano et al. 1990).

IL-6 is a potent stimulator of CRH production which leads to heightened HPA activity characterized by increasing ACTH and cortisol levels (Dentino et al. 1999). As IL-6 stimulates ACTH and cortisol levels well above the maximum level achieved by stimulation of CRH, it is thought that IL-6 may also stimulate parvicellular AVP and other ACTH secretagogues (Chrousos, 1995; Mastorakos et al. 1993; 1994). The manner in which pro-inflammatory cytokines cross the blood–brain barrier (BBB) to influence neurotransmission is unclear. Proposed methods include stimulating glial and endothelial cells to secrete IL-6, or the presence of a special transport system for inflammatory cytokines. Other methods proposed include an indirect route through stimulation of the central noradrenergic system (Chrousos, 1995; Chapman and Goodell, 1964) or entry where the BBB is deficient with the consequent stimulation of other messengers, for example, prostaglandins (Blatteis, 1990; Stitt and Cowen, 1997). Alternatively cytokines may affect the BBB by the induction of adhesion molecules, such as ICAM-1 and VCAM-1 in the brain endothelium, which increases the potential for circulating T lymphocytes to cross the BBB (Brown, 2001; Wichers and Maes, 2002). It is therefore possible that the hypercortisolaemia in melancholic depression arises from increased CRH secretion via pro-inflammatory cytokine stimulation.

Consequences of immune activation

Major depression is a pro-inflammatory state and as such can have profound consequences for physical well-being, especially cardiovascular health. It is well established from prospective studies that major depression increases the risk of a cardiovascular event by approximately threefold (Dinan, 1999). Minor elevations of CRP are predictive of cardiovascular events in patients with coronary artery disease (Haverkate et al. 1997). A large prospective cohort study involving 2 459 subjects and 3 969 matched controls was carried out in Reykjavik where a single CRP measurement was studied in relation to the 20-year incidence of CHD. Patients with a CRP greater than 2 mg/l had a relative risk of CHD OF 1.92 as compared to patients with CRP levels in the bottom third (Danesh et al. 2004). The precise mechanism underlying CRP levels and adverse outcomes is not clear. It has been suggested that statins, which are commonly used to lower cholesterol may reduce systemic inflammation and therefore reduce CRP by decreasing levels of atherogenic lipoproteins.

Immune-endocrine interaction

A recent study has shown that patients with major depressive disorder have impaired sensitivity of peripheral glucocorticoid receptors as demonstrated by reduced cutaneous vasoconstriction to topical steroids (Cotter et al. 2002). It has been hypothesized that the altered GR function in major depression occurs via ligand-independent mechanisms involving signal-transduction pathways driven by compounds unrelated to steroids such as cytokines (O'Malley et al. 1995). Studies indicate that GR function can be influenced by pro-inflammatory cytokines via inhibition of GR translocation from cytoplasm to nucleus (Miller et al. 1999) and inhibition of GR-mediated gene transcription (Pariante et al. 1999). The topical steroid vasoconstriction assay provides a convenient probe of peripheral GR function. We sought to assess the sensitivity of peripheral GRs in antidepressant resistant major depressives and investigate the association between GR sensitivity and circulating plasma cytokines (Fitzgerald et al. 2006). Nineteen antidepressant-resistant depressives together with age- and sex-matched healthy controls underwent the steroid vasoconstriction assay using three commercial preparations of corticosteroids containing clobetasol propionate 0.05%, betamethasone valerate 0.1%, and clobetasone butyrate 0.05%, corresponding to very potent, potent, and moderately potent steroid creams, respectively. The pro-inflammatory cytokines TNFα and IL-6 were measured. The severity of the depressive episode was assessed using the Hamilton Depression Scale (HAMD). Depressed subjects had a significantly reduced vasoconstriction response across all three strengths of steroid. They also had significantly higher concentrations of TNFα and IL-6. There was a significant inverse correlation between TNFα concentration and vasoconstriction response and also between the HAMD score and vasoconstriction response. These findings suggest that cutaneous GR function is abnormal in antidepressant-resistant depression, that circulating TNFα may play a significant role in this abnormality and that the efficacy of topical steroids in antidepressant-resistant depressives is reduced. A similar GR resistance has been reported in patients with bipolar disorder by Knijff et al. (2006) who examine the impact of dexamethasone on T cells. They suggest that the T-cell resistance to steroids is a trait marker in bipolar disorder. Pace et al. (2007) propose a molecular mechanism through which cytokines may induce glucocorticoid resistance via mitogen-activated protein kinases and NFκB.

Altered GR responsivity helps explain the abnormal negative feedback in HPA function in major depression and the inability to suppress peripheral inflammatory markers despite elevations in circulating cortisol. Data from Pariante et al. (1997) indicate that antidepressants inhibit steroid transporters localized on the BBB and in neurones, and thus increase the access of cortisol to the brain. In turn GR activation is facilitated by antidepressants and leads to an increased negative feedback by circulating glucocorticoids on the HPA axis. Several polymorphisms have been described in the glucocorticoid receptor gene and the findings support the view that variants of the GR gene might play a role in the pathophysiology of a major depression (van Rossum et al. 2006).

Limitations of immune studies

The pioneering work of Maes has resulted in a major focus on immune markers in major depression. Furthermore, the recent work of Miller and colleagues (Irwin and Miller, 2007) has increased our understanding of the manner in which cytokines may induce organic depression in those treated with interferon. However, there remain major gaps in our understanding of the immune anomalies in depression. The evidence that the disorder is associated with activation of innate immunity is now compelling (Dantzer et al. 2007). However, no studies have reported on the function of TLRs in major depression despite the fact that these are the gate keepers of innate responses. While major depression is not caused by viral or bacterial infections in the majority of cases it is possible that TLRs can be activated in other ways of relevance in depression. For example, in a recent study Shi et al. (2007) demonstrated that the TLR4 receptor can be activated by a fatty acid in the absence of lipolysaccharide. It is tempting to suggest that the activation in innate immunity seen in depression is mediated by a TLR stimulated by a fatty acid. This may be relevant given the fact that depression is associated with shifts in polyunsaturated fatty acids from the anti-inflammatory ω-3 series to the pro-inflammatory ω-6 series.

As well as the lack of studies on TLRs, to our knowledge no studies on the highly influential Tregs or Th17 cells has been conducted in depression or in other stress-related psychological disorders.

Conclusions

Major depression is frequently associated with both cortisol hypersecretion and immune activation. The extent to which these factors are core to the pathophysiology of major depression as opposed to being epiphenomena is still the subject of considerable debate. What is increasingly clear is that immune activation and elevations in cortisol have negative health consequences especially in terms of cardiovascular function, where depression is associated with an increased prevalence of heart disease. We propose that the HPA and immune activations observed in depression are sustained as a result of GR resistance.

References

Aguilera, G. and Rabadan-Diehl, C. (2000). Vasopressinergic regulation of the hypothalamic-pituitary-adrenal axis: implications for stress adaptation. *Regulatory Peptides*, **96**, 23–29.

Blatteis, C.M. (1990). Neuromodulative actions of cytokines. *Yale Journal of Biology and Medicine*, **63**, 133–146.

Boumpas, D.T., Chrousos, G.P., Wilder, R.L., Cupps, T.R., and Balow, J.E. (1993). Glucocorticoid therapy for immune mediated diseases: basic and clinical correlates. *Annals of Internal Medicine*, **119**, 1198–1208.

Brown, K.A. (2001). Factors modifying the migration of lymphocytes across the blood-brain-barrier. *International Immunopharmacology*, **1**, 2043–206.

Carrier, Y., Yuan, J., Kuchroo, V.K, and Weiner, H.L. (2006). Th3 cells in peripheral tolerance. 1: induction of Foxp3-positive regulatory T cells by Th3 cells derived from TGF-β T cell-transgenic mice. *Journal of Immunology*, **178**, 179–185.

Carroll, B.J., Feinberg, M., and Greden, J.F. (1981). Specific laboratory test for the diagnosis of melancholia: standardisation, validation and clinical utility. *Archives of General Psychiatry*, **38**, 15–22.

Chapman, L.F. and Goodell, H. (1964). The participation of the nervous system in the inflammatory reaction. *Annals New York Academy of Science*, **116**, 990–1017.

Chrousos, G.P. (1995). The hypothalamic-pituitary-adrenal axis and immune mediated inflammation. *New England Journal of Medicine*, **332**, 1351–1362.

Coleman, C.A., Muller-Trutwin, M.C., Apetrei, C., and Pandrea, I. (2007). T regulatory cells: aid or hindrance in the clearance of disease? *Journal of Cellular and Molecular Medicine*, **11**, 1291–1325.

Cotter, P., Mulligan, O., Landau, S., Papadopoulos, A., Lightman, S., and Checkley, S. (2002). Vasoconstrictor response to topical beclomethasone in major depression. *Psychoneuroendocrinology*, **27**, 475–487.

Danesh, J., Wheeler, J.G., Hirschfield, G.M. et al. (2004). C-reactive protein and other circulating markers of inflammation in the prediction of coronary heart disease. *New England Journal of Medicine*, **350**, 1387–1397.

Dantzer, R., O'Connor, J.C., Freund, G.C., Johnson, R.W., and Kelley, K.W. (2008). From inflammation to sickness and depression: when the immune system subjugates the brain. *Nature Reviews Neuroscience* **9**, 46–56.

Decker, D., Schondorf, M., Bidlingmater, F., Hirner, A., and Von Rueker, A.A. (1996). Surgical stress induces a shift in the type 1/type 2 T- helper cell balance suggesting down regulation of cell mediated and up regulation of antibody mediated immunity commensurate to the trauma. *Surgery*, **119**, 316–325.

Dentino, A.N., Pieper, C.F., Rao, K.M.K. et al.(1999). Association of interleukin-6 and other biological variables with depression in older people living in the community. *Journal of American Geriatric Society*, **47**, 6–11.

Dinan, T.G. (1999). Physical complications of depression. *British Medical Journal*, **318**, 826.

Dinan, T.G., Lavelle, E., Scott, L.V., Medbak, S., and Grossman, A. (1999). Desmopressin normalises the blunted ACTH response to corticotropin-releasing hormone in melancholic depression: evidence of enhanced vasopressinergic responsivity. *Journal of Clinical Endocrinology and Metabolism*, **84**, 2238–2246.

Dinan, T.G., Lavelle, E., and Scott, L.V. (2004). Further neuroendocrine evidence of enhanced V3 receptor responses in melancholic depression. *Psychological Medicine*, **34**, 169–172.

Dinan, T.G.and Scott, L.V. (2005). Anatomy of melancholia: focus on the hypothalamic-pituitary-adrenal axis overactivation and the role of vasopressin. *Journal of Anatomy*, **207**, 259–64.

Fitzgerald, P., O'Brien S., Scott LV, and Dinan, T.G. (2006). Cutaneous glucocorticoid receptor sensitivity and pro-inflammatory cytokine levels in antidepressant resistant depression. *Psychological Medicine*, **36**, 37–44.

Gold, P.W., Chrousos, G.P., and Kellner, C. (1984). Psychiatric implications of basic and clinical studies with CRF. *American Journal of Psychiatry*, **141**, 619–627.

Goldman, M. (2007). Translational mini review series on toll-like receptors: toll-like receptor ligands as novel pharmaceuticals for allergic disorders. *Clinical and Experimetnal Immunology*, **147**, 208–216.

Harrington, C. and Hall, P. (2008). Molecular and cellular themes in inflammation and immunology. *Journal of Pathology*, **214**, 123–125.

Haverkate, F., Thompson, S.G., Pyke, S.D., Gillimore, and J.R., Pepys, M.B. (1997). Production of C-reactive protein and risk of coronary events in stable and unstable angina. European Concerted Action on Thrombosis and Disabilities Angina Pectoris Study Group. *Lancet*, **349**, 462–466.

Hawlisch, H. and Kohl, J. (2006). Complement and toll-like receptors: key regulators of adaptive immune responses. *Molecular Immunology*, **43**, 13–21.

Herbert, T.B. and Cohen. S. (1993). Stress and immunity in humans: a meta-analytic review. *Psychosomatic Medicine*, **55**, 364–379.

Hirano, T., Akira, S., Taga, T., and Kisimoto, T. (1990). Biological and clinical aspects of interleukin-6. *Immunology Today*, **11**, 443–449.

Holsboer, F., Von Bardeleben, U., Gerken, A., Stalla, G.K., and Muller, O.A. (1984) Blunted corticotropin and normal cortisol response to human corticotropin-releasing factor in depression. *New England Journal of Medicine*, **311**, 1127.

Irwin, M.R. and Miller, A.H. (2007). Depressive disorders and immunity: 20 years of progress and discovery. *Brain Behavior and Immunity*, **21**, 374–383.

Kiecolt-Glaser, J.K. and Glaser, R. (2002). Depression and immune function: central pathways to morbidity and mortality. *Journal of Psychosomatic Research*, **53**, 873–876.

Knijff, E.M., Breunis, M.N., Van Geest, M.C. et al. (2006). A relative resistance of T cells to dexamethasone in bipolar disorder. *Bipolar Disorder*, **8**, 740–750.

Kushner, I. (1982). The phenomena of the acute phase response. *Annals of New York Academy Science*, **389**, 39–48.

Levine, J., Barak, Y., Chengappa, K.N, Rappoport, A., Rebey, M., and Barak, V. (1999). Cerebrospinal cytokine levels in patients with acute depression. *Neuropsychobiology*, **40**, 171–176.

Linkowski, P., Mendlewicz, J., Kerhofski, B. et al. (1987). 24-hour profiles of adrenocorticotropin, cortisol, and growth hormone in major depressive illness: effect of antidepressant treatment. *Journal of Clinical Endocrinology and Metabolism*, **65**, 141–152.

Maes, M. (1997). The immune pathophysiology of major depression: neurobiological, psychopathological and therapeutics Advances. In Honig, A. and Van Praag, H. (eds.), pp.197–215. Chichester, John Wiley.

Maes, M., Bosmans, K., de Johngh. R., Kenis, G., Vandoolaeghe, E., and Heels, H. (1997). Increased serum IL-6 and IL-1 receptor antagonist concentrations in major depression and treatment resistant depression. *Cytokine*, **9**, 853–858.

Maes, M. (1999). Major depression and activation of the inflammatory response system. *Advances in Experimental and Medical Biology*, **461**, 25–46.

Maes, M. (2001) The immunoregulatory effects of antidepressants. *Human Psychopharmacology*, **156**, 95–103.

Maes, M. (2001). Psychological stress and the inflammatory response system. *Clinical Science* (London), **101**, 193–194.

Mastorakos, G., Chrousos, G..P, and Weber, J.S. (1993). Recombinant interleukin-6 activates the hypothalamic-pituitary-adrenal axis in humans. *Journal of Clinical Endocrinology Metabolism*, **77**, 1690–1694.

Mastorakos, G., Weber, J..S, Magiakou, G.A., Gunn, H., Chrousos, G.P. (1994). Hypothalamic-pituitary-adrenal axis activation and stimulation of systemic vasopressin secretion by recombinant interleukin-6 in humans: potential implications for the syndrome of inappropriate vasopressin secretion. *Journal of Clinical Endocrinology Metabolism,* **79**, 934–939.

Mercado, A.M. and Glaser, R. (1995). Slowing of wound healing by psychological stress. *Lancet*, **346**, 1194–1196.

McCoy, C.E., and O'Neill, L.A.J. (2008). The role of toll-like receptors in macrophages. *Frontiers in Bioscience*, **13**, 62–70.

Miller, A.H., Pariante, C.M., and Pearce, B.D. (1999). Effects of cytokines on glucocorticoid receptor expression and function: glucocorticoid resistance and relevance to depression. *Advances in Experimental and Medical Biology*, **46**, 1107–1116.

Muller, M.B., Landgraf, R., and Keck, M. (2000). Vasopressin, major depression, and hypothalamic-pituitary-adrenocortical desensitization. *Biological Psychiatry*, **48**, 330–333.

Nemeroff, C.B, Widerlov, E., Bissette, G. et al. (1984). Elevated concentrations of CSF corticotropin-releasing factor-like immunoreactivity in depressed patients. *Science*, **226**, 1342–1344.

O'Brien, S., Scott, L.V, and Dinan T.G. (2006). Antidepressant therapy and C-reactive protein levels. *British Journal of Psychiatry*, **188**, 449–452

O'Brien, S., Scully, P., Fitzgerald, P., Scott, L.V, and Dinan, T.G. (2007). Plasma cytokine profiles in depressed patients who fail to respond to selective serotonin reuptake inhibitor therapy. *Journal of Psychiatric Research*, **41**, 326–331.

O'Malley, B.W., Schrader, W.T., Mani, S. et al. (1995). An alternative ligand-independent pathway for activation of steroid receptors. *Recent Progress in Hormone Research*, **50**, 333–347.

Pace, T.W.W, Hu, F., and Miller, A.H. (2007). Cytokine-effects on glucocorticoid receptor function: relevance to glucocorticoid resistance and the pathophysiology and treatment of major depression. *Brain Behavior Immunity*, **21**, 9–19.

Palsson-McDermott, E.M. and O'Neill L.A.J. (2007). Building an immune system from nine domains. *Biochemical Society Transactions,* **35**, 1437–1444.

Pariante, C.M., Pearce, B.D., Pisell, T.L., Owens, M.J., and Miller, A.H. (1997). Steroid-independent translocation of the glucocorticoid receptor by the antidepressant desipramine. *Molecular Pharmacology*, **52**, 571–581.

Pariante, C.M., Pearce, B.D., Pisell, T.L. et al. (1999). The proinflammatory cytokine, interleukin-1alpha, reduces glucocorticoid receptor translocation and function. *Endocrinology*, **140**, 4359–4366.

Raison, C.L., Gummick, J.F., and Miller, A.H. (2002). Neuroendocrine-Immune Interactions: Implications for health and Behaviour. In Pfaff, D.W, Arnold, A.P., Etgen, A.M., Fahrbach, S.E., and Rubin, R.T. (eds.). *Hormones Brain and Behaviour*, **5**, 209–262. New York, Academic Press.

Rubin, R.T. and Poland, R.E. (1984). Variability in cortisol level assay methods. *Archives of General Psychiatry*, **41**, 724–725.

Rubin, R., Poland, R.E., Lesser, I.M., Martin, D.J, Blodgett, A.L, and Winston, R.A. (1987). Neuroendocrine aspects of primary endogenous depression. III. Cortisol secretion in relation to diagnosis and symptom patterns. *Psychological Medicine*, **17**, 609–619.

Rubin, R., Dinan, T.G., and Scott, L.V. (2001). The neuroendocrinology of affective disorders. In Pfaff, D., Arnold, A.P., Etgen A.M., Fahrbach, S.E., Moss, R.L., Rubin, R.T. (eds.). *Hormones, Brain and Behaviour*. New York, Academic Press.

Schwarz, M.J., Chiang, S., Muller, N., and Ackenheill, M. (2001). T-helper-1 and T-helper-2 responses in psychiatric disorders. *Brain, Behavior and Immunity*, **15**, 340–370.

Shi, H., Kokoeva. M.V., Inouye, K., Tzamelli. I, Yin, T., and Flier, J.S. (2007). TLR4 links innate immunity and fatty acid-induced insulin resistance. *Journal of Clinical Investigation,* **116**, 3015–3025.

Smith, R.S. (1991). The macrophage theory of depression. *Medical Hypotheses*, **35**, 298–306.

Song, C., Dinan, T., and Leonard, B.E. (1994). Changes in immunoglobulin, complement and acute phase protein levels in the depressed patients and in healthy controls. *Journal of Affective Disorders*, **30**, 283–288.

Stitt, K.A. and Cowen, P.J. (1997). Serotonin and depression. In Honig, A. and van Praag, H.M. (eds.). *Depression: Neurobiological, Psychopathological and Therapeutic Advances*. Chichester, John Wiley and Sons.

Thompson, A. (1998). *The Cytokine Handbook*. 3rd Ed. San Diego, Academic Press.

Tilbrook, A.J., and Clarke, I.J. (2006). Neuroendocrine mechanisms of innate states of attenuated responsiveness of the hypothalamo-pituitary adrenal axis to stress. *Frontiers in Neuroendocrinology*, **27**, 285–307.

Turnbull, A.V., and Rivier, C.L. (1999). Regulation of the hypothalamic-pituitary-adrenal axis by cytokines: actions and mechanisms of action. *Physiology Reviews*, **79**, 1–71.

Vale, W., Spiess, J., Rivier, C., and Rivier, J. (1981) Characterisation of a 41 residue ovine hypothalamic peptide that stimulates secretion of the corticotropin and beta-endorphin. *Science*, **213**, 1394–1399.

van Bardeleben, U. and Holsboer, F. (1989). Cortisol response to a combined dexamethasone-human corticotropin-releasing hormone challenge in patients with depression. *Journal of Neuroendocrinology*, **1**, 489–488.

van Deventer, S.J.H., Buller, H.R, Carte, J.W, Aarden, L.A, Hack, C.E, Sturk, A. (1990). Experimental endotoxemia in humans: analysis of cytokine release and coagulation, fibrinolytic, and complement pathways. *Blood*, **76**, 2520–2526.

van Rossum, E.F., Binder, E.B., Majer, M. et al. (2006). Polymorphisms of the glucocorticoid receptor gene and major depression. *Biological Psychiatry*, **59**, 681–688.

Weber K.S., Miller, M.J., and Allen, P.M. (2008). Th17 cells exhibit a distinct calcium profile from Th1 and Th2 cells and have Th1-like motility and NF-AT nuclear localization. *Journal of Immunology*, **180**, 1442–1450.

Chapter 17

Neuropsychiatric effects of IFN-alpha: relevance to depression

Andrew H. Miller, Thaddeus W.W. Pace, and Charles L. Raison

Introduction

The notion that inflammation may represent a common mechanism of disease has gained widespread attention in a number of medical disorders including cardiovascular disease, diabetes, and cancer. In epidemiological studies, inflammatory biomarkers have been shown to predict the development or worsening of these disorders, and basic science investigations have revealed a multitude of clues regarding the relevant inflammatory mechanisms that may be involved (Aggarwal et al. 2006; Bisoendial et al. 2007; Bouzakri and Zierath, 2007; Pradhan and Ridker, 2002; Ridker, 2003). That inflammation and activation of the innate immune response may contribute to neuropsychiatric disorders is also receiving increasing interest. Studies in laboratory animals have revealed that administration of innate immune cytokines can lead to profound changes in behaviour, and the impact of cytokines on neuroendocrine and monoamine pathways as well as synaptic plasticity have been well described (Dantzer et al. 2008; Raison et al. 2006). Much attention has also been paid to how cytokine signals elaborated peripherally can access the brain including elucidation of cytokine passage through leaky regions in the blood–brain barrier, active transport via saturable transport molecules, activation of endothelial cells, and other cells lining the cerebral vasculature, and binding to cytokine receptors associated with peripheral afferent nerve fibres which then relay cytokine signals to key brain regions including the nucleus of the solitary tract and hypothalamus (Dantzer et al. 2008; Ericsson et al. 1994; Quan and Banks, 2007). Although much information has been gained through the investigation of laboratory animals, human studies in patients with neuropsychiatric disorders including major depression as well as patients undergoing treatment with the innate immune cytokine, interferon (IFN)-alpha have provided a complementary translational component to the investigation of the role of cytokines in the regulation of behaviour. This is the last of four chapters in this book that specifically discuss the role of inflammation in affective disorders, together with Chapters 10, 11, and 16.

Inflammation in depression

A large body of data has been amassed suggesting that activation of innate immune responses may play a role in the development of depression (Maes, 1995). Indeed, increased inflammatory markers including elevations in plasma and cerebrospinal fluid (CSF) cytokines and their soluble receptors as well as increases in acute phase reactants, chemokines, and adhesion molecules have been described in both medically ill and medically healthy depressed patients (Maes, 1995; Raison et al. 2006). Not only have mean differences in biomarkers of inflammation been reported in depressed versus non-depressed subjects, but also, significant correlations have been found between measures of inflammation and severity of depressive symptoms (Raison et al. 2006). In addition, associations between increased inflammatory makers and specific depressive symptoms such as fatigue and cognitive dysfunction have been described, especially in populations of medically ill patients, including patients with cancer and cancer survivors (Bower et al. 2002; Meyers et al. 2005). Increases in the cytokine, interleukin (IL)-6 and the acute phase protein, c-reactive protein (CRP – a downstream product of IL-6's action on the liver), are some of the most reliable indicators of inflammation in the context of depression (Mossner et al. 2007; Zorrilla et al. 2001), and in the case of IL-6, increases in plasma concentrations in depressed subjects have been found across the diurnal cycle (Alesci et al. 2005). In some, but not all, studies, innate immune cytokines also have been associated with antidepressant treatment responsiveness, with decreases in cytokines during treatment being associated with a positive response to therapy, and elevations in cytokines at baseline being associated with treatment resistance (Lanquillon et al. 2000; Raison et al. 2006).

Given the well-known association between psychosocial stress and the development of depression, data indicating that acute and chronic stress as well as early life stress is associated with increased innate immune cytokines and their signalling pathways have provided further support for a role of the immune system in depression. Indeed, healthy volunteers exposed to a public speaking and mental arithmetic task exhibited significant increases in DNA binding of nuclear factor kappa B (NF-kB), a lynchpin molecule in the initiation of the inflammatory response (Bierhaus et al. 2003). Acute stress-induced increases in NF-kB as well as IL-6 have been found to be exaggerated in depressed patients (Pace et al. 2006). Moreover, in patients with early life stress and depression, significant elevations in CRP have been found in comparison to depressed patients without early life stress as well as controls (Danese et al. 2008). Chronic caregiving stress has also been associated with increased activation of NF-kB responsive genes in peripheral blood mononuclear cells, a finding that was related to a decrease in genes with response elements for the glucocorticoid receptor (GR), indicating increased inflammatory and decreased anti-inflammatory (glucocorticoid) signalling as a function of chronic stress (Miller et al. 2008).

Studies in humans have indicated that by antagonizing cytokines there is improvement in measures of mood in patients with inflammatory disorders. For example, in a double-blind, placebo-controlled trial of the tumour necrosis factor antagonist, etanercept, in patients with psoriasis, participants who received etanercept exhibited significant improvement in depressive symptoms compared to placebo-treated subjects, an effect that was independent of improvement in disease activity (Tyring et al. 2006). These findings are consistent with recent studies in laboratory animals indicating that 'knocking out' the TNF-alpha receptor gene is associated with an antidepressant phenotype as well as reduced anxiety behaviour following viral infection (Simen et al. 2006; Silverman et al. 2007).

IFN-alpha as a translational vehicle

Given the rich database associating inflammation with behavioural changes such as depression, there has been considerable interest in examining the potential mechanisms involved. One approach to explore the pathways that may contribute to cytokine-induced depression in humans has been to study patients undergoing treatment with the innate immune cytokine, IFN-alpha (Capuron and Miller, 2004). IFN-alpha has both antiviral and antiproliferative activities, and is therefore used to treat infectious diseases such as hepatitis C virus (HCV) infection and cancer, including renal cell carcinoma and malignant melanoma (Dorr, 1993). Although an effective therapy for these conditions, IFN-alpha is notorious for causing significant depressive symptoms in 30–50% of subjects, depending on the dose (Capuron and Miller, 2004). Typical IFN-alpha-induced depressive symptoms include depressed mood, anhedonia, anxiety, irritability, fatigue, psycho-motor slowing, cognitive dysfunction, and sleep impairment (Capuron et al. 2002a). Of note, one of the strongest predictors of the development of depression during IFN-alpha treatment is the presence of depressive symptoms at baseline (Raison et al. 2005). Indeed, although a past history of depression is a significant predictor of depression during IFN-alpha therapy, the predictive power of past depression history is eliminated when baseline depressive symptoms are controlled for in the statistical analyses, indicating that a past history of depression may have its effect largely through increasing the odds that the subject will have significant depressive symptoms at baseline (Raison et al. 2005). Finally, it should be noted that administration of IFN-alpha to non-human primates (rhesus monkeys) has also been associated with anxiety and depressive-like behaviour (Felger et al. 2007).

Data examining the cytokine mechanisms involved in IFN-alpha-induced depression have revealed that baseline peripheral blood concentrations of the receptors for TNF-alpha and IL-6 are associated with increased depressive symptoms during IFN-alpha treatment (Friebe et al. 2007). Once IFN-alpha therapy has commenced, plasma IFN-alpha concentrations significantly correlate with measures of depression and fatigue as do plasma concentrations of TNF-alpha and its soluble receptor (Raison et al. 2008). Increases in IL-10 have also been associated with depressive symptoms during IFN-alpha treatment for cancer (Capuron et al. 2001b). In rhesus monkeys, increases in CSF cytokines, including IFN-alpha and IL-1, have been observed, indicating that IFN-alpha accesses the brain and/or stimulates cells of the blood–brain barrier to produce IFN-alpha within the brain (Felger et al. 2007). CNS IFN-alpha appears to, in turn, induce a central inflammatory response.

Effects of IFN-alpha on neuroendocrine function

Alterations in the functioning of the hypothalamic-pituitary-adrenal (HPA) axis in patients with major depression, including abnormal secretion of the glucocorticoid cortisol and decreased sensitivity to glucocorticoid-mediated feedback inhibition as reflected in the dexamethasone (DEX) suppression test (DST) and the DEX-corticotropin-releasing hormone (DEX-CRH) test, are some of the most reproducible findings in biological psychiatry (Pariante and Miller, 2001). Accordingly, the impact of IFN-alpha on the HPA axis and its relationship to depression has been the subject of investigation. Early studies indicated that the HPA axis response to the first injection of IFN-alpha was significantly higher in patients who went on to develop major depression during IFN-alpha therapy compared to individuals who did not develop depression during IFN-alpha treatment (Capuron et al. 2003b). Increases in both ACTH and cortisol following the first IFN-alpha injection were further correlated with symptoms of depression and anxiety after eight weeks of IFN-alpha administration (Capuron et al. 2003b). These data suggested that exaggerated HPA axis responses, possibly as a function of sensitized pathways involving CRH, a primary neuroregulatory peptide of the HPA axis, may represent a risk factor for the development of cytokine (IFN-alpha)-induced behavioural disturbances. Of relevance in this regard is that individuals exposed to early life stress have been found to exhibit sensitized CRH pathways and therefore may be at increased risk for the development of depression following exposure to inflammatory stimuli (Heim et al. 2000).

Interestingly, unlike studies examining acute exposure to IFN-alpha, studies examining patients after prolonged exposure to IFN-alpha have not revealed chronic elevations in ACTH or cortisol (Capuron et al. 2003b; Wichers et al. 2007). Nevertheless, in a recent study examining diurnal HPA-axis activity before and after IFN-alpha administration for 12 weeks in patients with HCV, significant IFN-alpha-induced flattening of the diurnal ACTH and cortisol curve was found as

Visit 1

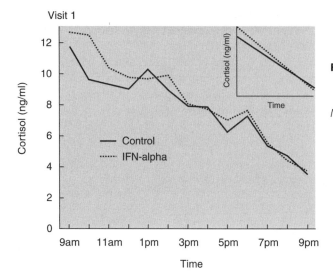

Visit 2

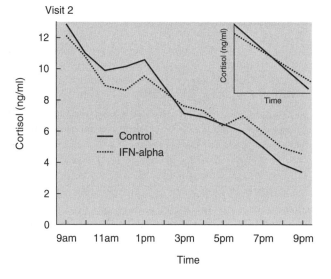

Fig. 17.1 Diurnal cortisol secretion during treatment with IFN–alpha.

Note: Patients who received interferon (IFN)–alpha treatment for 12 weeks exhibited significant flattening of the cortisol curve compared to non–IFN–alpha treated controls. Mean raw cortisol values from 9 a.m. to 9 p.m. in controls (blue line) versus subjects treated with interferon (IFN) alpha plus ribavirin (red line) at Visit 1 and Visit 2. Cortisol slopes from 9 a.m. to 9 p.m. in controls (blue line) versus subjects treated with interferon (IFN) alpha plus ribavirin (red line) at Visit 1 and Visit 2 are also depicted in inserts in each graph. Compared to control subjects, IFN–alpha/ ribavirin–treated patients exhibited a significantly flatter cortisol slope (p<0.05) and significantly higher evening cortisol values (p<0.05). (Reprinted with permission from Raison et al. 2008; Copyright 2008 Nature Publishing Group).

was a significant increase in evening plasma ACTH and cortisol concentrations (Raison et al. 2008) (Fig. 17.1). Flattening of the cortisol curve and increases in evening plasma cortisol concentrations were in turn correlated with the development of both depression and fatigue during IFN-alpha therapy (Raison et al. 2008). Flattening of the diurnal cortisol curve and increases in evening cortisol concentrations may represent decreased glucocorticoid sensitivity to feedback inhibition. Indeed, studies in cancer patients have revealed an association between fattening of the cortisol curve and non-suppression of cortisol on the DEX-CRH test (Spiegel et al. 2006).

Decreased sensitivity to feedback inhibition in the DST and DEX-CRH test is believed to be related in part to alterations in the receptors for glucocorticoids (Pariante and Miller, 2001). Relevant to the effects of IFN-alpha on the HPA axis, IFN-alpha has been shown to decrease GR expression in several cell lines (Cai et al. 2005) and decrease GR-mediated gene transcription and GR-DNA binding in hippocampal HT22 cells (Hu et al. unpublished observations). Moreover, IFN-alpha is known to activate both Janus kinases-signal transducers and activators of transcription (Jak-STAT) and p38 mitogen activated protein kinase (MAPK) pathways, both of which have been shown to disrupt GR signalling (Pace et al. 2007). Taken together, IFN-alpha inhibition of GR function may contribute to IFN-alpha effects on the HPA axis and behaviour.

Effects of IFN-alpha on monoamine metabolism

Given the role of monoamine systems in affect regulation and the impact of cytokines on monoamine metabolism in laboratory animals (Dantzer et al. 2008; Dunn et al. 1999), there has been considerable interest in the effects of IFN-alpha on monoamine neurotransmission in humans and non-human primates.

Serotonin

Probably the first evidence that serotonin may be involved in the effects of IFN-alpha on behaviour derived from studies showing that treatment with serotonin re-uptake inhibitors (SRI) could significantly reduce the development of depressive symptoms during IFN-alpha therapy and could improve depressive symptoms once they occurred (Hauser et al. 2000; 2002; Musselman et al. 2001). One study, based on a protocol developed in rodents (Yirmiya, 1996), demonstrated that pre-treatment of cancer patients with the SRI paroxetine was able to reduce IFN-alpha-induced depression by over fourfold, while also significantly reducing the number of subjects who discontinued IFN-alpha therapy (Musselman et al. 2001). A similar result was found in patients with HCV. However, the effect of paroxetine was only apparent in individuals whose depression scores at baseline were above the median of the study sample (Raison et al. 2007). These results indicate that identification of relevant risk factors may be especially important in identifying which individuals are likely to develop behavioural disturbances during cytokine exposure (e.g. during major surgery, chemotherapy, radiation, or cytokine treatment), and which patients are most likely to benefit from early treatment interventions. Relevant to serotonin in this regard, are recent data indicating that polymorphisms in the serotonin transporter gene, in conjunction with polymorphisms in the IL-6 gene, were found to be predictive of IFN-alpha-induced depression during treatment for HCV (Bull et al. 2008). Such identification of the genetic factors of risk will allow a personalized approach to managing and treating behavioural co-morbidities including depression in individuals with a variety of medical disorders associated with inflammation and increases in innate immune cytokines.

In addition to responses to SRI therapies, the effect of IFN-alpha on serotonin metabolism has also received considerable attention. IFN-alpha (as well as other cytokines) are capable of activating the enzyme indoleamine 2,3 dioxygenase (IDO), that metabolizes tryptophan (TRP) into kynurenine (KYN) which can then be broken down into kynurenic acid (KYNA) and quinolinic acid (QUIN) (Capuron and Miller, 2004; Dantzer et al. 2008). Given that TRP is the primary amino acid precursor for serotonin, increased IDO activity would serve to reduce the availability of serotonin. Data from IFN-alpha-treated patients have shown a correlation between IFN-alpha-induced decreases in TRP and increased depressive symptoms (Capuron et al. 2002b). Moreover, patients who developed depression on IFN-alpha therapy exhibited prolonged and accentuated decreases in TRP, in conjunction with increased plasma concentrations of KYN, indicating that activation of IDO pathways may be involved (Capuron et al. 2003a). Of note, inhibition of IDO activity has been shown to block the development of depressive-like behaviour in rodents following administration of the inflammatory stimuli, lipopolysaccharide (O'Connor et al. 2008). Although much emphasis has been given to the contribution of decreased

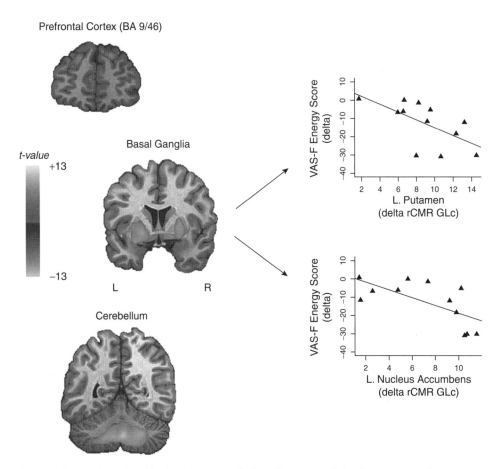

Fig. 17.2 Changes in regional brain glucose metabolism during IFN–alpha therapy. See colour plate section for colour version.

Note: Whole brain metabolic activity was assessed using positron emission tomography before and four weeks after IFN–alpha administration in 12 patients with malignant melanoma devoid of metastatic disease or pre–existing behavioural alterations. Whole brain glucose metabolism was estimated by fluorine–18–labeled–fluorodeoxyglucose uptake while subjects were at rest. Statistical threshold was set up at an experiment–wise alpha$<$0.05, with $p_{single-voxel} =0.0001$ and cluster size = 78 voxels. Images are displayed as coronal brain sections with blue regions repre-senting decreases in metabolic activity and yellow representing increases. L (left) and R (right) orientation of the images are indicated as are relevant Broadman areas (BA) in the prefrontal cortex. Correlations between changes (delta) in regional cerebral glucose metabolism (rCMRGLc) in the left putamen and left nucleus accumbens (relative to baseline) and changes (delta) in 'energy' subscale scores as measured by the Visual Analogue Scale of Fatigue (VAS–F) during IFN-alpha therapy ($R = -0.622$, $p = 0.03$ and $R = -0.669$, $p = 0.02$, respectively) are also depicted. Increased metabolic activity in these basal ganglia nuclei were associated with decreases in 'energy' subscale scores during IFN-alpha therapy. (Reprinted with permission from Capuron et al. 2007; Copyright 2007 Nature Publishing Group).

TRP to IFN-alpha-induced mood disturbances, there has been recent emphasis on the potential effects of more downstream products of the IDO pathway, including QUIN which is a NMDA agonist that has been associated with neuroendangerment through excitotoxicity in CNS inflammatory states (Muller and Schwarz, 2007; Wichers et al. 2005).

In addition to IDO pathways, activation of p38 MAPK by IFN-alpha and other cytokines may also influence the synaptic availability of serotonin. Indeed, stimulation of p38 MAPK has been shown to upregulate the expression and activity of the serotonin transporter (Zhu et al. 2005; 2006). Thus, IFN-alpha effects on both the synthesis and reuptake of serotonin may represent a 'double-hit' on synaptic serotonin availability during cytokine exposure.

Dopamine

IFN-alpha treatment leads to many behavioural features that are reflective of a hypodomaninergic state including anhedonia, fatigue, and psychomotor slowing (Capuron and Miller, 2004). Indeed, IFN-alpha-induced psychomotor slowing after five days has been shown to predict the development of depression after one month of IFN-alpha therapy (Capuron et al. 2001a). In addition, after 12 weeks of IFN-alpha treatment, psychomotor slowing is significantly correlated with both depression and fatigue (Majer et al. 2008). Consistent with the notion that dopamine (DA) pathways may be involved in these effects, stimulants, including the DA reuptake blocker, methylphenidate, has been shown to reduce IFN-alpha-associated fatigue in cancer patients (Meyers et al. 1998). Moreover, administration of the dopamine precursor, levodopa, has been shown to reverse IFN-alpha-induced akathisia, a syndrome of motor restlessness associated with DA blockade during the administration of antipsychotic medications (Sunami et al. 2000).

Imaging studies have also indicated that alterations in DA may be involved in the behavioural effects of IFN-alpha. IFN-alpha-treated patients have been shown in two studies to exhibit increased resting glucose metabolism in the basal ganglia, a brain region rich in DAergic neurons (Capuron et al. 2007; Juengling et al. 2000) (Fig. 17.2). Exaggerated metabolic activity in the basal ganglia has in turn been associated with IFN-alpha-induced symptoms of fatigue (Capuron et al. 2007). Increased basal ganglia metabolic activity has also been found in Parkinson's Disease (Eidelberg et al. 1994; Mentis et al. 2002; Spetsieris et al. 1995), a disease of DA depletion in which increased basal ganglia metabolic activity is believed to represent increased oscillatory burst activity secondary to disinhibition of DAergic inhibitory neurocircuits (Wichmann and DeLong, 1999). Relevant to the role of diminished DA availability in basal ganglia hyperactivity, levodopa infusion has been shown to reduce increased glucose metabolism in the basal ganglia in PD patients (Feigin et al. 2001).

Further consistent with the notion that DA is decreased in relevant brain regions following IFN-alpha administration, are decreases in the DA metabolite, homovanillic acid (HVA), that have been found in monkeys which exhibit depressive-like behaviour during IFN-alpha treatment (Felger et al. 2007). Specifically, monkeys who exhibited huddling behaviour had significantly lower CSF HVA in the IFN-alpha treatment condition versus the saline treatment condition than did animals that did not huddle (Felger et al. 2007). Interestingly, huddling behaviour, which is believed to be a depressive equivalent, was initially described by McKinney and colleagues in the Harlow Laboratories in rhesus monkeys who were chronically administered the monoamine depleting drug, reserpine (McKinney et al. 1971).

There are many pathways by which IFN-alpha and other cytokines may lead to reduced DA in the basal ganglia and other brain regions. First, IFN-alpha has been shown to influence the synthesis of DA through indirect effects on tyrosine hydroxylase (TH), the rate-limiting enzyme in DA synthesis. IFN-alpha has been found to decrease CNS concentrations of tetrahydrobiopterin (BH_4), an important enzyme co-factor for TH (Kitagami et al. 2003). IFN-alpha effects on BH_4 appear to be mediated by stimulation of nitric oxide (NO) (Kitagami et al. 2003). Of note, activation of an inflammatory response within the brain has been associated with increased NO production, suggesting that cytokine influences on BH_4 via NO may be a common mechanism for innate immune cytokines and inflammation to reduce DA availability in the basal ganglia. Another potential pathway which may lead to decreased synaptic availability of DA involves IFN-alpha activation of IDO and the downstream IDO metabolite KYNA. As noted previously, IFN-alpha treatment has been associated with increased plasma concentrations of KYN (Capuron et al. 2003a), which can be metabolized to KYNA in the brain by astrocytes. Of relevance to DA, intrastriatal administration of KYNA has been shown to reduce extracellular DA in the rat striatum, an effect mediated by inhibition of alpha7 nicotinic acetylcholine receptors (alpha7nAChR) on glutamatergic afferents, which ultimately serve to inhibit alpha7nAChR-stimulated striatal glutamate release (Wu et al. 2007). Glutamate in turn regulates tonic, impulse-independent, DAT-mediated DA release (Borland and Michael, 2004; Grace, 1991). Treatment with the alpha7nAChR agonist, galantamine, has been shown to reverse the effects of KYNA on extracellular DA levels in the striatum (Wu et al. 2007).

Another pathway by which the innate immune response may influence DA metabolism is through the activation of MAPK. As discussed above, MAPK pathways may play a role in the regulation of the expression of monoamine transporters, and in addition to effects on the serotonin transporter, activation of MAPK pathways, specifically ERK 1/2 have been found to increase the Vmax of the human DA transporter (hDAT), while increasing hDAT surface expression (Moron et al. 2003). Moreover, inhibition of MAPK signalling was found to decrease DA uptake in a dose- and time-dependent fashion in rat striatal synaptosome preparations and a human embryonic kidney (HEK) cell line (Moron et al. 2003).

Although decreased DA synthesis and/or increased DA re-uptake are plausible mechanisms for decreased DA neurotransmission, IFN-alpha may also paradoxically lead to decreased DAergic activity through chronic activation of DAergic neurons followed by downregulation of relevant postsynaptic DA receptors. For example, studies have shown that IFN-alpha binds to mu opioid receptors (Wang et al. 2006), which are expressed on basal ganglia DAergic neurons and can cause DA release (Di Chiara and Imperato, 1988; Ho et al. 1992).

IFN-alpha, anxiety, and alarm

Although much attention has been paid to the development of depressive symptoms following IFN-alpha administration, it should be noted that a significant percentage of IFN-alpha-treated individuals develop marked symptoms of anxiety, irritability, and hyperactivity. Indeed, clinical reports of IFN-alpha-treated patients have suggested that up to 50% of patients who develop clinically significant psychiatric symptoms during IFN-alpha therapy exhibit hypomanic, manic, or mixed states (Constant et al. 2005). These data are consistent with findings in IFN-alpha-treated rhesus monkeys where dominant animals tended to show increased locomotor activity while receiving IFN-alpha, in contrast to subordinate animals, who exhibited decreased activity (Felger et al. 2007).

In addition to increased anxiety, irritability, and locomotor activity, neuroimaging data suggests that IFN-alpha may also activate neural alarm systems. Using functional magnetic resonance imaging (fMRI) and a task of visuo-spatial attention, HCV patients receiving IFN-alpha were found to exhibit increased activation in the dorsal anterior cingulate cortex (dACC) [Broadman's Area (BA) 24], compared to non-IFN-alpha-treated HCV controls (Capuron et al. 2005) (Fig. 17.3). The dACC has been shown to play an important role in error detection, conflict monitoring and arousal

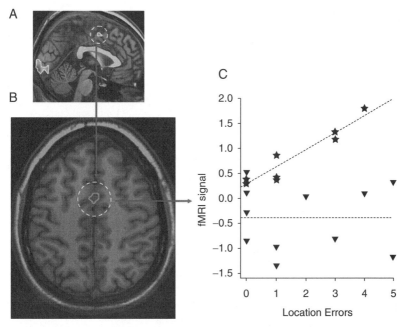

Fig. 17.3 Increased activation in the dACC of IFN-alpha-treated subjects. Reprinted by permission of Elsevier from Anterior cingulate activation and error processing during interferon-alpha treatment by Capuron, L et al. *Biological Psychiatry*, 58, 190-6 2005. See colour plate section for colour version.

Note: (A) Activation of the anterior cingulate cortex (ACC) in patients treated with interferon-alpha (IFN) (contrast 'location – detection'); (B) Activation of the ACC in patients treated with IFN-alpha compared to controls (CTRL) (contrast 'location – detection: IFN > CTRL'); (C) Relationship between ACC activation and the rate of errors within the location blocks in patients treated with IFN-alpha (red stars) (R = 0.954, p < 0.0001) and in controls (black triangles) (R = −0.018, p = 0.96). (Reprinted with permission from Capuron et al. 2005; Copyright 2005 Elsevier).

(Carter et al. 1998). Consistent with the finding of increased dACC activation in IFN-alpha-treated subjects, a much higher correlation was found between task-related error rates and dACC activation in patients treated with IFN-alpha versus control subjects (who showed no correlation between these variables) (Fig. 17.3). Increased activation of the dACC has been found in individuals with high-trait anxiety (especially at low error rates) as well as subjects with neuroticism and obsessive compulsive disorder, both of which are associated with increases in anxiety and arousal (Eisenberger et al. 2005; Paulus et al. 2004; Ursu et al. 2003). Activation of the dACC has also been seen in the context of social rejection, where it is correlated with emotional distress, consistent with the role of this brain region in the processing of social pain (Eisenberger and Lieberman, 2004). Combined with its role in error detection and conflict monitoring, the dACC's processing of social pain has been suggested to comprise a neural 'alarm system', which can both detect and respond to threatening environmental stimuli in the social domain (Eisenberger and Lieberman, 2004). On the basis of the neuroimaging data, it appears that IFN-alpha effects on neural circuits involving the dACC may in part mediate the potential impact of cytokines on arousal, anxiety, and alarm.

The combination of depressed mood, anhedonia, fatigue, and psychomotor slowing with the symptoms of anxiety and arousal, although ostensibly contradictory at first glance, may serve competing survival priorities which on the one hand satisfy organismic needs to conserve energy resources for fighting infection and healing wounds while at the same time maintaining vigilance against future attack.

Translational implications

Data from IFN-alpha studies on the impact of innate immune cytokines on the brain and behaviour and the mechanisms involved, reveal a number of potential therapeutic targets that may be relevant for both treating and preventing cytokine-induced behavioural alterations. Targeting cytokines themselves appears most logical, given direct relationships between IFN-alpha-induced TNF and the development of depressive symptoms. Regarding the neuroendocrine system, the effects of cytokines and their signalling pathways including MAPK and Jak-STAT on the GR is another point of potential intervention, especially with therapies that either block cytokine signalling pathways and/or increase GR function (which in turn can serve to feedback negatively on further cytokine release). Blockade of MAPK pathways also appears to be relevant to the effects of innate immune cytokines on both serotonin and DA pathways as would blockade of IDO, which would also inhibit the generation of potentially toxic downstream metabolites of KYN including KYNA and QUIN. Finally, given the role of psychosocial stress in the activation of innate immune responses as well as the contribution of baseline depressive symptoms and inflammatory markers to the development of depression following cytokine (IFN-alpha) exposure, psychotherapeutic strategies and/or complementary or alternative medicine approaches such as meditation which serve to reduce stress and/or inflammation may represent a viable preventative strategy, especially in individuals who have already been determined to be genetically vulnerable to cytokine-induced behavioural changes. Such preventative strategies might be most relevant for individuals participating in medical therapies with a high risk for innate immune system activation including major surgery, chemotherapy, radiation, or immune therapies with cytokines such as IFN-alpha.

Acknowledgements

This work was funded in part by grants from the National Institutes of Health (MH069124, MH069056, MH064619, MH070553, HL073921, MH58922, MH067990, and MH075102), a NIH/NCRR General Clinical Research Center grant (M01 RR00039), and support from the Centers of Disease Control and Prevention.

References

Aggarwal, B.B., Shishodia, S., Sandur, S.K., Pandey, M.K., and Sethi, G. (2006). Inflammation and cancer: how hot is the link? *Biochem Pharmacol*, **72**, 1605–1621.

Alesci, S., Martinez, P.E., Kelkar, S. et al. (2005). Major depression is associated with significant diurnal elevations in plasma interleukin-6 levels, a shift of its circadian rhythm, and loss of physiological complexity in its secretion: clinical implications. *J Clin Endocrinol Metabolism*, **90**, 2522–2530.

Bierhaus, A., Wolf, J., Andrassy, M. et al. (2003). A mechanism converting psychosocial stress into mononuclear cell activation. *Proc Natl Acad Sci. USA*, **100**, 1920–1925.

Bisoendial, R.J., Kastelein, J.J., and Stroes, E.S. (2007). C-reactive protein and atherogenesis: from fatty streak to clinical event. *Atherosclerosis*, **195**, e10–18.

Borland, L.M. and Michael, A.C. (2004). Voltammetric study of the control of striatal dopamine release by glutamate. *J Neurochem.*, **91**, 220–229.

Bouzakri, K. and Zierath, J.R. (2007). MAP4K4 gene silencing in human skeletal muscle prevents tumor necrosis factor-alpha-induced insulin resistance. J Biol Chem., **282**, 7783–7789.

Bower, J.E., Ganz, P.A., Aziz, N., and Fahey, J.L. (2002). Fatigue and proinflammatory cytokine activity in breast cancer survivors. *Psychosom Med.*, **64**, 604–611.

Bull, S.J., Huezo-Diaz, P., Binder, E.B. et al. (2008). Functional polymorphisms in the interleukin-6 and serotonin transporter genes, and depression and fatigue induced by interferon-alpha and ribavirin treatment. *Mol Psychiatry*, In press.

Cai, W., Khaoustov, V.I., Xie, Q., Pan, T., Le, W., and Yoffe, B. (2005). Interferon-alpha-induced modulation of glucocorticoid and serotonin receptors as a mechanism of depression. *J Hepatol.*, **42**, 880–887.

Capuron, L., Ravaud, A., and Dantzer, R. (2001a). Timing and specificity of the cognitive changes induced by interleukin-2 and interferon-alpha treatments in cancer patients. *Psychosom Med.*, **63**, 376–386.

Capuron, L., Ravaud, A., Gualde, N. et al. (2001b). Association between immune activation and early depressive symptoms in cancer patients treated with interleukin-2-based therapy. *Psychoneuroendocrinology*, **26**, 797–808.

Capuron, L., Gumnick, J.F., Musselman, D.L. et al. (2002a). Neurobehavioral effects of interferon-alpha in cancer patients: phenomenology and paroxetine responsiveness of symptom dimensions. *Neuropsychopharmacology*, **26**, 643–652.

Capuron, L., Ravaud, A., Neveu, P. J., Miller, A. H., Maes, M., and Dantzer, R. (2002b). Association between decreased serum tryptophan concentrations and depressive symptoms in cancer patients undergoing cytokine therapy. *Mol Psychiatry*, **7**, 468–473.

Capuron, L., Neurauter, G., Musselman, D.L. et al. (2003a). Interferon-alpha-induced changes in tryptophan metabolism: relationship to depression and paroxetine treatment. *Biol Psychiatry*, **54**, 906–914.

Capuron, L., Raison, C.L., Musselman, D.L., Lawson, D.H., Nemeroff, C.B., and Miller, A. H. (2003b). Association of exaggerated HPA axis response to the initial injection of interferon-alpha with development of depression during interferon-alpha therapy. *Am J Psychiatry*, **160**, 1342–1345.

Capuron, L. and Miller, A. H. (2004). Cytokines and psychopathology: lessons from interferon-alpha. *Biol Psychiatry*, **56**, 819–824.

Capuron, L., Pagnoni, G., Demetrashvili, M. et al. (2005). Anterior cingulate activation and error processing during interferon-alpha treatment. *Biol Psychiatry*, **58**, 190–196.

Capuron, L., Pagnoni, G., Demetrashvili, M.F. et al. (2007). Basal ganglia hypermetabolism and symptoms of fatigue during interferon-alpha therapy. *Neuropsychopharmacology*, **32**, 2384–92.

Carter, C.S., Braver, T.S., Barch, D.M., Botvinick, M.M., Noll, D., and Cohen, J.D. (1998). Anterior cingulate cortex, error detection, and the online monitoring of performance. *Science*, **280**, 747–749.

Constant, A., Castera, L., Dantzer, R. et al. (2005). Mood alterations during interferon-alfa therapy in patients with chronic hepatitis C: evidence for an overlap between manic/hypomanic and depressive symptoms. *J Clin Psychiatry*, **66**, 1050–1057.

Danese, A., Moffitt, T.E., Pariante, C.M., Ambler, A., Poulton, R., and Caspi, A. (2008). Elevated inflammation levels in depressed adults with a history of childhood maltreatment. *Arch Gen Psychiatry.*, **65**, 409–415.

Dantzer, R., O'Connor, J.C., Freund, G.G., Johnson, R.W., and Kelley, K.W. (2008). From inflammation to sickness and depression: when the immune system subjugates the brain. *Nat Rev Neurosci.*, **9**, 46–56.

Di Chiara, G. and Imperato, A. (1988). Opposite effects of mu and kappa opiate agonists on dopamine release in the nucleus accumbens and in the dorsal caudate of freely moving rats. *J Pharmacol Exp Ther.*, **244**, 1067–1080.

Dorr, R. T. (1993) Interferon-alpha in malignant and viral diseases: a review. Drugs, **45**, 177–211.

Dunn, A. J., Wang, J., and Ando, T. (1999). Effects of cytokines on cerebral neurotransmission. Comparison with the effects of stress. *Adv Exp Med Bio.*, **461**, 117–127.

Eidelberg, D., Moeller, J.R., Dhawan, V. et al. (1994). The metabolic topography of parkinsonism. *J Cereb Blood Flow Metab.*, **14**, 783–801.

Eisenberger, N.I. and Lieberman, M.D. (2004). Why rejection hurts: a common neural alarm system or physical and social pain. *Trends Cogn Sci.*, **8**, 294–300.

Eisenberger, N.I., Lieberman, M.D., and Satpute, A.B. (2005). Personality from a controlled processing perspective: an fMRI study of neuroticism, extraversion, and self-consciousness. *Cogn Affect Behav Neurosci.*, **5**, 169–181.

Ericsson, A., Kovacs, K.J., and Sawchenko, P.E. (1994). A functional anatomical analysis of central pathways subserving the effects of interleukin-1 on stress-related neuroendocrine neurons. *J Neurosci.*, **14**, 897–913.

Feigin, A., Fukuda, M., Dhawan, V. et al. (2001). Metabolic correlates of levodopa response in Parkinson's disease. *Neurology*, **57**, 2083–2088.

Felger, J.C., Alagbe, O., Hu, F. et al. (2007). Effects of interferon-alpha on rhesus monkeys: a nonhuman primate model of cytokine–induced depression. *Biol Psychiatry*, **62**, 1324–1333.

Friebe, A., Schwarz, M.J., Schmid-Wendtner, M. et al. (2007). Pretreatment levels of sTNF-R1 and sIL-6R are associated with a higher vulnerability for IFN-alpha-induced depressive symptoms in patients with malignant melanoma. *J Immunother.*, (1997), **30**, 333–337.

Grace, A. A. (1991). Phasic versus tonic dopamine release and the modulation of dopamine system responsivity: a hypothesis for the etiology of schizophrenia. *Neuroscience*, **41**, 1–24.

Hauser, P., Soler, R., Reed, S. et al. (2000). Prophylactic treatment of depression induced by interferon-alpha. *Psychosomatics*, **41**, 439–441.

Hauser, P., Khosla, J., Aurora, H. et al. (2002). A prospective study of the incidence and open-label treatment of interferon-induced major depressive disorder in patients with hepatitis C. *Mol Psychiatry*, **7**, 942–947.

Heim, C., Newport, D.J., Heit, S. et al. (2000). Pituitary-adrenal and autonomic responses to stress in women after sexual and physical abuse in childhood. *JAMA*, **284**, 592–597.

Ho, B.T., Huo, Y.Y., Lu, J.G., Tansey, L.W., and Levin, V.A. (1992). Opioid-dopaminergic mechanisms in the potentiation of d-amphetamine discrimination by interferon-alpha. *Pharmacol Biochem Behav.*, **42**, 57–60.

Juengling, F.D., Ebert, D., Gut, O. et al. (2000).Prefrontal cortical hypometabolism during low-dose interferon alpha treatment. *Psychopharmacology* (Berl), **152**, 383–389.

Kitagami, T., Yamada, K., Miura, H., Hashimoto, R., Nabeshima, T., and Ohta, T. (2003). Mechanism of systemically injected interferon-alpha impeding monoamine biosynthesis in rats: role of nitric oxide as a signal crossing the blood-brain barrier. *Brain Res.*, **978**, 104–114.

Lanquillon, S., Krieg, J.C., Bening-Abu-Shach, U., and Vedder, H. (2000). Cytokine production and treatment response in major depressive disorder. *Neuropsychopharmacology*, **22**, 370–379.

Maes, M. (1995). Evidence for an immune response in major depression: a review and hypothesis. *Prog Neuropsychopharmacol Biol Psychiatry*, **19**, 11–38.

Majer, M., Welberg, L.A., Capuron, L., Pagnoni, G., Raison, C.L., and Miller, A.H. (2008). IFN-alpha-induced motor slowing is associated with increased depression and fatigue in patients with chronic hepatitis C. *Brain Behav Immun.*, **22**, 870–880.

McKinney, W.T., Jr., Eising, R.G., Moran, E.C., Suomi, S.J., and Harlow, H.F. (1971). Effects of reserpine on the social behavior of rhesus monkeys. *Dis Nerv Syst.*, **32**, 735–741.

Mentis, M.J., McIntosh, A.R., Perrine, K. et al. (2002). Relationships among the metabolic patterns that correlate with mnemonic, visuospatial, and mood symptoms in Parkinson's disease. *Am J Psychiatry*, **159**, 746–754.

Meyers, C.A., Weitzner, M.A., Valentine, A.D., and Levin, V.A. (1998). Methylphenidate therapy improves cognition, mood, and function of brain tumor patients. *J Clin Oncol.*, **16**, 2522–2527.

Meyers, C.A., Albitar, M., and Estey, E. (2005). Cognitive impairment, fatigue, and cytokine levels in patients with acute myelogenous leukemia or myelodysplastic syndrome. *Cancer*, **104**, 788–793.

Miller, G.E., Chen, E., Sze, J. et al. (2008). A functional genomic fingerprint of chronic stress in humans: blunted glucocorticoid and increased NF-kappaB signaling. *Biol Psychiatry*.

Moron, J.A., Zakharova, I., Ferrer, J.V. et al. (2003). Mitogen-activated protein kinase regulates dopamine transporter surface expression and dopamine transport capacity. *J Neurosci.*, **23**, 8480–8488.

Mossner, R., Mikova, O., Koutsilieri, E. et al. (2007). Consensus paper of the WFSBP task force on biological markers: biological markers in depression. *World J Biol Psychiatry*, **8**, 141–174.

Muller, N. and Schwarz, M.J. (2007). The immune-mediated alteration of serotonin and glutamate: towards an integrated view of depression. *Mol Psychiatry.*, **12**, 988–1000.

Musselman, D.L., Lawson, D.H., Gumnick, J.F. et al. (2001). Paroxetine for the prevention of depression induced by high-dose interferon alfa. *N Eng J Med.*, **344**, 961–966.

O'Connor, J.C., Lawson, M.A., Andre, C. et al. (2008). Lipopolysaccharide-induced depressive-like behavior is mediated by indoleamine 2, 3-dioxygenase activation in mice. *Mol Psychiatry*.

Pace, T.W., Mletzko, T.C., Alagbe, O. et al. (2006). Increased stress-induced inflammatory responses in male patients with major depression and increased early life stress. *Am J Psychiatry*, **163**, 1630–1633.

Pace, T.W., Hu, F., and Miller, A.H. (2007). Cytokine-effects on glucocorticoid receptor function: relevance to glucocorticoid resistance and the pathophysiology and treatment of major depression. *Brain Behav Immun.*, **21**, 9–19.

Pariante, C.M. and Miller, A.H. (2001). Glucocorticoid receptors in major depression: relevance to pathophysiology and treatment. *Biol. Psychiatry*, **49**, 391–404.

Paulus, M.P., Feinstein, J.S., Simmons, A., and Stein, M.B. (2004). Anterior cingulate activation in high trait anxious subjects is related to altered error processing during decision making. *Biol Psychiatry*, **55**, 1179–1187.

Pradhan, A.D. and Ridker, P.M. (2002). Do atherosclerosis and type 2 diabetes share a common inflammatory basis? *Eur Heart J.*, **23**, 831–834.

Quan, N. and Banks, W.A. (2007). Brain-immune communication pathways. *Brain Behav Immun.*, **21**, 727–735.

Ridker, P.M. (2003). Clinical application of C-reactive protein for cardiovascular disease detection and prevention. *Circulation*, **107**, 363–369.

Raison, C.L., Borisov, A.S., Broadwell, S.D. et al. (2005). Depression during pegylated interferon-alpha plus ribavirin therapy: prevalence and prediction. *J Clin Psychiatry*, **66**, 41–48.

Raison, C.L., Capuron, L., and Miller, A.H. (2006). Cytokines sing the blues: inflammation and the pathogenesis of depression. *Trends Immunol.*, **27**, 24–31.

Raison, C.L., Woolwine, B.J., Demetrashvili, M.F. et al. (2007). Paroxetine for prevention of depressive symptoms induced by interferon-alpha and ribavirin for hepatitis C. *Aliment Pharmacol Ther.*, **25**, 1163–1174.

Raison, C.L., Borisov, A.S., Woolwine, B.J., Massung, B., Vogt, G., and Miller, A.H. (2008). Interferon-alpha effects on diurnal hypothalamic-pituitary-adrenal axis activity: relationship with proinflammatory cytokines and behavior. *Mol Psychiatry*, In press.

Silverman, M.N., Macdougall, M.G., Hu, F., Pace, T.W., Raison, C.L., and Miller, A.H. (2007). Endogenous glucocorticoids protect against TNF-alpha-induced increases in anxiety-like behavior in virally infected mice. *Mol Psychiatry*, **12**, 408–417.

Simen, B.B., Duman, C.H., Simen, A.A., and Duman, R.S. (2006). TNFalpha signaling in depression and anxiety: behavioral consequences of individual receptor targeting. *Biol Psychiatry.*, **59**, 775–785.

Spetsieris, P.G., Moeller, J.R., Dhawan, V., Ishikawa, T., and Eidelberg, D. (1995). Visualizing the evolution of abnormal metabolic networks in the brain using PET. *Comput Med Imaging Graph.*, **19**, 295–306.

Spiegel, D., Giese-Davis, J., Taylor, C.B., and Kraemer, H. (2006). Stress sensitivity in metastatic breast cancer: analysis of hypothalamic-pituitary-adrenal axis function. *Psychoneuroendocrinology*, **31**, 1231–1244.

Sunami, M., Nishikawa, T., Yorogi, A., and Shimoda, M. (2000). Intravenous administration of levodopa ameliorated a refractory akathisia case induced by interferon-alpha. *Clin Neuropharmacol.*, **23**, 59–61.

Tyring, S., Gottlieb, A., Papp, K. et al. (2006). Etanercept and clinical outcomes, fatigue, and depression in psoriasis: double-blind placebo-controlled randomised phase III trial. *Lancet*, **367**, 29–35.

Ursu, S., Stenger, V.A., Shear, M.K., Jones, M.R., and Carter, C.S. (2003). Overactive action monitoring in obsessive-compulsive disorder: evidence from functional magnetic resonance imaging. *Psycho Sci.*, **14**, 347–353.

Wang, J.Y., Zeng, X.Y., Fan, G.X., Yuan, Y.K., and Tang, J.S. (2006). mu- but not delta- and kappa-opioid receptor mediates the nucleus submedius interferon-alpha-evoked antinociception in the rat. *Neurosci Lett.*, **397**, 254–258.

Wichers, M.C., Koek, G.H., Robaeys, G., Verkerk, R., Scharpe, S., and Maes, M. (2005). IDO and interferon-alpha-induced depressive symptoms: a shift in hypothesis from tryptophan depletion to neurotoxicity. *Mol Psychiatry*, **10**, 538–544.

Wichers, M.C., Kenis, G., Koek, G.H., Robaeys, G., Nicolson, N.A., and Maes, M. (2007). Interferon-alpha-induced depressive symptoms are related to changes in the cytokine network but not to cortisol. *J Psychosom Res.*, **62**, 207–214.

Wichmann, T. and DeLong, M. R. (1999). Oscillations in the basal ganglia. *Nature*, **400**, 621–622.

Wu, H. Q., Rassoulpour, A., and Schwarcz, R. (2007). Kynurenic acid leads, dopamine follows: a new case of volume transmission in the brain? *J Neural Transm.*, **114**, 33–41.

Yirmiya, R. (1996). Endotoxin produces a depressive-like episode in rats. *Brain Res.*, **711**, 163–174.

Zhu, C.B., Blakely, R.D., and Hewlett, W.A. (2006). The proinflammatory cytokines interleukin–1beta and tumor necrosis factor-alpha activate serotonin transporters. *Neuropsychopharmacology*, **31**, 2121–2131.

Zhu, C.B., Carneiro, A.M., Dostmann, W.R., Hewlett, W.A., and Blakely, R.D. (2005). p38 MAPK activation elevates serotonin transport activity via a trafficking-independent, protein phosphatase 2A-dependent process. *J Biol Chem.*, **280**, 15649–15658.

Zorrilla, E.P., Luborsky, L., McKay, J.R. et al. (2001). The relationship of depression and stressors to immunological assays: a meta-analytic review. *Brain Behav Immun.*, **15**, 199–226.

Chapter 18

Depression and coronary heart disease

Andrew Steptoe

Investigation of the relationship between depression and coronary heart disease (CHD) is one of the most active fields of research at the intersection of psychiatry, physical medicine, and biological sciences, with important work being carried out using epidemiological, clinical, and experimental methods. Depression is relevant to many stages of CHD, including long-term aetiology, the acute triggering of cardiac events, prognosis following acute coronary syndromes (myocardial infarction and unstable angina), and rehabilitation. There are many possibilities for intervention and treatment, although the optimal management of depression in patients with CHD has yet to be established. Depression is also relevant to other cardiovascular disorders that are related to CHD, including heart failure (Rutledge et al. 2006) and stroke (Wouts et al. 2008).

Coronary heart disease is the product of the long-term accumulation of coronary atherosclerosis, a process that develops progressively over the life time. Risk factors such as smoking, high blood pressure, high blood cholesterol levels, adiposity, and family history contribute to aetiology, stimulating the endothelial dysfunction and inflammatory processes that result in macrophage infiltration into the intimal and medial layers of the coronary vessel wall, smooth muscle cell migration and proliferation, and the development of coronary plaque (Hansson, 2005). Acute coronary syndromes (ACS) such as myocardial infarction (MI) and unstable angina typically occur in people with advanced coronary atherosclerosis, and emerge through plaque disruption due to plaque rupture or erosion, coupled with inflammatory and haemostatic processes leading to thrombus formation (Steptoe and Brydon, 2007). Different mechanisms are relevant at various stages of this process, so the impact of depression may involve several mechanisms.

The literature relating depression and CHD has been thoroughly reviewed over recent years (Lett et al. 2006; Nicholson et al. 2006; Williams and Steptoe, 2007). This chapter will focus on recent developments in research and clinical management, concentrating on five topics: the role of depression in the aetiology of CHD, the involvement of depressed states in the triggering of acute cardiac events, depression and prognosis following ACS, the mechanisms relating depression with CHD, and the management of depression in patients with CHD. I will also address the issue of whether patients with CHD suffer from typical forms of depression, or whether their mood states are unusual, calling for innovative methods of management.

Depression in the aetiology of CHD

The strongest evidence to date for the contribution of depression to the aetiology of CHD comes from longitudinal observational cohort studies, in which depression is measured in large samples of healthy individuals who are then tracked over time for the development of disease. Multivariable statistical methods are used to establish whether depression predicts future CHD, and whether effects are independent of potential confounders such socio-economic status (SES) that are associated both with depression and CHD.

More than 30 studies of this type have been published over the past 30 years. A recent meta-analysis concluded that the relative risk of future CHD associated with depression was 1.90 (95% confidence intervals 1.48–2.42) after adjustment for conventional cardiovascular risk factors (Nicholson et al. 2006). The association is present both when depression is defined as a clinical syndrome, and as a continuous measure on a scale such as the Center for Epidemiologic Studies Depression scale (CES-D) or the Beck Depression Inventory (BDI). There is, however, wide variation in the quality of this literature, with few studies controlling adequately for all covariates, and not all questionnaire measures of depression perform equally well.

Another way of assessing the association is to analyse the rate of CHD in patients with clinical depression. A large-scale retrospective cohort study using the UK's General Practice Research Database showed that death rates from CHD were substantially increased in patients with severe mental illness, including depressive psychosis, after controlling for social deprivation, smoking and medication use (Osborn et al. 2007). We have recently analysed a nationally representative sample of men and women in Scotland, and found that over an average follow-up period of 8.5 years, the hazard ratio for death from cardiovascular disease was 1.82 (C.I. 1.19–2.78) for those who had a history of psychiatric episodes requiring hospitalization, after adjusting for age, gender, social and marital status, physical activity, smoking, and the presence of long-standing illness (Hamer et al. 2008).

An important issue is whether depression is associated with the progression of sub-clinical coronary artery disease, or only with clinical manifestations such as MI. Stewart et al. (2007) used carotid intima-media thickness as a surrogate marker of coronary atherosclerosis, and showed that individuals with higher scores on the BDI showed more rapid progression of atherosclerosis over three years after controlling for cardiovascular risk factors. Depression also predicts progression of coronary atherosclerosis following coronary artery bypass surgery, again independently of conventional risk factors (Wellenius et al. 2008).

These data indicate that depression appears to accelerate the disease process underlying CHD, and operates independently of smoking, high blood pressure, SES, and other risk factors. However, it should be emphasized that findings so far have been based on observational studies, and residual confounding is always a possibility. No intervention studies have been conducted to demonstrate that reducing depression in an otherwise healthy population will lead to a decrease in the incidence of CHD.

Depressed mood as a trigger of acute coronary syndromes

It used to be thought that acute MI occurred as the final stage of a process of blockage of the coronary vessels, when the walls of arteries became so thick that they completely blocked the lumen, preventing the passage of blood. It is now known that the key pathophysiological event in ACS is the disruption of coronary plaque and development of thrombus in the artery (Naghavi et al. 2003). Such acute events are unpredictable, and do not necessarily occur in people with the most advanced underlying disease. Acute events may occur spontaneously or be triggered by short-term physical and emotional stimuli (Steptoe and Brydon, 2009).

There is good evidence that episodes of anger and acute stress can act as triggers (Tofler and Muller, 2006). We have investigated the possible role of episodes of acute depression and sadness, using the case cross-methodology that has been developed to investigate acute triggers (Steptoe et al. 2006). We found that the odds of experiencing an ACS were significantly increased in people who reported moderate or severe depressed mood or sadness in the two hours before symptom onset. Triggering by depressed mood was not related to the extent of underlying disease, but was more common in lower SES patients, and in those who have experienced severe life stress in the previous four weeks. We have also found that patients who report triggering of ACS by acute depression or sadness show enhanced interleukin-6 (IL 6) responses to acute stress, suggesting a specific psychophysiological substrate for responses of this type (Steptoe and Brydon, 2009).

Depression and prognosis following acute coronary syndrome

Relatively high levels of depression are observed in people with CHD (Fan et al. 2008). Severe depression develops in 15–20% of patients within a few days of admission to hospital with an ACS, while a further 25% experience minor depression or dysphoria. A landmark study by Frasure-Smith and colleagues (1993) established that depression in ACS patients is not only a mental health concern but has fatal consequences by reducing survival. The association between depression following ACS and adverse cardiac prognosis has been confirmed numerous times, although not all studies have been positive (Lett et al. 2006; Nicholson et al. 2006). The pooled relative risk in a recent meta-analysis was 1.80 (C.I. 1.50–2.15). As in the work on primary aetiology, the association is not only with clinical depression, but also with elevated depressed mood within the normal range (Lespérance et al. 2002).

A major concern in this research is whether the association with depression is independent of the severity of the ACS and the underlying disease. It could be that people who are more ill become depressed, either because the medical staff give them a poor prognosis, or because the underlying disease stimulates inflammatory processes that in turn affect mood state. This issue has proved difficult to resolve, since detailed cardiac measures have not been available in all studies. Nicholson et al. (2006) showed that relative risk estimates were reduced to 1.53 (C.I. 1.11–2.10) in studies that took account of left ventricular function, a marker of cardiac health. However, other studies have shown that depression continues to predict death or recurrent MI even after left ventricular function, diabetes, and other factors are taken into account (Jaffe et al. 2006). A recent large study of patients with stable CHD showed that depression was not associated with very detailed cardiac function measures, suggesting that it was not related to underlying disease severity (Lett et al. 2008).

Depression is poorly recognized in patients with CHD (Rumsfeld and Ho, 2005). One study of more than 1 000 admissions found that while the prevalence of moderate or severe depressive symptoms was 17.6%, only one-quarter of these were recognized as probable cases of depression (Amin et al. 2006). Unrecognized cases were more likely to be from ethnic minorities, to be poorly educated, and to have poor cardiac function in terms of left ventricular ejection fraction. This under-recognition is partly because clinical medical staff have more immediate concerns in terms of ensuring survival and treating the disease, and partly because of the belief that feeling depressed is a natural reaction to ACS. Recognition by clinical staff will be greatly facilitated by the introduction of rapid and convenient assessment methods. This issue is being actively investigated, with comparisons between standard questionnaire measures, and the testing of very simple screening instruments, but no consensus has yet been reached (Doyle et al. 2006; Huffman et al. 2006).

Although the primary focus of research has been on depression as a predictor of poor cardiac outcomes, negative mood states soon after ACS are also related to long-term psychological adaptation and quality of life. Several studies have shown that depression and anxiety in the weeks after ACS predict poor long-term quality of life (Dickens et al. 2006; Lane et al. 2001). We have recently shown that depressed mood in the seven to ten days following ACS is an independent predictor of post-traumatic stress symptoms up to three years later (Wikman et al. 2008). Early depression is also a determinant of more objective indicators of adaptation such as a failure to return to work (Bhattacharyya et al. 2007).

As research with cardiac patients has evolved, the significance of depression at different stages of the experience of acute cardiac events has become apparent. Depression measured following ACS could be an emergent or incident response, or a continuation of a depressed state that was present before the cardiac event. If the episode of depression only begins after the ACS, it could be a recurrence of an established depressive illness, or a new state that the patient has never experienced before. A study of more than 450 patients in the Netherlands found that around half of the depression emerged post-MI (incident depression), while in the remainder it reflected ongoing or recurrent depression (de Jonge et al. 2006a). Interestingly, only incident depression was associated with new cardiac events over the next 2.5 years, while non-incident depression did not predict poor cardiac prognosis. This pattern has recently been confirmed in an eight-year follow-up of patients in northern England, where new onset depression following MI predicted cardiac mortality, while pre-MI depression did not (Dickens et al. 2008).

Results of this type suggest that the depression observed following ACS is of at least two types. The first may be a reflection of a depressive syndromes already established, while the second could be a new phenomenon associated specifically with the onset of acute heart disease. If only the latter is related to poor prognosis, then the question arises of whether its psychopathology and pathophysiology is different from depression in general. It may have particular biological characteristics that lead to increased risk to cardiac health. Another possibility is that cardiac disease severity is worse among patients with first-time incident depressive disorder. One small study has shown that underlying CAD is more severe in patients with incident rather than recurrent depression (Goodman et al. 2008). It is also possible that somatic and biological symptoms are more prominent in the depressive syndromes that predict future cardiac health (de Jonge et al. 2006b). Nevertheless, it must be acknowledged that not all studies have found differences in long-term cardiac health between incident and non-incident depression (Lespérance et al. 1996); so the issue is not yet resolved.

Mechanisms linking depression with coronary heart disease

There has been rapid development in the understanding of the mechanisms linking depression with CHD over the past decade. Two broad sets of processes are involved: direct biological pathways and behavioural or lifestyle factors. These are summarized in Fig. 18.1. Additionally, it is possible that there are shared genetic vulnerabilities for depression and CHD, involving processes related to serotonin metabolism and inflammation (Otte et al. 2007). Different processes may be

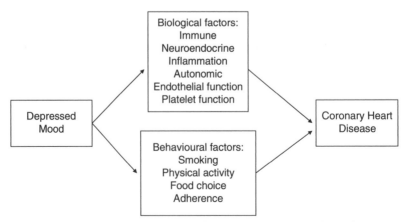

Fig. 18.1 Outline of processes potentially linking depression with coronary heart disease.

involved at various stages of coronary atherosclerosis and clinical CHD. Space prevents a detailed discussion of all these possibilities, so this chapter will only touch on some of the processes that have been implicated.

Endothelial dysfunction

The vascular endothelium plays a critical role in atherosclerosis, and impaired endothelial function is central to the development of CAD (Hansson, 2005). There is now evidence that depressed patients without CHD have impaired endothelial function. Broadley et al. (2005) showed not only that endothelial function is impaired in depressed patients, but also that the response could be reversed by metyrapone, a cortisol synthesis inhibitor. This suggests that the disturbances of vascular endothelium in depression may be driven in part by excess activation of the hypothalamic-pituitary-adrenocortical (HPA) axis. The selective serotonin re-uptake inhibitor (SSRI) citalopram has also been shown to improve endothelial function in depressed CHD patients (van Zyl et al. 2009). Since endothelial dysfunction is associated with the long-term development of atherosclerosis, it may be particularly important in linking depression with the primary aetiology of CHD.

Autonomic dysfunction

Heightened sympathetic nervous system activation and impaired parasympathetic control are involved in several stages of the development and prognosis of CHD. A high resting heart rate is a cardiovascular risk factor (Fox et al. 2007), while impaired heart rate variability (HRV) is indicative of abnormal parasympathetic control, and predicts future CHD and progression of subclinical disease (Huikuri et al. 1999). Impaired HRV is also associated with a poor prognosis following ACS (La Rovere et al. 1998).

Impaired HRV could be another process linking depression with CHD. A growing number of studies have assessed HRV in depressed individuals both with and without CHD. The literature was reviewed by Rottenberg (2007) who concluded that although depression appears to be associated with impaired HRV, effects are small and there is much variation between studies. Results in patients with CHD are inconsistent, with impaired HRV being recorded in some (Carney et al. 2001; 2005), but not other studies (Gehi et al. 2005; Martens et al. 2008). We recently showed that HRV over 24 hours was not associated with depressive symptoms assessed with a conventional measure (BDI), but was related to depressed mood measured over the period of electrocardiographic monitoring, suggesting quite immediate effects of mood (Bhattacharyya et al. 2008). There is also uncertainty about whether the relationship is causal. Carney et al. (2005) showed that altered HRV accounted in part for the reduced survival of depressed patients post-MI. By contrast, Drago et al. (2007) found that while depressed individuals had impaired HRV and higher heart rates than non-depressed post-MI patients, and depression was also associated with five year mortality, HRV did not mediate the association between depression and mortality. The role of autonomic processes in mediating the link between CHD and depression therefore requires further clarification.

Inflammatory processes

The central role of inflammatory processes in CHD has already been emphasized (Hansson, 2005; Steptoe and Brydon, 2007). Other chapters in this book have detailed the relationship between depression and inflammation (Chapters 10, 11, 16, and 17), and numerous epidemiological cohort studies have documented the association between depressed mood and elevations of C-reactive protein and interleukin 6 (IL-6), factors that are intimately involved in CHD (Penninx et al. 2003; Ranjit et al. 2007). Chronic low-level inflammation may therefore provide a link with CHD.

Unfortunately, studies of patients with CHD present a mixed picture. In the Heart and Soul Study, a prospective investigation of around 900 patients with established coronary artery disease, major depressive disorder was associated with low rather than high levels of CRP, fibrinogen, and IL-6 (Whooley et al. 2007). Another large study of patients following ACS showed that cardiac events over a two-year period were predicted both by depression and elevated C-reactive protein, but there was little additive risk in having both characteristics (Frasure-Smith et al. 2007). Vaccarino et al. (2007) monitored a sample of women with coronary ischaemia over 5.9 years, and found that major clinical events (MI, fatal CHD, etc.) were predicted by depression. Depressed individuals also had higher C-reactive protein; nevertheless, inflammation accounted only for a small proportion of variance in CHD associated with depression. It has to be said, however, that studies of CHD patients and high risk individuals are problematic, since many of the medications commonly prescribed (such as statins) have anti-inflammatory effects.

As noted in Chapters 10, 11, 16, and 17 of this book, the relationship between depression and inflammation is bidirectional. Acute coronary syndromes such as MI elicit very large inflammatory responses, and patients with greater inflammation in the days following hospital admission are at high risk (Koukkunen et al. 2001; Lindmark et al. 2001). This raises the intriguing possibility that the magnitude of acute inflammatory response during ACS is a determinant of the depressed mood that emerges in the early recovery period. This is not been directly investigated to date, but has important implications both for understanding pathophysiology and clinical management.

Platelet function and CHD

Another biological process that could link depression with CHD is disturbed platelet function. Nemeroff and Musselman (2000) proposed that enhanced platelet reactivity could predispose depressed individuals to thrombus formation, increasing risk for acute cardiac events. Experimentally, we have shown that patients whose ACS had been triggered by emotional distress display heightened platelet reactivity to standardized mental stress tests (Strike et al. 2006). SSRIs are also known to reduce platelet activation and aggregation. However, a systematic review of 34 studies argued that firm conclusions were difficult to draw because of the wide variation in measures and study quality, and substantial inconsistencies in the findings (von Kanel, 2004).

Behavioural processes

Depression is associated with maladaptive health behaviours such as smoking, physical inactivity, and adiposity that contribute to increased cardiovascular risk. Lifestyle factors may therefore be involved in the link between depression and CHD, although it is important to recall that most prospective studies have controlled statistically for smoking and body weight, and still showed positive associations between depression and CHD. It is unfortunate that the convention in the literature has been to control for behavioural variables, rather than examine their mediating role.

One behaviour that may be especially important is adherence to treatment. Patients with CHD are commonly prescribed several different medications, and are also advised about physical activity, nutrition, weight control, smoking, and stress management. Nonadherence is common in cardiac patients, and has been shown to increase risk of all cause and cardiovascular mortality (Rasmussen et al. 2007). Poor adherence both to medication and lifestyle advice is associated with factors such as poor social support and partner stress (DiMatteo, 2004; Molloy et al. 2008), and is also related to depression in CHD. Its role was elegantly demonstrated in two studies by Rieckmann (2006a, b). The first used electronic devices to monitor aspirin use in patients with ACS. Forty-two per cent of the persistently depressed individuals showed poor adherence, compared with 10.5% of non-depressed patients. In a later cross-panel analysis, these researchers found that improvement in depression led to greater medication adherence over the next two months, strongly implicating depression as a causal factor in this relationship.

Management of depression in patients with CHD

Two broad approaches to the management of depression are being investigated for patients with CHD. The first is pharmacotherapy, in which the treatment of choice has been SSRIs. The reason is that tricyclics and monoamine oxidase inhibitors both have some cardiotoxic effects, whereas SSRIs may not only be antidepressant but also have anti-inflammatory properties (Carney and Freedland, 2006). The second approach is psychotherapy using cognitive-behavioural or inter-personal techniques.

The trials of SSRIs published so far have focused on safety and efficacy for treating depression in CHD patients rather than effects on cardiac morbidity. These studies have been reviewed by von Ruden et al. (2008) who concluded that SSRIs were only moderately effective in reducing depression in CHD patients, and that their impact on CHD morbidity has not been convincingly demonstrated. In the recent Canadian Cardiac Randomized Evaluation of Antidepressant and Psychotherapy Efficacy (CREATE) trial, the SSRI citalopram did produce moderate effects on depression, while interpersonal therapy did not, but the study was not powered to assess cardiac endpoints (Lespérance et al. 2007). Analyses from the Myocardial Infarction and Depression-Intervention (MIND-IT) trial showed very little effect of the mixed serotonergic and noradren-ergic antidepressant mirtazapine in depressed post-MI patients, and there were no effects on cardiac prognosis (Honig et al. 2007).

The major trial to investigate cognitive-behavioural methods was the ENRICHD Study (Berkman et al. 2003). This failed to demonstrate favourable effects on survival following exten-sive cognitive-behavioural treatment for depression in post-MI patients. Many explanations for this failure have been put forward, including the fact that improvements in depression were modest, and that patients randomized to the comparison usual cardiological care group also demonstrated improvements in depression, reducing the differences between groups. Adherence to the psychotherapy was poor, with only half the patients randomized to intervention receiving the complete course of individual treatment sessions. Other cognitive-behavioural methods are currently being explored. For example, in Project COPES, problem-solving therapy is being applied, and patients are also being given a choice of psychotherapy and/ pharmacotherapy in their treatment (Burg et al. 2008). In the light of the evidence presented earlier in this chapter, it is also possible that conventional psychiatrically-orientated therapy may be less efficacious because it does not influence the biological and behavioural mediators of cardiovascular effects. This is a vigorous field of investigation, and it is as yet too early to present a consensus concerning the management of depression in patients with CHD.

Conclusions

Despite the intensive research on depression and CHD, findings in this field raise almost as many questions as they answer. The evidence relating depressive illness and depressed mood with the aetiology of CHD and with prognosis is abundant, but negative findings continue to be pub-lished. Some of these studies may be underpowered, but the inconsistency may also reflect the possibility that some aspects of the depressive experience relevant to CHD are idiosyncratic. There is also mixed evidence concerning all the putative mediating pathways that have been pro-posed to link depression with CHD. This may be resolved by larger sample sizes, clearer patient characterization, and attention to issues such as medication status. Nonetheless, the accumulated evidence is that depression is relevant to all stages of the coronary disease process. The challenge is to understand how best to manage depression so as to prevent future cardiovascular disease and enhance effective recovery and quality of life.

Acknowledgements

This research is supported by the British Heart Foundation.

References

Amin, A.A., Jones, A.M., Nugent, K., Rumsfeld, J.S., and Spertus, J.A. (2006). The prevalence of unrecognized depression in patients with acute coronary syndrome. *Am Heart J.*, **152**, 928–934.

Berkman, L.F., Blumenthal, J., Burg, M. et al. (2003). Effects of treating depression and low perceived social support on clinical events after myocardial infarction: the Enhancing Recovery in Coronary Heart Disease Patients (ENRICHD) Randomized Trial. *JAMA*, **289**, 3106–3116.

Bhattacharyya, M.R., Perkins-Porras, L., Whitehead, D.L., and Steptoe, A. (2007). Psychological and clinical predictors of return to work after acute coronary syndrome. *Eur Heart J.*, **28**, 160–165.

Bhattacharyya, M.R., Whitehead, D.L., Rakhit, R., and Steptoe, A. (2008). Depressed mood, positive affect and heart rate variability in patients with suspected coronary artery disease. *Psychosom Med*, **70**, 1020–1027.

Broadley, A.J., Korszun, A., Abdelaal, E. et al. (2005). Inhibition of cortisol production with metyrapone prevents mental stress-induced endothelial dysfunction and baroreflex impairment. *J Am Coll Cardiol.*, **46**, 344–350.

Burg, M.M., Lesperance, F., Rieckmann, N., Clemow, L., Skotzko, C., and Davidson, K.W. (2008). Treating persistent depressive symptoms in post-ACS patients: the project COPES phase-I randomized controlled trial. *Contemp Clin Trials*, **29**, 231–240.

Carney, R.M., Blumenthal, J.A., Stein, P.K. et al. (2001). Depression, heart rate variability, and acute myocardial infarction. *Circulation*, **104**, 2024–2028.

Carney, R.M., Blumenthal, J.A., Freedland, K.E. et al. (2005). Low heart rate variability and the effect of depression on post-myocardial infarction mortality. *Arch Intern Med.*, **165**, 1486–1491.

Carney, R.M. and Freedland, K. (2006). The management of depression in patients with coronary heart disease. In Steptoe, A. (ed.), *Depression and Physical Illness*, pp. 109–124. Cambridge, Cambridge University Press.

de Jonge, P., van den Brink, R.H., Spijkerman, T.A., and Ormel, J. (2006a). Only incident depressive episodes after myocardial infarction are associated with new cardiovascular events. *J Am Coll Cardiol.*, **48**, 2204–2208.

de Jonge, P., Ormel, J., van den Brink, R.H. et al. (2006b). Symptom dimensions of depression following myocardial infarction and their relationship with somatic health status and cardiovascular prognosis. *Am J Psychiatry*, **163**, 138–144.

Dickens, C., McGowan, L., Percival, C. et al. (2008). New onset depression following myocardial infarction predicts cardiac mortality. *Psychosom Med.*, **70**, 450–455.

Dickens, C.M., McGowan, L., Percival, C. et al. (2006). Contribution of depression and anxiety to impaired health-related quality of life following first myocardial infarction. *Br J Psychiatry*, **189**, 367–372.

DiMatteo, M.R. (2004). Social support and patient adherence to medical treatment: a meta-analysis. *Health Psychol.*, **23**, 207–218.

Doyle, F., McGee, H.M., De La Harpe, D., Shelley, E., and Conroy, R. (2006). The hospital anxiety and depression scale depression subscale, but not the beck depression inventory-fast scale, identifies patients with acute coronary syndrome at elevated risk of 1-year mortality. *J Psychosom Res.*, **60**, 461–467.

Drago, S., Bergerone, S., Anselmino, M. et al. (2007). Depression in patients with acute myocardial infarction: influence on autonomic nervous system and prognostic role. Results of a five-year follow-up study. *Int J Cardiol.*, **115**, 46–51.

Fan, A.Z., Strine, T.W., Jiles, R., and Mokdad, A. H. (2008). Depression and anxiety associated with cardiovascular disease among persons aged 45 years and older in 38 states of the United States, 2006. *Prev Med.*, **46**, 445–450.

Fox, K., Borer, J.S., Camm, A.J. et al. (2007). Resting heart rate in cardiovascular disease. *J Am Coll Cardiol.*, **50**, 823–830.

Frasure-Smith, N., Lespérance, F., and Talajic, M. (1993). Depression following myocardial infarction: impact on 6-month survival. *JAMA*, **270**, 1819–1825.

Frasure-Smith, N., Lespérance, F., Irwin, M.R., Sauve, C., Lesperance, J., and Theroux, P. (2007). Depression, C-reactive protein and two-year major adverse cardiac events in men after acute coronary syndromes. *Biol Psychiatry*, **62**, 302–308.

Gehi, A., Mangano, D., Pipkin, S., Browner, W.S., and Whooley, M.A. (2005). Depression and heart rate variability in patients with stable coronary heart disease: findings from the Heart and Soul Study. *Arch Gen Psychiatry*, **62**, 661–666.

Goodman, J., Shimbo, D., Haas, D.C., Davidson, K.W., and Rieckmann, N. (2008). Incident and recurrent major depressive disorder and coronary artery disease severity in acute coronary syndrome patients. *J Psychiatr Res.*, **42**, 670–675.

Hamer, M., Stamatakis, E., and Steptoe, A. (2008). Psychiatric hospital admissions, behavioural risk factors, and all cause mortality: The Scottish Health Survey. *Arch Intern Med.*, **168**, 2474–2479.

Hansson, G.K. (2005). Inflammation, atherosclerosis, and coronary artery disease. *N Engl J Med*, **352**, 1685–1695.

Honig, A., Kuyper, A.M., Schene, A.H. et al. (2007). Treatment of post-myocardial infarction depressive disorder: a randomized, placebo-controlled trial with mirtazapine. *Psychosom Med.*, **69**, 606–613.

Huffman, J.C., Smith, F.A., Blais, M.A., Beiser, M.E., Januzzi, J.L., and Fricchione, G.L. (2006). Recognition and treatment of depression and anxiety in patients with acute myocardial infarction. *Am J Cardiol.*, **98**, 319–324.

Huikuri, H.V., Jokinen, V., Syvanne, M. et al. (1999). Heart rate variability and progression of coronary atherosclerosis. *Arterioscler Thromb Vasc Biol.*, **19**, 1979–1985.

Jaffe, A.S., Krumholz, H.M., Catellier, D.J. et al. (2006). Prediction of medical morbidity and mortality after acute myocardial infarction in patients at increased psychosocial risk in the Enhancing Recovery in Coronary Heart Disease Patients (ENRICHD) study. *Am Heart J.*, **152**, 126–135.

Koukkunen, H., Penttila, K., Kemppainen, A. et al. (2001). C-reactive protein, fibrinogen, interleukin-6 and tumour necrosis factor-alpha in the prognostic classification of unstable angina pectoris. *Ann Med.*, **33**, 37–47.

La Rovere, M.T., Bigger, J.T., Jr., Marcus, F.I., Mortara, A., and Schwartz, P.J. (1998). Baroreflex sensitivity and heart-rate variability in prediction of total cardiac mortality after myocardial infarction. ATRAMI (Autonomic Tone and Reflexes After Myocardial Infarction) Investigators. *Lancet*, **351**, 478–484.

Lane, D., Carroll, D., Ring, C., Beevers, D.G., and Lip, G.Y. (2001). Mortality and quality of life 12 months after myocardial infarction: effects of depression and anxiety. *Psychosom Med.*, **63**, 221–230.

Lespérance, F., Frasure-Smith, N., and Talajic, M. (1996). Major depression before and after myocardial infarction: its nature and consequences. *Psychosom Med.*, **58**, 99–110.

Lespérance, F., Frasure-Smith, N., Talajic, M., and Bourassa, M.G. (2002). Five-year risk of cardiac mortality in relation to initial severity and one-year changes in depression symptoms after myocardial infarction. *Circulation*, **105**, 1049–1053.

Lespérance, F., Frasure-Smith, N., Koszycki, D. et al. (2007). Effects of citalopram and interpersonal psychotherapy on depression in patients with coronary artery disease: the Canadian Cardiac Randomized Evaluation of Antidepressant and Psychotherapy Efficacy (CREATE) trial. *JAMA*, **297**, 367–379.

Lett, H., Ali, S., and Whooley, M. (2008). Depression and cardiac function in patients with stable coronary heart disease: findings from the heart and soul study. *Psychosom Med.*, **70**, 444–449.

Lett, H.S., Sherwood, A., Watkins, L., and Blumenthal, J. A. (2006). Depression and prognosis in cardiac patients. In Steptoe, A. (ed.), *Depression and Physical Illness*, pp. 87–108. Cambridge, Cambridge University Press.

Lindmark, E., Diderholm, E., Wallentin, L., and Siegbahn, A. (2001). Relationship between interleukin 6 and mortality in patients with unstable coronary artery disease: effects of an early invasive or noninvasive strategy. *JAMA*, **286**, 2107–2113.

Martens, E.J., Nyklicek, I., Szabo, B.M., and Kupper, N. (2008). Depression and anxiety as predictors of heart rate variability after myocardial infarction. *Psychol Med.*, **38**, 375–383.

Molloy, G.J., Perkins-Porras, L., Strike, P.C., and Steptoe, A. (2008). Social networks and partner stress as predictors of adherence to medication, rehabilitation attendance, and quality of life following acute coronary syndrome. *Health Psychol*, **27**, 52–58.

Naghavi, M., Libby, P., Falk, E. et al. (2003). From vulnerable plaque to vulnerable patient: a call for new definitions and risk assessment strategies: Part I. *Circulation*, **108**, 1664–1672.

Nemeroff, C.B. and Musselman, D.L. (2000). Are platelets the link between depression and ischemic heart disease? *Am Heart J.*, **140**, 57–62.

Nicholson, A., Kuper, H., and Hemingway, H. (2006). Depression as an aetiologic and prognostic factor in coronary heart disease: a meta-analysis of 6362 events among 146 538 participants in 54 observational studies. *Eur Heart J.*, **27**, 2763–2774.

Osborn, D.P., Levy, G., Nazareth, I., Petersen, I., Islam, A., and King, M.B. (2007). Relative risk of cardio-vascular and cancer mortality in people with severe mental illness from the United Kingdom's general practice research database. *Arch Gen Psychiatry*, **64**, 242–249.

Otte, C., McCaffery, J., Ali, S., and Whooley, M.A. (2007). Association of a serotonin transporter polymorphism (5-HTTLPR) with depression, perceived stress, and norepinephrine in patients with coronary disease: the heart and soul study. *Am J Psychiatry*, **164**, 1379–1384.

Penninx, B.W., Kritchevsky, S.B., Yaffe, K. et al. (2003). Inflammatory markers and depressed mood in older persons: results from the health, aging and body composition study. *Biol Psychiatry*, **54**, 566–572.

Ranjit, N., Diez-Roux, A.V., Shea, S. et al. (2007). Psychosocial factors and inflammation in the multi-ethnic study of atherosclerosis. *Arch Intern Med.*, **167**, 174–181.

Rasmussen, J.N., Chong, A., and Alter, D.A. (2007). Relationship between adherence to evidence-based pharmacotherapy and long-term mortality after acute myocardial jnfarction. *JAMA*, **297**, 177–186.

Rieckmann, N., Gerin, W., Kronish, I. M. et al. (2006a). Course of depressive symptoms and medication adherence after acute coronary syndromes: an electronic medication monitoring study. *J Am Coll Cardiol.*, **48**, 2218–2222.

Rieckmann, N., Kronish, I.M., Haas, D. et al. (2006b). Persistent depressive symptoms lower aspirin adherence after acute coronary syndromes. *Am Heart J.*, **152**, 922–927.

Rottenberg, J. (2007). Cardiac vagal control in depression: a critical analysis. *Biol Psychol.*, **74**, 200–211.

Rumsfeld, J.S. and Ho, P.M. (2005). Depression and cardiovascular disease: a call for recognition. *Circulation*, **111**, 250–253.

Rutledge, T., Reis, V.A., Linke, S.E., Greenberg, B.H., and Mills, P.J. (2006). Depression in heart failure a meta-analytic review of prevalence, intervention effects, and associations with clinical outcomes. *J Am Coll Cardiol.*, **48**, 1527–1537.

Steptoe, A., Strike, P.C., Perkins-Porras, L., McEwan, J.R. and Whitehead, D.L. (2006). Acute depressed mood as a trigger of acute coronary syndromes. *Biol Psychiatry*, **60**, 837–842.

Steptoe, A. and Brydon, L. (2007). Psychosocial factors and coronary heart disease: the role of psychoneuroimmunological processes. In Ader, R. (ed.), *Psychoneuroimmunology*, 4th Edition, pp. 945–974. San Diego, Elsevier.

Steptoe, A. and Brydon, L. (2009) Emotional triggering of cardiac events. *Neurosci Biobehav Rev.*, **33**, 63–70.

Stewart, J.C., Janicki, D.L., Muldoon, M.F., Sutton-Tyrrell, K., and Kamarck, T.W. (2007). Negative emotions and 3-year progression of subclinical atherosclerosis. *Arch Gen Psychiatry*, **64**, 225–233.

Strike, P. C., Magid,K., Whitehead, D.L., Brydon, L., Bhattacharyya, M.R., and Steptoe, A. (2006). Pathophysiological processes underlying emotional triggering of acute cardiac events. *Proc Natl Acad Sci USA*, **103**, 4322–4327.

Tofler, G.H. and Muller, J.E. (2006). Triggering of acute cardiovascular disease and potential preventive strategies. *Circulation*, **114**, 1863–1872.

Vaccarino, V., Johnson, B.D., Sheps, D.S. *et al.* (2007). Depression, inflammation, and incident cardio-vascular disease in women with suspected coronary ischemia: the National Heart, Lung, and Blood Institute-sponsored WISE study. *J Am Coll Cardiol.*, **50**, 2044–2050.

van Zyl, L.T., Lespérance, F., Frasure-Smith, N. *et al.* (2009) Platelet and endothelial activity in comorbid major depression and coronary artery disease patients treated with citalopram: the Canadian Cardiac Randomized Evaluation of Antidepressant and Psychotherapy Efficacy Trial (CREATE) biomarker sub-study. *J Thromb Thrombolysis*, **27**, 48–56.

von Kanel, R. (2004). Platelet hyperactivity in clinical depression and the beneficial effect of antidepressant drug treatment: how strong is the evidence? *Acta Psychiatr Scand.*, **110**, 163–177.

von Ruden, A.E., Adson, D.E., and Kotlyar, M. (2008). Effect of selective serotonin reuptake inhibitors on cardiovascular morbidity and mortality. *J Cardiovasc Pharmacol Ther.*, **13**, 32–40.

Wellenius, G.A., Mukamal, K.J., Kulshreshtha, A., Asonganyi, S., and Mittleman, M.A. (2008). Depressive symptoms and the risk of atherosclerotic progression among patients with coronary artery bypass grafts. *Circulation*, **117**, 2313–2319.

Whooley, M. A., Caska, C. M., Hendrickson, B. E., Rourke, M. A., Ho, J. and Ali, S. (2007). Depression and inflammation in patients with coronary heart disease: findings from the heart and soul study. *Biol. Psychiatry*, **62**, 314–320.

Wikman, A., Bhattacharyya, M.R., Perkins-Porras, L., and Steptoe, A. (2008). Persistence of posttraumatic stress symptoms 12 and 36 months after acute coronary syndrome. *Psychosom Med.*, **70**, 764–772.

Williams, E. D. and Steptoe, A. (2007). The role of depression in the etiology of acute coronary syndrome. *Curr Psychiatry Rep.*, **9**, 486–492.

Wouts, L., Oude Voshaar, R.C., Bremmer, M.A., Buitelaar, J.K., Penninx, B.W., and Beekman, A.T. (2008). Cardiac disease, depressive symptoms, and incident stroke in an elderly population. *Arch. Gen. Psychiatry*, **65**, 596–602.

Chapter 19

Does depression induce pain and fatigue?

Antony J. Cleare

In the past decade depression has emerged as a condition affecting both body and mind, and indeed exemplifying *par excellence* the indivisibility of body and mind. An explosion of research has demonstrated the adverse effects of depression on the body, much of which is reviewed elsewhere, throughout most of the chapters in this book. The focus of this chapter will be on the commonest of the bodily symptoms: pain and fatigue.

Interrelationship between depression, fatigue, and pain

Fatigue as a symptom is extremely common in the general population. Between 20% and 50% of the population report to be suffering from fatigue (depending on the definition), while 10% of those in primary health care have fatigue of six months or more duration (Wessely et al. 1998). A smaller group can be shown to have significant disability resulting from their fatigue. Chronic pain is also common: one recent large community study found that 17% of people had suffered six months or more of pain sufficient to require medical consultation (Ohayon and Schatzberg, 2003).

The classic work of Kroenke and colleagues showed that the overwhelming majority of patients presenting with pain and fatigue have no identifiable organic disease that can explain these symptoms (Kroenke and Mangelsdorff, 1989). Thus, other explanations for the frequent occurrence of these symptoms need to be sought.

Such unexplained fatigue can be of varying severity and is probably dimensionally distributed (Pawlikowska et al. 1994). The far end of the spectrum has been operationalized as chronic fatigue syndrome (Fukuda et al. 1994) although there remains uncertainty as to the best way to define such a condition (Reeves et al. 2003), and there remains great controversy as to whether there are any discrete identifiable conditions among patients with disabling chronic fatigue (Wessely et al. 1998). At the present time, an understanding of chronic fatigue akin to that of hypertension appears best to fit the epidemiology of the condition (Wessely et al. 1998).

There are a number of important observations surrounding patients with medically unexplained chronic fatigue. First, statistical analysis of the pattern of symptom reporting suggests that there are two broad groups of patients. On one hand there are those who complain of a relatively constrained group of symptoms of which fatigue is the most prominent, and on the other there is a group who complain of a multitude of other physical symptoms (Hickie et al. 1995). These other symptoms are often themselves severe and disabling and can meet criteria for other somatic syndromes. For example, Aaron and colleagues (Aaron et al. 2000) compared patients with chronic fatigue to their non-fatigued twins and found hugely increased rates of other pain syndromes (fibromyalgia, odds ratio 21.5; chronic pelvic pain, odds ratio 5.8; chronic lower back pain odds ratio 3.3), as well as other conditions such as irritable bowel syndrome (odds ratio 9.0) and multiple chemical sensitivities (odds ratio 7.5). Over 70% of those with chronic fatigue also reported a history of chronic widespread pain sufficient for a diagnosis of fibromyalgia.

In this context there is a wealth of data finding a close correlation between the number of somatic symptoms a person experiences and a number of psychological symptoms (Wessely et al. 1998). The direction of causality appears to be in both directions: in many patients the physical symptoms predate the depression, while in many others the depression predates the physical symptoms (Hotopf et al. 1998). Rates of diagnosable depression are high in patients who experience chronic fatigue syndrome (Wessely and Powell, 1989) or fibromyalgia (McBeth and Silman, 2001) and appear to be higher still in those with several somatic syndromes. The overlap in many of the features of the various somatic syndromes has led some to suggest that the current classification of such syndromes into individual symptom groups is erroneous and that their similarities outweigh their differences (Wessely et al. 1999).

Figure 19.1 shows a schematic representation of these overlaps based on the conceptualizations of Fukuda et al. (1994) and using the data from a study of psychiatric comorbidity in a group of CFS patients in tertiary care (Wessely and Powell, 1989).

Fatigue in depression

Within the ICD-10 classification system, fatigue is a core symptom of depression, alongside low mood and anhedonia. The DSM-IV classification does not recognize fatigue as a core symptom, although it is one of the seven non-core features of the depressive syndrome.

Atypical depression

More profound feelings of fatigue – specifically a feeling of 'leaden paralysis' – form part of the syndrome of atypical depression, which is included as an illness specifier in the DSM-IV. In atypical depression, the subject fills the usual criteria for a depressive episode, but with the following specific features:

(a) reversed biological symptoms (i.e. hypersomnia, hyperphagia, weight gain, and diurnal mood variation better in the morning)

(b) preserved mood reactivity

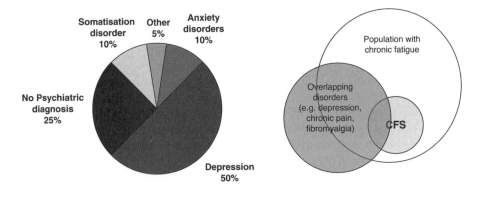

Psychiatric diagnoses in a tertiary care sample of patients with CFS (data from Wessley and Powell 1989)

Overlap of depression, fatigue and pain in the community

Fig. 19.1 Psychiatric disorder, fatigue and chronic fatigue syndrome.

(c) extreme (leaden) anergia

(d) chronic interpersonal rejection sensitivity.

In general, patients with atypical depression tend to have an earlier onset, a higher proportion of females, increased comorbidity with dysthymia, substance misuse and sociopathy, and have a higher incidence of atypical depression in their relatives.

Sullivan and colleagues used data from the large US National Comorbidity Survey, and using latent class analysis identified six syndromes, two of which corresponded to mild atypical depression and severe atypical depression, respectively (Sullivan et al. 1998). Atypicality was associated with decreased syndrome consequences, comorbid conduct disorder and social phobia, higher interpersonal dependency and lower self-esteem, and parental alcohol/drug use disorder. This study confirmed earlier epidemiological findings from other samples that the concept of atypical depression does have validity. For example, a study of 1 000 female twin pairs suggested that there was a syndrome of atypical depression characterized by increased eating, hypersomnia, frequent, relatively short episodes, and a proclivity to obesity (Kendler et al. 1996). Furthermore, individuals with recurrent episodes tended to have the same syndrome on each occasion. The members of twin pairs concordant for depression had the same depressive syndrome more often than expected by chance and this resemblance was greater in monozygotic than in dizygotic pairs.

Chronic fatigue syndrome and depression

Depression can commonly be diagnosed in patients suffering from chronic fatigue syndrome. Rates vary depending on the instruments used and the patient sample studied, but commonly a third to a half of patients will meet criteria for depression (Anon, 1996). A number of explanations are put forward as to why depression can so readily be diagnosed in these patients. One explanation is that of overlapping symptoms and, indeed, a number of symptoms contained within the diagnostic criteria for depression, notably fatigue, concentration problems and sleep problems, are contained both within the DSM-IV criteria for depression and the Fukuda et al. consensus criteria for chronic fatigue syndrome. Nevertheless, even if one excludes overlapping symptoms from definitions, it seems that many of the other depressive symptoms remain more common in patients with chronic fatigue syndrome than the general population.

Another explanation postulated has been that depression is a reaction to the severity of symptoms and disability in chronic fatigue syndrome. While chronic fatigue syndrome is undoubtedly a distressing and disabling condition and this may partly explain the association, it is certainly not the whole story. A number of studies have compared rates of depression and other psychiatric disorder between patients with CFS and patients with similarly distressing and disabling conditions, such as rheumatoid arthritis, multiple sclerosis, and myasthenia gravis, and found several-fold higher rates in patients with CFS (Cleare and Wessely, 2001).

Instead there appears to be something more integral between a tendency to experience depressive illness and a tendency to experience chronic fatigue. First, there appears to be some shared genetic vulnerability to these two diatheses. Recent studies suggest that while there is a genetic propensity to suffer from chronic fatigue, with the concordance between monozygotic twins more than twice that of dizygotic twins (Farmer et al. 1999; Hickie et al. 1999), part of this vulnerability is conferred through the genetic tendency to suffer from anxiety or depression (Hickie et al. 1999).

Second, a number of studies have shown that those with past history of depression are more at risk of developing chronic fatigue in response to the classical triggers for fatigue. For example, many patients develop prolonged fatigue following severe viral infections. Studies from Matthew Hotopf and colleagues have shown that patients with a prior history of depression or other psychiatric disorder have around a fivefold higher rate of developing chronic fatigue following viral meningitis (Hotopf et al. 1996), and similar results have been found for other severe viral infections.

Pain in depression

Cross-sectionally, pain is a very common feature of depression. A large recent study found that 43% of those with major depression in the community also report chronic pain, a figure four times that of non-depressed individuals (Ohayon and Schatzberg, 2003). This held across a range of different sites and types of pain (Fig. 19.2). Generally research suggests that between two-fifths and two-thirds of depressed patients report painful physical symptoms (Peveler et al. 2006).

Similarly, the rates of depression in chronic pain conditions, such as fibromyalgia, are significantly higher than expected in the general population (Epstein et al. 1999; McBeth and Silman, 2001). One study found that 57% of patients with fibromyalgia suffered from concurrent depression (Okifuji, 2000) and another that a quarter had a current depressive episode and two-thirds a prior depressive episode (Epstein et al. 1999).

Longitudinally, just as with fatigue, there is evidence that depression is a risk factor for the subsequent development of chronic pain. A number of studies have shown that depression can predate the onset of chronic pain syndromes. Von Korff et al. found that depression at baseline predicted the onset of headache and chest pain after three years (Von Korff et al. 1993), while in another study depression was associated with the onset of new episodes of neck, back, hip, or knee pain lasting greater than one month (Magni et al. 1994). The *onset* of the widespread pain of fibromyalgia has also been found prospectively associated with depression (Forseth et al. 1999), while depression has also been show to be associated with *persistence* of chronic pain

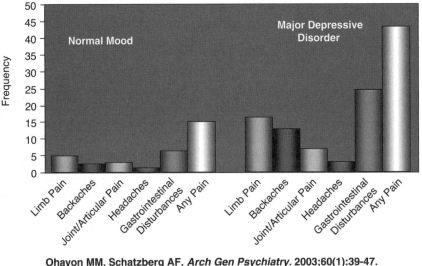

Ohayon MM, Schatzberg AF. *Arch Gen Psychiatry*. 2003;60(1):39-47.

Fig. 19.2 Prevalence of pain of at least six months duration requiring medical consultation in different bodily areas in patient with no depressive symptoms and those with major depressive disorder (Ohayon and Schatzberg, 2003).

(McBeth et al. 2001). Epidemiological studies suggest that depression predicts the outcome of chronic muskuloskeletal pain (Magni et al. 1993).

One factor postulated as a potential link between pain and depression is that of childhood abuse. A history of childhood sexual assault is an established risk factor both for adulthood depression (Heim et al. 2004) and for broadly defined somatoform disorders (Ehlert et al. 1999; Imbierowicz and Egle, 2003; Lampe et al. 2003) including chronic pelvic pain (Walker et al. 1988). It is also notable that adult sexual and/or physical assault is an additional factor that increases the risk of chronic pain (Walker et al. 1988; 1997). Recent studies have also linked childhood abuse to later chronic fatigue, odds ratios varying from 2.9 for emotional abuse to 9 for sexual abuse (Heim, 2006).

Other attempts to explain the concurrence of depression and pain point to similarities in neurochemical pathways such as those involving serotonin and noradrenaline (Blier and Abbott, 2001). Emerging brain imaging techniques such as functional MRI may be able to shed light on any overlap in the regions activated by emotional and physical pain.

HPA axis in depression, fatigue, and chronic pain

A wide variety of potential candidates explaining the overlap of depression, fatigue, and pain have been put forward. One of the most widely studied has been the hypothalamo-pituitary-adrenal axis (HPA axis). This section will summarize research on the HPA axis in these various conditions. The role of the HPA axis in affective disorders and other stress-related conditions is discussed also in several other Chapters of this book (Chapters 5, 7–9, 11, 15, 16, 21, and 26).

HPA axis in chronic fatigue syndrome and classical depression

In CFS, most, but not all, of the better-quality studies using serial samples of blood or saliva, or 24-hour urinary collections, have found reduced basal cortisol output, the reverse of that seen in classical major depression (Cleare, 2003a). Studies of the circadian rhythm suggest a blunted early morning rise of corticotrophin (ACTH) in CFS (DiGiorgio et al. 2005), which is paralleled by the findings of an impaired ACTH or cortisol response to a variety of challenges to the HPA axis, including CRH, AVP, synacthen, insulin, naloxone, exercise, and social stress (Cleare, 2003a). A non-invasive challenge to the axis – the salivary cortisol response to awakening – is blunted in CFS (Roberts, 2004) and enhanced in depression (Bhagwagar et al. 2005). There is also evidence of heightened negative feedback and glucocorticoid receptor function in CFS (Cleare, 2003a). However, there is no evidence for a unique or uniform dysfunction of the HPA axis. Given the many factors that may impinge on the HPA axis in CFS, such as inactivity, sleep disturbance, psychiatric comorbidity, medication, and ongoing stress, it seems likely that HPA axis disturbance in CFS is heterogeneous and of multifactorial aetiology (Cleare, 2004).

One of the problems with the above work is that it has been largely undertaken on samples of patients ill for several years, and the relevance of these HPA axis changes to the onset of illness is unknown. Prospective studies of groups at high risk of developing chronic fatigue (post-EBV infection and post-surgery) have found that the development of fatigue six months later was not associated with any HPA axis changes (Candy et al. 2003; Rubin et al. 2005). Thus, at present it would appear that HPA axis changes are not important during the early stages of the genesis of fatiguing illnesses.

HPA axis and treatment

It seems that the low cortisol levels that may develop at a later stage of the illness could be of clinical relevance and contribute to symptom maintenance in CFS. Thus, one placebo controlled trial found that supplementation with a low dose of hydrocortisone (5–10 mg daily) was able to improve fatigue in up to a third of the patients (Cleare et al. 1999), although this has yet to be replicated. A successful response to hydrocortisone replacement also led to a normalization of the HPA axis changes demonstrable prior to treatment. Furthermore, there is now evidence that HPA axis changes in CFS can be reversed by modifying behavioural features of the illness such as inactivity, deconditioning, and sleep disturbance: using cognitive behavioural therapy to treat CFS led to a significant rise in cortisol levels across the day (Roberts et al. 2008). There is also preliminary evidence that a more disrupted HPA axis predicts a poorer response to CBT in CFS (Cleare, 2003b).

In major depression, there is also some evidence that a more disrupted HPA axis predicts a poorer response to psychological therapy in major depression (Thase et al. 1996). We have recently shown that treatment resistance in depression is associated with marked HPA axis dysregulation and that greater dysregulation is associated with an overall poorer response to treatment (Juruena et al. 2007). Remission of depression is associated with a reduction in the HPA axis overdrive. Some suggest that antidepressants themselves act via the HPA axis (Juruena et al. 2003) and there is also evidence that antiglucocorticoid treatment strategies have shown some promise in treating depression associated with hypercortisolism (Gallagher et al. 2008).

The contrast between the state of the HPA axis in CFS and depression is summarized in Table 19.1.

HPA axis in fibromyalgia

Studies to date in patients with fibromyalgia have shown several similarities to those in CFS, including reduced 24-hour urinary free cortisol (Crofford et al. 1994; Lentjes et al. 1997; McCain and Tilbe, 1989). As in CFS, other studies find normal UFC levels (Maes et al. 1998) or raised salivary cortisol levels (Catley et al. 2000). A recent study that looked at ACTH and cortisol across a 24-hour period in both CFS and FM found subtle differences, with a higher evening cortisol in FM and a lower early morning cortisol in CFS (Crofford et al. 2004). Further similarities between CFS and FM include the findings of blunted cortisol responses to a variety of challenges, including exhaustive physical exercise (van Denderen et al. 1992), exogenous CRH (Crofford et al. 1994), exogenous ACTH (Kirnap et al. 2001), and the IST (Adler et al. 1999; Kirnap et al. 2001).

Table 19.1 HPA axis in CFS and classical major depression

◆ In CFS
- Reduced HPA axis function
- Lower HPA function associated with poorer treatment response
- Improving HPA axis function associated with treatment response
- Can enhance HPA pharmacologically or through CBT/graded exercise

◆ In Depression
- Enhanced HPA axis function
- Higher HPA function associated with poorer treatment response
- Reducing HPA axis function associated with treatment response
- Can reduce HPA directly or indirectly
  - Antidepressants
  - Combination therapy/CBT
  - Novel methods being trialled e.g. Block synthesis – metyrapone, ketoconazole; Reduce central drive – CRH receptor antagonists; Use antagonistic adrenal steroids – e.g. DHEA

However, several studies have found exaggerated ACTH responses to stimulation (Crofford et al. 1994; Griep et al. 1993; 1998), something not seen in CFS, and another difference between CFS and fibromyalgia. Demitrack suggests that these different ACTH responses may in fact represent differences in AVP tone: whereas in CFS, AVP levels were found to be low (Bakheit et al. 1993), in fibromyalgia they were found to be high compared to controls, in response to postural challenge (Crofford et al. 1994). Since AVP acts in synergy with CRH to release ACTH, a difference in AVP levels would be consistent with the differences demonstrated in ACTH responses for the two syndromes (Crofford et al. 2004).

HPA axis in atypical depression

While hypercortisolaemia is present in at least 50% of patients with classical major depression, more so in more severe or psychotic illnesses, several studies have now suggested that the opposite pattern of hypocortisolaemia is prevalent in atypical depression. Gold and colleagues have suggested that, while typical major depression can be characterized by an excessive activation of both the physiological stress systems, the locus ceruleus-noradrenergic system and the HPA axis, the opposite changes are present in atypical depression (Gold et al. 1995). Some support for this is provided by studies showing that the control of noradrenergic function is relatively preserved in atypical compared to typical depression (Asnis et al. 1995; McGinn et al. 1996). Gold and colleagues suggest that it is diminished CRH activity that is specifically related to the symptoms of hypoarousal (hypersomnia, hyperphagia, lethargy, fatigue, and relative apathy) of the syndrome (Gold and Chrousos, 1999). Support that it is low CRH rather than low cortisol that is related to the atypical symptoms comes from one detailed study of Cushing's syndrome patients. In this syndrome, cortisol is high and CRH low. Dorn and colleagues found that atypical depression was the predominant depressive syndrome, affecting 17 out of a group of 33 patients (Dorn et al. 1995). This suggests that it is the CRH status that is more closely linked to these symptoms than the cortisol status.

Linking HPA axis to symptoms

One hypothesis that may link the HPA axis findings across these disorders is that there are common components to the illnesses that may be linked to the common HPA axis changes. Thus the prominence of fatigue may be linked to the particular disturbance to the HPA axis in response to a stressor. Alternatively, common behavioural changes (altered sleep or reduced physical activity) that are common to the disorders may affect the HPA axis in similar ways. It might be possible to tease out a possible specific symptom link by focussing on subjects that have CFS but not muscle pain, fibromyalgia but not fatigue, atypical depression but not fatigue, and so on, in order to determine this.

Relevance to treatment and prognosis

The presence of pain or fatigue in patients with depression has a number of implications for treatment.

The presence of pain may be associated with a poorer response to antidepressant treatments and with greater overall costs of care (Greenberg et al. 2003). Similarly, the presence of residual symptoms after treatment of depression, including pain and fatigue, is a strong predictor of early relapse in patients with major depression (Judd et al. 1998). It is also important to be aware that chronic pain is an independent risk factor for suicide (Fishbain, 1999). The converse is also true: if treating patients with chronic pain/fibromyalgia or chronic fatigue syndrome then the presence of depression is a poor prognostic factor (Cairns, 2005).

It seems likely that where there is significant pain or fatigue associated with depression, then treating depression alone is likely to result in less favourable outcomes. Similarly, if patients with CFS or FM are left with untreated depression, improvement is less likely. A full review of the evidence-based therapies available is beyond the scope of this chapter, but the following principles hold.

There is now evidence for the efficacy of specialized psychological therapies in the management of both chronic pain (Morley et al. 1999) and chronic fatigue (Reid et al. 2005). In patients fulfilling criteria for atypical depression, tricyclics are generally ineffective (McGrath et al. 1992), whereas there may be a preferential response to irreversible monoamineoxidase inhibitors such as phenelzine (Liebowitz et al. 1988). The evidence for the use of an SSRI or moclobemide remains poorer than that for phenelzine at present. The NIMH study suggested that CBT and interpersonal psychotherapy are both effective in atypical depression.

Patients with chronic pain do respond to tricyclic antidepressants, which can also help with associated sleep disturbance (Richards and Cleare, 2000). Recent evidence also suggests that newer antidepressants acting on both serotonin and noradrenaline re-uptake may also have efficacy in reducing pain associated with depression (Goldstein et al. 2004) and in treating fibromyalgia (Arnold et al. 2007).

There is sparse evidence to suggest which antidepressants might be preferred in patients with CFS and comorbid depression (Reid et al. 2005).

Multidisciplinary treatments in which both pain/fatigue and depression are targeted are advisable; good examples being the pain management programmes incorporating both pain relief, rehabilitation, and psychological therapies (Williams et al. 1993). A 'stepped care' approach would also seem sensible, in which clinicians commence with simple, straightforward approaches, usually taking place in primary care, and gradually involve more complex treatment modalities when or if patients fail to respond. Multidimensional assessment tools such as those developed for CFS (Sharpe et al. 1997) can be invaluable in understanding and directing therapeutic strategies.

Summary

Depression has a complex interrelation with pain and fatigue. Depression can be seen as both a cause and a consequence of pain and fatigue, but the relationship is perhaps best understood if pain and fatigue are seen as an integral part of depression. In this way body and mind are not split, and the great commonalities in the pathways to an individual's experience of depression, pain, and fatigue – genetic, childhood environment, neurobiology – can be best appreciated. Much further work is needed to understand more specifically some of the unique underpinnings of the range of presentations in clinical practice, with the aim of translating this into improved targeting of existing therapies and, we hope, the development of new therapeutic strategies in the future. In the meantime, an appreciation of the importance of looking for, and treating appropriately, pain and fatigue in depressed patients remains a vital clinical priority.

References

Aaron, L.A., Herrell, R., Ashton, S. et al. (2001). Comorbid clinical conditions in chronic fatigue: a co-twin control study. *Journal of General Internal Medicine*, **16**, 24–31.

Adler, G.K., Kinsley, B.T., Hurwitz, S., Mossey, C.J., and Goldenberg, D.L. (1999). Reduced hypothalamic-pituitary and sympathoadrenal responses to hypoglycemia in women with fibromyalgia syndrome. *American Journal of Medicine*, **106**, 534–543.

Anon. (1996). *Chronic Fatigue Syndrome: Report of a Committee of the Royal Colleges of Physicians, Psychiatrists and General Practitioners*. London, Royal Colleges of Physicians.

Arnold, L.M., Pritchett, Y.L., D'Souza, D.N., Kajdasz, D.K., Iyengar, S., and Wernicke, J.F. (2007). Duloxetine for the treatment of fibromyalgia in women: pooled results from two randomized, placebo-controlled clinical trials. *Journal of Women's Health*, **16**, 1145–1156.

Asnis, G.M., McGinn, L.K., and Sanderson, W.C. (1995). Atypical depression: clinical aspects and noradrenergic function. *American Journal of Psychiatry*, **152**, 31–36.

Bakheit, A.M., Behan, P.O., Watson, W.S., and Morton, J.J. (1993). Abnormal arginine-vasopressin secretion and water metabolism in patients with postviral fatigue syndrome. *Acta Neurol Scand.*, **87**, 234–238.

Bhagwagar, Z., Hafizi, S., and Cowen, P.J. (2005). Increased salivary cortisol after waking in depression. *Psychopharmacology*, **182**, 54–57.

Blier, P. and Abbott, F.V. (2001). Putative mechanisms of action of antidepressant drugs in affective and anxiety disorders and pain. *Journal of Psychiatry and Neuroscience*, **26**, 37–43.

Cairns, R. and Hotopf, M. (2005). A systematic review describing the prognosis of chronic fatigue syndrome. *Occupational Medicine*, **55**, 20–31.

Candy, B., Chalder, T., Cleare, A. et al. (2003). Predictors of fatigue following the onset of infectious mononucleosis. *Psychological Medicine*, **33**, 847–853.

Catley, D., Kaell, A.T., Kirschbaum, C., and Stone, A.A. (2000). A naturalistic evaluation of cortisol secretion in persons with fibromyalgia and rheumatoid arthritis. *Arthritis Care and Research*, **13**, 51–61.

Cleare, A., Heap, E., Malhi, G., Wessely, S., O'Keane, V., and Miell, J. (1999). Low-dose hydrocortisone in chronic fatigue syndrome: a randomised crossover trial. *Lancet*, **353**, 455–458.

Cleare, A.J. and Wessely, S. (2001). Chronic fatigue syndrome. In *Encyclopædia of Life Sciences*. John Wiley and Sons Ltd., www.els.net, pp. 1–10.

Cleare, A. (2003a). The neuroendocrinology of chronic fatigue syndrome. *Endocrine Reviews*, **24**, 236–252.

Cleare, A.J. (2003b). The neuroendocrinology of chronic fatigue syndrome. *Endocrine Abstracts*, **5**, S35.

Cleare, A. (2004). The HPA axis and the genesis of chronic fatigue syndrome. *Trends In Endocrinology And Metabolism*, **15**, 55–59.

Crofford, L., Pillemer, S., Kalogeras, K. et al. (1994). Hypothalamic-pituitary-adrenal axis perturbations in patients with fibromyalgia. *Arthritis and Rheumatism*, **37**, 1583–1592.

Crofford, L.J., Young, E.A., Engleberg, N.C. et al. (2004). Basal circadian and pulsatile ACTH and cortisol secretion in patients with fibromyalgia and/or chronic fatigue syndrome. *Brain, Behavior, and Immunity*, **18**, 314–325.

DiGiorgio, A., Hudson, M., Jerjes, W., and Cleare, A.J. (2005). Circadian pattern of pituitary hormones in chronic fatigue syndrome. *Psychosomatic Medicine*, **67**, 433–440.

Dorn, L.D., Burgess, E.S., Dubbert, B. et al. (1995). Psychopathology in patients with endogenous Cushing's syndrome: 'atypical' or melancholic features. *Clinical Endocrinology*, **43**, 433–442.

Ehlert, U., Heim, C., and Hellhammer, D.H. (1999). Chronic pelvic pain as a somatoform disorder. *Psychotherapy and Psychosomatics*, **68**, 87–94.

Epstein, S., Kay, G., Clauw, D. et al. (1999). Psychiatric disorders in patients with fibromyalgia: a multicenter investigation. *Psychosomatics*, **40**, 57–63.

Farmer, A., Scourfield, J., Martin, N., Cardno, A., and McGuffin, P. (1999). Is disabling fatigue in childhod influenced by genes? *Psychological Medicine*, **29**, 279–282.

Fishbain, D.A. (1999). The association of chronic pain and suicide. *Seminars in Clinical Neuropsychiatry*. **4**, 221–227.

Forseth, K.O., Husby, G., Gran, J.T., and Forre, O. (1999). Prognostic factors for the development of fibromyalgia in women with self-reported musculoskeletal pain: a prospective study. *J Rheumatol.* **26**, 2458–2467.

Fukuda, K., Straus, S., Hickie, I., Sharpe, M., Dobbins, J., and Komaroff, A. (1994). The chronic fatigue syndrome: a comprehensive approach to its definition and study. *Annals of Internal Medicine*, **121**, 953–959.

Gallagher, P., Malik, N., Newham, J., Young, A.H., Ferrier, I. N., and Mackin, P. (2008). Antiglucocorticoid treatments for mood disorders. *Cochrane Database of Systematic Reviews*, CD005168.

Gold, P.W., Licinio, J., Wong, M.L., and Chrousos, G.P. (1995). Corticotropin releasing hormone in the pathophysiology of melancholic and atypical depression and in the mechanism of action of antidepressant drugs. *Annals of the NewYork Academy of Sciiences*, **771**, 716–729.

Gold, P.W. and Chrousos, G. P. (1999). The endocrinology of melancholic and atypical depression: relation to neurocircuitry and somatic consequences. *Proceedings of the Association of American Physicians*, **111**, 22–34.

Goldstein, D.J., Lu, Y., Detke, M.J., Hudson, J., Iyengar, S., and Demitrack, M.A. (2004). Effects of duloxetine on painful physical symptoms associated with depression. *Psychosomatics*, **45**, 17–28.

Greenberg, P.E., Leong, S.A. and Birnbaum, H.G. et al. (2003). The economic burden of depression with painful symptoms. *Journal of Clinical Psychiatry*, **64**, 17–23.

Griep, E., Boersma, J., and de Kloet, R. (1993). Altered reactivity of the hypothalamic-pituitary adrenal axis in the primary fibromyalgia syndrome. *Journal of Rheumatology*, **20**, 469–474.

Griep, E.N., Boersma, J.W., Lentjes, E.G. (1998). Function of the hypothalamic-pituitary-adrenal axis in patients with fibromyalgia and low back pain. *Journal of Rheumatology*, **25**, 1374–1381.

Heim, C., Plotsky, P.M., and Nemeroff, C. (2004). Importance of studying the contribution of early adverse experience to neurobiological findings in depression. *Neuropsychopharmacology*, **29**, 641–648.

Heim, C., Dieter Wagner, Maloney, E., Papanicolaou, D.A. et al. (2006). Early adverse experience and risk for chronic fatigue syndrome results from a population-based study. *Archives of General Psychiatry*, **63**, 1258–1266.

Hickie, I., Lloyd, A., Hadzi-Pavlovic, D., Parker, G., Bird, K., and Wakefield, D. (1995). Can the chronic fatigue syndrome be defined by distinct clinical features? *Psychological Medicine*, **25**, 925–935.

Hickie, I., Bennett, B., Lloyd, A., Heath, A., and Martin, N. (1999). Complex genetic and environmental relationships between psychological distress, fatigue and immune functioning: a twin study. *Psychological Medicine*, **29**, 269–277.

Hotopf, M., Noah, N., and Wessely, S. (1996). Chronic fatigue and minor psychiatric morbidity after viral meningitis: a controlled study. *Journal of Neurology Neurosurgery and Psychiatry*, **60**, 504–509.

Hotopf, M., Mayou, R., Wadworth, M., and Wessely, S. (1998). Temporal relationships between physical symptoms and psychiatric disorder: results from a national birth cohort. *British Journal of Psychiatry*, **173**, 255–261.

Imbierowicz, K. and Egle, U.T. (2003). Childhood adversities in patients with fibromyalgia and somatoform pain disorder. *European Journal of Pain*, **7**, 113–119.

Judd, L.L., Akiskal, H.S., Maser, J.D. et al. (1998). Major depressive disorder: a prospective study of residual subthreshold depressive symptoms as predictor of rapid relapse. *Journal of Affective Disorders*, **50**, 97–108.

Juruena, M.F., Cleare, A.J., Bauer, M.E., and Pariante, C.M. (2003). Molecular mechanisms of glucocorticoid receptor sensitivity and relevance to affective disorders. *Acta Neuropsychiatrica*, **15**, 354–367.

Juruena, M.F., Cleare, A.J., Papadopoulos, A. et al. (2007). Prednisolone suppression test as a predictor of outcome in treatment resistant depression. *European Neuropsychopharmacology* **17**, S186–S187.

Kendler, K.S., Eaves, L.J., Walters, E.E., Neale, M.C., Heath, A.C., and Kessler, R.C. (1996). The identification and validation of distinct depressive syndromes in a population-based sample of female twins. *Archives of General Psychiatry*, **53**, 391–399.

Kirnap, M., Colak, R., Eser, C., Ozsoy, O., Tutus, A., and Kelestimur, F. (2001). A comparison between low-dose (1 microg), standard-dose (250 microg) ACTH stimulation tests and insulin tolerance test in the evaluation of hypothalamo-pituitary-adrenal axis in primary fibromyalgia syndrome. *Clinical Endocrinology*, **55**, 455–459.

Kroenke, K. and Mangelsdorff, D. (1989). Common symptoms in ambulatory care: Incidence, evaluation, therapy and outcome. *American Journal of Medicine*, **86**, 262–266.

Lampe, A., Doering, S., Rumpold, G. et al. (2003). Chronic pain syndromes and their relation to childhood abuse and stressful life events. *Journal of Psychosomatic Research*, **54**, 361–367.

Lentjes, E.G., Griep, E.N., Boersma, J.W., Romijn, F.P., and de Kloet, E.R. (1997). Glucocorticoid receptors, fibromyalgia and low back pain. *Psychoneuroendocrinology*, **22**, 603–614.

Liebowitz, M., Quitkin, F., Stewart, J. et al. (1988). Antidepressant specificity in atypical depression. *Archives of General Psychiatry*, **45**, 129–137.

Maes, M., Lin, A., Bonaccorso, S. et al. (1998). Increased 24-hour urinary cortisol excretion in patients with post-traumatic stress disorder and patients with major depression, but not in patients with fibromyalgia. *Acta Psychiatrica Scandinavica*, **98**, 328–335.

Magni, G., Marchetti, M., Moreschi, C., Merskey, H., and Luchini, S.R. (1993). Chronic musculoskeletal pain and depressive symptoms in the National Health and Nutrition Examination. I. Epidemiologic follow-up study. *Pain*, **53**, 163–168.

Magni, G., Moreschi, C., Rigatti-Luchini, S., and Merskey, H. (1994). Prospective study on the relationship between depressive symptoms and chronic musculoskeletal pain. *Pain*, **56**, 289–297.

McBeth, J., Macfarlane, G.J., Hunt, I.M., and Silman, A.J. (2001). Risk factors for persistent chronic widespread pain: a community-based study. *Rheumatology International*, **40**, 95–101.

McBeth, J. and Silman, A.J. (2001). The role of psychiatric disorders in fibromyalgia *Current Rheumaology Reports*, **3**, 157–164.

McCain, G. and Tilbe, K. (1989). Diurnal hormone variation in fibromyalgia syndrome: a comparison with rheumatoid arthritis. *Journal of Rheumatology*, **16** (Suppl 19), 154–157.

McGinn, L.K., Asnis, G.M., and Rubinson, E. (1996). Biological and clinical validation of atypical depression. *Psychiatry Research*, **60**, 191–198.

McGrath, P.J., Stewart, J.W., Harrison, W.M. et al. (1992). Predictive value of symptoms of atypical depression for differential drug treatment outcome. *Journal of Clinical Psychopharmacology*, **12**, 197–202.

Morley, S., Eccleston, C., and Williams, A. (1999). Systematic review and meta-analysis of randomized controlled trials of cognitive behaviour therapy and behaviour therapy for chronic pain in adults, excluding headache. *Pain*, **80**, 1–13.

Ohayon, M.M. and Schatzberg, A.F. (2003). Using chronic pain to predict depresive morbidity in the general population. *Archives of General Psychiatry*, **60**, 9–47.

Okifuji, A. e. a. (2000). Evaluation of the relationship between depression and fibromyalgia syndrome: why aren't all paitents depressed? *Journal of Rheumatology*, **27**, 212–219.

Pawlikowska, T., Chalder, T., Hirsch, S., Wallace, P., Wright, D., and Wessely, S. (1994). A population based study of fatigue and psychological distress. *British Medical Journal*, **308**, 743–746.

Peveler, R., Katona, C., Wessely, S., and Dowrick, C. (2006). Painful symptoms in depression: under-recognised and under-treated? *British Journal of Psychiatry*, **188**, 202–203.

Reeves, W., Lloyd, A., Vernon, S. et al. (2003). Identification of ambiguities in the 1994 chronic fatigue syndrome research case definition and recommendations for resolution. *BioMed Central Health Services Research*, **3**, 25.

Reid, S., Chalder, T., Cleare, A., Hotopf, M., and Wessely, S. (2005). Chronic fatigue syndrome. *Clinical Evidence*, **14**, 1366–1378.

Richards, S. and Cleare, A. J. (2000). Treating fibromyalgia. *Rheumatology International*, **39**, 343–346.

Roberts, A.D.L., Papadopoulos, A.S., Wessely, S., Chalder, T., and Cleare, A.J. (2008). Salivary cortisol output before and after cognitive behavioural therapy for chronic fatigue syndrome. *Journal of Affective Disorders* , doi: 10.1016/j.jad.2008.09.013.

Roberts, A.W.S., Chalder T, Papadopolous A., and Cleare A.J, (2004). Salivary cortisol response to awakening in chronic fatigue syndrome. *British Journal of Psychiatry*, **184**, 136–141.

Rubin, G.J., Hotopf, M., Papadopoulos, A., and Cleare, A.J. (2005). Salivary cortisol as a predictor of postoperative fatigue. *Psychosomatic Medicine*, **67**, 441–447.

Sharpe, M., Chalder, T., Palmer, I., and Wessely, S. (1997). Chronic fatigue syndrome: a practical guide to assessment and management. *General Hospital Psychiatry*, **19**, 195–199.

Sullivan, P.F., Kessler, R.C., and Kendler, K.S. (1998). Latent class analysis of lifetime depressive symptoms in the national comorbidity survey. *American Journal of Psychiatry,* **155**, 1398–1406.

Thase, M.E., Dube, S., Bowler, K. et al. (1996). Hypothalamic-pituitary-adrenocortical activity and response to cognitive behavior therapy in unmedicated, hospitalized depressed patients. *American Journal of Psychiatry,* **153**, 886–891.

van Denderen, J., Boersma, J., Zeinstra, P., Hollander, A., and van Neerbos, B. (1992). Physiological effects of exhaustive physical exercise in primary fibromyalgia syndrome (PFS): is PFS a disorder of neuroendocrine reactivity? *Scandinavian Journal of Rheumatology,* **21**, 35–37.

von Korff, M., Le Resche, L., and Dworkin, S.F. (1993). First onset of common pain symptoms: a prospective study of depression as a risk factor. *Pain,* **55**, 251–258.

Walker, E.A., Keegan, D., Gardner, G., Sullivan, M., Bernstein, D., and Katon, W.J. (1997). Psychosocial factors in fibromyalgia compared with rheumatoid arthritis: II. Sexual, physical, and emotional abuse and neglect. *Psychosomatic Medicine,* **59**, 572–577.

Walker, E., Katon, W., Harrop Griffiths, J., Holm, L., Russo, J. and Hickok, L.R. (1988). Relationship of chronic pelvic pain to psychiatric diagnoses and childhood sexual abuse. *Am J Psychiatry,* **145**, 75–80.

Wessely, S. and Powell, R. (1989). Fatigue syndromes: a comparison of chronic 'postviral' fatigue with neuromuscular and affective disorder. *Journal of Neurology Neurosurgery and Psychiatry,* **52**, 940–948.

Wessely, S., Hotopf, M., and Sharpe, M. (1998). *Chronic Fatigue and its Syndromes.* Oxford University Press: Oxford.

Wessely, S., Nimnuan, C., and Sharpe, M. (1999). Functional somatic syndromes: one or many? *Lancet,* **354**, 936–939.

Williams, A.C., Nicholas, M.K., Richardson, P.H. et al. (1993). Evaluation of a cognitive behavioural programme for rehabilitating patients with chronic pain. *British Journal of General Practice,* **43**, 513–518.

Chapter 20

Explaining the association between depression and mortality: a life course epidemiology approach

Matthew Hotopf and Max Henderson

Introduction

There is an increasingly convincing literature demonstrating in general population samples that individuals with psychiatric disorders have increased mortality (Harris and Barraclough, 1998). This applies not just for depression, but even more starkly for psychotic disorders, eating disorders, and substance use disorders. Much of this excess is accounted for by suicide (Saha et al. 2007), self-neglect, and severe adversity such as homelessness, all of which arise directly out of mental disorder. Exposure to known physical health risk factors (e.g. smoking, intravenous drug use) or – in eating disorders – directly to starvation (Keel et al. 2003), may account for the very poor outcome of many psychiatric disorders.

People with depression die younger than the non-depressed (Ganguli et al. 2002; Hoyer et al. 2000; Mykletun et al. 2007; Takeshita et al. 2002; Wulsin et al. 1999b;). Because of study heterogeneity it is difficult to gain a clear global estimate of the excess mortality associated with depression, but one systematic review suggested that the better studies indicated a relative risk of approximately 1.7, indicating a 70% increase in mortality rates (Wulsin et al. 1999a). Although this excess risk at the individual level may not be as high as the mortality associated with other mental disorders, the high prevalence of depression in the population means that – assuming a causal relationship exists – depression may contribute to more deaths than other psychiatric disorders. Comparable population-based data for other health conditions is hard to come by, mainly due to the lack of suitable cohorts. Occupational cohorts, albeit with caveats like the healthy worker effect (Howe et al. 1988) provide the best approximation; for example, in the GAZEL study, a prospective occupational cohort of 13 077 men and 4 871 women aged 37–51 from the National Gas and Electricity Company, France, the hazard ratio for death (adjusted for age, sex, and socio-economic position) was 5.2 for cancer, 1.4 for diabetes, 1.8 for chronic bronchitis, and 2.1 for coronary heart disease (Kivimaki et al. 2008)

More dramatic associations exist between depression and adverse health outcomes in people with established physical disease. Patients with acute physical illness seem to survive less long if they also have depression (Arfken et al. 1999; Herrmann et al. 2000; Silverstone, 1990). The disease most closely studied has been acute myocardial infarction (MI) where depression, if present shortly after the time of the infarct is associated with further cardiovascular events (Frasure-Smith et al. 1993; 2000). However the association is not confined to acute MI and depression, when comorbid with other physical diseases such as stroke (House et al. 2001; Morris et al. 1993; Williams et al. 2004), HIV/AIDS (Patterson et al. 1996), renal disease (Peterson et al. 1991), and cancer (Schulz et al. 1996), has been observed to be associated with higher mortality, in most, though not all case series.

In the population studies on depression and mortality, it is difficult to rule out that the association is confounded by the presence of physical disease, which is a powerful risk factor for depression and would be predicted to be associated with increased mortality. In Wulsin's systematic review, it is remarkable how few studies control for the presence of physical disease (Wulsin et al. 1999a), but the association tends to persist even when they do. In individuals with established physical disease, the association between depression and poor outcomes does not seem to be accounted for by measures of disease severity, so in Frasure Smith and colleagues' seminal study (Frasure-Smith et al. 1993) on mortality following MI, analyses were controlled for cardiac function and still found substantial impacts of depression.

Depression as a cause of cardiac disease

If we accept that these associations exist, and are not merely confounded by disease severity, how best do we account for them? We suggest that there are three broad pathways (Fig. 20.1). The first two are explored by Andrew Steptoe, in Chapter 18 of this book. One such pathways suggest that depression is directly 'toxic', whether due to increased platelet aggregation (Musselman et al. 1996; 2000), altered autonomic function (Broadley et al. 2005; Carney et al. 2000; 2005), or immune dysregulation (Pasic et al. 2003). These physical consequences of depression ultimately lead to increased risk of cardiovascular disease (Lett et al. 2004). The usual pathophysiological explanations given for these mechanisms are the observed changes to HPA function, immune dysregulation, or alterations to serotonergic pathways all of which have been observed in depression (Carney et al. 2005; Evans et al. 2005; Musselman et al. 1998). (Several chapters in this book

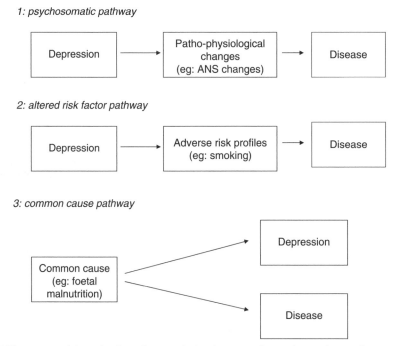

Fig. 20.1 Three potential mechanisms for association between depression and mortality.

discuss in details some of these biological mechanisms.) One implication of this pathway is that by preventing or treating depression, we might be able to reverse the underlying mechanisms involved and reduce cardiovascular mortality (Carney et al. 1999).

Depression and cardiac risk factors

A second set of explanations is that depression – like other mental disorders – marks out individuals who are likely to have a range of adverse physical health risk factors. Thus patients with depression are more likely to smoke (Ismail et al. 2000), less likely to take exercise (Hassmen et al. 2000), and more likely to be obese (Roberts et al. 2000; Simon et al. 2006), all of which are recognized risk factors for coronary heart disease. In studies of cohorts of patients with established physical disease, depression may also influence outcome via its impact on treatment adherence or participation in rehabilitation (Ades et al. 1992). Many studies which have assessed the impact of depression on cardiovascular disease have failed to control for multiple such risk factors in a single model, although when they do, there still tends to be a relatively strong independent impact of depression (Surtees et al. 2008). Given that depression is a chronic, relapsing and remitting disorder, often present over many years, the cumulative impact of exposure to such risk factors may require longitudinal measures, which are rarely available. Controlling for life style risk factors in a single 'snap shot' is unlikely fully to control for risk factors like smoking. In summary, although it is highly plausible that the association between depression and physical disease incidence or mortality could be explained by such mechanisms, and although many previous studies have not controlled for such pathway variables adequately, those studies which do control for them tend to find the association persists.

If this second set of mechanisms was to blame for the association between depression and mortality, it might also imply that strategies to reduce prevalence of depression would impact on cardiovascular disease incidence, and in clinical samples the identification and treatment of depression would reduce mortality. Although the association with depression is not direct, depression is still acting in a presumably reversible way, to worsen physical health. The following section briefly reviews the ambitious trials which have sought to improve physical health outcomes following acute MI by treating depression.

Treatment of depression in acute MI

A few large, well-conducted, randomized controlled trials in samples of patients with depression following MI have now been reported, and this area of research is also discussed in Chapter 18 of this book. The Enhancing Recovery in Cardiac Disease study (ENRICHD) (Writing Committee for the ENRICHD Investigators, 2003) randomized 2 481 post-MI patients with low perceived social support or depression to receive cognitive therapy with antidepressants (usually sertraline) when indicated versus usual care. While the trial showed that the intervention was an effective treatment for depression and perceived low social support, there were no differences in cardiac event free survival, the primary cardiac outcome, over a long follow-up period. Subsequent subgroup analyses have suggested that the patients in the intervention group whose symptoms were refractory to the intervention were at greater risk of cardiac events (Carney et al. 2004) and that treatment with selective serotonin re-uptake inhibitors appeared to confer some benefit against future cardiac events (Taylor et al. 2005). In SADHART patients with acute MI and major depressive disorder were randomized to receive sertraline or placebo. Over the 24-week follow-up period there were no statistically significant benefits of sertraline in terms of cardiac outcomes, although most such outcomes (including death from cardiac causes) were less common in the sertraline treated group. The trial had an unexpectedly weak impact on depression symptoms, with no difference in total change score on the Hamilton Rating Scale for Depression, although some benefits in other depression related outcomes. In the MIND-IT study (van Melle et al. 2007) acute MI patients with depression were randomized either to receive antidepressants (with mirtazepine as first choice, but some latitude in the physician's ability to choose) versus care as usual (which could include antidepressants). The intervention had no impact either on depressive symptoms or on cardiac events. These trials as a group are impressive and ambitious endeavours, but their results sadly suggest that treating depression in acute MI is difficult (i.e. treatments for depression which in other contexts are well proven have been ineffective) and that the treatment has no impact on the primary cardiac outcomes under study.

While these results are disappointing, two points should be borne in mind. First, these results do not imply treatment of depression in these contexts is pointless – they generally found that the interventions were effective in treating the symptoms of depression, and this is clearly a valid end in itself. Secondly, the failure to find an improvement in event-free survival does not disprove the pathways described above. However it does suggest that treating depression in this population is unlikely to have the anticipated benefits on cardiac survival.

'Common cause' explanations

The final set of explanations for the impact of depression on mortality are our main focus in this chapter. We suggest that the relationship may be explained by the pleiotropic effects of early risk factors which may impact both on depression, and on physical health. The observed association between depression and heart disease is therefore confounded by these 'upstream' risk factors. If this explanation was correct, population-based approaches to prevention or treatment of depression would be unlikely to impact on incidence of, or mortality from, physical diseases. In the remaining part of this chapter, we shall speculate on how some of these pathways derived from life course epidemiology may explain the increased mortality associated with depression.

Life course epidemiology

Kuh and colleagues define life course epidemiology as the following:

> [T]he study of long term effects on later health or disease risk of physical or social exposures during gestation, childhood, adolescence, young adulthood and later adult life. The aim is to elucidate biological, behavioural, and psychosocial processes that operate across an individual's life course, or across generations, to influence the development of disease risk.
>
> (Kuh and Ben-Shlomo, 2004)

While psychologists and psychiatrists have understood the importance of developmental perspectives to the origins of mental disorders since before Freud, life course approaches in general epidemiology are a more recent development. This came about partly due to a dissatisfaction with the prevailing risk factor approach to chronic disease epidemiology. In the 1940s and 1950s the epidemiologists studying chronic diseases concentrated on finding risk factors or exposures measured in the middle years of adult life and typically associated with life-style, such as smoking, obesity, or hypercholestrolaemia. This approach proved immensely fruitful, particularly in identifying smoking as a powerful risk factor for many diseases, but it became increasingly apparent that many risk factors could be traced back in time to adolescence or childhood. Famous studies of post-mortem findings of US Armed Forces personnel killed in the Korean and Vietnam wars indicated that atheroma was already present in young men long before any clinical indication of heart disease (Enos et al. 1953; McNamara et al. 1971). Clearly it was necessary to go back in time to understand why many of these men killed in prime physical health were already showing signs of cardiovascular disease.

A second impetus for understanding developmental origins of disease came from social epidemiology, and particularly from the study of powerful variation in mortality, and the realization from studies such as the original Whitehall cohort and Whitehall II that social class and disadvantage had important impacts on hard physical health outcomes. Mortality among the lowest grades of civil servants was approximately 1.5–3 times that of the highest (Marmot and Shipley, 1996), and this difference was not accounted for by smoking, cholesterol, or hypertension (Smith et al. 1990). If low social status and social deprivation are risk factors for CHD, they presumably exert their impact over a prolonged period of time, and need to be seen in a longitudinal context, possibly extending back to childhood.

Two broad approaches to understanding the impact of early risk factors on later ones have been studied (Kuh and Ben-Shlomo, 2004; Kuh et al. 2003). The first – that of programming in critical development – is a familiar concept in neuroscience, where it is well established that vicissitudes at key stages of development can have relatively specific impacts on the development of functions such as vision or cognition. In life course epidemiology, the approach has been championed by David Barker, with a number of elegant studies demonstrating how babies of low birthweight grow up to be adults with high blood pressure (Barker and Barker, 2006; Barker et al. 2002; 2006), type II diabetes (Barker and Barker, 1999) and coronary heart disease (Barker et al. 1993). The Barker hypothesis suggests that the foetal environment has a key function in programming later development.

The second approach is that of accumulation of risk through the life course (Kuh et al. 1997). This model does not emphasize the importance of an event taking place during a critical period, but rather that adversity may beget further adversity. Growing up in a deprived environment may affect life chances in many ways, including direct biological mechanisms owing to a range of risk factors such as poor nutrition, greater exposure to accidents, passive smoke. Less direct mechanisms may also have considerable impact, such as the impact of early adversity on educational participation and attainment, early child-rearing, lower status occupational roles, crime, and so on. While such trajectories are not pre-determined, in a probabilistic manner individuals who are exposed to early disadvantage may accumulate a wide range of adverse risk factors over a life course.

If the association between depression and cardiovascular disease is due to shared 'upstream' risk factors, what might these be, and how might we go about exploring the association further?

Genetic mechanisms

The first possibility is shared genes. The details of such a mechanism are outside the scope of this chapter, but are reviewed by McCaffery and colleagues (McCaffery et al. 2006). There are a number of theoretical reasons why genes which convey risk for coronary heart disease might also increase risk of depression. Candidate genes identified included genes involved in inflammation or serotonin regulation. Although there are a range of candidate mechanisms, there is very little direct evidence to support these suppositions. The McCaffery review identified only one large (2 731 pairs) twin study that overlap in depression, and cardiovascular disease was due to shared genes, with approximately 20% of the overlap being explained by this mechanism (Scherrer et al. 2003). Another small (173 twin pairs) study has found the reverse – that the phenotypic overlap between depression and metabolic syndrome phenotypes was mainly due to shared environmental pathways and not to genes (McCaffery et al. 2003). Further twin studies could potentially determine whether the same or different genes are likely to be responsible. The genetics of affective disorders is specifically discussed in Chapters 4, 5, 6, and 23 of this book.

Foetal programming

The second possibility is that depression, like cardiovascular disease, is associated with low birthweight. It is not necessary here to review the weight of evidence indicating that in affluent Western populations at least, low birthweight is associated with a range of physical health outcomes, including type 2 diabetes, coronary heart disease, and hypertension. Is low birthweight also associated with an increased risk of depression? Table 20.1 summarizes some of the studies to have addressed this issue, including results from the three British birth cohorts. These three studies, representing individuals born in 1946, 1958, and 1970, each consisting of population samples followed over many years, and with multiple ascertainment of depressive symptoms over the lifespan, find associations between low birthweight and depression, albeit with somewhat inconsistent results in the 1970 cohort. The Hertfordshire cohort – used for much of Barker's seminal work on cardiovascular disease, showed an impact of low birthweight on depressive symptoms at follow-up, as well as a suggestion that slow growth in early life was associated with increased risk of later suicide. The Aberdeen Children of the 1950s cohort and the Norwegian Hunt study have found broadly similar results, although in both these studies the impact of low birthweight was limited to individuals who were small despite full-term gestation. Results from the Dutch famine cohort studies indicated that individuals exposed in the second and third trimesters to (maternal) starvation were more likely over the course of their adult life to be admitted to hospital with severe depression. Thus, the observational studies available indicate that there is an association, albeit a small to moderate one. The main studies have also been able to control for a wide variety of potential confounders, such as maternal smoking, parental social class, and adult physical disease.

If small babies are at risk of depression and metabolic syndrome, what could the mechanism be? One promising candidate is hypothalamic pituitary adrenal axis reactivity. In an analysis of three samples (including the Hertfordshire cohort), Phillips and colleagues showed a consistent association between low birthweight and increased fasting plasma cortisol taken as a single measurement.[57] The association could not be accounted for by smoking, social class, or obesity. Further, plasma cortisol levels were also associated with adult hypertension, giving some credence to the idea that the HPA axis may be involved in the pathogenic pathway between low birthweight and hypertension. Similar findings have been reported by others, although the relationship has not always been replicated, so in one study a more sensitive measure of 24-hour salivary cortisol not associated with birthweight,[59] and in another a more complex inverted u relationship existed between HPA activity and birthweight (Rautanen et al. 2006). Put together, the literature on HPA axis function and birthweight is not yet conclusive, but is certainly strongly suggestive. Given the well-known association between HPA axis function and depression, it is possible that HPA axis reactivity may be one mechanism for potential common pathways between low birthweight on the one hand and depression and cardiovascular disease risk factors on the other. The role of the HPA axis in programming is specifically discussed in Chapter 8 of this book, while the HPA axis is discussed throughout several other chapters.

Social causes

While proponents of the Barker hypothesis sees foetal and neonatal development as a critical period in which certain metabolic pathways are programmed, proponents of early life social causes of disease would see disadvantages as having a cumulative impact, with the build up of

Table 20.1 Studies on low birthweight and subsequent depression

Reference	Sample (N for the analyses presented)	Exposure	Outcome	Variables controlled for	Results
Colman et al. 2007	MRC National Survey of Health and Development (1946 Birth Cohort) $N = 4627$	Birthweight	Six latent longitudinal classes of individuals with different patterns of depressive symptoms over the life-course	Gender, father's social class, number of people in the home, parental separation and divorce, parental education	Low birthweight associated with worsening course of depressive symptoms across lifespan
Cheung et al. 2002	National Child Development Survey (1958 Birth Cohort). Population-based birth cohort. $N = 9731$	Birthweight Growth to age 7	Depressive symptoms on Rutter Malaise Inventory at 23, 33, and 42	Social class, maternal smoking	Low birthweight and slow growth to age 7 was associated with higher scores Malaise Inventory
Gale and Martyn 2004	British Cohort Study (1970 Birth Cohort). Population-based prospective birth cohort. $N = 8292$	Birthweight	General Health Questionnaire 12, at 16 years; Rutter Malaise Inventory at 26 years	Father's social class, gestational age, maternal smoking in pregnancy, maternal depression, maternal separations, parental divorce	Moderate effect of low birthweight on depression for men, but not women at 16, and women but not men at 26.
Osler et al. 2005	Population-based cohort study of men born in Copenhagen in 1953, linked to registry data on psychiatric service use ($N = 10753$)	Birthweight and Ponderal index	Psychiatric admissions for depression aged 15–49 years	Paternal social class and parental marital status	No association observed between birthweight and hospitalization
Berle et al. 2006	Norwegian population-based cross-sectional study (Nord-Trondelag Health Study: HUNT) with record linkage to birth records ($N = 7806$)	Gestational length, birthweight, being small for gestational age	Depression measured on the Hospital Anxiety and Depression Scale	Educational attainment and socio-economic status (adult)	Small effect of being small for gestational age. No impact of birthweight per se.
Wiles et al. 2005	Aberdeen Children of the 1950s study – a retrospective cohort study $N = 5572$	Gestational length and birthweight	Four items from the General Health Questionnaire-12	Multiple birth, maternal age, father's social class, gender, adult social class and marital status, IQ and childhood neurotic traits	No impact of birthweight or gestational age, but low birthweight babies born at full term had higher risk of depressive symptoms.

(continued)

Table 20.1 (Continued) Studies on low birthweight and subsequent depression

Reference	Sample (N for the analyses presented)	Exposure	Outcome	Variables controlled for	Results
Thompson et al. 2001	Hertfordshire cohort. Retrospective cohort study using historical data on birthweight and early growth N = 882	Birthweight and weight at one year	Depression measured at age 68 on the Geriatric Depression Scale	Physical illness and social class at birth current social class, recent bereavement	For men but not women there was a substantial impact of low birthweight on depression symptoms.
Barker et al. 1995	Hertfordshire cohort 10 141 boys and 5 585 girls born 1911–1930	Birthweight and weight at age one	Death from suicide	Social class	No impact of birthweight on suicide, but babies who did not gain weight from birth to one year had substantially higher suicide rate.
Brown et al. 1995	Dutch famine cohort. Cohort of individuals born around the time of the Dutch Hunger winter of 1944	Trimester of pregnancy during which mother likely to be exposed to severe food deprivation	Admission with ICD-9 depressive psychosis	Sex, season of birth	Exposure during the second trimester was associated with increased risk of incident depression in men, but not women
Brown et al. 2000	Expanded version of (Brown et al.1995)	Trimester of pregnancy during which mother likely to be exposed to severe food deprivation	Admission with ICD-9 depressive psychosis		Exposure in second and third trimesters was associated with moderate increased risk of depression on men and women
Patton et al. 2004	Case control study nested in a study of adolescent health. N = 63 cases of depression and 112 controls	Birthweight and gestational age recalled by parent	CIS-R and CIDI depression	Gender, maternal smoking, parental education, separation, history of depression, serious illness in first year of life	Substantial association between depression and prematurity or low birthweight

what has been called 'health capital' (Kuh et al. 1997). To see how this might happen, it is worth considering a single life event in childhood, namely parental divorce. Work from the various British birth cohorts indicates that parental divorce in childhood and adolescence has a range of impacts in later life. Thus in the 1946 birth cohort parental divorce – which then was a relatively rare event – was associated with increased bed-wetting throughout childhood, poorer educational attainment (even taking account of socio-economic status), and lower income in adult life (Kuh et al. 1990; Wadsworth et al. 1990). It was also associated with poorer cognitive performance in adolescence (Richards et al. 2004), shorter adult trunk length (Wadsworth et al. 2002), poorer mental health, and greater alcohol consumption in later life (Kuh et al. 1990; Power et al. 1990; Rodgers et al. 1997). While physical health outcomes have not been examined in as much depth, it seems likely that an exposure which has such diverse impacts could affect physical disease risk behaviours and physical health. It is no doubt true that the 'exposure' of parental divorce is more complex than typical risk behaviours like smoking or diet, as it probably represents a wide range of adversities and as such is probably better seen as a marker for parental conflict, family disruption, and (usually) paternal separation. These component adversities are likely then to impact on proximal variables such as educational attainment or early sexual activity, which then may impact on occupational status and so on.

Parental divorce illustrates how just one social factor in childhood may have important impacts on both later physical and mental health. Childhood abuse and neglect is a much broader (and harder to measure) category, which might plausibly have a similar impact. There is no question that abuse and neglect have powerful impact on later mental health outcomes, including depression and anxiety, substance misuse and other externalizing traits. There are relatively few high-quality cohort studies on the impact of childhood adversity on physical health. It is also necessary to take account of 'softer' physical health outcomes, such as physical symptoms or illness behaviours related to minor physical illness, since these variables may not reflect physical disease itself and may be strongly influenced by personality. However, there is some evidence that children who have been abused have more objectively measurable adverse physical health outcomes, relevant to cardiovascular disease. Thus several studies have found an association between childhood victimhood and adult obesity (Alvarez et al. 2007; Lissau et al. 1994; Williamson et al. 2002; Whitaker et al. 2007), hypertension (Ekeberg et al. 1990), type 2 diabetes (Thomas et al. 2008) and coronary heart disease itself (Dong et al. 2004), even after controlling for socio-economic status.

It is still a matter of speculation as to how childhood adversity might bring about such long-term physical health problems. Repetti and colleagues (Repetti et al. 2002) in a detailed review discussed potential pathophysiological pathways which might account for the association between childhood adversity on the one hand, and physical or mental health outcomes on the other. They identified three main pathways, including the serotonin system, sympathetic adrenomedullary activity, and the HPA. Given the well-established relationship between depression and the HPA and the multiple physiological impacts of glucocorticoids on metabolism (Whitworth et al. 2000), it is tempting to suggest that – as in the literature relating to the Barker hypothesis – the HPA provides a common pathophysiological pathway from early experience of abuse and neglect to physical and mental disorders, and there is indeed evidence that early adversity is associated with altered HPA function, even in the absence of depression (e.g. Heim et al. 1998). It remains to be seen whether the pleiotropic impacts of childhood maltreatment is a sufficient explanation for the relationship between depression and physical disease, although it is intriguing that maltreatment in early life is associated with raised inflammatory markers in early adult life (Danese et al. 2007) an association which implies wider pleiotropic impacts of adversity than heart disease and depression.

Conclusions

We suggest then that to understand comorbidity, and in particular the apparent negative impact of depression on mortality, it is necessary to take account of the pleiotropic impact of both genes and early environment. To study this further, we suggest that behavioural genetic studies using twin designs may be helpful in determining whether there could be common genetic risk factors for depression and coronary heart disease (or more likely related phenotypes such as dyslipidaemia, obesity, hypertension, and insulin resistance). Further, life course epidemiological studies using large birth cohorts may be able to determine whether early environmental factors such as low birthweight or social adversities also have pleiotropic impacts.

Acknowledgement

Hotopf is funded by the South London and Maudsley NHS Foundation Trust, King's College London NIHR Biomedical Research Centre. Henderson is funded by the UK Medical Research Council.

References

Ades, P.A., Waldmann, M.L., McCann, W.J., and Weaver, S.O. (1992). Predictors of cardiac rehabilitation participation in older coronary patients, *Arch Intern Med.* **152**, 1033–1035.

Alvarez, J., Pavao, J., Baumrind, N. et al. (2007). The relationship between child abuse and adult obesity among California women. *American Journal of Preventive Medicine*, **33**, 28–33.

Arfken, C.L., Lichtenberg, P.A., and Tancer, M.E. (1999).Cognitive impairment and depression predict mortality in medically ill older adults. *Journal of Gerontology*, **54** A, M152–M156. Ref Type: Generic

Barker, D.J.P., Gluckman, P.D., Godfrey, K.M., Harding, J.E., Owens, J.A., and Robinson, J. S. (1993), Fetal nutrition and cardiovasular disease in adult life, *Lancet*, **341**, 938–941.

Barker, D.J.P., Osmond, C., Rodin, I., Fall, C.H.D., and Winter, P.D. (1995), Low weight gain in infancy and suicide in adult life, *British Medical Journal*, **311**, 1203.

Barker, D.J. and Barker, D.J. (1999). The fetal origins of type 2 diabetes mellitus. *Annals of Internal Medicine*, **130** Pt 1, 322–324.

Barker, D.J., Forsen, T., Eriksson, J.G. et al. (2002). Growth and living conditions in childhood and hypertension in adult life: a longitudinal study. *Journal of Hypertension*, **20**, 1951–1956.

Barker, D.J. and Barker, D.J.P. (2006). Birth weight and hypertension. *Hypertension*, **48**, 357–358.

Barker, D.J., Bagby, S.P., Hanson, M.A. et al. (2006). Mechanisms of disease: in utero programming in the pathogenesis of hypertension. *Nature Clinical Practice Nephrology*, **2**, 700–707.

Berle, J.O., Mykletun, A., Daltveit, A.K. et al. (2006). Outcomes in adulthood for children with foetal growth retardation: a linkage study from the Nord-Trondelag Health Study (HUNT) and the Medical Birth Registry of Norway. *Acta Psychiatrica Scandinavica*, **113**, 501–509.

Broadley, A.J.M., Frenneaux, M.P., Moskvina, V., Jones, C.J.H., and Korszun, A. (2005). Baroreflex Sensitivity Is Reduced in Depression. *Psychosomatic Medicine*, **67**, 648–651.

Brown, A.S., Susser, E.S., Lin, S.P., Neugebauer, R., and Gorman, J.M. (1995). Increased risk of affective disorders in males after second trimester prenatal exposure to the Dutch hunger winter of 1944–1945. *The British Journal of Psychiatry*, **166**, 601–606.

Brown, A.S., van Os,J., Driessens, C., Hoek, H.W., and Susser, E.S. (2000). Further evidence of relation between prenatal famine and major affective disorder. *American Journal of Psychiatry*, **157**,190–195.

Carney, R.M., Freedland, K.E., Veith, R.C., and Jaffe, A.S. (1999). Can treating depression reduce mortality after an acute myocardial infarction? *Psychosomatic Medicine*, **61**, 666–675.

Carney, R.M., Freedland, K.E., Stein, P.K., Skala, J.A., Hoffman, P., and Jaffe, A. S. (2000), Change in heart rate and heart rate variability during treatment for depression in patients with coronary heart disease. *Psychosomatic Medicine*, **62**, 639–647.

Carney, R.M., Blumenthal, J.A., Freedland, K.E. et al. (2004). Depression and late mortality after myocardial infarction in the Enhancing Recovery in Coronary Heart Disease (ENRICHD) Study. *Psychosomatic Medicine*, **66**, 466–474.

Carney, R.M., Freedland, K.E., and Veith, R.C. (2005). Depression, the autonomic nervous system, and coronary heart disease. *Psychosomatic Medicine*, **67** Suppl 1, S29–S33.

Cheung, Y.B., Khoo, K.S., Karlberg, J., and Machin, D. (2002). Association between psychological symptoms in adults and growth in early life: longitudinal follow up study. *British Medical Journal*, **325**, 749.

Colman, I., Ploubidis, G.B., Wadsworth, M.E., Jones, P.B., and Croudace, T.J. (2007), A longitudinal typology of symptoms of depression and anxiety over the life course. *Biological Psychiatry*, **62**, 1265–1271.

Danese, A., Pariante, C.M., Caspi, A. et al. (2007). Childhood maltreatment predicts adult inflammation in a life-course study. *Proceedings of the National Academy of Sciences of the United States of America*, **104**, 1319–1324.

Dong, M., Giles, W.H., Felitti, V.J. et al. (2004). Insights into causal pathways for ischemic heart disease: adverse childhood experiences study. *Circulation*, **110**, 1761–1766.

Ekeberg, O., Kjeldsen, S.E., Eide, I. et al. (1990). Childhood traumas and psychosocial characteristics of 50-year-old men with essential hypertension. *Journal of Psychosomatic Research*, **34**, 643–649.

Enos, M.W.F., Holmes, L.C.R.H., and Beyer, C.J. (1953). Coronary disease among United States soldiers killed in action in Korea. *Journal of the American Medical Association*, **152**, 1090–1093.

Evans, D.L., Charney, D.S., Lewis, L. et al. (2005), Mood disorders in the medically ill: scientific review and recommendations. *Biological Psychiatry*, **58**, 175–189.

Frasure-Smith, N., Lesperance, F., and Talajic, M. (1993). Depression following myocardial infarction: impact on 6-month survival. *JAMA*, **270**, 1819–1825.

Frasure-Smith, N., Lesperance, F., Gravel, G. et al. (2000). Social support, depression, and mortality during the first year after myocardial infarction. *Circulation*, **101**, 1919–1924.

Gale, C. R. and Martyn, C. N. (2004), Birth weight and later risk of depression in a national birth cohort. *The British Journal of Psychiatry*, **184**, 28–33.

Ganguli, M., Dodge, H.H., and Mulsant, B. H. (2002). Rates and predictors of mortality in an aging, rural, community-based cohort: the role of depression. *Archives of General Psychiatry*, **59**, 1046–1052.

Harris, E. C. and Barraclough, B. (1998). Excess mortality of mental disorder. *British Journal of Psychiatry*, **173**, 11–53.

Hassmen, P., Koivula, N., and Uutela, A. (2000). Physical exercise and psychological well-being: a population based study in Finland. *Preventive Medicine*, **30**, 17–25.

Heim, C., Ehlert, U., Hanker, J.P., and Hellhammer, D.H. (1998). Abuse related posttraumatic stress disroder and alterations of the hypothalamic-pituitary-adrenal axis in women with chronic pelvic pain. *Psychosomatic Medicine*, **60**. 309–318.

Herrmann, C., Brand-Driehorst, S., Kaminsky, B., Leibing, E., Staats, H., and Ruger, U. (2000). Diagnostic Groups and depressed mood as predictors of 22-month mortality in medical inpatients. *Psychosomatic Medicine*, **60**, 570–577.

House, A., Knapp, P., and Bamford, J. (2001). Mortality at 12 and 24 months after stroke may be associated with depressive symptoms at 1 month. *Stroke*, **32**, 696–701.

Howe G, Chiarelli A, and Lindsay J. (1988). Components and modifiers of the healthy worker effect: evidence from three occupational cohorts and implications for industrial compensation. *Am J Epidem.* **128**, 1364–1375.

Hoyer, E.H., Mortensen, P.B., and Olesen, A.V. (2000). Mortality and causes of death in a total national sample of patients with affective disorders admitted for the first time between 1973 and 1993. *British Journal of Psychiatry*, **176**, 76–82.

Ismail, K., Sloggett, A., and De, S.B. (2000). Do common mental disorders increase cigarette smoking? Results from five waves of a population-based panel cohort study. *American Journal of Epidemiology*, **152**, 651–657.

Keel, P.K., Dorer, D.J., Eddy, K.T., Franko, D., Charatan, D.L., and Herzog, D.B. (2003). Predictors of mortality in eating disorders. *Archives of General Psychiatry*, **60**, 179–183.

Kivimaki, M., Head, J., Ferrie, J. et al. (2008). Sickness absence as a prognostic marker for common chronic conditions: analysis of mortality in the GAZEL study. *Occ Environ Med*, **65**, 820–826.

Kuh, D. and Ben-Shlomo, Y. (2004). *A Life Course Approach to Chronic Disease Epidemiology: Tracing the Origins of Ill-Health from Early to Adult Life*, 2nd Edition. Oxford, Oxford University Press.

Kuh, D., Ben-Shlomo, Y., Lynch, J., Hallqvist, J., and Power, C. (2003). Life course epidemiology. *Journal of Epidemiology and Community Health*, **57**, 778–783.

Kuh, D., Maclean, M., Kuh, D., and Maclean, M. (1990). Women's childhood experience of parental separation and their subsequent health and socioeconomic status in adulthood. *Journal of Biosocial Science*, **22**, 121–135.

Kuh, D., Power, C., Blane, D., and Bartley, M. (1997). Social pathways between childhood and adult health. In Kuh, D. and Ben-Shlomo, Y. (eds.), *A life course approach to chronic disease epidemiology*, 1st Edition, pp. 169–198. Oxford, Oxford University Press.

Lett, H.S., Blumenthal, J.A., Babyak, M.A. et al. (2004). Depression as a risk factor for coronary artery disease: evidence, mechanisms, and treatment. *Psychosomatic Medicine*, **66**, 305–315.

Lissau, I., Sorensen, T.I., Lissau, I., and Sorensen, T.I. (1994). Parental neglect during childhood and increased risk of obesity in young adulthood. *Lancet*, **343**, 324–327.

Marmot, M.G. and Shipley, M. (1996). Do socioeconomic differences in mortality persist after retirement? 25 Year follow up of civil servants from the first Whitehall study. *British Medical Journal*, **313**, 1177–1180.

McCaffery, J.M., Frasure-Smith, N., Dube, M.P., Theroux, P. et al. (2006). Common genetic vulnerability to depressive symptoms and coronary artery disease: a review and development of candidate genes related to inflammation and serotonin. *Psychosomatic Medicine*, **68**, 187–200.

McCaffery, J.M., Niaura, R., Todaro, J.F. et al. (2003). Depressive symptoms and metabolic risk in adult male twins enrolled in the National Heart, Lung, and Blood Institute twin study. *Psychosomatic Medicine*, **65**, 490–497.

McNamara, M.J.J., Molot, M. M.A., Stremple, M.J.F., and Cutting, R. T. (1971). Coronary artery disease in combat casualties in Vietnam. *Journal of the American Medical Association*, **216**, 1185–1187.

Morris, P.L.P., Robinson, R.G., and Samuels, J. (1993). Depression, introversion and mortality following stroke. *Australian and New Zealand Journal Psychiatry*, **27**, 443–449.

Musselman, D.L., Marzec, U.M., Manatunga, A. et al. (2000).Platelet reactivity in depressed patients treated with paroxetine: preliminary findings. *Archives of General Psychiatry*, **57**, 875–882.

Musselman, D.L., Tomer, A., Manatunga, A.K. et al. (1996). Exaggerated platelet reactivity in major depression. *American Journal of Psychiatry*, **153**, 1313–1317.

Musselman, D.L., Evans, D.L., and Nemeroff, C. B. (1998). The relationship of depression to cardiovascular disease: epidemiology, biology, and treatment. *Archives of General Psychiatry*, **55**, 580–592.

Mykletun, A., Bjerkeset, O., Dewey, M., Prince, M., Overland, S., and Stewart, R. (2007). Anxiety, depression, and cause-specific mortality: The HUNT Study. *Psychosomatic Medicine*, **69**, 323–331.

Osler, M., Nordentoft, M., Andersen, A.M., Osler, M., Nordentoft, M., and Andersen, A.M.N. (2005). Birth dimensions and risk of depression in adulthood: cohort study of Danish men born in 1953. *British Journal of Psychiatry*, **186**, 400–403.

Pasic, J., Levy, W.C., and Sullivan, M.D. (2003). Cytokines in Depression and Heart Failure. *Psychosomatic Medicine*, **65**, 181–193.

Patterson, T.L., Shaw, W.S., Semple, S.J. et al. (1996). Relationship of psychosocial factors to HIV disease progression. *Ann.Behav.Med.*, **18**, 30–39.

Patton, G.C., Coffey, C., Carlin, J.B., Olsson, C.A., and Morley, R. (2004). Prematurity at birth and adolescent depressive disorder. *The British Journal of Psychiatry*, **184**, 446–447.

Peterson, R.A., Kimmel, P.L., Sacks, C.R. et al. (1991). Depression, perception of illness and mortality in patients with end-stage renal disease. *International Journal of Psychiatry in Medicine*, **21**, 343–354.

Power, C., Estaugh, V., Power, C., and Estaugh, V. (1990). The role of family formation and dissolution in shaping drinking behaviour in early adulthood. *British Journal of Addiction*, **85**, 521–530.

Rautanen, A., Eriksson, J.G., Kere, J. et al. (2006). Associations of body size at birth with late-life cortisol concentrations and glucose tolerance are modified by haplotypes of the glucocorticoid receptor gene. *Journal of Clinical Endocrinology and Metabolism*, **91**, 4544–4551.

Repetti, R.L., Taylor, S.E., and Seeman, T.E. (2002). Risky families: family and social environments and the mental and physical health of offspring. *Psychological Bulletin*, **128**, 330–366.

Richards, M., Wadsworth, M.E., Richards, M., and Wadsworth, M.E.J. (2004). Long term effects of early adversity on cognitive function. *Archives of Disease in Childhood*, **89**, 922–927.

Roberts, R.E., Kaplan, G.A., Shema, S.J., and Strawbridge, W. (2000). Are the obese at greater risk of depression? *Am.J.Epidemiol*, **152**, 163–170.

Rodgers, B., Power, C., Hope, S., Rodgers, B., Power, C., and Hope, S. (1997). Parental divorce and adult psychological distress: evidence from a national birth cohort: a research note. *Journal of Child Psychology and Psychiatry and Allied Disciplines*, **38**, 867–872.

Saha, S., Chant, D., and McGrath, J. (2007). A systematic review of mortality in schizophrenia: is the differential mortality gap worsening over time? *Archives of General Psychiatry*, **64**, 1123–1131.

Scherrer, J.F., Xian, H., Bucholz, K.K. J. et al. (2003). A twin study of depression symptoms, hypertension, and heart disease in middle-aged men. *Psychosomatic Medicine*, **65**, 548–557.

Schulz, R., Bookwala, J., Knapp, J.E., Scheier, M., and Williamson, G.M. (1996). Pessimism, age, and cancer mortality. *Psychology and Aging*, **11**, 304–309.

Silverstone, P.H. (1990). Depression increases mortality and morbidity in acute life-threatening medical illness. *Journal of Psychosomatic Research*, **34**, 651–657.

Simon, G.E., Von Korff, M., Saunders, K., Miglioretti, D.L., Crane, P.K., van Belle, G. et al. (2006). Association between obesity and psychiatric disorders in the us adult population. *Archives of General Psychiatry*, **63**, 824–830.

Smith, G.D., Shipley, M.J., and Rose, G. (1990). Magnitude and causes of socioeconomic differentials in mortality: further evidence from the Whitehall Study. *Journal of Epidemiology and Community Health*, **44**, 265–270.

Surtees, P.G., Wainwright, N.W. J., Luben, R.N., Wareham, N.J., Bingham, S.A., and Khaw, K.T. (2008). Depression and ischemic heart disease mortality: evidence from the EPIC-Norfolk United Kingdom Prospective Cohort Study. *American Journal of Psychiatry*, **165**, 515–523.

Takeshita, J., Masaki, K., Ahmed, I. et al. (2002). Are depressive symptoms a risk factor for mortality in elderly japanese american men? The Honolulu-Asia Aging Study. *American Journal of Psychiatry*, **159**, 1127–1132.

Taylor, C.B., Youngblood, M.E., Catellier, D. et al. (2005). Effects of antidepressant medication on morbidity and mortality in depressed patients after myocardial infarction. *Archives of General Psychiatry*, **62**, 792–798.

Thomas, C., Hypponen, E., Power, C., Thomas, C., Hypponen, E., and Power, C. (2008). Obesity and type 2 diabetes risk in mid adult life: the role of childhood adversity. *Pediatrics*, **121**, e1240–e1249.

Thompson, C.H.R.I., Syddall, H.O.L.L., Rodin, I.A.N., Osmond, C.L.I.V., and Barker, D.J.P. (2001). Birth weight and the risk of depressive disorder in late life. *The British Journal of Psychiatry*, **179**, 450–455.

van Melle, J.P., De, J.P., Honig, A. et al. (2007). Effects of antidepressant treatment following myocardial infarction. *British Journal of Psychiatry*, **190**, 460–466.

Wadsworth, M., Maclean, M., Kuh, D. et al. (1990). Children of divorced and separated parents: summary and review of findings from a long-term follow-up study in the UK. *Family Practice*, 7, 104–109.

Wadsworth, M.E., Hardy, R.J., Paul, A.A., Marshall, S.F., Cole, T.J., Wadsworth, M.E.J. et al.(2002). Leg and trunk length at 43 years in relation to childhood health, diet and family circumstances; evidence from the 1946 national birth cohort.[see comment]. *International Journal of Epidemiology*, **31**, 383–390.

Whitaker, R.C., Phillips, S.M., Orzol, S. M., Burdette, H. L. (2007). The association between maltreatment and obesity among preschool children. *Child Abuse and Neglect*, **31**, 1187–1199.

Whitworth, J.A., Mangos, G.J., and Kelly, J.J. (2000). Cushing, Cortisol, and Cardiovascular Disease. *Hypertension*, **36**, 912–916.

Wiles, N.J., Peters, T.J., Leon, D.A. et al. (2005). Birth weight and psychological distress at age 45-51 years: results from the Aberdeen Children of the 1950s cohort study. *British Journal of Psychiatry*, **187**, 21–28.

Williams, L.S., Ghose, S.S., and Swindle, R.W. (2004). Depression and other mental health diagnoses increase mortality risk after ischemic stroke. *American Journal of Psychiatry*, **161**, 1090–1095.

Williamson, D.F., Thompson, T.J., Anda, R.F. et al. (2002). Body weight and obesity in adults and self-reported abuse in childhood. *International Journal of Obesity and Related Metabolic Disorders: Journal of the International Association for the Study of Obesity*, **26**, 1075–1082.

Writing Committee for the ENRICHD Investigators. (2003). Effects of Treating Depression and Low Perceived Social Support on Clinical Events After Myocardial Infarction: The Enhancing Recovery in Coronary Heart Disease Patients (ENRICHD) Randomized Trial. *JAMA*, **289**, 3106–3116.

Wulsin, L.R., Vaillant, G.E., and Wells, V.E. (1999a). A systematic review of the mortality of depression. *Psychosomatic Medicine*, **61**, 6–17.

Wulsin, L.R., Vaillant, G.E., and Wells, V.E. (1999b). A systematic review of the mortality of depression. *Psychosomatic Medicine*, **61**, 6–17.

Chapter 21

Depression: unipolar or bipolar, what's the difference (and what does it matter anyway)?

Allan H. Young

Introduction

The word depression is fraught with problems; not the least of these being that it is widely used but only rarely exactly defined. In different areas of human activity, depression may be applied in the context of meteorology, nerve cell function, stock market activity, and indeed a multiplicity of other settings. Even when depression is clearly used to refer to a mood state, confusion frequently arises. There is, of course, the problem of differentiating between a depressed mood as part of normal experience, 'well founded moodiness of health', and pathological mood states. However, this chapter is only concerned with overt clinical depression and the problems inherent in the split between 'unipolar' and 'bipolar' forms of malignant sadness. Although some have argued that there are clearly detectable differences between these two forms of clinical depression, I will argue that the key differentiator is the presence of pathological mood elevation, particularly mania. The clinical value of making a distinction based on less clearly pathological states such as hypomania and subsyndromal degrees of mood elevation is less well founded. It is notable that there is a wide variation between different countries in the prevalence of unipolar disorder and much less variation internationally for bipolar disorder, suggesting at the very least that bipolar disorder is less influenced by transcultural factors. An argument will be advanced that depression research (both aetiopathogenic and therapeutic trials) should therefore be primarily focused, at least initially, on the diagnostic category defined by the occurrence of mania. Because bipolar one disorder arguably has greater transcultural integrity than other closely related disorders, for example, bipolar two disorder, such a strategy would be likely to optimize the heuristic utility of research. Subsequent elaboration of research findings gained from initial studies in bipolar one disorder should then take place into more heterogeneous disorders including bipolar two, bipolar spectrum, and unipolar mood disorders and even related conditions such as schizophrenia. This is the second chapter to discuss the differences and similarities between depression and bipolar disorder, together with Chapters 6, 22, and 26.

Unipolar and bipolar depression

Mood disorders are leading causes of ill health worldwide (Prince et al. 2007). The fundamental division into unipolar (major depressive disorder) and bipolar mood disorders is an evolution of the more venerable concept of manic-depressive illness (Angst and Marneros, 2001). Although mania and melancholia have been described in the medical literature since antiquity, it was not until the end of the nineteenth century that Emil Kraepelin consolidated the diagnoses corresponding to affective disorders under the rubric of manic-depressive insanity as distinguished from dementia praecox. Subsequently, Kraepelin's unitary concept of mood disorder was adopted into psychiatric nosologies worldwide. In the 1960s, however, work by Professors Jules Angst, Carlo Perris, and George Winokur independently demonstrated that there were important clinical, familial, and course characteristics validating the distinction between unipolar and bipolar disorders (Angst and Marneros, 2001). The validity of these observations remains unchallenged and forms the bedrock of the current diagnostic dichotomy of unipolar and bipolar disorders. Notably, thinking about unipolar and bipolar disorders has further advanced in the last three decades: important developments include renewed interest into both Kraepelin's mixed states and Kahlbaum's and Hecker's cyclothymia and related affective temperaments; the concept of soft bipolar spectrum (Akiskal, 2007); and the distinction of schizoaffective disorders into unipolar and bipolar forms (Angst and Marneros, 2001). Indeed, some have argued that shared genetic vulnerability may make us fundamentally rethink our classification of psychiatric disease (Craddock and Owen, 2007).

Despite these recent advances, notable problems remain with the practical aspects of these diagnoses, particularly with regards to the heterogeneity within the category of unipolar (major depressive) disorders and the overlap between major depression and some bipolar disorders.

Problems with major depression

Major depressive disorder (MDD) is a highly prevalent, persistent, and often seriously impairing condition (Kessler et al. 2007). MDD, perhaps not surprisingly for such a common illness, undoubtedly contains a heterogeneous mix of different aetiologies, disease processes, and outcomes. Although the percentage of people with mood disorders in treatment has increased substantially since the early 1990s, a majority of cases remain either untreated or undertreated. An especially serious concern is the misdiagnosis of depressive episodes due to bipolar disorder (BPD) as being due to MDD. Particular concern has been raised about this with regard to bipolar two (BP-II) and bipolar spectrum disorders (BPS) and the question arises as to whether there are distinguishing symptoms or patterns of symptoms which may help us differentiate these two closely related forms of depression. Data derived from the French National EPIDEP study was used to examine this issue by Hantouche and Akiskal (Hantouche and Akiskal, 2005). Their data indicate greater psychomotor retardation, stability and uniformity in the clinical picture of strictly defined MDD. By contrast, BP-II depressions appeared to be characterized, despite the hypersomnic tendency, by psychomotor activation. This can be taken to indicate greater degree of mixed features than those observed in MDD. Moreover, in BP-II, there was less agreement between clinicians than between self-ratings on the presence of various features of depression. Taken together, these findings may explain why episodes of BP-II depression present clinicians with diagnostic problems. The symptomatic profiles of unipolar and bipolar depression have also been examined recently by Forty et al. (Forty et al. 2008), who compared clinical course variables and depressive symptom profiles in a large sample of individuals with major depressive disorder ($n = 593$) and bipolar disorder ($n = 443$). The proportions of women in the major depression group and the bipolar group were 70.2% and 71.3%, respectively. The median age at interview was 49 years for the major depression group and 47 years for the bipolar group. Forty-six per cent of the major depression group was recruited systematically, compared with 37% of the bipolar group. The median illness duration was 19 years for the major depression group and 20 years for the bipolar group. Clinical characteristics associated with a bipolar course included the presence of psychosis, diurnal mood variation, and hypersomnia during depressive episodes, and a greater number of shorter depressive episodes. The authors concluded that such features should alert a clinician to a possible bipolar course. However, it must be stressed that none of the features, which the authors concluded were potentially indicative of bipolar disorder (psychosis, diurnal mood variation, hypersomnia, and a greater number of shorter depressive episodes) were particularly rare in the MDD group and the differences, although statistically significant, were not always numerically great. For example, the three most statistically 'significant' differences were for psychotic features (present in 10.5% of MDD; 30.2% of BPD); diminished libido (present in 63.5% of MDD; 34.8% of BPD), and the duration of the longest episode of depression (MDD median 69 weeks; BPD median 26 weeks). Goldberg and Harrow (Goldberg and Harrow, 2004) also found that (young) depressed inpatients with psychotic features may be at especially high risk for eventually developing mania. These authors noted that the probability for developing a bipolar spectrum disorder increased in linear fashion for patients at risk for polarity conversion during the first 10–15 years after an index depressive episode. From even this brief review of the extensive literature on this subject it seems clear that although certain clinical features of depression may raise a clinician's index of suspicion for bipolar disorder, none are powerfully predictive enough to be definitive. Detection of symptoms of pathological mood elevation does, of course, allow the diagnosis of bipolar disorder to be made. Issues related to this will now be discussed.

Bipolar disorder

Bipolar disorder has recently been convincingly argued to comprise the 'heartland of psychiatry' (Goodwin and Geddes, 2007). Furthermore, bipolar disorder encompasses all of the clinical and scientific challenges that presently face psychiatry, a number of which are pungently discussed by these authors. Bipolar disorder is a severe, long-term illness characterized by cyclical episodes of mania/hypomania and depression. By convention, bipolar disorder is defined as being bipolar one disorder (BPD-I) in subjects who have suffered at least one episode of mania, whereas bipolar two disorder (BPD-II) refers to patients who have experienced pathological mood elevation only to the extent of hypomania. Subsyndromal BPD is designated bipolar spectrum (BPDS). The lifetime prevalence of BPD-I/BPD-II combined is approximately 2% (Merikangas et al. 2007), with a similar lifetime prevalence for subsyndromal forms. The impact of bipolar disorder on the patient is highly significant, such that bipolar disorder leads to 2% of all disability-adjusted life years associated with non-communicable disease worldwide (Prince et al. 2007). It should be noted, however, that this figure does not include subsyndromal forms. In a landmark paper, Angst and Sellaro (Angst and Sellaro, 2000) reviewed two centuries' literature on the natural history of bipolar disorder, including modern naturalistic studies and new data from a lifelong follow-up study of 220 bipolar patients, part of the famous 'Zurich Longitudinal Cohort', carried out by Professor Angst and colleagues. From this review, Angst and Sellaro reached the following conclusions: the findings of modern follow-up studies are closely compatible with those studies conducted before the introduction of modern medications such as antidepressant and mood-stabilizing treatments, and that bipolar disorder has always been highly recurrent and considered to have a poor prognosis. For example, bipolar patients who have been hospitalized spend about 20% of their lifetime from the onset of their disorder in episodes. Fifty percent of bipolar episodes last between two and seven months (median three months). The intervals between the first few episodes tend to shorten; later the episodes return at an irregular rhythm of about 0.4 episodes per year with high inter-individual variability. Switches from mania into mild depression and from depression into hypomania were frequently reported in the nineteenth century and the first half of the twentieth, well before the introduction of modern pharmacotherapy. Antidepressant and antimanic drugs have to be given as long as the natural episode lasts, although some medications (both mood stabilizers and antipsychotics) now have data supportive of longer term treatment

(Smith et al. 2007). Angst and Sellaro further recommend that – given the poor outcome of bipolar disorders found in naturalistic follow-up studies and in their lifelong investigation – intensive antidepressant, antimanic, and mood-stabilizing treatments are required in most cases. Despite modern treatments, the outcome into old age is still poor, full recovery without further episodes rare, recurrence of episodes with incomplete remission the rule, and the development of chronicity and suicide still frequent. Although bipolar disorder is defined by the occurrence of pathological mood elevation in the form of mania (bipolar one) or hypomania (bipolar two), at some point in the longitudinal history of the illness, it is now clear that the greater part of the burden imposed by these illnesses is consequent upon the depressed phase.

Bipolar depression

The degree of disability associated with episodes of bipolar depression is disproportionately greater compared with episodes of bipolar mania (Post et al. 2003), and patients with bipolar depression experience significantly greater psychosocial impairment (Judd et al. 2005) and as few as one-third of BPD patients achieve full social and occupational functional recovery to their own premorbid levels (Huxley and Baldessarini, 2007). A recent finding of particular importance is that patients with bipolar one disorder are likely to experience depressive symptoms approximately three times more frequently than symptoms of mania and the predominance of depressed symptomatology is even more pronounced in bipolar two disorder. (Judd et al. 2002; Kupka et al. 2007). Furthermore, beyond the high frequency of episodes, bipolar depression is a major cause of suicide, such that the lifetime prevalence of a suicide attempt is approximately 29% in these patients (Vieta et al. 1997). Angst et al. (Angst et al.2005) examined the variation in the suicide risk over lifetime and on the suicide-preventive effect of the long-term treatment of mood-disorder patients with antidepressants and neuroleptics. This research examined data on 186 MDD, 60 BPD-II, 130 BPD-I, and 30 preponderantly manic patients (again BPD-I under conventional classifications) that were followed up from 1963 to 2003. By 2003, 45 (11.1%) of the 406 patients had committed suicide. Suicide rates were highest among MDD patients (Standardized Mortality Ratio, SMR = 26.4) and then declined from BPD-I (SMR = 13.6), BPD-II (SMR = 10.6) with the lowest rates among the predominantly manic patients (SMR = 4.7). The different outcomes for the predominantly manic patients from the rest of the BPD-I group suggest that this subdivision may have predictive validity, at least for death rates from suicide. Prospectively, the suicide rate decreased over the 44 years' follow-up; the use of lithium, antipsychotics and antidepressants reduced suicides significantly. Long-term treatment also reduced overall mortality, and combined treatments proved more effective than mono-therapy.

Diagnosing bipolar disorder

The considerable impact and frequency of episodes of bipolar depression emphasizes the importance of effectively managing depressive symptoms to achieve the ultimate goal of mood stabilization. However, a key challenge in bipolar disorder is the accurate diagnosis of the illness. Factors that confound the diagnosis and treatment of bipolar disorder include a considerable symptomatic overlap with other psychiatric illnesses, an incomplete medical history of the patient, and lack of patient insight. Treatment is complicated further by the high prevalence of comorbidities such as anxiety disorders and substance use disorders in these patients. These comorbidities can have a detrimental effect on the disease course, including an increase in the number of suicide attempts (Keller, 2006; Perlis, 2005; Pollack et al. 2000; Vieta et al. 2001). A combination of these factors can lead to bipolar disorder being under-diagnosed or misdiagnosed as major depressive disorder, anxiety disorder, or schizophrenia with reported rates of misdiagnosis as high as 69% (Hirschfeld et al. 2003). Inaccurate diagnosis can result in inappropriate treatment being implemented, which can ultimately compromise long-term outcomes. Potential steps that could be taken in order to improve diagnosis of bipolar disorder include investigating the presence of manic/hypomanic, psychotic, or reverse vegetative symptoms in every patient presenting with depressive symptoms and also establishing whether there is a family history of bipolar disorder. An additional issue regarding the diagnosis of bipolar depression is some degree of controversy regarding the lack of accepted diagnostic criteria. In order to address this, a 'probabilistic' approach to the diagnosis of bipolar one depression has recently been proposed (Mitchell et al. 2008). This approach focuses on the most commonly reported symptoms in patients with bipolar depression, such as hypersomnia, increased weight, and manic symptoms, compared with those symptoms most commonly reported in patients with major depression, such as reduced sleep and weight loss. These recommendations propose that the combination of four to five or more of these defined symptoms should increase the likelihood of diagnosis of either bipolar or major depression.

Weissman and colleagues (Weissman et al. 1996) have contrasted large cross-national differences in prevalence of depression with relatively uniform prevalence rates for bipolar disorder. Epidemiological studies of schizophrenia also show generally similar prevalence and symptom patterns across a wide range of culture and economic development (Sartorius et al. 1986). Two quite different explanations have been advanced to account for this contrast. First, social or environmental factors may have a stronger influence on depression than on more severe disorders such as bipolar disorder or schizophrenia. Alternatively, depression measures may be more difficult to apply across a range of cultures than are measures of bipolar or psychotic disorders. The defining characteristics of mania or psychosis (e.g. pressured speech, agitation, hallucinations) may be more easily distinguished from everyday experience than the defining characteristics of depression (e.g. feeling down or depressed most of the day nearly every day). Evidence for variability in diagnostic thresholds varying with cultural background and how this may influence the perception of psychiatric symptoms was examined by Mackin et al. (Mackin et al. 2006). These authors examined the effects of cultural biases on the identification of manic symptoms using the Young Mania Rating Scale. Two video interviews, each with an American person with mania, were shown to psychiatrists from three countries (United States, United Kingdom, and India). Total scores on the scale differed significantly between the United States and United Kingdom ($P < 0.001$) and between India and United Kingdom ($P < 0.001$) rater groups. Overall, differences between India and United States rater groups were less marked ($P = 0.28$). These differences suggest that cultural biases influence the interpretation of manic symptoms. Various screening tools have been developed which allow more sensitive detection of hypomanic symptoms (Parker et al. 2007). Use of these tools may potentially guide both clinical practice and research. For example, Angst's HCL-32 is being used currently in a large, transnational study to determine the amount of BPDS present in routine 'unipolar' samples (Angst et al. 2005).

Some colleagues have argued for a return to the practice of classifying recurrent depression with bipolar disorder as a remedy for contemporary diagnostic confusion; indeed the subtitle of the most recent edition of the definitive textbook in the field, *Bipolar Disorders and Recurrent Depression*, reflects this (Goodwin and Jamieson, 2007). Although this argument may seem well founded, we must guard against exporting the problems that bedevil the current approach to unipolar disorder into bipolar disorders. The heuristic utility of diagnostic subtypes is of crucial importance. Bipolar one disorder (being based on a diagnosis of mania) is one of the most reliable diagnostic categories in psychiatry. There is a strong argument for the integrity of bipolar one disorder to remain uncompromised. Notwithstanding this, there is also a pressing need for clarity on the relationship and valid boundary between bipolar one and bipolar two subtypes and also between bipolar two and bipolar spectrum. Future research may indeed need to even refine the concept of bipolar one further to take greater measure of features such as psychosis, neurocognitive impairment, age of onset, and comorbidities. Defining subtypes of bipolar disorder solely on rather arbitrary duration or severity of symptoms may be discarded in the future in favour of a typology based on these or other factors. At present however, in terms of reliability, and also possible validity, bipolar one disorder is as good as it gets.

The role of treatment

Although unrecognized bipolarity in depression clearly matters, it is perhaps not widely recognized that this may be just as important for our understanding of unipolar as bipolar illnesses. In the largest placebo-controlled trial conducted thus far, acute bipolar depression (both one and two subtypes) did not respond to a therapeutic dose of paroxetine over the course of an eight-week treatment period to a significantly greater extent than placebo (McElroy et al. 2008). This lends weight to the notion that unrecognized bipolar two and bipolar spectrum depressions may be diluting samples in supposed unipolar studies and perhaps reducing the signal of therapeutic efficacy of selective serotonin reuptake inhibitors (SSRIs). Another important finding from the work of McElroy et al. was that the rates of manic switch on paroxetine were not significantly higher than those on placebo. This is evidence against the notion that SSRIs are destabilizing drugs in bipolar one and two depressions. Notably, similar large placebo-controlled studies have not yet been carried out in bipolar spectrum disorders. This recent trial has added to other recent evidence (Sachs et al. 2007). In this study it was found that the use of adjunctive, standard antidepressant medication, as compared with the use of mood stabilizers, was not associated with increased efficacy or with increased risk of treatment-emergent affective switch. Clearly, both of these studies suggest that although using treatments such as paroxetine in bipolar depression may be less dangerous than some might have feared, it is also less helpful than we might have hoped. There are also important implications for our understanding of the use of antidepressants in unipolar disorders. Recent meta-analyses of antidepressant medications have reported only modest benefits over placebo treatment, and some authors have suggested that when unpublished trial data are included, the benefit falls below accepted criteria for clinical significance (Kirsch et al. 2008). However, the issue of unrecognized bipolar patients in these supposedly 'unipolar samples' has received little comment, although clearly this may be an important factor and raises the possibility that the signal of efficacy for certain antidepressant treatments may have been underestimated by the inclusion of these patients.

Implications for research

Chapter 6 in this volume examines the genetic relationship between unipolar and bipolar mood disorders. These authors also echo recent calls for a more dimensional approach to the classification of mood disorders. Although it is difficult to envisage a dimensional approach doing anything in the near future but supplementing our current categories in a workday clinical setting, for research efforts such an approach may be vitally important. Rather inconsiderately, genes and indeed other important biological factors, appear not to have read our textbooks or indeed to respect our carefully arrived-at categories contained within. As discussed by Smith et al., examination of the role of genes across diagnostic boundaries is currently already underway. Indeed, such research may make many of our debates about classification eventually redundant and may allow us to formulate our thinking about bipolar disorders in a new way, one that will hopefully aid us in our treatment choices. As mentioned above, other biological factors are found to be not entirely respectful of the unipolar/bipolar split. An example of this is dysfunction of the hypothalamic-pituitary-adrenal (HPA) axis, which is also discussed in several other chapters of this book. Function of the HPA axis has long been suspected to be abnormal in mood disorders. However, recent work has shown that this varies with subtype. Although there is good evidence that the HPA axis function is abnormal in bipolar disorder (Watson et al. 2004) and in melancholic/psychotic depression (Carroll et al. 2007) this is not so in chronic depression (Watson et al. 2002). A recent meta-analysis has also confirmed that anti-glucocorticoid treatments may show some utility in both bipolar and unipolar disorders (Gallagher et al. 2008) although the findings so far appear to be unpromising in schizophrenia (Gallagher et al. 2005).

Conclusions

Depression may occur as part of a primary mood disorder that is either unipolar or bipolar. The separation into these subtypes is well founded. Certain symptom patterns and characteristics should make the clinician suspect that the depression belongs to a bipolar illness rather than a unipolar illness. However, the only definitive way to tell is to ascertain a history of pathological mood elevation. For bipolar one disorder, looking for mania is relatively straightforward. Bipolar two disorder and subsyndromal states pose greater difficulties even with the use of new research instruments. To compound these difficulties there is a continuing risk that unipolars will 'switch' into a bipolar illness by developing pathological mood elevation. For this reason it has been argued that research should be focused on bipolar one disorder. This subtype has the most clear-cut and reliable diagnosis and aetiopathogenic factors overlap with both unipolar disorders as well as with schizophrenia. Examination of aetiopathogenic factors in bipolar one disorder could then be elaborated into unipolar disorder and other psychiatric illnesses such as schizophrenia. Relatively few large randomized placebo-controlled trials have been conducted in bipolar one disorder compared to unipolar disorder. However, those that have (e.g. McElroy et al. 2008), have not shown evidence of the same inflated placebo response and weak therapeutic signal that has become increasingly evident in trials in unipolar disorder. If bipolar disorder is the heartland of psychiatry, it should be the principal target of our efforts to understand mood disorders.

References

Akiskal, H.S. (2007). The emergence of the bipolar spectrum: validation along clinical-epidemiologic and familial-genetic lines. *Psychopharmacol Bull.*, **40**, 99–115.

Angst, J. and Sellaro, R. (2000). Historical perspectives and natural history of bipolar disorder. *Biol Psychiatry*, Sep 15; **48**, 445–457.

Angst, J. and Marneros, A. (2001). Bipolarity from ancient to modern times: conception, birth and rebirth. *J Affect Disord.*, Dec; **67**, 3–19.

Angst, J., Adolfsson, R., Benazzi, F. et al. (2005). The HCL-32: towards a self-assessment tool for hypomanic symptoms in outpatients. *J Affect Disord.*, Oct; **88**, 217–33.

Angst, J., Angst, F., Gerber-Verder, R., and Gamma, A. (2005). Suicide in 406 mood-disorder patients with and without long-term medication: a 40 to 44 years' follow-up. *Arch Suicide Res.*, **9**, 279–300.

Carroll, B.J., Cassidy, F., Naftolowitz, D. et al. (2007). Pathophysiology of hypercortisolism in depression. *Acta Psychiatr Scand Suppl.*, 90–103.

Craddock, N. and Owen, M.J. (2007). Rethinking psychosis: the disadvantages of a dichotomous classification now outweigh the advantages. *World Psychiatry*, Jun; **6**, 84–91.

Forty, L., Smith, D., Jones, L. et al. (2008). Clinical differences between bipolar and unipolar depression. *Br J Psychiatry*, **192**, 388–389.

Gallagher, P., Watson, S., Smith, M.S., Ferrier, I.N., and Young, A.H. (2005). Effects of adjunctive mifepristone (RU-486) administration on neurocognitive function and symptoms in schizophrenia. *Biol Psychiatry.*, Jan 15; **57**, 155–61.

Gallagher, P., Malik, N., Newham, J., Young, A.H., Ferrier, I.N., and Mackin, P. (2008). Antiglucocorticoid treatments for mood disorders. *Cochrane Database Syst Rev.*, Jan **23**; CD005168.

Goldberg, J.F. and Harrow, M. (2004). Consistency of remission and outcome in bipolar and unipolar mood disorders: a 10-year prospective follow-up. *J Affect Disord.*, Aug; **81**, 123–31.

Goodwin, F.K. and Jamison, K.R. (2007). *Manic-Depressive Illness: Bipolar Disorders and Recurrent Depression, 2nd Edition.* New York, Oxford University Press.

Goodwin, G.M. and Geddes, J.R. (2007). What is the heartland of psychiatry? *Br J Psychiatry*, **191**, 189–191.

Hantouche, E.G. and Akiskal, H.S. (2005). Bipolar II vs. unipolar depression: psychopathologic differentiation by dimensional measures. *J Affect Disord.*, Feb; **84**, 127–32.

Hirschfeld, R.M., Lewis, L., and Vornik, L.A. (2003). Perceptions and impact of bipolar disorder: how far have we really come? Results of the national depressive and manic-depressive association 2000 survey of individuals with bipolar disorder. *J Clin Psychiatry*, **64**, 161–174.

Huxley, N. and Baldessarini, R.J. (2007). Disability and its treatment in bipolar disorder patients. *Bipolar Disord.*, Feb–Mar; **9**, 183–96.

Judd, L.L., Akiskal, H.S., Schettler, P.J. et al. (2005). Psychosocial disability in the course of bipolar I and II disorders: a prospective, comparative, longitudinal study. *Arch Gen Psychiatry*, **62**, 1322–1330.

Judd, L.L., Akiskal, H.S., Schettler, P.J. et al. (2002). The long-term natural history of the weekly symptomatic status of bipolar I disorder. *Arch Gen Psychiatry*, **59**, 530–537.

Keller, M.B. (2006). Prevalence and impact of comorbid anxiety and bipolar disorder. *J Clin Psychiatry*, **67** Suppl 1, 5–7.

Kessler, R.C., Merikangas, K.R., and Wang, P.S. (2007). Prevalence, comorbidity, and service utilization for mood disorders in the United States at the beginning of the twenty-first century. *Annu Rev Clin Psychol.*, **3**, 137–158.

Kirsch, I., Deacon, B.J., Huedo-Medina, T.B. et al. (2008). Initial severity and antidepressant benefits: a meta-analysis of data submitted to the Food and Drug Administration. *PLoS Med.*, Feb; **5**, 260–268.

Kupka, R.W., Altshuler, L.L., Nolen, W.A. et al. (2007). Three times more days depressed than manic or hypomanic in both bipolar I and bipolar II disorder. *Bipolar Disord.*, **9**, 531–535.

Mackin, P., Targum, S.D., Kalali, A., Rom, D., and Young, A.H. (2006). Culture and assessment of manic symptoms. *Br J Psychiatry*, Oct; **189**, 379–80.

McElroy, S., Young, A.H., Carlsson, A., et al. (2008). A double-blind, placebo–controlled study with acute and continuation phase of quetiapine and paroxetine in adults with bipolar depression (EMBOLDEN II). *Bipolar Disord.*, Feb; **10**, 59.

Merikangas, K.R., Akiskal, H.S., Angst, J. et al. (2007). Lifetime and 12-month prevalence of bipolar spectrum disorder in the national comorbidity survey replication. *Arch Gen Psychiatry*, **64**, 543–552.

Mitchell, P.B., Goodwin, G.M., Johnson, G.F., and Hirschfeld, R.M. (2008). Diagnostic guidelines for bipolar depression: a probabilistic approach. *Bipolar Disord.*, 10, 144–152.

Parker, G., Fletcher, K., Barrett, M. et al. (2007). Screening for bipolar disorder: The utility and comparative properties of the MSS and MDQ measures. *J Affect Disord.*, Jul; **109**, 83–9.

Perlis, R.H. (2005). Misdiagnosis of bipolar disorder. *Am J Manag Care*, 11, S271–S274.

Pollack, L.E., Cramer, R.D., and Varner, R.V. (2000). Psychosocial functioning of people with substance abuse and bipolar disorders. *Subst Abus.*, **21**, 193–203.

Post, R.M., Denicoff, K.D., Leverich, G.S. et al. (2003). Morbidity in 258 bipolar outpatients followed for 1 year with daily prospective ratings on the NIMH life chart method. *J Clin Psychiatry*, **64**, 680–690.

Prince, M., Patel, V., Saxena, S., Maj, M., Maselko, J., Phillips, M.R., and Rahman, A. (2007). No health without mental health. *Lancet*, **370**, 859–877.

Sachs, G.S., Nierenberg, A.A., Calabrese, J.R. et al. (2007). Effectiveness of adjunctive antidepressant treatment for bipolar depression. *N Engl J Med.*, **356**, 1711–1722.

Sartorius, N., Jablensky, A., Korten, A. et al. (1986). Early manifestations and first-contact incidence of schizophrenia in different cultures. A preliminary report on the initial evaluation phase of the WHO Collaborative Study on determinants of outcome of severe mental disorders. *Psychol Med.*, Nov; **16**, 909–928.

Smith, L.A., Cornelius, V., Warnock, A., Bell, A., and Young, A.H. (2007). Effectiveness of mood stabilizers and antipsychotics in the maintenance phase of bipolar disorder: a systematic review of randomized controlled trials. *Bipolar Disorders.*, Jun; **9**, 394–412.

Vieta, E., Benabarre, A., Colom, F. et al. (1997). Suicidal behavior in bipolar I and bipolar II disorder. *J Nerv Ment Dis.*, **185**, 407–409.

Vieta, E., Colom, F., Corbella, B. et al. (2001). Clinical correlates of psychiatric comorbidity in bipolar I patients. *Bipolar Disord.*, **3**, 253–258.

Watson, S., Gallagher, P., Del-Estal, D., Hearn, A., Ferrier, I.N., and Young, A.H. (2002). Hypothalamic-pituitary-adrenal axis function in patients with chronic depression. *Psychol Med.*, Aug; **32**, 1021–1028.

Watson, S., Gallagher, P., Ritchie, J.C., Ferrier, I.N., and Young, A.H. (2004). Hypothalamic-pituitary-adrenal axis function in patients with bipolar disorder. *Br J Psychiatry*, Jun; **184**, 496–502.

Weissman, M.M., Bland, R.C., Canino, G.J. et al. (1996). Cross-national epidemiology of major depression and bipolar disorder. *JAMA*, Jul 23–31; **276**, 293–299.

Chapter 22

Can neuroimaging help distinguish bipolar depression from major depressive disorder?

Matthew T. Keener and Mary L. Phillips

Introduction

Bipolar disorder (BP) and major depressive disorder (MDD) are among the ten most debilitating illnesses worldwide (Kessler et al. 2003; Murray and Lopez, 1996), with a prevalence of at least 1% and 15%, respectively. Bipolar disorder type I (BPI) in particular is associated with a poor clinical and functional outcome, a high suicide rate (Baldessarini and Tondo, 2003), and a huge societal cost (Wyatt and Henter, 1995). One reason for this poor prognosis of BPI is the frequent misdiagnosis or late diagnosis of the disorder (e.g. Bowden and Tondo, 2001; 2005), leading to unnecessary delays in the initiation of appropriate treatment. Indeed, while depression is the more common presentation in BPI, and a cause of greater psychosocial disruption than the manic episodes (e.g. Calabrese et al. 2004), BPI depression continues to be frequently misdiagnosed and inappropriately treated as MDD depression in individuals without a clear previous history of manic episodes (e.g. Ghaemi et al. 2002; Hirschfeld et al. 2003; Lish et al. 1994; Manning et al. 2003). BP depression shows a relatively poor response to antidepressants alone or even in combination treatment (Fagiolini et al. 2002; Ghaemi et al. 2003; Sachs et al. 2007), which can additionally elicit manic upswings in patients with a bipolar diathesis.

Bipolar disorder type II (BPII) is characterized by multiple, protracted depressive episodes and hypomania rather than mania (DSM_IV). For those individuals presenting during a depressive episode, it is just as difficult to identify as BPI and may be more common. The reported lifetime prevalence of BPII, for example, ranges from 0.5% (Regier et al. 1993) to 11% (Angst et al. 2003). BPII may therefore affect 2 to 3 times as many individuals as BPI, and may be almost as common as MDD. Even the most conservative estimates would mean that 1.5 million American individuals suffer from this disorder (Reiger et al. 1993). Furthermore, accumulating evidence indicates that BPII is at least as disabling – some would suggest more disabling – than BPI (Maina et al. 2007): with an increased risk for suicide (Balazs et al. 2003; Rihmer et al. 1999) relative to individuals suffering from MDD or BPI, and experiencing a more chronic course of illness with a lower interepisode probability of returning to premorbid levels of functioning (Judd et al. 2003). Identifying BPII is, therefore, just as important – and perhaps more important – a challenge as identification of the more traditional BPI in individuals during depressed episode.

There are emerging data which show that there may be differences in the presentation of depression between BP and MDD depression, with the former being more commonly associated with psychosis, atypical features, and diurnal mood variation in a large clinical sample (e.g. Forty et al. 2008). These differences in presentation of BP versus MDD depression at a population level, however, do not directly translate into accurately diagnosing the depression within a given individual. A major challenge for psychiatrists working with depressed patients is to find new ways to improve the accuracy of diagnosing BP, both BPI and BPII, versus MDD as early as possible in depressed patients, especially those who present without a clear history of mania or hypomania. Bipolar depression which regularly begins in late adolescence (McMahon, 1994) commonly goes on for a decade prior to being correctly diagnosed (Lish, 1994). Early diagnosis would therefore have a major impact on initiating appropriate treatment. In doing so, we could decrease the number of years lived with symptom burden, as well as possibly improve quality of life, occupational, and social function, in patients with depressive disorders (DePaulo, 2006). This is the third chapter to discuss the differences and similarities between depression and bipolar disorder, together with Chapter 6, 21, and 26.

Meeting the challenge of diagnosis: the search for diagnostically relevent endophenotypes of BP and MDD depression

The recent research agenda for developing the fifth edition of the *Diagnostic and Statistical Manual for Psychiatric Diagnosis* (DSM-V) has emphasized a need to translate research findings from basic and clinical neuroscience into a new psychiatric classification system based upon pathophysiological and etiological processes (Hasler et al. 2004; 2006; Kupfer et al. 2002; Phillips and Frank, 2006). These pathophysiological processes involve complex relationships between genetic variables, abnormalities in brain systems and psychological mechanisms that give rise to symptom expression (e.g. Kraemer et al. 2002). An endophenotype is an objective biomarker that is more closely related to the genetic vulnerability and underlying pathophysiology of a disorder than the 'fuzzy' psychiatric symptomatology of the condition (Gottesman and Gould, 2003). Endophenotypes should be selectively associated with the disorder of interest, but should also be observable in groups at high risk for developing the disorder, like first-degree relatives. These biomarkers should be present in both depression and remission, rather than specific to either illness phase. Measurement in individuals with BPI and BPII of brain system abnormalities underlying characteristic behavioural impairments that are common to depression and remission is therefore a first step towards identification of future potential biomarkers of bipolar illness (Kupfer, 2005; Swann, 2006). A second step towards this goal is the identification of brain system abnormalities that are specific to BPI and BPII depression and not common to the depression of MDD. The identification of differential endophenotypic markers for BP depression would then aid diagnosis earlier on in illness history and would also revolutionize treatment choice in patients presenting with a first episode of depression, as individuals with an underlying bipolar diathesis would be prescribed mood stabilizers rather than antidepressant monotherapy, for example.

Brain imaging techniques, such as magnetic resonance imaging (MRI) and positron emission tomography (PET), can be used to directly quantify the neural system abnormalities that are associated with MDD and BP depression and when used in concert with targeted neurocognitive paradigms may also provide insights into the ways that the underlying pathophysiology interacts with psychological mechanisms of symptom formation and may be employed as a first stage towards identifying endophenotypes associated with depression in MDD and BP.

In this chapter, we examine data from neuroimaging studies that primarily examine the evidence for disorder-specific abnormalities in neural systems linked with *core domains of pathology* in MDD and in BP depression. These findings are a first stage towards the search for endophenotypes to aid the diagnosis of MDD and BP depression.

Core domains of pathology in emotional processing and executive control

Major depressive disorder and BP are increasingly recognized as multisystem disorders involving disturbances across several symptom domains (e.g. Grote and Frank, 2003; Phillips and Frank, 2006). Mood instability is a core domain of pathology in these disorders, which appears to arise from the disruption of brain mechanisms involved in normal emotional processing. This domain is associated with mood variability in depression (e.g. diurnal variation) as well as other aspects of affective lability including irritability or anxiety. In BP, the mood instability domain also gives rise to hypomanic, manic, and mixed affective states. The second core domain of pathology common to the depression of both disorders is impaired executive control. Executive control refers to a collection of higher level psychological processes that enable the flexible organization of complex behaviour, including planning, working memory, inhibitory control, strategy development, and cognitive flexibility (Stuss and Levine, 2002). Deficits in executive control in depression give rise to symptoms including the inability to concentrate and difficulty in decision-making; they may also impact upon other cognitive domains including memory (Deckersbach et al. 2004). Executive dysfunction is likely to impact upon patients' ability to successfully carry out activities of daily living including work-related activities, and impacts more broadly upon quality of life. Executive deficits are also likely to further impair the ability to control or regulate mood (e.g. Keener and Phillips, 2007; Phillips et al. 2003). The combination of these domains of pathology most probably underlies the mood dysregulation apparent in BP and to some extent MDD depression.

Neural systems subserving core domains of pathology

Existing data from functional neuroimaging studies in healthy individuals point towards distinguishable neural systems for emotional processing and executive control. Normal emotion processing, as measured by tasks assessing the processing of emotional facial expressions, for example, has been mapped to a neural system centred on subcortical limbic regions including the amygdala, the ventral striatum, the subgenual cingulate gyrus and ventromedial prefrontal cortex (VMPFC) (e.g. Knutson and Cooper, 2005; Phillips et al. 2003; Price, 2003). Executive control, in contrast, has been mapped to a lateral prefrontal cortical system, comprising dorsolateral (DLPFC) and ventrolateral prefrontal cortices (VLPFC) (Robbins, 1998), which act in concert with striatal mechanisms involved in response selection, and the hippocampus, important for memory encoding and retrieval (Zola-Morgan et al. 1991). Appropriate emotion *regulation*, in addition to relying on the engagement of the above two neural systems, additionally involves anterior cingulate (ACG), orbitofrontal (OFC), and dorsomedial prefrontal (MdPFC) cortices. The OFC and ACG are the regions of the prefrontal cortex that are the most densely connected with the amygdala and other subcortical limbic and paralimbic regions (Öngür et al. 2000) and, in addition to outcome-based appraisal (Oschner and Gross et al. 2007) and decision-making (Delgado et al. 2005), are implicated overall in automatic cognitive change processes involved in emotion regulation (Phillips et al. 2008b).

We will now examine the extent to which existing studies using functional neuroimaging measures have provided direct evidence for functional abnormalities in neural systems underlying these two domains of pathology in MDD and BP depression. Some of the experimental evidence underlying these ideas is presented in Chapter 12 of this book, while Chapter 13 specifically also discusses the neurobiological substrates of emotional processing.

Neuroimaging measures

Major depressive disorder

The majority of functional neuroimaging studies of MDD individuals pre- and post-remission after treatment with pharmacological and psychological interventions have been performed during resting state and *not* during performance of specific emotion processing or attentional tasks (e.g. Baxter et al. 1989; Goldapple et al. 2004; Goodwin et al. 1993; Holthoff et al. 2004; Kennedy et al. 2001; Martin et al. 2001; Mayberg et al. 2000; Vlassenko et al. 2004). There are discrepant findings from these studies. Some studies report increases in dorsal and ventral prefrontal cortical activity (e.g. Baxter et al. 1989; Martinot et al. 1990; Mayberg et al. 2000; Vlassenko et al. 2004), or decreases in subcortical and ventral prefrontal cortical activity (Holthoff et al. 2004), in MDD depressed individuals and in mixed groups of individuals with MDD and BPI depression after depression improvement with pharmacological intervention. Other studies suggest decreases in DLPFC and VLPFC activity and metabolism after successful psychological and pharmacological interventions (e.g. Goldapple et al. 2004; Kennedy et al. 2007; Tutus et al. 1998), or relative increases only in subcortical, limbic regions after both types of intervention in MDD depressed individuals (Martin et al. 2001). Studies have also reported an inverse relationship between depression severity and dorsal prefrontal cortical and anterior cingulate gyral activity in depressed MDD individuals at rest (e.g. Baxter et al. 1989; Kimbrell et al. 2002). Overall, the findings at rest do not yet demonstrate a consistent pattern of activation. What does arise however are demonstrated alterations in neural systems involving prefrontal as well as subcortical limbic cortices, and an emerging number of studies are attempting to use paradigms to examine the neural systems of interest during specific task-related processing.

Emotion processing

Regarding neural activity during performance of emotion processing tasks, abnormally increased amygdala activity has been demonstrated by MDD depressed individuals to negative, but either not or less so to positive, emotional faces, for example, (Anand et al. 2007; Dannlowski et al. 2007; Fales et al. 2008; Fu et al. 2004; 2007; Neumeister et al. 2006; Sheline et al. 2001; Surguladze et al. 2005). Decreased ventromedial prefrontal activity during sad mood induction compared with healthy individuals has also been reported in MDD remitted and depressed individuals (Liotti et al. 2002).

Impaired executive control

Decreased DLPFC activity relative to healthy individuals has been reported in depressed MDD individuals during trials of working memory and attention (e.g. Elliott et al. 1997; Goethals et al. 2005; Okada et al. 2003). Fewer studies have shown increased DLPFC activity during working memory in MDD depression (e.g. Harvey et al. 2005). In most studies in MDD, an amelioration of abnormal neural activity has been shown after remission. For example, abnormally increased amygdala activity to negative emotional faces in depressed MDD individuals (Fu et al. 2004; Sheline et al. 2001; Surguladze et al. 2005) significantly reduces after remission induced by antidepressant medication (Anand et al. 2007; Sheline et al. 2001; Fu et al. 2004). Increases after remission in insular and anterior cingulate gyral activity to negative versus neutral scenes have also been reported (Davidson et al. 2003).

Emotion regulation

Regarding neuroimaging studies that have employed paradigms to directly examine neural systems underlying emotion regulation in individuals with MDD depression, the findings indicate decreased DLPFC activity relative to healthy individuals during working memory trials following negative stimuli (Siegle et al. 2002), during attempts to ignore negative stimuli (e.g. Fales et al. 2008), and during both unattended and attended emotional judgement (Grimm et al. 2008). In a probabilistic reversal learning task that required subjects to ignore misleading negative feedback, MDD depressed patients showed reduced activation of VLPFC during reversal, and failed to suppress amygdala activity during receipt of negative feedback, consistent with deficient top-down control of limbic circuitry by the prefrontal cortex (Taylor-Tavares et al. 2006).

Bipolar depression

Emotion processing

We will begin by examining the findings in the few studies that have examined neural activity to emotional challenges in remitted euthymic BP. These demonstrated increased subcortical (amygdala and ventral striatal) activity to mild happy (Lawrence et al. 2004) and intense fearful expressions (Lawrence et al. 2004; Yurgelun-Todd et al. 2000), while another study demonstrated increased amygdala activity to happy expressions in a mixed group of remitted and symptomatic BP (Blumberg et al. 2005).

Decreased blood flow was reported in medial prefrontal cortex during sad mood induction relative to baseline in remitted and depressed patients with BP (type 1; Kruger et al. 2003), but this study did not include a group of healthy individuals for comparison.

Interestingly, other studies utilizing emotional words as opposed to faces have demonstrated widespread decreases in subcortical as well as in prefrontal cortical neural activity in remitted individuals with BPI (Malhi et al. 2005), which suggests that emotional facial expressions may be processed distinctly from other emotional stimuli for remitted individuals with BPI, and may be particularly salient as socially relevant environmental stimuli.

Turning to BP depression, the few neuroimaging studies to date have demonstrated increased subcortical limbic activity to emotional facial expressions in stable BP individuals with subsyndromal depression (Blumberg et al. 2005; Lawrence et al. 2004) and to visualized scenes (captioned photographs) in depressed BP individuals (Blumberg et al. 2003) compared with healthy controls. Increased subcortical limbic activity (predominantly in the amygdala) has also been demonstrated in depressed and remitted BP patients (approximately 50% type 1) studied at rest (Drevets et al. 2002; Bauer et al. 2005). In addition, increased subcortical limbic activity has been demonstrated to positive stimuli such as happy faces (Chen et al. 2006) in depressed BP when compared to manic BP and healthy controls. The latter pattern of increased subcortical limbic activity to positive emotional stimuli may distinguish BPI from MDD depressed individuals, as discussed below.

Impaired executive control

The majority of neuroimaging studies in BP have focused on an examination of euthymic individuals. Here, findings have indicated poor task performance on executive measures such as the Stroop task (Strakowski et al.2005), and reduced activity in dorsal and ventral prefrontal cortical (Blumberg et al. 2003; Monks et al. 2004) as well as dorsal cingulate gyral (Gruber et al. 2004) activity when compared to healthy controls on working memory tasks.

There is a small number of studies examining neural activity during executive function in BP depression. One study examining remitted subjects with subsyndromal depression during an attentional task (Kronhaus et al. 2006) found decreased VLPFC activity with depression severity correlating negatively with the magnitude of VLPFC decrease, that is, greater depression severity was associated with more normalized VLPFC activity. Similarly, a study (Blumberg et al. 2003) comparing neural activity during performance of an attentional Stroop task in euthymic versus depressed individuals with bipolar disorder showed relative increases in VLPFC activity in bipolar depressed compared with euthymic individuals. These studies suggest a more complex pattern of functional abnormality in lateral PFC that may distinguish BP depression from BP remission, with BP depression showing more normalized VLPFC activity.

Emotion regulation

A small number of neuroimaging studies have employed paradigms to directly examine neural systems underlying emotion regulation in individuals with BP. Tasks such as the emotional Stroop and the affective Go/NoGo are often utilized to examine this area of interface. To date, however, studies have focused on an examination of remitted rather than depressed BP individuals. One recent study employed an affective Go/NoGo paradigm to examine neural activity during voluntary attentional control of emotion in BD remission (Wessa et al. 2007). Here, despite intact task performance, remitted BD adults demonstrated abnormally increased activity in bilateral OFC and left dorsal ACG, in addition to increased activity in different subcortical limbic regions implicated in emotion processing, when inhibiting responses to emotional relative to neutral distractors. Two studies employing an emotional Stroop paradigm demonstrated decreased left OFC activity in euthymic BD adults (Lagopoulis et al. 2007; Malhi et al. 2005) that was associated with slower task performance (Malhi et al. 2005).

In summary, the few studies to date indicate that BP remission and BP depression are both associated with increased activity in subcortical limbic regions to positive and negative emotional stimuli. While BP remission is associated with decreased activity in DLPFC/VLPFC and hippocampus, during executive control and memory tasks, BP depression may be associated with relative increases in DLPFC/VLPFC activity during these tasks in comparison with BP remission.

Abnormal neural activity in BPII depressed individuals

There has been an emergent literature focusing on the comparison of BPI and BPII as well as BPII versus MDD depressed individuals on neurocognitive task performance (e.g. Simonsen et al. 2008; Taylor-Tavares et al. 2007), however only one neuroimaging study to date focused on the examination of BPII depressed individuals (Mah et al. 2007). Here, abnormally increased metabolism was shown in different subcortical limbic regions (amygdala, ventral striatum, anterior insula) and ventral prefrontal cortex in medicated BPII depressed versus healthy individuals, indicating patterns of abnormal neural activity similar to those demonstrated by BPI depressed individuals.

Functional neuroimaging studies in MDD versus BP depression: towards diagnostic biomarkers?

Findings from studies employing emotional challenge paradigms suggest that, similar to individuals with BP, MDD depressed individuals show increased amygdala and subcortical activity to emotional stimuli (Surguladze et al. 2005; Fu et al. 2004) and decreased lateral prefrontal activity in response to cognitive control tasks relative to healthy individuals (Elliott et al. 1997), as well as following exposure to emotional stimuli (Siegle et al. 2002). There are, however, three findings from neuroimaging studies that may distinguish BP from MDD.

First, in MDD there appears to be a state dependence of functional neural abnormalities in that an amelioration of abnormal neural activity has been shown after remission. For example, abnormally increased amygdala activity to negative emotional faces in MDD individuals (Fu et al. 2004;

Sheline et al. 2001; Surguladze et al. 2005) significantly reduces in remission after antidepressant medication (Fu et al. 2004; Sheline et al. 2001).

Secondly, in UPD, unlike BPI, findings suggest that abnormalities in limbic subcortical activation may occur to some negative, but not positive, emotional stimuli (Surguladze et al. 2005). Only one functional neuroimaging study to date has directly compared BP and MDD individuals (Lawrence et al. 2004) and here subsyndromal BP depression was distinguished from MDD depression by amygdala and ventral striatal activity to positive emotional stimuli in the former but not the latter.

Thirdly, to date studies indicate, predominantly, a pattern of decreased DLPFC activity during cognitive challenge paradigms in both MDD and BP depressed patients; however depressed BP individuals display increased lateral PFC activity relative to BP individuals in remission during executive control tasks (Blumberg et al. 2003; Kronhaus et al. 2006). It is unclear, however, as to whether this is the case in depressed relative to recovered individuals with MDD. Some longitudinal studies, albeit during at rest rather than during emotion processing or executive control tasks (Mayberg et al. 2000), suggest a pattern of increased DLPFC activity in recovery relative to the depressed state in MDD. The nature of the differential pattern of DLPFC activity during executive control tasks in depression versus recovery may, therefore, distinguish BP and MDD individuals.

Potential confounds of neuroimaging studies of BP and MDD depression: medication effects

In healthy individuals, acute and subacute administration of SRI class antidepressant medication has been associated with decreased amygdala activity to fearful facial expressions and aversive scenes (Del-Ben et al. 2005; Harmer et al. 2006; Takahashi et al. 2005), while benzodiazepine dose inversely correlates with amygdala activity to facial expressions (Paulus et al. 2005). Mood-stabilizing medications, including divalproex sodium and lithium, have been reported as either decreasing prefrontal cortical blood flow (Gaillard et al. 1996; Leiderman et al. 1991), or having no effect (Oliver et al. 1998; Theodore, 2000). In examining the atypical antipsychotics, sultopride has been associated with decreased amygdala activity to aversive compared with neutral scenes in healthy individuals (Takahashi et al. 2005).

Findings from longitudinal studies in MDD suggest that antidepressant medications may reduce amygdala activity to emotional stimuli (Davidson, 2003; Fu, 2004; Sheline, 2001), and either increase PFC (e.g. Baxter et al. 1989; Kennedy et al. 2001; Martinot et al. 1990; Mayberg et al. 2000; Vlassenko et al. 2004) or decrease PFC (Brody et al. 2001; Holthoff et al. 2004; Kennedy et al. 2007; Saxena et al. 2002; Tutus et al. 1998) cortical activity in MDD depressed individuals.

We recently reviewed the evidence for potential effects of medication on neural activity in BPI individuals (Phillips et al. 2008a). In depressed BPI individuals, antidepressant medication has been associated with increased PFC metabolism at rest (Baxter et al. 1989). Mood stabilizers have been associated with decreased amygdala activity in remitted BP individuals (50% type 1) at rest (Drevets et al. 2002) and decreased amygdala activity in a mixed group of remitted and unwell BP individuals to emotional facial expressions (Blumberg et al. 2005). Other studies have shown a significant positive correlation between antipsychotic medication dose (in chlorpromazine equivalents) and activity in rostral ACG and DLPFC in remitted, euthymic individuals with BPI (Gruber et al. 2004), and increased DLPFC activity in medicated versus unmedicated euthymic individuals with BPI (Strakowski et al. 2005) during Stroop task performance, although no significant effect of any psychotropic medication was reported in individuals with BPI during a working memory task (Adler et al. 2004). Long-term psychotropic medication use (Nugent et al. 2006) and antidepressant exposure (Lopez-Larson et al. 2002) have been associated with decreased ventral prefrontal cortical grey matter volume in bipolar individuals, but long-term effects of psychotropic medication upon regional structural volumes remain unclear (Harrison, 2002; Manji et al. 2001; Sassi et al. 2002). BPII depressed individuals taking lithium or sodium valproate show increased subcortical metabolism versus healthy individuals (Mah et al. 2007).

Taken together, these findings indicate effects of mood stabilizers in BPI, antidepressants in depressed MDD (and healthy), and benzodiazepines in healthy populations in reducing amygdala activity to emotional stimuli, but additional effects of antipsychotic medications in increasing DLPFC activity during an attention task in BPI. Medicated more than unmedicated depressed individuals show decreased subcortical limbic activity during emotion processing, and increased dorsal prefrontal cortical activity during cognitive control paradigms, that is, levels of activity in these regions resembling those of healthy individuals. These reports suggest that functional neural abnormalities observed in depressed individuals likely reflect pathophysiologic processes that may be ameliorated by, rather than abnormalities that are secondary to, psychotropic medication. No studies have yet examined the impact of total psychotropic medication load, reflecting medication dose and variety, upon neural activity in depression, which therefore, remains a major limitation of current neuroimaging studies to date.

Summary

To date, unfortunately, there is no one pathognomonic neuroimaging finding that can diagnose either major depressive disorder or bipolar disorder in any one individual at rest. Emerging evidence, however, is demonstrating that by utilizing specific targeted neurocognitive paradigms, MDD and BP depression may be distinguished by direct measures of abnormal activity in subcortical limbic and lateral prefrontal neural systems. These abnormalities may underlie, respectively, the mood instability and impaired cognitive control of emotion, the core domains of pathology that are observed clinically in both disorders. Increased subcortical limbic activity to happy stimuli may, in particular, be an important pathophysiologic process distinguishing the depression associated with BP from that associated with MDD.

It is clear that at this point diagnostic functional neuroimaging is in its infancy. In the future, however, studies employing these newly developed functional neuroimaging techniques and paradigms may be able to draw us closer to meeting the critical challenges of early and accurate diagnosis of both MDD and BP depression, not only at a group level but at the level of the individual. This should also prevent relapse and facilitate return to work as well as restoring quality of life in patients with depressive disorders. In tandem, a major future challenge will be to identify endophenotypic markers in order to identify not only those affected, but those at-risk individuals prior to clinical onset of psychiatric disorders.

References

Adler, C.M., Holland, S.K., Schmithorst, V. et al. (2004). Changes in neuronal activation in patients with bipolar disorder during performance of a working memory task. *Bipolar Disord.*, **6**, 540–549.

Anand, A., Li, Y., Wang, Y. et al. (2005). Antidepressant effect on connectivity of the mood-regulating circuit: an FMRI study. *Neuropsychopharmacol*, **30**, 1334–1344.

Angst, J., Gamma, A., Benazzi, F., Ajdacic, V., Eich, D., and Rossler, W. (2003). Toward a re-definition of subthreshold bipolarity: epidemiology and proposed criteria for bipolar-II, minor bipolar disorders and hypomania. *J Affect Disord.*, **73**, 133–146.

Balazs. J., Lecrubier, Y., Csiszer, N., Kosztak, J., and Bitter (2003). Prevalence and comorbidity of affective disorders in persons making suicide attempts in Hungary: importance of the first depressive episodes and of bipolar II diagnoses. *J Affect Disord.*, **76**, 113–119.

Baldessarini, R.J. and Tondo, L. (2003). Suicide risk and treatments for patients with bipolar disorder. *JAMA*, **290**, 1517–1519.

Bauer, M., London, E.D., Rasgon, N. et al. (2005). Supraphysiological doses of levothyroxine alter regional cerebral metabolism and improve mood in bipolar depression. *Mol Psychiatry*, **10**, 45–469.

Baxter, L.R., Jr, Schwartz, J.M., Phelps, M.E., et al. (1989). Reduction of prefrontal cortex glucose metabolism common to three types of depression. *Arch Gen Psychiatry*, **46**, 243–250.

Blumberg, H.P., Leung, H.C., Skudlarski, P., Lacadie, C.M., Fredericks, C.A., Harris, B.C. et al. (2003). A functional magnetic resonance imaging study of bipolar disorder: State- and trait-related dysfunction in ventral prefrontal cortices. *Arch Gen Psychiatry*, **60**, 601–609.

Blumberg, H.P., Donegan, N.H., Sanislow, C.A., Collins, S., Lacadie, C., Skudlarski, P. et al. (2005). Preliminary evidence for medication effects on functional abnormalities in the amygdala and anterior cingulate in bipolar disorder. *Psychopharmacology*, **183**, 308–313.

Bowden, C.L. (2001). Strategies to reduce misdiagnosis of bipolar depression. *Psychiatric Services*, **52**, 51–55.

Bowden, C.L. (2005). A different depression: clinical distinctions between bipolar and unipolar depression. *J Affect Disord.*, **84**, 117–125.

Brody, A.L., Saxena, S., Stoessel, P. et al. (2001). Regional brain metabolic chances in patients with major depression treated with either paroxetine or interpersonal therapy: preliminary findings. *Arch Gen Psychiatry*, **58**, 631–640.

Calabrese, J.R., Hirschfeld, R.M., Frye, M.A., and Reed, M.L. (2004). Impact of depressive symptoms compared with manic symptoms in bipolar disorder: results of a U.S. community-based sample. *J Clin Psychiatry*, **65**,1499–1504.

Chen, C.H., Lennox, B., Jacob, R. et al. (2006). Explicit and implicit facial affect recognition in manic and depressed states of bipolar disorder: a functional magnetic resonance imaging study. *Biol Psychiatry*, **59**, 31–39.

Dannlowski, U., Ohrmann P., Bauer, J. et al. (2007). Amygdala reactivity to masked negative faces is associated with automatic judgmental bias in major depression: a 3 T fMRI study. *J Psychiatry Neurosci.*, **32**, 423–429.

Davidson, R.J., Irwin, W., Anderle, M.J., and Kalin, N.H. (2003). The neural substrates of affective processing in depressed patients treated with venlafaxine. *Am J Psychiatry,* **160**, 64–75.

Deckersbach, T., Savage, C.R., Reilly-Harrington, N., Clark, L., Sachs, G., and Rauch, S.L. (2004). Episodic memory impairment in bipolar disorder and obsessive-compulsive disorder: the role of memory strategies. *Bipolar Disord.*, **6**, 233–244.

Del-Ben, C.M., Deakin, J.F., McKie, S. et al. (2005). The effect of citalopram pretreatment on neuronal responses to neuropsychological tasks in normal volunteers: an FMRI study. *Neuropsychopharmacol*, **30**, 1724–1734.

Delgado, M.R., Frank, R.H., and Phelps, E.A. (2005). Perceptions of moral character modulate the neural systems of reward during the trust game. *Nat Neurosci.*, Nov; **8**(11), 1611–1618.

DePaulo, R.J. (2006). Bipolar disorder treatment: an evidence-based reality check. *Am J Psychiatry*, **163**, 175–176.

Drevets, W.C., Price, J.L., Bardgett, M.E., Reich, T., Todd, R.D., and Raichle, M.E. (2002). Glucose metabolism in the amygdala in depression: relationship to diagnostic subtype and plasma cortisol levels. *Pharmacol Biochem Behav.*, **71**, 431–447.

Elliott, R., Baker, S.C., Rogers, R.D. et al. (1997). Prefrontal dysfunction in depressed patients performing a complex planning task: a study using positron emission tomography. *Psychol. Med.*, **27**, 931–942.

Fagiolini, A., Frank, E., Cherry, C.R. et al. (2002). Clinical indicators for the use of antidepressants in the treatment of bipolar I depression. *Bipolar Disord.*, **4**(5), 277–282.

Fales, C.L., Barch, D.M., Rundle, M.M. et al. (2008). Altered emotional interference processing in affective and cognitive-control brain circuitry in major depression. *Biol Psychiatry*, **15**, 63, 377–384.

Forty, L., Smith, D., Jones, L. et al. (2008). Clinical differences between bipolar and unipolar depression. *Br J Psych.*, **192**, 388–389.

Fu, C.H., Williams, S.C., Cleare, A.J. et al. (2004). Attenuation of the neural response to sad faces in major depression by antidepressant treatment: a prospective, event-related functional magnetic resonance imaging study. *Arch Gen Psychiatry*, **61**, 877–889.

Fu, C.H., Williams, S.C., Brammer, M.J. et al. (2007). Neural responses to happy facial expressions in major depression following antidepressant treatment. *Am J Psychiatry*, Apr; **164**(4), 599–607.

Gaillard, W.D., Zeffiro, T., Fazilat, S., DeCarli, C., and Theodore, W.H. (1996). Effect of valproate on cerebral metabolism and blood flow: an 18F-2-deoxyglucose and ^{15}O water positron. *Epilepsia*, **37**, 515–521.

Ghaemi, S.N., Ko, J.Y., and Goodwin, F.K. (2002). "Cade's disease" and beyond: misdiagnosis, antidepressant use, and a proposed definition for bipolar spectrum disorder. *Can Jl Psychiatry*, **47**, 125–134.

Ghaemi, S.N., Hsu, D.J., Soldani, F., and Goodwin, F.K. (2003). Antidepressants in bipolar disorder: the case for caution. *Bipolar Disord.*, **5**(6), 421–433.

Goethals, I., Audenaert, K., Jacobs, F. et al. (2005). Blunted prefrontal perfusion in depressed patients performing the Tower of London task. *Psychiatry Res.*, **139**, 31–40.

Goodwin, G.M., Austin, M.P., Dougall, N. et al. (1993). State changes in brain activity shown by the uptake of 99mTc-exametazime with single photon emission tomography in major depression before and after treatment. *J Affect Disord.*, **29**, 243–253.

Goldapple, K., Segal, Z., Garson, C. et al. (2004). Modulation of cortical-limbic pathways in major depression: treatment-specific effects of cognitive behavior therapy. *Arch Gen Psychiatry*, **6**, 34–41.

Gottesman, I.I. and Gould, T.D. (2003). The endophenotype concept in psychiatry: etymology and strategic intentions. *Am J Psychiatry*, **160**, 636–645.

Grimm, S., Beck, J., Schuepbach, D. et al. (2008). Imbalance between left and right dorsolateral prefrontal cortex in major depression is linked to negative emotional judgment: an fMRI study in severe major depressive disorder. *Biol Psychiatry*, **15**, **63**, 369–376.

Grote, N.K. and Frank, E. (2003). Difficult-to-treat depression: the role of contexts and comorbidities. *Biol Psychiatry*, **53**(8), 660–670.

Gruber, S.A., Rogowska, J., and Yurgelun-Todd, D.A. (2004). Decreased activation of the anterior cingulate in bipolar patients: an fMRI study. *J Affect Disord.*, **82**, 191–201.

Harmer, C.J., Mackay, C.E., Rein, C.B., Cowen, P.J., and Goodwin, G.M. (2006). Antidepressant drug treatment modifies the neural processing of nonconscious threat cues. *Biol Psychiatry*, **59**, 816–821.

Harrison, P.J. (2002). The neuropathology of primary mood disorder. *Brain*, **125**, 1428–1449.

Harvey, P.O., Fossati, P., Pochon, J.B. et al. (2005). Cognitive control and brain resources in major depression: an fMRI study using the n-back task. *Neuroimage*, **26**, 860–869.

Hasler, G., Drevets, W.C., Manji, H.K., and Charney, D.S., (2004). Discovering endophenotypes for major depression. *Neuropsychopharmacol.*, **29**(10), 1765–1781.

Hasler, G., Drevets, W.C., Gould, T.D., Gottesman, I.I., and Manji, H.K. (2006). Toward constructing an endophenotype strategy for bipolar disorders. *Biol Psychiatry*, **60**, 93–105.

Hirschfeld, R.M., Lewis, L., and Vornik, L.A. (2003). Perceptions and impact of bipolar disorder: how far have we really come? Results of the National Depressive and Manic-depressive Association 2000 survey of individuals with bipolar disorder. *J Clin Psychiatry*, **64**, 161–174.

Holthoff, V.A., Beuthien-Baumann, B. et al. (2004). Changes in brain metabolism associated with remission in unipolar major depression. *Acta Psychiat Scand.*, **10**, 184–194.

Judd, L.L., Akiskal, H.S., Schettler, P.J. et al. (2003). The comparative clinical phenotype and long term longitudinal episode course of bipolar I and II: a clinical spectrum or distinct disorders? *J Affect Disord.*, **73**, 19–32.

Keener, M.T. and Phillips, M.L. (2007). Neuroimaging in bipolar disorder: a review of current findings. *Curr Opin Psychiatr.*, **9**, 512–520.

Kennedy, S.H., Evans, K.R., Kruger, S. et al. (2001). Changes in regional brain glucose metabolism measured with positron emission tomography after paroxetine treatment of major depression. *Am J Psychiatry*, **158**, 899–905.

Kessler, R.C., Berglund, P., Demler, O. et al. (2003). The epidemiology of major depressive disorder: results from the National Comorbidity Survey Replication. *JAMA*, **23**, 3095–3105.

Kimbrell, T.A., Ketter, T.A., George, M.A. et al. (2002). Regional cerebral glucose utilization in patients with a range of severities of unipolar depression. *Biol Psychiatry.*, **51**(3), 237–252.

Knutson, B. and Cooper, J.C. (2005). Functional magnetic resonance imaging of reward prediction. *Curr Opin Neurol.*, **18**, 411–417.

Kraemer, H.C., Schultz, SK., and Arndt, S. (2002). Biomarkers in psychiatry: methodological issues. *Am J Geriat Psychiat.*, **10**, 653–659.

Kronhaus, D.M., Lawrence, N.S., Williams, A.M. et al. (2006). Stroop performance in bipolar disorder: further evidence for abnormalities in the ventral prefrontal cortex. *Bipolar Disord.*, **8**, 28–39.

Kruger, S., Seminowicz, D., Goldapple, K., Kennedy, S.H., and Mayberg, H.S. (2003). State and trait influences on mood regulation in bipolar disorder: blood flow differences with an acute mood challenge. *Biol Psychiatry*, **54**, 1274–1283.

Kupfer, D.J., First, M.B., and Regier, D.A. (eds.) (2002). *A Research Agenda for DSM-V* American Psychiatric Association: Washington, D.C.

Kupfer, D.J. (2005). The increasing medical burden in bipolar disorder. *JAMA*, **293**, 2528–2530.

Lawrence, N.S., Williams, A.M., Surguladze, S. et al. (2004). Subcortical and ventral prefrontal cortical neural responses to facial expressions distinguish patients with bipolar disorder and major depression. *Biol Psychiatry*, **55**, 578–587.

Leiderman, D.B., Balish, M., Bromfield, E.B., and Theodore, W.H (1991). Effect of valproate on human cerebral glucose metabolism. *Epilepsia*, **32**, 417–422.

Liotti, M., Mayberg, H.S., McGinnis, S., Brannan, S.L., and Jerabek, P. (2002). Unmasking disease-specific cerebral blood flow abnormalities: mood challenge in patients with remitted unipolar depression. *Am J Psychiatry*, **159**, 1830–1840.

Lish, J.D., Dime-Meenan, S., Whybrow, P.C., Price, R.A., and Hirschfeld, R.M. (1994). The National Depressive and Manic-depressive Association (DMDA) survey of bipolar members. *J Affect Disord.*, **31**, 281–294.

Lopez-Larson, M.P., DelBello, M.P., Zimmerman, M.E., Schwiers, M.L., Strakowski, S.M. (2002). Regional prefrontal gray and white matter abnormalities in bipolar disorder. *Biol Psychiatry*, **52**, 93–100.

Mah, L., Zarate, C.A., Jr., Singh, J. et al. (2007) Regional cerebral glucose metabolic abnormalities in bipolar II depression. *Biol Psychiatry*, **61**, 765–75.

Maina,G., Albert, U., Bellodi, L. et al. (2007). Health-related quality of life in euthymic bipolar disorder patients: differences between bipolar I and II subtypes. *J Clin Psychiatry*, **68**, 207–212.

Malhi, G.S., Lagopoulos, J., and Sachdev, P.S. et al. (2005). An emotional Stroop functional MRI study of euthymic bipolar disorder. *Bipol Disord.*, **7**, 58–69.

Manji, H.K., Drevets, W.C., and Charney, D.S. (2001) The cellular neurobiology of depression. *Nat Medicine.*, **7**, 541–547.

Manning, J.S. (2003). Bipolar disorder in primary care. *J Fam Pract.*, **3** (Suppl), S6–9.

Martin, S.D., Martine, E., Rai, S.S., Richardson, M.A., and Royall, R. (2001). Brain blood flow changes in depressed patients treated with interpersonal psychotherapy or venlafaxine hydrochloride: preliminary findings. *Arch Gen Psychiatry*, **58**, 641–648.

Martinot, J.L., Hardy, P., Feline, A. et al. (1990). Left prefrontal glucose hypometabolism in the depressed state: a confirmation. *Am J Psychiatry*, **147**, 1313–1317.

Mayberg, H.S., Brannan, S.K., Mahurin, R.K. et al. (2000). Regional metabolic effects of fluoxetine in major depression: serial changes and relationship to clinical response. *Biol Psychiatry*, **48**, 30–843.

McMahon, F.J., Stine, O.C., Chase, G.A., Meyers, D.A., Simpson, S.G., and DePaulo, J.R. Jr. (1994). Influence of clinical subtype, sex, and lineality on age at onset of major affective disorder in a family sample. *Am J Psychiatry*, **151**, 210–215.

Monks, P.J., Thompson, J.M., Bullmore, E.T. et al. (2004). A functional MRI study of working memory task in euthymic bipolar disorder: evidence for task-specific dysfunction. *Bipolar Disord.*, **6**, 550–564.

Murray, C.J.L. and Lopez, A.D. (1996). The Global Burden of Disease: A Comprehensive Assessment of Mortality and Disability from Disease, Injuries and Risk Factors in 1990 and project to 2020. Harvard School of Public Health on behalf of the World Health Organization and the World Bank. Cambridge, MA, Harvard University Press.

Neumeister, A., Drevets, W.C., Belfer, I. et al. (2006). Effects of a alpha 2C-adrenoreceptor gene polymorphism on neural responses to facial expressions in depression. *Neuropsychopharmacol.*, **31**,1750–1756.

Nugent, A.C., Milham, M.P., Bain, E.E. et al. (2006). Cortical abnormalities in bipolar disorder investigated with MRI and voxel-based morphometry. *Neuroimage*, **30**, 485–497.

Ochsner K.N. and Gross, J.J. (2007)..The neural architecture of emotion regulation. In Gross, J.J. (ed.) pp. 87–109. *Handbook of Emotion Regulation*. New York, Guilford Press.

Oliver, D.W. and Dormehl, I.C. (1998). Cerebral blood flow effects of sodium valproate in drug combinations in the baboon model. *Arzneimittelforschung*, **48**, 1058–1063.

Okada, G., Okamoto, Y., Morinobu, S., Yamawaki, S., and Yokota, N. (2003). Attenuated left prefrontal activation during a verbal fluency task in patients with depression. *Neuropsychobiology*, **47**, 21–26.

Öngür, D. and Price, J.L. (2000). The organization of networks within the orbital and medial prefrontalcortex of rats, monkeys and humans. *Cereb Cortex.*, **10**, 206–219.

Paulus, M.P., Feinstein, J.S., Castillo, G., Simmons, A.N., and Stein, M.B. (2005). Dose-dependent decrease of activation in bilateral amygdala and insula by lorazepam during emotion processing. *Arch Gen Psychiatry*, **62**, 282–288.

Phillips, M.L., Drevets, W.C., Rauch, S.L., and Lane, R.D., (2003). The neurobiology of emotion perception I: towards an understanding of the neural basis of normal emotion perception. *Biol Psychiatry*, **54**, 504–514.

Phillips, M.L. and Frank, E. (2006). Redefining bipolar disorder: toward DSM-V. *Am J Psychiatry*, **163**, 1135–1136.

Phillips, M.L. (2007). The emerging role of neuroimaging in psychiatry: characterizing treatment-relevant endophenotypes. *Am J Psychiatry*, **164**, 697–699.

Phillips, M.L., Travis, M.J., Fagiolini, A., and Kupfer, D.J. (2008a). Medication effects in neuroimaging studies of bipolar disorder. *Am J Psychiatry*, **165**, 313–320.

Phillips, M.L., Ladouceur, C.D., and Drevets, W.C. (2008b). A neural model of voluntary and automatic emotion regulation: implications for understanding the pathophysiology and neurodevelopment of bipolar disorder. *Mol Psychiatry,* (In Press).

Price, J.L. (2003). Comparative aspects of amygdala connectivity. *Ann N Y Acad Sci.*, **985**, 50–58.

Regier, D.A., Farmer, M.E., Rae, D.S. et al. (1993). One-month prevalence of mental disorders in the United States and sociodemographic characteristics: the Epidemiologic Catchment Area study. *Acta Psychiatrica Scandinavica.*, **88**, 35–47.

Rihmer, Z. and Pestality, P. (1999). Bipolar II disorder and suicidal behavior. *Psychiatr Clin North America.*, **22**, 667–673.

Robbins, T.W. (1998). Dissociating executive functions of the prefrontal cortex. In Roberts, A.C., Robbins, T.W. and Weiskrantz, L.R. (eds.) *The Prefrontal Cortex: Executive and Cognitive Functions.* New York, Oxford University Press.

Sachs, G.S., Nierenberg, A.A., Calabrese, J.R. et al. (2007). Effectiveness of adjunctive antidepressant treatment for bipolar depression. *NEJM*, **356**, 1711–1722.

Sassi, R.B., Brambilla, P., Hatch, J.P. et al. (2004). Reduced left anterior cingulate volumes in untreated bipolar patients. *Biol Psychiatry*, **56**, 467–475.

Saxena, S., Brody, A.L., Ho, M.L., Zohrabi, N., Maidment, K.M., and Baxter, L.R. (2003). Differential brain metabolic predictors of response to paroxetine in obsessive-compulsive disorder versus major depression. *Am J Psychiatry*, **160**, 522–532.

Sheline, Y.I., Barch, D.M., Donnelly, J.M., Ollinger, J.M., Snyder, A.Z., and Mintun, M.A. (2001). Increased amygdala response to masked emotional faces in depressed subjects resolves with antidepressant treatment: An fMRI study. *Biol Psychiatry*, **50**, 651–658.

Siegle, G.J., Steinhauer, S.R., Thase, M.E., Stenger, V.A., and Carter, C.S. (2002). Can't shake that feeling: fMRI assessment of sustained amygdala activity in response to emotional information in depressed individuals. *Biol Psychiatry*, **51**, 693–707.

Simonsen, C., Sundet, K., Vaskinn, A. et al. (2008). Neurocognitive profiles in bipolar I and bipolar II disorder: differences in pattern and magnitude of dysfunction. *Bipolar Disorder*, **10**, 245–255.

Strakowski, S.M., Adler, C.M., Holland, S.K. et al. (2005). Abnormal FMRI brain activation in euthymic bipolar disorder patients during a counting Stroop interference task. *Am J Psychiatry*, **162**(9), 1697–1705.

Stuss, D.T. and Levine, B. (2002). Adult clinical neuropsychology: lessons from studies of the frontal lobes. *Ann Rev Psychol.*, **53**, 401–433.

Surguladze, S., Brammer, M., Keedwell, P. et al. (2005). A differential pattern of neural response towards sad versus happy facial expressions in major depressive disorder. *Biol Psychiatry*, **57**, 201–209.

Swann, A. (2006). What is bipolar disorder? *Am J Psychiatry*, **163**, 177–179.

Takahashi, H., Yahata, N., Koeda, M. et al. (2005). Effects of dopaminergic and serotonergic manipulation on emotional processing: a pharmacological fMRI study. *Neuroimage*, **27**, 991–1001.

Taylor-Tavares, J.V., Clark, L., Williams, G.B., Furey, M.L., Sahakian, B.J., and Drevets, W.C. (2006). Neural correlates of oversensitivity to misleading negative feedback in unipolar and bipolar depression. *Neuroimage*, **31** (Suppl 1), S143.

Theodore, W.H. (2000). PET: cerebral blood flow and glucose metabolism – pathophysiology and drug effects. *Adv Neurol.*, **83**,121–130.

Tutus, A., Simsek, A., Sofuoglu, S. et al. (1998). Changes in regional cerebral blood flow demonstrated by single photon emission computed tomography in depressive disorders: comparison of unipolar vs. bipolar subtypes. *Psychiat Res.*, **83**, 169–177.

Vlassenko, A., Sheline, Y.I., Fischer, K., and Mintun, M.A. (2004). Cerebral perfusion response to successful treatment of depression with different serotonergic agents. *J Neuropsych Clinl Neurosci.*, **16**, 360–363.

Wyatt, R.J. and Henter, I. (1995). An economic evaluation of manic-depressive illness – 1991. *Soc Psychaitry Psychiatr Epidemiol.*, **30**, 213–219.

Wessa, M., Houenou, J., Paillere-Martinot, M.L. et al. (2007). Fronto-striatal overactivation in euthymic bipolar patients during an emotional go/nogo task. *Am J Psychiatry.*, **164**, 638–646.

Yurgelun-Todd, D.A., Gruber, S.A., Kanayama, G., Killgore, W.D., Baird, A.A., and Young, A.D., (2000). fMRI during affect discrimination in bipolar affective disorder. *Bipolar Disord.*, **2**, 237–248.

Zola-Morgan, S., Squire, L.R., Alvarez-Royo, P., and Clower, R.P. (1991). Independence of memory functions and emotional behavior: separate contributions of the hippocampal formation and the amygdale. *Hippocampus*, **1**, 207–220.

Chapter 23

Pharmacogenetics of antidepressant response

Bhanu Gupta*, Robert Keers*, Rudolf Uher, Peter McGuffin, and Katherine J. Aitchison

Introduction

In the treatment of depression, there is substantial individual variability in both the response to medication and in the incidence and severity of adverse drug reactions (ADRs). It has been estimated that between 30 % and 50% of people do not respond to the first antidepressant they are prescribed (Fava, 2003) and ADRs frequently interfere with treatment. Pharmacogenetic research is concerned with the role of genetic factors in predicting both response to, and potential adverse effects of, medication. The terms pharmacogenetics and pharmacogenomics have been used to refer to hypothesis-based studies in this field investigating candidate genes and hypothesis-free studies using the whole genome or its expressed counterparts, respectively (Aitchison and Gill, 2002), but are now often used interchangeably (see e.g. www.pharmgkb.org). This is the last of four chapters in this book that discuss the genetics of affective disorders, together with Chapter 4, 5, 6, and 23. Moreover, this and the last chapters in this book (Chapter 24, 25, 26, and 27) specifically discuss the more recent developments in the treatment of affective disorders.

Response to medication is a complex phenotype that, like other phenotypes in psychiatry, is likely to result not only from a number of genetic, but also environmental factors. In the study of complex phenotypes it is important to consider not only both genetic and environmental factors, but also the interplay between them (Rutter et al. 2006). A good example of this in relation to depression is the interaction between genotype at the serotonin transporter linked polymorphic region (5-HTTLPR) and stressful life events (reviewed in Uher and McGuffin, 2008). In addition, complex clinical factors such as personality and temperament have also been shown to interact with both environmental (Mazure et al. 2000) and genetic factors (Ishii et al. 2007) in predicting response to antidepressants.

In this chapter we review the most promising emerging genetic, environmental, and clinical predictors of response to antidepressants. Using the GENDEP study as an example (Uher et al. 2008), we then outline methodology for investigating both genetic and environmental factors and the interplay between them in predicting response to antidepressants, and novel methodology for investigating clinical response in general.

Genetic factors leading to interindividual variability in drug response can be considered at the level of pharmacokinetics (affecting drug absorption, metabolism, and excretion) and pharmacodynamics (affecting response at the level of the target organ). Potential candidate genes for pharmacogenetic studies therefore include those that encode drug metabolizing

---

* These two authors contributed equally to this work.

enzymes (DMEs, e.g. cytochrome P450 enzymes), neuronal drug transporters (e.g. the serotonin transporter), neurotransmitter targets (e.g. serotonin receptor subtypes), enzymes involved in neurotransmitter synthesis, and other candidates with good a priori rationale for study in relation to the phenotype of interest. Several such candidates already investigated in pharmacogenetic studies of antidepressant treatment have been previously reviewed (Basu and Aitchison 2005; Serretti and Artioli, 2004; Serretti et al. 2008).

The environmental factors that have been best studied in relation to response to antidepressants are stressful life events (Mazure et al. 2000; Monroe et al. 1983) and the best-studied clinical factors are personality or temperament (Joyce et al. 1994).

Drug metabolizing enzymes

Cytochrome P450 (CYP) enzymes comprise a large family of DMEs shown to play a critical role in drug metabolism. A number of studies have investigated the impact of genetic variation in genes encoding the CYPs on drug metabolism and efficacy and/or ADRs. CYPs are among the most polymorphic genes, with polymorphisms ranging from single nucleotide substitutions (SNPs) to several nucleotide insertions or deletions, and even deletions of the complete coding sequence of a gene and copy number variants (CNVs), in which multiple copies of a functional coding sequence result in increased enzyme activity (www.cypalleles.ki.se). In addition, microRNAs (non-coding RNAs that typically decrease expression of mRNAs) and pharmacoepigenetic phenomena (such as DNA methylation) have also been shown to affect the expression of the CYP genes (Rountree et al. 2001). It estimated that the outcome of therapy to 20–25% of all drugs is affected by CYP gene expression levels (Ingelman-Sundberg et al. 2007). For medications used in the treatment of depression, the most relevant CYPs for which there are identified polymorphisms affecting enzyme activity are CYP2D6 and CYP2C19.

CYP2D6

The *CYP2D6* gene is located on chromosome 22q13.1. There are over 70 allelic variants (www.cypalleles.ki.se) associated with four major phenotypes: ultrarapid metabolizers (UM), extensive metabolizers (EM), intermediate metabolizers (IM) and poor metabolizers (PM). An increased risk of ADRs has been associated with CYP2D6 PM status and an increase incidence of inadequate therapeutic response or therapeutic resistance with UMs (Ingelman-Sundberg et al. 2007). PMs have functionally inactive copies of both alleles, IMs have one reduced activity allele and one non-functional allele or two reduced activity alleles, EMs have at least one active allelic variant, and UMs show increased enzyme activity, for example, due to gene duplication (e.g. *CYP2D6*1xN or CYP2D6*2xN*). The alleles also show variation in their frequency by ethnicity, for example, in Ethiopians up to 29% of individuals are UMs based on their genotype, while only 1% of Asians are PMs (Aitchison et al. 2000).

Dalen et al. (1998) reported that approximately 40% of the variance in the logarithm of the dose-corrected nortriptyline level was accounted for by the number of functional copies of *CYP2D6*. Similar findings have been reported for other antidepressants also metabolized by CYP2D6, namely the serotonin-norepinephrine reuptake inhibitor (SNRI) venlafaxine (Otton et al. 1996), and the selective serotonin reuptake inhibitor (SSRI) paroxetine (Brosen et al. 1993). Single dose experiments have shown that for individuals having only one copy of the gene, a therapeutic plasma level may be attained with a starting dose in the recommended range, with levels outside the normal range with an initiation dose at the upper end of the normal range (Bertilsson et al. 2002). On the other hand, for individuals who are UMs, doses at the upper limit of the recommended prescribed range may not be sufficient to reach therapeutic drug levels (Bertilsson et al. 1993). For venlafaxine, a relationship between PM status and increased occurrence of cardiovascular ADRs or even toxicity has been reported (Lessard et al. 1999). Specific dose recommendations based on *CYP2D6* and *CYP2C19* phenotype have been put forward by Kircheiner et al. (2004), for example, with the dose of TCAs being halved for CYP2D6 PMs. Therapeutic drug monitoring of TCAs and venlafaxine has been recommended by a European Consortium (Baumann et al. 2004).

CYP2C19

The CYP2C19 gene is located on chromosome 10q24. CYP2C19 plays a significant role in the demethylation of tertiary amines including amitriptyline, and in the metabolism of some SSRIs including citalopram. Amitriptyline is demethylated to nortriptyline by CYP2C19 and other CYPs, and both amitriptyline and nortriptyline are hydroxylated by CYP2D6. Nortriptyline is an active metabolite and indeed is prescribed as an antidepressant in its own right (the ratio of affinity for the noradrenaline transporter to the serotonin transporter is higher for nortriptyline than for amitriptyline). A combination of high CYP2C19 activity and low CYP2D6 activity has been shown to confer the highest risk of ADRs to amitriptyline (Steimer et al. 2005). CYP2C19 preferentially metabolizes the S-enantiomer of citalopram (Herrlin et al. 2003; von Moltke et al. 2001) which has an allosteric modulatory effect at the serotonin transporter whereby the binding of the first molecule of S-citalopram is enhanced by the binding of a second molecule (Chen et al. 2005). A functional gene dosage effect has been shown for citalopram and S-citalopram, with a difference in dose-corrected serum concentration and dose-corrected serum metabolite concentration and between individuals carrying one or two functionally active *CYP2C19* alleles (Rudberg et al. 2006). A retrospective analysis of ten years of genotyping for *CYP2D6* variants in depressed patients at the Karolinska Institute revealed an excess of ADRs in *CYP2D6* PMs, with an excess of inadequate response to treatment or treatment-resistance in *CYP2D6* UMs (Sjoqvist and Eliasson, 2007; Steimer et al. 2005).

GENDEP is a multicentre European study that was specifically designed as a pharmacogenetic study of antidepressant response. Participants were randomized to either escitalopram or nortriptyline, with clinician override of the randomization being permitted for clinical reasons. Using data from this study, we have recently reported the first association between *CYP2C19* genotype and steady state serum level of a drug in a prospective study, in this case, escitalopram (logarithm, dose-corrected; (Huezo-Diaz et al. submitted). Our report essentially replicates and strengthens of the finding of Rudberg et al. (2008), of an association between *CYP2C19* genotype and dose-corrected escitalopram level in a retrospective analysis of therapeutic drug monitoring data. There is already available a microarray test (the AmpliChip CYP450 Test®, Roche Diagnostics, USA) which can identify 33 *CYP2D6* allelic variants and two *CYP2C19* variants and is approved for clinical diagnostic use. In addition, there are other methods of genotyping for these enzymes (reviewed in de Leon, 2006).

Drug transporters

The serotonin transporter

The serotonin transporter is the main site of action for SSRIs and the gene encoding the transporter (*SLC6A4*) is the best-studied candidate gene in pharmacogenetic studies of antidepressants to date (reviewed in Serretti et al. 2008). SLC6A4 is located on chromosome 17q -11.1q-12, spans 31 kb and includes 14 exons. There are two functional polymorphisms in this gene that have been associated with response to antidepressants to date: the *5-HTTLPR* and *STin2* (reviewed in Aitchison et al. 2002). The *5-HTTLPR* (serotonin transporter linked polymorphic region) is a variable number imperfect tandem repeat (VNTR) located about 1 kb upstream of the transcription start site, comprising a GC rich 20–23 base pair repeat element that is repeated 14 or 16 times in the two commonest allelic variants, known as 'short' or 'S' and 'long' or 'L' alleles, respectively. The first functional investigation of these variants showed that the 'S' variant was associated with lower expression of the serotonin transporter in in vitro assays (Heils et al. 1996) than 'L' variant. There are other rare (<5%) allelic variants, for example, with more than 16 repeats, which have been described in Japanese and African Americans (Delbruck et al. 1997; Gelernter et al. 1997). In addition, sequence variation of the 20–23 repeat element was described as early as 1999 by Nakamura et al. (1999). More recently, one such variant in the sixth repeat element (rs25531) G>A has been investigated for associations with expression level of the serotonin transporter and clinical response (Hu et al. 2007). In addition, there is a SNP in the first intron, rs2020933, which has been shown to be responsible for more of the variance in allelic expression imbalance than rs25531 in a recent analysis (Martin et al. 2007).

The 'L' allele has been associated with better response to SSRIs in Caucasians in most studies (Serretti et al. 2007). The recent STAR*D study initially reported no association with the *5-HTTLPR* and response to citalopram (Kraft et al. 2007). However, on reanalysis, stratifying the sample population by ethnicity, the *5-HTTLPR* was associated with remission (Mrazek et al. 2009). An effect in the opposite direction has been seen in Asian populations, with several studies reporting a better outcome with the 'S' allele (Kim et al. 2006; Yu et al. 2002). This may be due to the higher frequency of sequence variation within the *5-HTTLPR* in Asians (Nakamura et al. 1999), and perhaps to the different allele frequencies within ethnic groups (the 'L' allele frequency being lower in Asians than in Caucasians).

In Caucasians, the 'S' allele has been associated with not only a relatively poor response to SSRIs but also a worse illness course, characterized by rapid cycling (Rousseva et al. 2003). Given the apparent functionality of rs25531 described by Hu et al. (2006), the *5-HTTLPR* in some subsequent analyses was been treated as a tri-allelic locus: La/La; any heterozygote combination; and S/S or Lg/Lg; where La represents the A allele of rs25531 on a background of the L allele and Lg the G variant of rs25531 on an L allele background, and similarly with the S allele (S/S denotes the S allele with either variant of rs25531, as in the work of Hu et al. (2006) – these two variants were functionally approximately equivalent on an S allele background. However, more recent work has focused on rs2020933 identified by Martin et al. (2007), which is in linkage disequilibrium with the *5-HTTLPR*.

In the GENDEP study, we have recently reported that the *5-HTTLPR* moderated response to escitalopram, with patients with the L allele improving more than those homozygous for the S allelle. A significant three-way interaction between *5-HTTLPR* genotype, drug and gender indicated that the effect of 5-HTTLPR was concentrated in male patients treated with escitalopram (Huezo-Diaz et al. in press).

The *STin2* polymorphism is also a VNTR with the most common allelic variants being 9, 10, or 12 copies of a 16–17 base pair element (*STin2.9*, *STin2.10*, and *STin2.12*, respectively). There is some evidence to suggest that this polymorphism is functional. A study by Mackenzie et al. (1999) showed that the region was a significant positive regulator of 5HTT expression in embryonic mouse development, an effect which was significantly stronger in the *STin2.12* when compared to *STin2.10*. There have been some promising findings regarding STin2 polymorphism and antidepressant response. Kim et al. (2000) reported that individuals homozygous for *STin2.12* showed a better response to fluoxetine, although Ito et al. (2002) failed to replicate this finding. A later study by Kim et al. (2006) identified an association of *STin2.12* and better response to fluoxetine and sertraline. In the same study, an interaction between *5HTTLPR* and *STin2* in predicting response was also found.

The noradrenaline transporter

The noradrenaline transporter (NAT, also known as the norepinephrine transporter, or NET) is also a primary target of a number of antidepressants, especially secondary amine tricyclics (Gillman, 2007). Like the serotonin transporter, the role of NAT is to transport released neurotransmitter (noradrenaline) back into the presynaptic terminal of noradrenergic neurones (a fully functional NAT in this manner 'recycles' at least 90% of the released noradrenaline (Schomig et al. 1989). Thus inhibition of NAT increases the concentration of noradrenaline in the synapse.

Patients with major depression have shown reduced levels of NAT in the locus coeruleus when compared to controls (Klimek et al. 1997). It has therefore been hypothesized that NAT is a good aetiological candidate for the pathophysiology of depression and, like the serotonin transporter, in addition, for response to relevant antidepressants (Leonard, 1997; Ressler and Nemeroff, 1999). NAT is encoded by the gene *SLC6A2* on chromosome 16q12.2 and includes 15 exons spanning 48 kb (Porzgen et al. 1998). The 5' region of NAT has been studied up to 4.6 kb upstream, and shown to contain several important cis-acting transcription elements (Kim et al. 1999).

A number of studies have investigated the association between genetic variation in *SLC6A2* and antidepressant response. Kim et al. (2006) investigated the effects of the G1287A polymorphism on antidepressant response in Korean patients with late-onset major depression. In this study, the response to both SSRIs (fluoxetine or sertraline) and a secondary amine TCA (nortriptyline) was compared with variation in both *SLC6A2* and *SLC6A4*. The response to nortriptyline was significantly associated with the G1287G genotype in *SLC6A2*. A study by Yoshida et al. (2004) reported that response to the SNRI milnacipran was associated with both the G1287A and T-1287C polymorphisms in *SLC6A2*.

P-glycoprotein

P-glycoprotein, also known as multidrug resistance protein 1 (encoded in man by the gene *ABCB1*) is one of the best-studied drug transporter proteins. It is found in the intestine, liver, kidney, and on the luminal membranes of the endothelial capillaries that form the blood–brain barrier. For drugs for which it has a significant affinity, p-glycoprotein therefore plays a critical role in regulating the concentration of these drugs in the brain. Indeed, experiments in mice have shown that the bio-availability of various antidepressants, including TCAs, SSRIs (citalopram and paroxetine), and the SNRI venlafaxine, is regulated by this transporter. However, fluoxetine and mirtazapine are not substrates for p-glycoprotein. Uhr et al. (2008) have recently shown that variation in the *ABCB1* gene predicts the treatment course and outcome in patients treated with antidepressants that are ABCB1 transporter substrates.

Neurotransmitter receptors

The serotonin 2A receptor gene (HTR2A)

The *HTR2A* gene encodes the serotonin$_{2A}$ receptor (5-HT$_{2A}$), which has previously been associated with antidepressant response (Choi et al. 2005; Cusin et al. 2002; Peters et al. 2004). STAR*D is a large multicentre antidepressant trial in the USA, which used a split sample design to genotype 768 SNPs in 68 genes in 1 953 subjects treated with citalopram in the first level of the study. A significant association between treatment outcome and a marker in *HTR2A* (rs7997012) was reported in both the first and the second subsamples genotyped (McMahon, 2006). Participants homozygous for the A allele at this SNP had an 18% reduction in risk of non-response to treatment when compared to those homozygous for the other allele (McMahon et al. 2006). The A allele was six times more frequent in white than in black subjects, with treatment being less effective in black subjects In addition, an association was found between a SNP (rs1954787) in the GRIK4 gene (encoding a kainic acid glutamate receptor, KA1) and response to treatment in the STAR*D cohort. Subjects who were homozygous for both of the alleles associated with response in HTR2A and GRIK4 were 23% less likely to experience non-response to treatment (Paddock et al. 2007).

Enzymes involved in synthesis of neurotransmitters

The tryptophan hydroxylases (TPH1 and TPH2)

The tryptophan hydroxylase-1 gene (*TPH1*) is located on chromosome 11p14–15.3 and codes for tryptophan hydroxylase-1 (TPH1), a rate-limiting enzyme in serotonin biosynthesis. The best-studied *TPH1* variants are two polymorphisms in intron 7, A779C, and A218C, which are in strong linkage disequilibrium. In studies of the latter, the minor allele (A218) has been shown to be associated with decreased 5-HT synthesis. Serretti et al. (2001a, b) also reported an association between the A218C polymorphism and response to treatment with either fluvoxamine or paroxetine in Caucasians, in which the A218 allele was associated with a reduced rate of response to paroxetine (without pindolol augmentation) or to fluvoxamine (again, without pindolol), in comparison to subjects with CC genotype. Some studies of the A218C polymorphism in Asian samples have been negative (Ham et al. 2005; Hong et al. 2006; Yoshida et al. 2002). However, the latest study by Ham et al. found that the rate of remission on treatment with citalopram was poor in those with *TPH1* AA or AC genotypes (Ham et al. 2007)

A second tryptophan hydroxylase gene (TPH2) has been identified, which has been found to be expressed in the brain (Austin and O'Donnell, 1999), and studied in relation to antidepressant response (Peters et al. 2004).

Other moderators of drug response

Circadian rhythm genes

Given the disturbance in circadian rhythm that may be found in depression (e.g. early morning wakening), genes encoding proteins that regulate this are also rational candidates for antidepressant response, especially in regard to insomnia symptoms. The Circadian Locomotor Output Cycles Kaput (*CLOCK*) gene (on 4q12) encodes a protein that is expressed in the suprachiasmatic nucleus of the hypothalamus and is a key regulator of the sleep–wake cycle. A SNP at position 3111 in the 3' flanking region of *CLOCK* has been identified which affects the stability and half-life of the expressed mRNA. Serretti et al. (2005) reported that the efficacy of two SSRIs (fluvoxamine and paroxetine) in the treatment of sleep disturbance symptomatology was moderated by variation in *CLOCK*. In this study, individuals homozygous for the C allele showed significantly more sleep disturbance symptoms throughout the trial.

Another circadian rhythm gene, PERIOD3 (*PER3*) has also been studied in relation to antidepressant response. Artioli et al. (2007) reported that *PER3* was associated with not only time to response to SSRIs, but also with age of onset, and with diurnal variation in mood severity.

Hypothalamo-pituitary-adrenal (HPA) axis candidates

There is considerable evidence to date in support of the involvement of the hypothalamo-pituitary-adrenal (HPA) axis in both the aetiology of depression and in response to antidepressants. In a recent study, young females at high and low risk of depression by virtue of their family history were genotyped and exposed to HPA axis tests. Girls homozygous for the 'S' allele of the *5-HTTLPR* showed a more marked and more prolonged cortisol response to stress than those with the 'L'allele (Gotlib et al. 2008).

Clinical response has been associated with normalization of hypothalamic pituitary adrenal axis hypersensitivity (HPA) and glucocorticoid receptor resistance (Barden et al. 1995; Holsboer and Barden, 1996). An association of a three SNP haplotype with response to fluoxetine or desipramine in the corticotrophin-releasing hormone receptor 1 (*CRHR1*) gene has been reported (Licinio et al. 2004). Similarly, a polymorphism in the glucocorticoid receptor gene has been shown to be associated with partial glucocorticoid receptor resistance (van Rossum et al. 2006). FKBP5 is a glucocorticoid receptor chaperone protein; Binder et al. (2007) reported an association between a polymorphism in *FKBP5* and response to antidepressants, where patients homozygous for the minor allele of the associated SNP responded more than ten days earlier than non-homozygotes and the effect was independent of class of antidepressant (TCA, SSRI, or mirtazapine). See also Chapter 5 in this book for the genetic regulation of the stress response.

The influence of personality and life events on response to antidepressants

Personality

Personality characteristics and the presence or absence of personality disorder have been shown to be important predictors of response to treatment in depression (Mulder et al. 2006). Cloninger has proposed a biosocial theory of personality based on dimensions of temperament being linked to (genetically determined) neurotransmitter systems in the brain (Cloninger, 1986; 1987; 1999; Keller et al. 1992; Lee and Murray, 1988). He initially developed the Tridimensional Personality Questionnaire (TPQ), which measured three dimensions: novelty seeking (NS), harm avoidance (HA), and reward dependence (RD). Following this, he developed the Temperament and Character Inventory (TCI), and the revised form (the TCI-R), both of which have seven dimensions (Cloninger, 1999; Cloninger et al. 1993).

Drug metabolizing enzymes are found not only in the liver and other peripheral organs, but also in the brain (Niznik et al. 1990). It has therefore been postulated that they play a role in the metabolism of endogenous compounds including neurotransmitters. In the case of CYP2D6, endogenous substrates have been identified: 5-methoxyindolethylamines (Yu et al. 2003). A recent study reported that *CYP2C19* genotype was associated with specific personality traits in females but not in males. Using the Temperament and Character Inventory (TCI), scores on reward dependence (RD), cooperativeness (CO), and self-transcendence (ST) were lower in *CYP2C19* PM individuals, suggesting that such individuals could be described as practical, relatively socially insensitive or 'tough' (Ishii et al. 2007). The results of this study were in contrast to another study which found that harm avoidance (HA) scores were lower in EM individuals versus PM. This would imply that PMs may have a tendency to increased fear, social inhibition, and pessimism (Yasui-Furukori et al. 2006). Two studies found that *CYP2D6* PMs were more anxiety prone and less successfully socialized than EM while two newer studies concluded that PMs were less harm avoidant and less careful than EMs (Bertilsson et al. 1989; Llerena et al. 1993; Kirchheiner et al. 2006; Roberts et al. 2004). These interesting findings to date merit further investigation.

Joyce et al. (1994) carried out a six-week study in which 84 patients with major depressive disorder completed a double blind trial with clomipramine or desipramine. They concluded that temperament predicted 35% of the variance in outcome. Women with high RD responded better to clomipramine, and men and women with high HA responded better to desipramine

(Tome et al. 1997; Joyce et al. 1994). Since then, several studies have attempted to replicate these findings. Joffe et al. (1993) found that high baseline HA predicted poor response to imipramine or desipramine, while a recent study by Mulder et al. (2006) showed that HA scores predicted poor response to fluoxetine and nortriptyline. Other studies have reported good treatment response to maprotiline in patients with high baseline self-directedness (SD), and cooperativeness (CO), or to paroxetine and pindolol in patients with high baseline NS and low HA (Sato et al. 1999; Tome et al. 1997)

Life events

Monroe et al. (1983) assessed the effect of adverse life events on response to amitriptyline. Life events were measured at baseline, after 6 and 12 weeks, and 6 and 12 months of treatment. The study reported that antecedent positive or 'entrance' events significantly predicted good outcome at 6 weeks, while outcome at 6 months was predicted by negative life events. In contrast, *concurrent* life events (i.e. those occurring during the treatment period) had no effect on treatment response at any of the measured weeks.

Interestingly, however, a later study by Monroe et al. (1992) reported contradictory findings. In this study, patients who reported more antecedent life stressors (including both desirable and undesirable life events, and serious difficulties) showed a poorer response to treatment with imipramine and psychotherapy. In the same study, concurrent (occurring within 6 weeks of treatment) desirable and undesirable life events also predicted poorer response.

More recently, Mazure et al. (2000) measured life events as the frequency of adverse interpersonal events including adverse *achievement* events. Poor outcome at six weeks of antidepressant treatment was predicted by the baseline frequency of adverse achievement life events, controlling for sex, age, socio-economic status, ethnicity, baseline depression severity, and drug type. By contrast, adverse *interpersonal* life events were a significant predictor of good outcome. One possible explanation for these contrasting effects is that those who experienced adverse *interpersonal* life events may have larger networks and may therefore experience more social support.

Mazure and colleagues also reported a number of interesting interactions between cognitive style, personality, and life events as predictors of outcome following antidepressant treatment. For example, there was a significant interaction between the frequency of interpersonal life events and 'sociotropy' (high levels of dependence and excessive need to please others) in predicting poorer outcome following treatment. In addition, there was a significant interaction between the occurrence of adverse *achievement* life events and the 'need for control' in predicting poorer outcome following treatment. Although in this study the overall frequency of adverse life events significantly predicted the onset of depression, this measure was not a significant predictor of outcome following antidepressant treatment.

Investigating the influence of life events and personality in pharmacogenetic studies

Although there have been several studies assessing both clinical factors (such as personality type) and environmental factors (such as the occurrence of stressful life events) as predictors of antidepressant response, there are no studies to date in which genetic, environmental, and clinical factors have all been investigated. Of note, Wilhelm et al. (2006), investigated the interaction between stressful life events, *5-HTTLPR* genotype, and baseline severity of depression in a longitudinal follow-up study, and found that individuals with the short allele had a greater likelihood of depression when following one or more adverse life events.

The reason for this may well be sample size constraints in previous studies. In GENDEP, we have recruited over 900 subjects, and of these, over 100 have crossed over (i.e. have data on treatment with one drug, followed by the other), giving a total number of informative longitudinal treatment paths of over 1 000. We have applied the TCI-R at baseline, week 12, and week 26 and the Brief Life Events Questionnaire (BLEQ) at baseline, week 8, and week 26. The BLEQ is a measure of negative life events and is based on the list of threatening experiences proposed by Brugha et al. (1985), adapted to include childbirth and the subjective severity of each item (Farmer et al. 2004). Response to treatment has been assessed weekly using the Montgomery Asberg Depression Rating Scale (MADRS), the 17-item Hamilton Depression Rating Scale (HDRS-17), and the Beck Depression Inventory (BDI) up to the twelfth week of treatment, with a further assessment point at 26 weeks (Uher et al. 2008). Candidate genes in all of the above groups have been genotyped, and in addition, the sample is being subjected to genome-wide association analysis. The GENDEP study has therefore provided a sample in which both a longitudinal analysis of environmental factors in relation to outcome and the interplay between environmental and genetic factors may be assessed as predictors of response.

Novel methodology for measuring clinical response

The validity of the findings of pharmacogenetic studies predicates upon accurate and internally consistent measures of response to treatment. The measures most commonly used in studies of depression are the three that we have used in GENDEP; however, GENDEP is the first study to have employed all three in a large, longitudinal study. These measures have inherent differences. For example, they emphasize different groups of symptoms; moreover, the MADRS and HDRS-17 are clinican-rated, while the BDI is self-reported. In the first analysis of these measures of response in GENDEP, item response theory and factor analysis were used to evaluate the psychometric properties of the three measures (Uher et al. 2008). The MADRS and BDI were found to provide internally consistent but mutually distinct estimates of depression severity. The HDRS-17 was less internally consistent and included items which were not discriminating for outpatients consenting to a study (e.g. the insight item – the HDRS was originally developed for inpatients with depression). Three dimensions were derived from factor analysis of the data: 'observed mood and anxiety', 'cognitive', and 'neurovegetative'/ 'somatic.'

In a subsequent analysis of GENDEP data (when the sample size had reached 811), the two study medications did not separate out in terms of efficacy when longitudinal change in the scores of the original measures was used in a mixed effect model. However, longitudinal analysis of the symptom dimensions in such a model revealed that the 'observed mood and anxiety' and 'cognitive' dimensions improved significantly ($P = 0.002$ and 0.034, respectively) more with escitalopram than nortriptyline, while the 'neurovegetative' dimension improved significantly more ($P = 0.01$) with nortriptyline. Although such results may seem to a clinician as would be expected, they are nonetheless scientifically very interesting, as it is the first time that difference in such symptom dimensions between these drugs has been demonstrated. Using measures such as the MADRS or HDRS, it is notoriously difficult for a new antidepressant to show superior efficacy to placebo (Kirsch et al. 2008), and even harder for antidepressants to show differential efficacy in comparison to each other. Employment of more than one response measure, item response theory and factor analysis might well prove fruitful in other clinical trials, not just those seeking to delineate pharmacogenetic/pharmacogenomic factors affecting clinical response.

Further analysis of GENDEP data using genetic and environmental factors as predictors of the longitudinal change of these symptom dimensions, as well as of change in the MADRS is in progress.

Conclusion

This field is now at an exciting stage. Some replications of genetic factors predicting response to antidepressants have been achieved using standard methodologies (e.g. the 5-HTTLPR polymorphism in the serotonin transporter gene; Serretti et al. 2007). Reasons for the relative paucity of replicated findings and suggestions for improved methodologies have been made (Serretti et al. 2007). Such reasons include the fact that many early pharmacogenetic studies have used either a relatively low powered approach such as logistic regression on a dichotomized outcome variable based on a threshold percentage change in score of a clinical outcome variable, or at best linear regression models, as opposed to mixed effect models. True associations may also have been masked by hidden population stratification (Aitchison and Gill, 2002), studies not previously being adequately powered to assess environmental as well as genetic factors, and gene–gene as well as gene–environment interactions. Nonetheless, we already have one readily translatable finding, which is replication of *CYP2C19* genotype as a predictor of escitalopram level.

In recent years, two large studies of antidepressant response in which genetic information is available have been conducted (STAR*D and GENDEP). Novel approaches to the phenotypic analysis of GENDEP are yielding informative results. It is hoped that as these are combined with the candidate gene, environmental and complex clinical factors, and genome-wide association studies (GWAS), and integrated with other relevant datasets, that increased insight regarding the genetic, environmental, and clinical factors relevant to the clinical response to the treatment of depression including ADRs and to the aetiology of depression will be gained.

Summary of key findings

Drug metabolizing enzymes

- About 20–25% of all antidepressant drug therapy is affected by the drug metabolizing enzymes CYP2D6 and CYP2C19.

- Variation in the genes encoding these enzymes results in four distinct phenotypes: ultrarapid metabolizers (UM), extensive metabolizers (EM), intermediate metabolizers (IM), and poor metabolizers (PM). While PMs have an apparent increased risk of adverse drug reactions (ADRs), UMs often show inadequate responses to medication.

- These findings are already being translated to clinical practice. Guidelines for dose adjustment according to *CYP2D6* and *CYP2C19* genotype are now available and the microarray Amplichip CYP450 Test® (Roche diagnostics, USA) has been approved for the identification of *CYP2D6* and *CYP2C19* metabolizer status.

Drug transporters

- *SLC6A4* encodes the serotonin transporter, the main site of action of SSRIs. A functional polymorphism exists in the promoter region of this gene (*5-HTTLPR*) and comprises two allelic variants known as 'short' ('S') or 'long' ('L').

- While the 'S' type has been associated with a relatively poor response to SSRIs and worse illness course, the 'L' type has been associated with a better response in Caucasians.

- In some Asian populations (with different characteristics of the *5-HTTLPR*), a relationship in the opposite direction has been reported.

Neurotransmitter receptors

♦ *HTR2A* gene encodes the serotonin$_{2A}$ receptor (5-HT$_{2A}$). A number of variants in this gene have been associated with response to SSRIs.

♦ In the largest pharmacogenetic study to date (STAR*D), a strong association was reported for the marker rs7997012 and antidepressant response. Subjects homozygous for 'A' allele at this marker showed a more favourable response to SSRIs.

Personality

♦ Temperament can predict a high degree of variance in antidepressant treatment outcome.

♦ High baseline neuroticism or harm avoidance predicts poor response while high cooperativeness and self-directedness predicts a more favourable response to antidepressants.

Life events

♦ The occurrence of stress both prior and during treatment has been shown to affect antidepressant response.

♦ The most consistent finding is that the occurrence of stress prior to treatment predicts a more favourable outcome to both SSRIs and TCAs.

References

Aitchison, K.J. and Gill, M. (2002). Pharmacogenetics in the postgenomic era. in R. Plomin, J. DeFries, I. Craig, and P. McGuffin (eds) *Behavioral Genetics in the Postgenomic Era*, pp. 235–361. Washington DC, APA books.

Aitchison, K.J., Jordan, B.D., and Sharma, T. (2000). The relevance of ethnic influences on pharmacogenetics to the treatment of psychosis. *Drug Metabol. Drug Interact.*, **16**, 15–38.

Artioli, P., Lorenzi, C., Pirovano, A. et al. (2007). How do genes exert their role? Period 3 gene variants and possible influences on mood disorder phenotypes. *Eur.Neuropsychopharmacol.*, **17**, 587–594.

Austin, M.C. and O'Donnell, S.M. (1999). Regional distribution and cellular expression of tryptophan hydroxylase messenger RNA in postmortem human brainstem and pineal gland. *J.Neurochem.*, **72**, 2065–2073.

Barden, N., Reul, J.M., and Holsboer, F. (1995). Do antidepressants stabilize mood through actions on the hypothalamic-pituitary-adrenocortical system? *Trends Neurosci.*, **18**, 6–11.

Basu, A. and Aitchison, K. J. (2005). Pharmacogenetics: antidepressant drug response. *Psychiatry*, **4**, 30–34.

Baumann, P., Hiemke, C.,Ulrich, S. et al. (2004). The AGNP-TDM expert group consensus guidelines: therapeutic drug monitoring in psychiatry. *Pharmacopsychiatry*, **37**, 243–265.

Bertilsson, L., Alm, C., De Las, C.C., Widen, J., Edman, G., and Schalling, D. (1989). Debrisoquine hydroxylation polymorphism and personality. *Lancet*, **1**, 555.

Bertilsson, L., Dahl, M.L., Dalen, P., and Al-Shurbaji, A. (2002). Molecular genetics of CYP2D6: clinical relevance with focus on psychotropic drugs. *Br J Clin Pharmacol.*, **53**, 111–122.

Bertilsson, L., Dahl, M.L., Sjoqvist, F. et al. (1993). Molecular basis for rational megaprescribing in ultrarapid hydroxylators of debrisoquine. *Lancet*, **341**, 63.

Binder, E.B. (2007). The co-chaperone FKBP5, stress hormone system regulation and antidepressant drug response. *Biological Psychiatry*, **61**, 106S.

Brosen, K., Hansen, J.G., Nielsen, K.K., Sindrup, S.H., and Gram, L.F. (1993). Inhibition by paroxetine of desipramine metabolism in extensive but not in poor metabolizers of sparteine. *Eur J Clin Pharmacol.*, **44**, 349–355.

Brugha, T., Bebbington, P., Tennant, C., and Hurry, J. (1985). The list of threatening experiences: a subset of 12 life event categories with considerable long-term contextual threat. *Psychol Med.*, **15**, 189–194.

Chen, F., Larsen, M.B., Sanchez, C., and Wiborg, O. (2005). The S-enantiomer of R,S-citalopram, increases inhibitor binding to the human serotonin transporter by an allosteric mechanism. Comparison with other serotonin transporter inhibitors. *Eur.Neuropsychopharmacol.*, **15**, 193–198.

Choi, M.J., Kang, R.H., Ham, B.J., Jeong, H.Y., and Lee, M.S. (2005). Serotonin receptor 2A gene polymorphism (-1438A/G) and short-term treatment response to citalopram. *Neuropsychobiology*, **52**, 155–162.

Cloninger, C.R. (1986). A unified biosocial theory of personality and its role in the development of anxiety states. *Psychiatr Dev.*, **4**, 167–226.

Cloninger, C.R. (1987). A systematic method for clinical description and classification of personality variants. A proposal. *Arch Gen Psychiatry*, **44**, 573–588.

Cloninger, C.R. (1999). The Temperament and Character Inventory . (Revised Edition) Centre for Psychobiology of Personality, St. Louis, MO, Washington University.

Cloninger, C.R., Svrakic, D.M., and Przybeck, T.R. (1993). A psychobiological model of temperament and character. *Arch Gen Psychiatry*, **50**, 975–990.

Cusin, C., Serretti, A., Zanardi, R. et al. (2002). Influence of monoamine oxidase A and serotonin receptor 2A polymorphisms in SSRI antidepressant activity. *Int J Neuropsychopharmacol.*, **5**, 27–35.

Dalen, P., Dahl, M. L., Bernal Ruiz, M. L., Nordin, J., and Bertilsson, L. (1998). 10-Hydroxylation of nortriptyline in white persons with 0, 1, 2, 3, and 13 functional CYP2D6 genes. *Clin Pharmacol Ther.*, **63**, 444–452.

De Leon, J. (2006). AmpliChip CYP450 test: personalized medicine has arrived in psychiatry. *Expert Rev Mol Diagn.*, **6**, 277–286.

Delbruck, S.J., Wendel, B., Grunewald, I. et al. (1997). A novel allelic variant of the human serotonin transporter gene regulatory polymorphism. *Cytogenet Cell Genet.*, **79**, 214–220.

Farmer, A., Breen, G., Brewster, S. et al. (2004). The Depression Network (DeNT) Study: methodology and sociodemographic characteristics of the first 470 affected sibling pairs from a large multi-site linkage genetic study. *BMC Psychiatry*, **4**, 42.

Fava, M. (2003). Diagnosis and definition of treatment-resistant depression. *Biol Psychiatry*, **53**, 649–659.

Gelernter, J., Kranzler, H., and Cubells, J.F. (1997). Serotonin transporter protein (SLC6A4) allele and haplotype frequencies and linkage disequilibria in African- and European-American and Japanese populations and in alcohol-dependent subjects. *Hum.Genet.*, **101**, 243–246.

Gillman, P.K. (2007). Tricyclic antidepressant pharmacology and therapeutic drug interactions updated. *Br J Pharmacol.*, **151**, 737–748.

Gotlib, I.H., Joormann, J., Minor, K.L., and Hallmayer, J. (2008). HPA axis reactivity: a mechanism underlying the associations among 5-HTTLPR, stress, and depression. *Biol Psychiatry*, **63**, 847–851.

Ham, B.J., Lee, B.C., Paik, J.W. et al. (2007). Association between the tryptophan hydroxylase-1 gene A218C polymorphism and citalopram antidepressant response in a Korean population. *Prog Neuropsychopharmacol Biol Psychiatry*, **31**, 104–107.

Ham, B.J., Lee, M.S., Lee, H.J. et al. (2005). No association between the tryptophan hydroxylase gene polymorphism and major depressive disorders and antidepressant response in a Korean population. *Psychiatr Genet.*, **15**, 299–301.

Heils, A., Teufel, A., Petri, S. et al. (1996). Allelic variation of human serotonin transporter gene expression. *J Neurochem.*, **66**, 2621–2624.

Herrlin, K., Yasui-Furukori, N., Tybring, G., Widen, J., Gustafsson, L. L., and Bertilsson, L. (2003). Metabolism of citalopram enantiomers in CYP2C19/CYP2D6 phenotyped panels of healthy Swedes. *Br J Clin Pharmacol.*, **56**, 415–421.

Holsboer, F. and Barden, N. (1996). Antidepressants and hypothalamic-pituitary-adrenocortical regulation. *Endocr Rev.*, **17**, 187–205.

Hong, C.J., Chen, T.J., Yu, Y.W., and Tsai, S.J. (2006). Response to fluoxetine and serotonin 1A receptor (C-1019G) polymorphism in Taiwan Chinese major depressive disorder. *Pharmacogenomics J.*, **6**, 27–33.

Hu, X.Z., Lipsky, R.H., Zhu, G. et al. (2006). Serotonin transporter promoter gain-of-function genotypes are linked to obsessive-compulsive disorder. *Am J Hum Genet.*, **78**, 815–826.

Hu, X.Z., Rush, A.J., Charney, D. et al. (2007). Association between a functional serotonin transporter promoter polymorphism and citalopram treatment in adult outpatients with major depression. *Arch Gen Psychiatry.*, **64**, 783–792.

Huezo-Diaz, P., Perroud, N., Spencer, E. et al. (2008a). Effect of CYP2C19 genotype on steady-state escitalopram level: a prospective study. *Submitted.*

Huezo-Diaz, P., Uher, R., Smith, R. et al. (2008b). Moderation of antidepressant response by the serotonin transporter gene in the GENDEP study. *British Journal of Psychiatry*, in press.

Ingelman-Sundberg, M., Sim, S.C., Gomez, A., and Rodriguez-Antona, C. (2007). Influence of cytochrome P450 polymorphisms on drug therapies: pharmacogenetic, pharmacoepigenetic and clinical aspects. *Pharmacol Ther.*, **116**, 496–526.

Ishii, G., Suzuki, A., Oshino, S., Shiraishi, H., and Otani, K. (2007). CYP2C19 polymorphism affects personality traits of Japanese females. *Neurosci Lett.*, **411**, 77–80.

Ito, K., Yoshida, K., Sato, K., et al. (2002). A variable number of tandem repeats in the serotonin transporter gene does not affect the antidepressant response to fluvoxamine. *Psychiatry Res.*, **111**, 235–239.

Joffe, R.T., Bagby, R.M., Levitt, A.J., Regan, J.J., and Parker, J.D. (1993). The tridimensional personality questionnaire in major depression. *Am J Psychiatry*, **150**, 959–960.

Joyce, P.R., Mulder, R.T., and Cloninger, C.R. (1994). Temperament predicts clomipramine and desipramine response in major depression. *J Affect Disord.*, **30**, 35–46.

Keller, M.B., Lavori, P.W., Mueller, T.I. et al. (1992). Time to recovery, chronicity, and levels of psychopathology in major depression. A 5-year prospective follow-up of 431 subjects. *Arch Gen Psychiatry*, **49**, 809–816.

Kim, C.H., Kim, H.S., Cubells, J.F., and Kim, K.S. (1999). A previously undescribed intron and extensive 5' upstream sequence, but not Phox2a-mediated transactivation, are necessary for high level cell type-specific expression of the human norepinephrine transporter gene. *J Biol Chem.*, **274**, 6507–6518.

Kim, D.K., Lim, S.W., Lee, S. et al. (2000). Serotonin transporter gene polymorphism and antidepressant response. *Neuroreport*, **11**, 215–219.

Kim, H., Lim, S.W., Kim, S. et al. (2006a). Monoamine transporter gene polymorphisms and antidepressant response in koreans with late-life depression. *JAMA*, **296**, 1609–1618.

Kirchheiner, J., Lang, U., Stamm, T., Sander, T., and Gallinat, J. (2006). Association of CYP2D6 genotypes and personality traits in healthy individuals. *J Clin Psychopharmacol.*, **26**, 440–442.

Kirchheiner, J., Nickchen, K., Bauer, M. et al. (2004). Pharmacogenetics of antidepressants and antipsychotics: the contribution of allelic variations to the phenotype of drug response. *Mol Psychiatry.*, **9**, 442–473.

Kirsch, I., Deacon, B.J., Huedo-Medina, T.B., Scoboria, A., Moore, T.J., and Johnson, B.T. (2008). Initial severity and antidepressant benefits: a meta-analysis of data submitted to the Food and Drug Administration. *PLoS.Med.*, **5**, e45.

Klimek, V., Stockmeier, C., Overholser, J. et al. (1997). Reduced levels of norepinephrine transporters in the locus coeruleus in major depression. *J Neurosci.*, **17**, 8451–8458.

Kraft, J.B., Peters, E.J., Slager, S.L. et al. (2007). Analysis of association between the serotonin transporter and antidepressant response in a large clinical sample. *Biological Psychiatry*, **61**, 734–742.

Lee, A.S. and Murray, R.M. (1988). The long-term outcome of Maudsley depressives. *Br J Psychiatry*, **153**, 741–751.

Leonard, B.E. (1997). The role of noradrenaline in depression: a review. J Psychopharmacol., 11, S39–S47.

Lessard, E., Yessine, M.A., Hamelin, B.A., O'Hara, G., LeBlanc, J., and Turgeon, J. (1999). Influence of CYP2D6 activity on the disposition and cardiovascular toxicity of the antidepressant agent venlafaxine in humans. *Pharmacogenetics*, 9, 435–443.

Licinio, J., O'Kirwan, F., Irizarry, K. et al. (2004). Association of a corticotropin-releasing hormone receptor 1 haplotype and antidepressant treatment response in Mexican-Americans. *Mol Psychiatry.*, 9, 1075–1082.

Llerena, A., Edman, G., Cobaleda, J., Benitez, J., Schalling, D., and Bertilsson, L. (1993). Relationship between personality and debrisoquine hydroxylation capacity. Suggestion of an endogenous neuroactive substrate or product of the cytochrome P4502D6. *Acta Psychiatr Scand.*, 87, 23–28.

MacKenzie, A. and Quinn, J. (1999). A serotonin transporter gene intron 2 polymorphic region, corre-lated with affective disorders, has allele-dependent differential enhancer-like properties in the mouse embryo. *Proc Natl Acad Sci USA*, 96, 15251–15255.

Martin, J., Cleak, J., Willis-Owen, S.A., Flint, J., and Shifman, S. (2007). Mapping regulatory variants for the serotonin transporter gene based on allelic expression imbalance. *Mol Psychiatry.*, 12, 421–422.

Mazure, C.M., Bruce, M.L., Maciejewski, P.K., and Jacobs, S.C. (2000). Adverse life events and cognitive-personality characteristics in the prediction of major depression and antidepressant response. *Am J Psychiatry*, 157, 896–903.

McMahon, F. (2006). Pharmacogenetics of treatment outcome and side effects in the STAR star D cohort. *Neuropsychopharmacology*, 31, S38–S39.

McMahon, F.J., Buervenich, S., Charney, D. et al. (2006). Variation in the gene encoding the serotonin 2A receptor is associated with outcome of antidepressant treatment. *Am J Hum Genet.*, 78, 804–814.

Monroe, S.M., Bellack, A.S., Hersen, M., and Himmelhoch, J.M. (1983). Life events, symptom course, and treatment outcome in unipolar depressed women. *J Consult Clin Psychol.*, 51, 604–615.

Monroe, S.M., Kupfer, D.J., and Frank, E. (1992). Life stress and treatment course of recurrent depression: 1. Response during index episode. *J Consult Clin Psychol.*, 60, 718–724.

Mrazek, D.A., Rush, A.J., Biernacka, J.M. et al. (2008). SLC6A4 variation and citalopram response. *Am J Med Genet B Neuropsychiatr Genet.*, 150B, 341–351.

Mulder, R.T., Joyce, P.R., Frampton, C.M., Luty, S.E., and Sullivan, P.F. (2006). Six months of treatment for depression: outcome and predictors of the course of illness. *Am J Psychiatry*, 163, 95–100.

Nakamura, T., Matsushita, S., Nishiguchi, N., Kimura, M., Yoshino, A., and Higuchi, S. (1999). Association of a polymorphism of the 5HT2A receptor gene promoter region with alcohol dependence. *Mol Psychiatry*, 4, 85–88.

Niznik, H.B., Tyndale, R.F., Sallee, F.R. et al. (1990). The dopamine transporter and cytochrome P45OIID1 (debrisoquine 4-hydroxylase) in brain: resolution and identification of two distinct [3H]GBR-12935 binding proteins. *Arch Biochem Biophys.*, 276, 424–432.

Otton, S.V., Ball, S.E., Cheung, S.W., Inaba, T., Rudolph, R.L., and Sellers, E.M. (1996). Venlafaxine oxida-tion in vitro is catalysed by CYP2D6. *Br J Clin Pharmacol.*, 41, 149–156.

Paddock, S., Laje, G., Charney, D. et al. (2007). Association of GRIK4 with outcome of antidepressant treat-ment in the STAR*D cohort. *Am J Psychiatry*, 164, 1181–1188.

Peters, E.J., Slager, S.L., McGrath, P.J., Knowles, J.A., and Hamilton, S.P. (2004). Investigation of seroton-in-related genes in antidepressant response. *Mol Psychiatry*, 9, 879–889.

Porzgen, P., Bonisch, H., Hammermann, R., and Bruss, M. (1998). The human noradrenaline transporter gene contains multiple polyadenylation sites and two alternatively spliced C-terminal exons. *Biochim Biophys Acta.*, 1398, 365–370.

Ressler, K.J. and Nemeroff, C.B. (1999). Role of norepinephrine in the pathophysiology and treatment of mood disorders. *Biol Psychiatry*, 46, 1219–1233.

Roberts, R.L., Luty, S.E., Mulder, R.T., Joyce, P.R., and Kennedy, M.A. (2004). Association between cytochrome P450 2D6 genotype and harm avoidance. *Am J Med Genet B Neuropsychiatr Genet.*, **127B**, 90–93.

Rountree, M.R., Bachman, K.E., Herman, J.G., and Baylin, S.B. (2001). DNA methylation, chromatin inheritance, and cancer. *Oncogene*, **20**, 3156–3165.

Rousseva, A., Henry, C., van den, B. D. et al. (2003). Antidepressant-induced mania, rapid cycling and the serotonin transporter gene polymorphism. *Pharmacogenomics J*, **3**, 101–104.

Rudberg, I., Hendset, M., Uthus, L.H., Molden, E., and Refsum, H. (2006). Heterozygous mutation in CYP2C19 significantly increases the concentration/dose ratio of *racemic* citalopram and escitalopram (S-citalopram). *Ther Drug Monit.*, **28**, 102–105.

Rutter, M., Moffitt, T.E., and Caspi, A. (2006). Gene-environment interplay and psychopathology: multiple varieties but real effects. *J Child Psychol Psychiatry*, **47**, 226–261.

Sato, T., Hirano, S., Narita, T. et al. (1999). Temperament and character inventory dimensions as a predictor of response to antidepressant treatment in major depression. *J Affect Disord.*, **56**, 153–161.

Schomig, E., Fischer, P., Schonfeld, C.L., and Trendelenburg, U. (1989). The extent of neuronal re-uptake of 3H-noradrenaline in isolated vasa deferentia and atria of the rat. *Naunyn Schmiedebergs Arch Pharmacol.*, **340**, 502–508.

Serretti, A. Zanardi, R., Cusin, C., Rossini, D., Lorenzi, C., and Smeraldi, E. (2001a). Tryptophan hydroxylase gene associated with paroxetine antidepressant activity, *Eur. Neuropsychopharmacol*, **11,** 375–380.

Serretti, A., Zanardi, R., Rossini, D., Cusin, C., Lilli, R., and Smeraldi, E. (2001b). Influence of tryptophan hydroxylase and serotonin transporter genes on fluvoxamine antidepressant activity, *Mol. Psychiatry*, **6**, 586–592.

Serretti, A. and Artioli, P. (2004). The pharmacogenomics of selective serotonin reuptake inhibitors. *Pharmacogenomics J.*, **4**, 233–244.

Serretti, A., Cusin, C., Benedetti, F. et al. (2005). Insomnia improvement during antidepressant treatment and CLOCK gene polymorphism. *Am J Med Genet B Neuropsychiatr Genet.*, **137B**, 36–39.

Serretti, A., Kato, M., De, R.D., and Kinoshita, T. (2007). Meta-analysis of serotonin transporter gene promoter polymorphism (5-HTTLPR) association with selective serotonin reuptake inhibitor efficacy in depressed patients. *Mol Psychiatry*, **12**, 247–257.

Serretti, A., Kato, M., and Kennedy, J.L. (2008). Pharmacogenetic studies in depression: a proposal for methodologic guidelines. *Pharmacogenomics J.*, **8**, 90–100.

Sjoqvist, F. and Eliasson, E. (2007). The convergence of conventional therapeutic drug monitoring and pharmacogenetic testing in personalized medicine: focus on antidepressants. *Clin Pharmacol Ther.*, **81**, 899–902.

Steimer, W., Zopf, K., von Amelunxen, S. et al. (2005). Amitriptyline or not, that is the question: pharmacogenetic testing of CYP2D6 and CYP219 identifies patients with low or high risk for side effects in amitriptyline therapy. *Clinical Chemistry*, **51**, 376–385.

Tome, M.B., Cloninger, C.R., Watson, J.P., and Isaac, M.T. (1997). Serotonergic autoreceptor blockade in the reduction of antidepressant latency: personality variables and response to paroxetine and pindolol. *J Affect Disord.*, **44**, 101–109.

Uher, R., Farmer, A., Maier, W. et al. (2008). Measuring depression: comparison and integration of three scales in the GENDEP study. *Psychol Med.*, **38**, 289–300.

Uher, R. and McGuffin, P. (2008). The moderation by the serotonin transporter gene of environmental adversity in the aetiology of mental illness: review and methodological analysis. *Mol Psychiatry*, **13**, 131–146.

Uhr, M., Tontsch, A., Namendorf, C. et al. (2008). Polymorphisms in the drug transporter gene ABCB1 predict antidepressant treatment response in depression. *Neuron*, **57**, 203–209.

van Rossum, E.F., Binder, E.B., Majer, M. et al. (2006). Polymorphisms of the glucocorticoid receptor gene and major depression. *Biol Psychiatry*, **59**, 681–688.

von Moltke, L.L., Greenblatt, D.J., Giancarlo, G.M., Granda, B.W., Harmatz, J.S., and Shader, R.I. (2001). Escitalopram (S-citalopram) and its metabolites in vitro: cytochromes mediating biotransformation, inhibitory effects, and comparison to R-citalopram. *Drug Metab Dispos*, **29**, 1102–1109.

Wilhelm, K., Mitchell, P.B., Niven, H. et al. (2006). Life events, first depression onset and the serotonin transporter gene. *Br J Psychiatry*, **188**, 210–215.

Yasui-Furukori, N., Saito, M., Nakagami, T., Kaneda, A., Tateishi, T., and Kaneko, S. (2006). Association between multidrug resistance 1 (MDR1) gene polymorphisms and therapeutic response to bromperidol in schizophrenic patients: a preliminary study. *Prog Neuropsychopharmacol Biol Psychiatry*, **30**, 286–291.

Yoshida, K., Naito, S., Takahashi, H. et al. (2002). Monoamine oxidase: a gene polymorphism, tryptophan hydroxylase gene polymorphism and antidepressant response to fluvoxamine in Japanese patients with major depressive disorder. *Prog Neuropsychopharmacol Biol Psychiatry*, **26**, 1279–1283.

Yoshida, K., Takahashi, H., Higuchi, H. et al. (2004). Prediction of antidepressant response to milnacipran by norepinephrine transporter gene polymorphisms. *Am J Psychiatry*, **161**, 1575–1580.

Yu, A.M., Idle, J.R., Herraiz, T., Kupfer, A., and Gonzalez, F.J. (2003). Screening for endogenous substrates reveals that CYP2D6 is a 5-methoxyindolethylamine O-demethylase. *Pharmacogenetics*, **13**, 307–319.

Yu, Y.W., Tsai, S.J., Chen, T.J., Lin, C.H., and Hong, C.J. (2002). Association study of the serotonin transporter promoter polymorphism and symptomatology and antidepressant response in major depressive disorders. *Mol Psychiatry*, **7**, 1115–1119.

Chapter 24

Can the EEG be used to predict antidepressant response?

R. Hamish McAllister-Williams and
Grzegorz Wisniewski

Introduction

The pharmacological management of depression presents a number of challenges. Most notably in randomized controlled trials only around 60–70% of patients show a response to a particular antidepressant over an eight-week treatment trial (Fawcett and Barkin, 1997). In naturalistic practice, response rates appear to be even lower (Trivedi et al. 2006). Further we have a larger variety of treatment options than in other areas of psychiatry, with numerous pharmacological groups of drugs (albeit that currently these all act on monoaminergic systems). Interestingly, response rates to serotonin-selective and noradrenergic-selective drugs are similar. Clinical experience suggests that some patients respond to serotonergic but not noradrenergic antidepressants, or vice versa, though some will respond to either. This presents a prescribing problem. How do you predict, first, if a patient will respond and secondly to what sort of antidepressant? At present the best that can be done is to undertake treatment trials with patients. As each of these takes time what is required is a biomarker that helps predict both the likelihood of response and which drug is more likely to be effective. There are several potential lines of investigation into biomarkers of antidepressant response, for example, pharmacogenetics (for reviews see, Perlis, 2007 and Serretti et al. 2005), imaging (Evans et al. 2006; Dougherty and Rauch, 2007; Miller et al. 2008), and neuroendocrine (e.g. Ising et al. 2007). This chapter reviews the evidence regarding the potential use of electroencephalographic (EEG) to predict response to antidepressants. Some of the experimental and clinical evidence relevant to the ideas presented here are also discussed in Chapters 12 and 13 of this book. Moreover, this and the last chapters in this book (Chapter 23, 25, 26, and 27) specifically discuss the more recent developments in the treatment of affective disorders.

The first report of EEG recording from a mammal was made more than one century ago (Caton, 1875) and the first human recording over 65 years ago (Berger, 1929). However, EEG techniques in recent years have tended to 'play second fiddle' to neuroimaging methodologies. This stems largely from the technique not delivering important findings after years of study, with but a few notable exceptions such as the diagnosis of epilepsy and sleep disorders. However, EEG and event-related potential (ERP) techniques still have much to offer in the further elucidation of the pathophysiology of mood disorders and potentially as biomarkers of treatment response, if used in appropriate ways often utilizing novel computational analysis. The EEG (together with magneto-encephalography [MEG]) has a great strength above any other form of functional imaging, such as functional magnetic resonance imaging (fMRI) or positron emission tomography (PET), in that it records signals that are the direct result of electrical activity of neurones, rather than some 'down-stream' consequence such as changes in oxygen utilization or blood flow.

Partly as a result of this, EEG and MEG have temporal resolutions that are generally an order of magnitude better than fMRI or PET. EEG also has an advantage of being relatively inexpensive, easy to conduct, and well tolerated compared to both fMRI and PET, and does not require the use of radio-ligands as in PET. This facilitates multiple recordings in subjects, such as in cross-over or longitudinal studies. The EEG does have some downsides, most notably problems of spatial resolution. However, the relative low cost and ease of use of EEG means that it has greater potential utility for everyday clinical practice than is the case for many neuroimaging methodologies.

This chapter is a selective review of the evidence that EEG and ERP data may be able to predict antidepressant response in depressed patients. The review primarily covers evidence around the use of antidepressants in relation to unipolar depression. We have confined ourselves to awake EEG data and do not discuss the potential use of sleep-EEG analysis (Kupfer and Frank 2001; Kupfer et al. 1976) . While there is a wealth of data regarding the EEG effects of antidepressant administration to depressed patients and healthy subjects, we will focus on evidence that baseline EEG data (i.e. before treatment initiation), or changes in the EEG early on in treatment (within the first two weeks), predict response. There may be research interest, but no clinical utility, in findings of EEG changes in responders versus non-responders occurring after four or eight weeks treatment. Such data is not reviewed here.

We divide the chapter into two main sections. First, evidence relating to resting EEG data and secondly the use of ERPs. The chapter is written with the non-EEG specialist reader in mind.

The resting EEG as a predictor of antidepressant response

The EEG is generated by inhibitory and excitatory postsynaptic potentials at cortical neuronal synapses. These postsynaptic potentials summate in the cortex and can be recorded at the scalp as EEG. Action potentials probably do not contribute significantly to the EEG because there is little penetration of these into extracellular space and hence transmission to the scalp. Rather scalp EEG electrodes record the summation of postsynaptic potentials of large areas of pyramidal neurones in the underlying cortex. For a signal to be detectable these neurones must be firing synchronously with the cells orientated in parallel at 90° to the plane of the scalp. The challenge to the EEG researcher is in 'decoding' the wealth of information contained within the recordings. This can be potentially done in a number of ways. One of these is exploring the rhythmic activity contained within the EEG. This can be done, for example, using a Fast Fourier Transformation (FTT) of the time series data to obtain the signal power against frequency (Fig. 24.1). The resultant data is often described in relation to certain frequency bands. The definition of these bands does vary but approximately 0–3 Hz is defined as Delta. This is seen in young children but decreases with age. In adulthood it is mainly seen over frontal scalp during slow wave sleep or secondary to a variety of pathological conditions (e.g. subcortical lesions, encephalitis). Theta is defined as 4–7 Hz and tends to be a sign of drowsiness or again various pathological conditions. Alpha, occurring between 8 Hz and 12 Hz, is found over posterior scalp bilaterally though in higher amplitude over the dominant hemisphere. It increases in amplitude when the eyes are shut or during relaxation. This band is probably the most widely studied in different theoretical contexts due to it being believed that alpha reflects cognitive and memory processes (Klimesch, 1999; Knyazev, 2007), bioelectrical cortical asymmetry (Henriques and Davidson, 1991), and is as a reliable EEG measure of physiological state of vigilance and arousal (Bruder et al. 2008; Ulrich et al. 1984). Beta, 12–30 Hz, tends to be symmetrical and frontally distributed. It increases when concentrating or thinking. Lastly, in recent years there has been an increasing attention paid to the gamma band between 30 Hz and 100 Hz which appears to relate to a variety of cognitive processes. The power within each band can be described in absolute terms or relative to the total

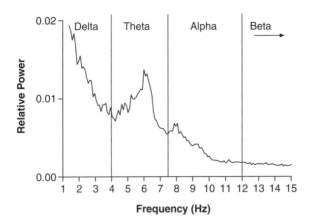

Fig. 24.1 Fast Fourier Transformation (FFT) of resting EEG, eyes open, recorded from 14 healthy male subjects. The graph illustrates relative power plotted against frequency. Relative power has been calculated by dividing the absolute power at any given frequency by the total power between 0 Hz and 30 Hz for each individual subject. This decreases inter-subject variation due to total spectral power differences; for example, due to differences in signal transduction through individuals skull, scalp, and EEG electrodes. Delta, theta, alpha, and beta frequency bands are marked. Note that there is considerable variability in the exact ranges of these bands between research groups. (Data adapted from McAllister-Williams and Massey, 2003).

EEG spectral power. Calculation of the spectral power is sometimes referred to as 'quantitative EEG' or QEEG.

A challenge for researchers and reviewers alike is that there is a wealth of variables within QEEG, with various bands, absolute and relative measures, all recorded at numerous EEG electrode sites across the scalp. Coupled with many of the published studies being of a small number of patients risking both type one and two errors, and a variety of different antidepressant drugs studied, the literature can be somewhat confusing and inconsistent. This is particularly the case when examining straightforward spectral power data. In recent years more complex, sometimes theoretically driven, analysis techniques have been developed which may be more sensitive and hence the reported findings are more consistent.

EEG spectral analysis

Suggestions that the awake EEG contains information that may predict antidepressant response have been around for over two decades. The group of Ulrich reported in 1984 that in-patients with endogenous depression clinically defined responders and non-responders differed in their average EEG power spectra recorded over the left occipital lobe, the responders having higher alpha power though the main finding reported was that in responders there was a greater decrease in alpha power after four weeks of treatment comparing to the baseline recording (Ulrich et al. 1984) This data from 20 patients treated with amitriptyline or pirlindol was further analysed suggesting that non-response was associated with alpha power being less than 50% of total spectral power (Ulrich and Frick, 1986). However in a larger study of 45 patients treated with either clomipramine or maprotiline, there were few clear pre-treatment differences between responders and non-responders to either drug (Ulrich et al. 1988). Rather it appeared that non-responders were characterized by a greater decrease in alpha than responders two hours after the first dose of medication was administered. There is no other data examining alpha power a few hours after treatment commencement to confirm or refute this observation though a single dose of paroxetine is reported not to alter any spectral power band in depressed patients (Knott et al. 2002). A study in 29 patients treated with imipramine did examine baseline alpha power but was only able to detect a trend for increased alpha in responders (Knott et al. 1996) in line with Ulrich and colleagues' initial findings but this did not reach statistical significance. Thus it is unclear if simple measures of baseline alpha power predict antidepressant response.

Three others studies have investigated the predictive potential of baseline alpha power using a particular analysis method referred to as 'neurometric EEG mapping'. This mapping is in two-dimensions and involves EEG data being initially transformed into spectral power using the FFT (as in others studies described above). The FFT data from whole groups of patients are then z-transformed against population norms for age and log-transformed for normalization of distribution. This method was first used to classify different psychiatric disorders in 1980s (John et al. 1988). In their naturalistic, prospective study of 54 patients with unipolar or bipolar depression, Suffin and Emory recorded EEG before starting six months of treatment with a tricyclic antidepressant (TCA) or a selective serotonin re-uptake inhibitor (SSRI). Of 35 responders, 30 (86%) had an excess of relative alpha power frontally and to a lesser extent in occipital regions (Suffin and Emory, 1995). The most obvious limitation of this study was that almost half of all patients were teenagers (with a mean age of 13.4 years). The other two studies that have utilized the neurometrics technique have used it to investigate antidepressant responses in obsessive compulsive disorder (OCD). In the first of these 27 patients with OCD were treated with SSRIs. Response was associated with increased relative power in alpha at baseline, while non-responders exhibited higher relative theta power, especially in frontal and frontotemporal regions (Prichep et al. 1993). The reported accuracy rates for the determination of responders and non-responders were 82.4% and 80%, respectively. In the second study in OCD, 20 patients with no concurrent depression were treated with paroxetine 40–80 mg for at least 12 weeks. Responders were reported as having a significant excess of absolute and relative alpha power especially in the frontopolar, frontal, and posterior temporal regions (Hansen et al. 2003) essentially replicating the initial findings. These OCD studies are consistent with those in depressed patients and hence pre-treatment alpha power may reflect the likelihood of antidepressants having a biological effect rather than treating a particular pathological condition.

A possible alternative alpha power predictor of antidepressant response is asymmetry, following the observations of Ulrich and colleagues that the best baseline predictor of response was alpha power in the left, but not right, occipital lobe (Ulrich et al. 1984). Hemispheric asymmetry is a well-described observation in depression. In general, the findings are of greater alpha power (indicating reduced activity) over right frontal sites seen in both the resting EEG (Henriques and Davidson, 1991) and during cognitive tasks (Alhaj et al. 2007). It may reflect certain depressive symptoms, such as rumination and self-esteem (Putnam and McSweeney, 2008) and/or be a result of the hypercortisolaemia often seen in depression (Alhaj et al. 2008). The situation is, however not clear-cut since the opposite pattern of alpha laterality (though over parietal sites) has been reported in depressed (Reid et al. 1998) and recovered patients (Henriques and Davidson, 1990). The actual pattern of asymmetry seen may be determined by the presence of anxiety symptoms (Bruder et al. 1997). Psychophysics investigations have also been used to assess asymmetry and its impact on antidepressant response; in particular dichotic listening tests, in which words, syllables, or tones are simultaneously presented to the two ears and the difference in accuracy for reporting right- and left-ear items can be used to provide a measure of perceptual asymmetry. Bruder and colleagues have reported that medication-free depressed patients who subsequently responded to fluoxetine had a greater right ear (left hemisphere) advantage for dichotic words and less left ear (right hemisphere) advantage for complex tones when compared with treatment non-responders (Bruder et al. 1996). As a result this group explored the predictive power of pre-treatment EEG alpha asymmetry on antidepressant response. In a study of 53 patients treated with fluoxetine (34 responders and 19 non-responders), non-responders showed an alpha asymmetry indicative of overall greater activation (i.e. less alpha power) of the right hemisphere than the left, whereas responders did not (Bruder et al. 2001). This was, however, evident only in women but not in men. Despite this, the group were able to replicate their finding in just 18 patients, only 5 of whom were women, with no apparent effect of gender on the prediction of response which had a sensitivity of 64% and specificity of 71% (Bruder et al. 2008). The findings of this group appear to have been replicated by a Russian team (based on the English translation of their abstract; Bochkarev et al. 2004).

An alternative power spectrum band that has been explored extensively regarding its possible predictive value with regard to antidepressant response is the theta band. Knott et al. reported the response to imipramine in 29 patients and described the responders as having significantly *less* baseline, but a greater *increase* three hours after the first dose of treatment, of theta than non-responders (Knott et al. 1996). This group have replicated their findings in a group of 70 male patients treated with paroxetine, 51 of whom completed 6 weeks treatment. A negative correlation was found between baseline frontal theta and decrease in Hamilton Depression Rating Scale (HDRS) score (Knott et al. 2002). These findings are consistent with more sophisticated investigations of theta using localization techniques (see below) and the one neurometrics study in depressed patients where frontal theta excess was identified in 5 of 7 non-responders (Suffin and Emory, 1995).

Anterior cingulate theta

It has been hypothesized that activity/metabolic rate in the rostral (pregenual) anterior cingulate cortex (rACC) predicts antidepressant response (Mayberg, 1997). This is based on observations that subjects with higher metabolic rates respond better to sleep deprivation (Ebert et al. 1994; Smith et al. 1999; Wu et al. 1999) as well as paroxetine (Brody et al. 1999; Saxena et al. 2003), sertraline (Buchsbaum et al. 1997), and venlafaxine (Davidson et al. 2003). In addition a meta-analysis of PET studies shows that responders differ from non-responders in a network of regions including limbic areas and rACC (Seminowicz et al. 2004) and deep brain stimulation of this area is reported to be beneficial in treatment-resistant depression (Mayberg et al. 2005). It should be noted that the higher rACC activity in treatment responders is in contrast to the *lower* activity seen in *dorsal* ACC in depression generally (Drevets, 1999).

While the EEG does not provide good spatial resolution, source analysis can be employed to localize the origin of various activity. One such technique that has been employed is Low Resolution Electromagnetic Tomography (LORETA) (Pascual-Marqui et al. 1994). This method localizes EEG activity to 2 394 voxels in a standardized brain space based on digitized MRI from the Brain Imaging Centre, Montreal Neurologic Institute (Pascual-Marqui et al. 1999). Because there is no unique solution to the localization of electrical activity recorded at the scalp, all source analysis techniques need to make assumptions to obtain a solution. LORETA's assumption is that the activity in any one voxel is close to the activity of its neighbouring voxels and that activity is constrained to grey matter and hippocampus. This is in essence a physiological constraint since for activity to be evident at the scale it must result from a large collection of synchronous neurones. The result of the assumption is that LORETA solutions produce a 'blurred' localization of a point source (Fig. 24.2). While of a lower spatial resolution, a close relationship to simultaneous acquired fMRI has been reported (Mulert et al. 2004a). In addition it has been reported that there is a correlation between rACC theta activity measured using LORETA and PET glucose metabolism (Pizzagalli et al. 2003).

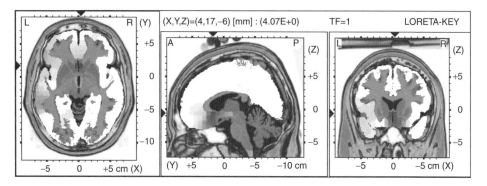

Fig. 24.2 LORETA image of anterior cingulate activity. Note that the figure is to illustrate the nature of LORETA images and its ability to localize neural activity to the anterior cingulate. In this case, data was obtained from 24 healthy male subjects undertaking a recollection memory task. The LORETA localization is of subtracted EEG activity following dehydroepiandrosterone and placebo administration. Maximal activation is seen in Broadman Area 25. (Data adapted from Alhaj et al. 2006).

Two independent research groups have reported the use of LORETA to assess rACC theta activity in depressed patients' pre-treatment. In the first of these Pizzagalli and colleagues (2001) investigated 18 depressed patients. All had been medication free for at least 4 weeks prior to treatment with nortiptyline with monitoring of plasma concentrations. Sixteen of the 18 patients showed a response over 4–6 months, averaging a 63% improvement in Beck Depressive Inventory (BDI) score. All 18 patients were divided into those with a better and those with a worse response around the median BDI improvement. Comparisons between these two groups across all frequency bands revealed a significant difference only for theta and this was confined to rACC. The 'better' responders exhibited higher theta power than the 'less-good responders'. Further there was a significant correlation between rACC theta power and improvement in BDI (Pizzagalli et al. 2001).

The findings of Pizzagalli et al. have been replicated in a group of 20 patients randomized to either citalopram or reboxetine for 4 weeks (Mulert et al. 2007b). Again responders had higher rACC theta than non-responders with a Cohen's effect size of 1.33. The effect was confined to rACC and not seen in the dorsal ACC. Subgroup analysis found a significant effect only for the reboxetine and not the citalopram responders. However there was a positive correlation between rACC theta and decrease in HDRS for both treatment groups. LORETA localization of rACC has also been conducted by a Brazilian group investigating 17 patients with OCD who reported lower beta activity in responders (Fontenelle et al. 2006). In this instance it may be that response to antidepressant in different conditions is predicted by different measures of rACC activity (theta in depression and beta in OCD), though this question requires further research.

Theta cordance

Electroencephalographic Cordance is an analysis procedure developed at the University of California in Los Angeles (UCLA). It combines information from both absolute and relative power from the EEG spectrum, as well as information from neighbouring electrodes for each scalp electrode (Leuchter et al. 1994). It has been reported to have a stronger correlation with cerebral perfusion than standard spectral analysis (Leuchter et al. 1999). Further cordance is less influenced by age, gender, and severity of baseline depression that simple spectral power

(Morgan et al. 2005). The analysis algorithm produces two measures – a categorical value (concordant versus discordant) and a numerical value. An electrode is reported as concordant if both the relative and absolute power of the EEG recorded from it are either above or below the mean value for all electrodes, and discordant if one is above and the other below. The group have mainly confined their research to an analysis of the theta band. The first indication that cordance might predict antidepressant outcome came from data from 24 patients randomized to fluoxetine (13) or placebo (11). The 13 fluoxetine-treated patients were divided by their pre-treatment EEG into concordant or discordant groups with less than or more than 30% of electrodes discordant across the whole scalp. While 7 out of 8 in the concordant group achieved remission (HDRS ≤ 10) none of the discordant group did so (Cook et al. 1999).

Since this first publication, the UCLA group have published extensively on the Cordance method and its predictive ability in depression. The data that they analyse comes from two placebo-controlled randomized trials of fluoxetine (the 24 patients reported in the Cook et al. 1999 paper) and venlafaxine ($n = 27$ patients). In general the group have focused on theta cordance at frontal electrode sites, on the basis that this reflects ACC theta (Cook et al. 2002). In addition they have examined the change in cordance from baseline following 48 hours, one or two weeks of treatment, because subsequent analysis of both RCTs found no baseline cordance measures predicting response (Leuchter et al. 2002). However the decrease in frontal theta cordance at 48 hours (a trend) and at one week (significantly) predicts response with a sensitivity of 69% and sensitivity of 75% (Cook et al. 2002). There is no difference between response to fluoxetine or venlafaxine and the final HDRS score correlates with cordance at week one (Cook et al. 2002). Placebo responders are reported to show a significant *increase* in prefrontal theta cordance while both medication and placebo non-responders showed no change (Leuchter et al. 2002). Further, it is not just change during active treatment that is important. In both studies patients had a one-week placebo run in before randomization. Decreased frontal cordance during this time is also associated with lower final HDRS score (Hunter et al. 2006). Interestingly, just in the venlafaxine data set, there was a negative correlation between change in cordance and side effects after one week of placebo lead in and two weeks of active treatment (Hunter et al. 2005).

The UCLA group have also shown similar findings for electroconvulsive therapy (ECT) treatment (Stubbeman et al. 2004) and have conducted a pilot study in 12 depressed patients who had failed at least 6 weeks of SSRI monotherapy. Cordance was measured before and around one week after these patients either had their SSRI augmented or they were switched to another anti-depressant. Five out of 6 responders, compared to 2 out of 6 non-responders, showed a decrease in prefrontal theta cordance (Cook et al. 2005). This has been replicated by work from a Czech group, first in 17 inpatients with treatment-resistant depression in which all 5 responders showed a decrease frontal theta cordance over one week, compared to just 2 out of 12 non-responders (Bares et al. 2007). In the most recent study from this group, again in treatment-resistant patients ($n = 25$) a similar finding predicted response to 4 weeks treatment with venlafaxine (Bares et al. 2008). Apart from a study of homeopathic remedies in fibromyalgia (Bell et al. 2004), this is the only replication of the use of cordance as a biomarker of treatment response outside of the UCLA so far published, as far as we are aware.

ERPs as predictors of antidepressant response

A method of obtaining extra information from the EEG is to record this while a subject is performing a particular cognitive task. The EEG record is subsequently divided into epochs, time locked to the presentation of a stimulus or the subjects response. Several epochs associated with particular stimuli and/or responses can then be averaged together. This is what is meant by 'event-related potentials' (ERPs). By doing this 'noise' (unrelated EEG activity) is averaged out, leaving just the electrical activity that relates to the task the subject was performing. Over the years there have been a number of ERP paradigms developed using visual or verbal stimuli such as the 'P300' and 'miss-match negativity'.

P300 ERPs

Perhaps the most studied conventional ERP paradigm in depression is the auditory evoked P300 (or 'P3'). This usually involves presentation of auditory tones to subjects, the majority of which are identical with random deviant tones occurring at a low frequency (perhaps 1 in 10 tones). When the ERPs related to the standard tones are compared to those related to deviant ones, the 'deviant ERPs' show a large positive going deflection occurring around 300 ms following the onset of the tone. These 'P300' deflections reflect multiple cognitive processes including attention and higher auditory processing and originate from multiple cortical areas (Mulert et al. 2004b; Volpe et al. 2007). In depression, there are reports of a delay in the latency of the P300 component (Bruder et al. 1991) compared to that seen in healthy subjects (Blackwood et al. 1996; O'Donnell et al. 2004; Souza et al. 1995) and a decrease in the current density in right hemisphere on LORETA analysis (Kawasaki et al. 2004), in line with right-sided hypoactivity.

The precise neurobiological basis of the P300 is unknown but the finding that its latency correlates with the prolactin response to the 5-HT_{1A} agonist flesinoxan (Hansenne and Ansseau, 1999) does make it of interest with regard to antidepressants given the hypothesized importance of these receptors in the therapeutic action of at least some antidepressants (Blier and de Montigny, 1994). However, there is very little published data on the relationship of P300 and antidepressants beyond findings that its latency normalizes after 4 weeks treatment (Hetzel et al. 2005) and a 'normal' P300 amplitude predicts response to ECT (Ancy et al. 1996).

Error processing ERPs

Another ERP of potential interest is that relating to error processing. This is the neuropsychological activity that compares the actual responses made to internal representations of correct responses (Falkenstein et al. 2000; Ruchsow et al. 2002). It is associated with characteristic ERPs when errors are made during forced choice tasks. Two main ERP components are seen (Fig. 24.3). These have been termed error negativity (Ne), a negative peak occurring around 0~160 ms after an incorrect response, and error positivity (Pe), a positive wave with an onset approximately 200 ms following an incorrect response and lasting for around 300 ms (Falkenstein et al. 2000). It is generally argued that Ne reflects error detection (Falkenstein et al. 2000; Vidal et al. 2000) while Pe may represent a post-error detecting component that is independent of Ne (Falkenstein et al. 2000). Ne is largest in frontal-central areas whereas Pe is maximal at posterior regions (Falkenstein et al. 2000). ERP source analysis has suggested that Ne originates from neural activity located in the anterior cingulate cortex (Dehaene et al. 2002; Ruchsow et al. 2002), a finding supported by a functional magnetic resonance imaging (fMRI) study showing increased blood flow in the anterior cingulate cortex when an error-processing-related task is performed (Carter et al. 1998). This makes the task of interest in depression.

Again, there is little data relating to error processing ERPs in depressed patients. However a recent study in medication-free patients found that, relative to comparison subjects, depressed patients had larger Ne, and higher current density in the rACC and medial prefrontal cortex 80 ms after committing an error (Holmes and Pizzagalli, 2008). A study using an emotional go-nogo paradigm with response locked ERPs has reported that remaining symptomatic 8 weeks after treatment with escitalopram in 12 elderly depressed patients is associated with a larger Ne and smaller Pe (Alexopoulos et al. 2007).

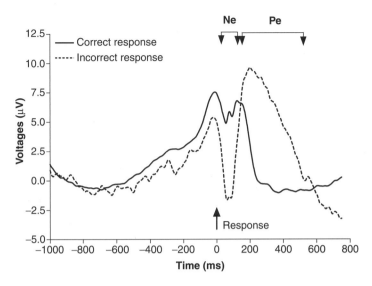

Fig. 24.3 Error processing ERPs recorded from 14 healthy male volunteers. The ERPs have been recorded at the FCz electrode site and associated with correct and incorrect responses made during a Stroop task. An arrow indicates the onset of subjects' responses (0 ms). Error negativity (Ne) and positivity (Pe) is indicated. This is quantified by subtracting the correct ERP data from the incorrect ERP. (Data adapted from Hsu et al. 2003).

Loudness dependency of auditory evoked potentials (LDAEPs)

Hegerl and Juckel (1993) have suggested that a potential method for investigating serotonergic function in man is the examination of the loudness dependency of auditory event related potentials (LDAEPs). A characteristic EEG waveform can be seen following an auditory stimulus of a single tone. An early negative deflection, N1, and positive deflection P2, occur between 100 ms and 200 ms post-stimulus and their peak-to-peak amplitude depends partially on the loudness of the stimulus (Fig. 24.4). Hegerl and Juckel suggest that the slope of a plot of N1/P2 amplitude against loudness, the amplitude/stimulus intensity function (ASF-slope), inversely correlates with serotonergic activity (Hegerl and Juckel, 1993). The most convincing evidence for this hypothesis comes from animal studies showing that direct injection of a 5-HT$_{1A}$ agonist into the dorsal raphe nucleus of cats increased the ASF-slope (Juckel et al. 1999), an effect presumed to occur due to somatodendritic 5-HT$_{1A}$ autoreceptor activation decreasing the firing rate of raphe neurones and so reducing 5HT release in cortex. However the evidence supporting the hypothesis in man is more circumstantial. For example, the ASF-slope is reported to negatively correlate with plasma 5-HT concentrations following fluvoxamine (a selective serotonin re-uptake inhibitor; SSRI) administration, but only in depressed patients and not controls (see Hegerl et al. 2001). However acute administration of SSRIs may actually decrease overall central serotonergic activity due to increased 5-HT activating somatodendritic 5-HT$_{1A}$ autoreceptors (Hjorth and Auerbach, 1994). Direct manipulation of human central 5-HT using the tryptophan depletion paradigm (Moore et al. 2000; Reilly et al. 1997) appears to have no effect on either N1/P2 amplitude (Phillips et al. 2000) or LDAEP (Dierks et al. 1999; Debener et al. 2002; Massey et al. 2004). A recent review has thus concluded that the LDAEP is not a good index of central 5-HT function (O'Neill et al. 2008).

While the LDAEP is reported to be no different in depressed patients compared with controls (Linka et al. 2007), O'Neill and colleagues (2008) argue that the LDAEP does have significant

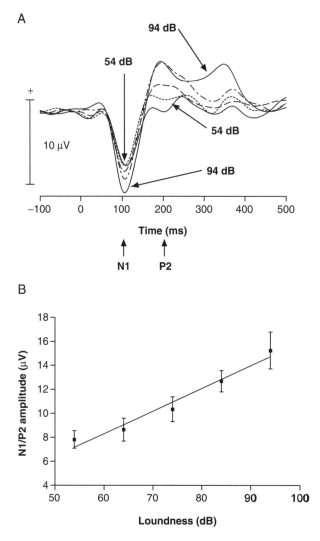

Fig. 24.4 A. Loudness dependency of auditory-evoked potentials (LDAEPs). Auditory-evoked potentials recorded from 14 healthy male volunteers associated with 5 different loudness intensities recorded at the Cz electrode. The smallest (solid line) were recorded associated with 54 dB tones, and largest (also solid lines) with 94 dB tones, as indicated. The intermediate-sized potentials were recorded associated with 64 dB (dotted lines), 74 dB (dashed lines), and 84 dB (dot-dash lines) tones, respectively. B. Auditory-evoked potential amplitude stimulus function. The peak-to-peak amplitudes between the N1 and P2 components (means ± standard errors) is plotted against loudness of the auditory stimuli. A linear regression line has been fitted to the data using GraphPad Prism version 3.02. (Data adapted from Massey et al. 2004).

promise as a potential biomarker of antidepressant response. The reason for their optimism is that the ability to predict antidepressant response has been replicated by more groups than for any other EEG method described above, and included more patients than any other technique. In addition there is a suggestion that it might be able to differentially predict response to antidepressants from different pharmacological classes. The one point of inconsistency is how the LDAEP is measured. The group of Juckel and Hegerl who originally introduced the technique have argued that the greatest sensitivity is derived from dipole source localization of the N1/P2 ERP components into primary and secondary auditory cortex (Gallinat et al. 2000; Juckel et al. 1997). This is on the basis that the highest concentration of serotonin, and the highest synthesis rates, have been found in the primary sensory cortices, especially the primary auditory cortex (Azmitia and Gannon, 1986). The source reflecting mainly the activity of the primary auditory cortex is termed the 'tangential' dipole on the base of its spatial orientation and it is argued this is the best predictor for response to serotonergic antidepressants (Gallinat et al. 2000). However, not all groups use the dipole source localization method and simply measure the peak-to-peak amplitude of the N1/P2 complex, while others just examine the N1 or P2 components separately to calculate the ASF-slope. Little is known as to how these, perhaps subtle, differences in analysis influences the reliability of the putative biomarker.

The first published study using the LDAEP to predict antidepressant response was not from the Juckle and Hegerl group. Paige and colleagues studied the predictive power of the LDAEP (using just the P2 component) in 17 depressed patients treated with a variety of antidepressant but mainly SSRIs (12 of the 17). The response after 4–8-weeks treatment correlated with the ASF-slope and all those who responded to an SSRI had a baseline ASF-slope greater than the median (Paige et al. 1994). This group have subsequently shown a similar result for the pharmacologically different antidepressant bupropion (Paige et al. 1995). The group of Juckel and Hegerl subsequently published a study of 29 patients treated for 4 weeks with SSRIs using the dipole source localization of the N1/P2 ERP complex technique (Gallinat et al. 2000). They divided the patients into two groups around the median value for the ASF-slope. Those with higher slopes showed a significantly greater reduction in HDRS. Response rates (decrease in HDRS ≥ 50%) for the high and low slope groups were 9 out of 15 patients and 3 out of 14, respectively, and responders overall had significantly greater ASF-slopes. The largest replication of these findings comes from a Chinese group who treated 100 patients with fluoxetine (Lee et al. 2005). Again patients were divided around the median ASF-slope (N1/P2 peak-to-peak amplitude). After 4 weeks treatment those above the median had a 44% decrease in HDRS versus 34% for those below median.

Intriguingly, the LDAEP may differentially predict response to antidepressants with differing pharmacologies. Linka and colleagues have replicated the findings described above (though only in relation to N1 amplitude and not P2 or N1/P2 peak-to-peak amplitudes) in 16 inpatients with depression treated with the SSRI citalopram (Linka et al. 2004). Conversely they report that there is an opposite relationship between ASF-slope and response to the noradrenergic uptake blocker, reboxetine (Linka et al. 2005). This finding has been replicated by Juckel and colleagues in 35 inpatients again treated with either citalopram or reboxetine (Juckel et al. 2007).

Combined techniques

As described above a number of different EEG techniques have been explored as potential biomarkers of antidepressant response with several being of potential utility. Two groups have attempted to combine more than one measure together to increase the sensitivity and specificity in terms of response prediction.

Focusing on pre-treatment alpha spectral power, Bruder and colleagues combined global alpha power (sensitivity 73% and specificity 58%) and alpha asymmetry (sensitivity 64% and specificity 71%) giving an overall sensitivity of 83% and specificity of 68% (Bruder et al. 2008). The relatively small increase in sensitivity and specificity when combining these measures may relate to the fact that a correlation ($r = 0.34$) existed between them. Of perhaps even more interest is a report combining theta activity localized to rACC with LORETA and the LDAEP technique – two methods with very different theoretical bases and that do not correlate one with another (Mulert et al. 2007a). The combination of the two techniques significantly discriminated responders from non-responders in 20 patients randomized to either citalopram or reboxetine for 4 weeks with a large Cohen's effect size of 1.41.

Conclusions

Electroencephalographic methods in general are often considered to not have the cache of other functional-imaging techniques. However they are cheap and easy to perform. This alone is an important starting point when considering whether the EEG could have utility as a potential biomarker of antidepressant response. A reasonable number of studies have explored this question using a variety of techniques. Generally studies have been rather small, the methodologies used have been inconsistent and many findings have not been widely replicated in labs beyond those where the techniques were developed. Nevertheless there is some consistency suggesting that baseline alpha, alpha asymmetry, or theta activity, or change in theta early in treatment, may have predictive value. The cordance-analysis technique is of interest in this regard but requires more replications. Of even more theoretical interest is the utilization of localization techniques to explore theta activity specifically in rACC and how this may predict antidepressant response, as would be predicted from a wide body of literature regarding the pathophysiology of the condition. It would be of interest to further examine the predictive power of neuropsychological tasks that activate the ACC, such as error processing, possibly in combination with measures of theta activity. The most widely replicated EEG technique that may predict antidepressant response is the LDAEP, though the original assumption that the ASF-slope is a simple index of central serotonergic function seems increasingly untenable. Perhaps the most exciting developments in the field are the combination of more than one technique together to improve the precision of prediction. More research is needed and certainly justified in this area. For example such work could investigate the sensitivity and specificity of combining some of the most promising individual measures, such as alpha asymmetry, theta activity in rACC, and LDAEP analysis.

References

Alexopoulos, G.S., Murphy, C.F., Gunning-Dixon, F.M. et al. (2007). Event-related potentials in an emotional go/no-go task and remission of geriatric depression. *Neuroreport*, **18**, 217–221.

Alhaj, H.A., Massey, A.E., and McAllister-Williams, R.H. (2006). Effects of DHEA administration on episodic memory, cortisol and mood in healthy young men: a double-blind, placebo-controlled study. *Psychopharm.*, **188**, 541–551.

Alhaj, H.A., Massey, A.E., and McAllister-Williams, R.H. (2007). A study of the neural correlates of episodic memory and HPA axis status in drug-free depressed patients and healthy controls. *J Psychiatr Res.*, **41**, 295–304.

Alhaj, H.A., Massey, A.E., and McAllister-Williams, R.H. (2008). Effects of cortisol on the laterality of the neural correlates of episodic memory. *J Psychiatr Res.*

Ancy, J., Gangadhar, B.N., and Janakiramaiah, N. (1996). 'Normal' P300 amplitude predicts rapid response to ECT in melancholia. *J Affect Disord.*, **41**, 211–215.

Azmitia, E.C. and Gannon, P.J. (1986). The primate serotonergic system: a review of human and animal studies and a report on Macaca fascicularis. *Adv Neurol.*, **43**, 407–468.

Bares, M., Brunovsky, M., Kopecek, M. et al. (2007). Changes in QEEG prefrontal cordance as a predictor of response to antidepressants in patients with treatment resistant depressive disorder: a pilot study. *J Psychiat Res.*, **41**, 319–325.

Bares, M., Brunovsky, M., Kopecek, M. et al. (2008). Early reduction in prefrontal theta QEEG cordance value predicts response to venlafaxine treatment in patients with resistant depressive disorder. *Eur Psychiatry.*

Bell, I.R., Lewis, D.A., Schwartz, G.E. et al. (2004). Electroencephalographic cordance patterns distinguish exceptional clinical responders with fibromyalgia to individualized homeopathic medicines. *Journal of Alternative & Complementary Medicine*, **10**, 285–299.

Berger, H. (1929). Uber das Elektrenkephalogramm des Menschen. *Arch Psychiat Nervenkr.*, **87**, 527–570.

Blackwood, D.H., Sharp, C.W., Walker, M.T., Doody, G.A., Glabus, M.F., and Muir, W.J. (1996). Implications of comorbidity for genetic studies of bipolar disorder: P300 and eye tracking as biological markers for illness. *Brit J Psychiatry*, **168**, 85–92.

Blier, P. and de Montigny, C. (1994). Current advances in the treatment of depression. *Trends Pharmacol.*, **15**, 220–226.

Bochkarev, V.K., Avedisova, A.S., and Liupaeva, N.V. (2004). [Placebo to antidepressant effects ratio by electroencephalographic data]. [Russian]. Zhurnal Nevrologii i Psikhiatrii Imeni S S. Korsakova. **104**, 42–48.

Brody, A.L., Saxena, S., Silverman, D.H. et al. (1999). Brain metabolic changes in major depressive disorder from pre- to post-treatment with paroxetine. *Psychiatry Res.*, **91**, 127–139.

Bruder, G.E., Towey, J.P., Stewart, J.W., Friedman, D., Tenke, C., and Quitkin, F.M. (1991). Event-related potentials in depression: influence of task, stimulus hemifield and clinical features on P3 latency. *Biol Psychiatry*, **30**, 233–246.

Bruder, G.E., Otto, M.W., McGrath, P.J. et al. (1996). Dichotic listening before and after fluoxetine treatment for major depression: relations of laterality to therapeutic response. *Neuropsychopharm.*, **15,** 171–179.

Bruder, G., Fong, R., Tenke, C.E. et al. (1997). Regional brain asymmetries in major depression with or without an anxiety disorder: A quantitative electroencephalographic study. *Biol Psychiatry*, **41**, 939–948.

Bruder, G.E., Stewart, J.W., Tenke, C.E. et al. (2001). Electroencephalographic and perceptual asymmetry differences between responders and nonresponders to an SSRI antidepressant. *Biol Psychiatry*, **49**, 416–425.

Bruder, G.E., Sedoruk, J.P., Stewart, J.W. et al. (2008). Electroencephalographic alpha measures predict therapeutic response to a selective serotonin reuptake inhibitor antidepressant: pre- and post-treatment findings. *Biol Psychiatry*, **63**, 1171–1177.

Buchsbaum, M.S., Wu, J., Siegel, B.V. et al. (1997). Effect of sertraline on regional metabolic rate in patients with affective disorder. *Biol Psychiatry*, **41**, 15–22.

Kupfer, D.J. and Frank, E. (2001). Sleep and treatment response in depression: new findings using power spectral analysis. *Psychiatry Res.*, **103**, 51–67.

Carter, C.S., Braver, T.S., Barch, D.M., Botvinick, M.M., Noll, D., and Cohen, J.D. (1998). Anterior cingulate cortex, error detection, and the online monitoring of performance. *Science*, **280**, 747–749.

Caton, R. (1875). The electric currents of the brain. *Brit Med J.*, **2**, 278.

Cook, I.A., Leuchter, A.F., Witte, E. et al. (1999). Neurophysiologic predictors of treatment response to fluoxetine in major depression. *Psychiatry Res.*, **85**, 263–273.

Cook, I.A., Leuchter, A.F., Morgan, M. et al. (2002). Early changes in prefrontal activity characterize clinical responders to antidepressants. *Neuropsychopharm*, **27**, 120–131.

Cook, I.A., Leuchter, A.F., Morgan, M.L., Stubbeman, W., Siegman, B., and Abrams, M. (2005). Changes in prefrontal activity characterize clinical response in SSRI nonresponders: a pilot study. *J Psychiat Res.*, **39**, 461–466.

Davidson, R.J., Irwin, W., Anderle, M.J., and Kalin, N.H. (2003). The neural substrates of affective processing in depressed patients treated with venlafaxine. *Am J Psychiatry*, **160**, 64–75.

Debener, S., Strobel, A., Kurschner, K. et al. (2002). Is auditory evoked potential augmenting/reducing affected by acute tryptophan depletion? *Biol Psychology*, **59**, 121–133.

Dehaene, S., Posner, M.I., and Tucker, D.M. (2002). Localization of a neural system for error detectionand compensation. *Psychol Sci.,* **5**, 303–305.

Dierks, T., Barta, S., Demisch, L. et al. (1999). Intensity dependence of auditory evoked potentials (AEPs) as biological marker for cerebral serotonin levels: effects of tryptophan depletion in healthy subjects. *Psychopharm.,* **146**, 101–107.

Dougherty, D.D. and Rauch, S.L. (2007). Brain correlates of antidepressant treatment outcome from neuroimaging studies in depression. *Psychiatr Clin North Am.,* **30**, 91–103.

Drevets, W.C. (1999). Prefrontal cortical-amygdalar metabolism in major depression. *Ann N Y Acad Sci.,* **877**, 614–637.

Ebert, D., Feistel, H., Barocka, A. and Kaschka, W. (1994). Increased limbic blood flow and total sleep deprivation in major depression with melancholia. *Psychiatry Res.,* **55**, 101–109.

Evans, K.C., Dougherty, D.D., Pollack, M.H., and Rauch, S.L. (2006). Using neuroimaging to predict treatment response in mood and anxiety disorders. *Ann Clin Psychiatry,* **18**, 33–42.

Falkenstein, M., Hoormann, J., Christ, S., and Hohnsbein, J. (2000). ERP components on reaction errors and their functional significance: a tutorial. *Biol Psychology,* **51**, 87–107.

Fawcett, J. and Barkin, R.L. (1997). Efficacy issues with antidepressants. *J Clin Psychiatry,* **58** Suppl 6, 32–39.

Fontenelle, L.F., Mendlowicz, M.V., Ribeiro, P., Piedade, A., and Versiani, M. (2006). Low-resolution electromagnetic tomography and treatment response in obsessive-compulsive disorder. *Int J Neuropsychopharmacol.,* **9**, 89–94.

Gallinat, J., Bottlender, R., Juckel, G. et al. (2000). The loudness dependency of the auditory evoked N1/ P2-component as a predictor of the acute SSRI response in depression. *Psychopharm,* **148**, 404–411.

Hansen, E.S., Prichep, L.S., Bolwig, T.G., and John, E.R. (2003). Quantitative electroencephalography in OCD patients treated with paroxetine. *Clin Electroencephalogr.,* **34**, 70–74.

Hansenne, M. and Ansseau, M. (1999). P300 event-related potential and serotonin-1A activity in depression. *European Psychiatry: the Journal of the Association of European Psychiatrists,* **14**, 143–147.

Hegerl, U. and Juckel, G. (1993). Intensity dependence of auditory evoked potentials as an indicator of central serotonergic neurotransmission: a new hypothesis. *Biol Psychiatry,* **33**, 173–187.

Hegerl, U., Gallinat, J., and Juckel, G. (2001). Event-related potentials. Do they reflect central serotonergic neurotransmission and do they predict clinical response to serotonin agonists? *J Affect Disord.,* **62**, 93–100.

Henriques, J.B. and Davidson, R.J. (1990). Regional brain electrical asymmetries discriminate between previously depressed and healthy control subjects. *J Abnorm Psychol.,* **99**, 22–31.

Henriques, J.B. and Davidson, R. (1991). Left Frontal Hypoactivation in Depression. *J Abnorm Psychol.,* **100**, 535–545.

Hetzel, G., Moeller, O., Evers, S. et al. (2005). The astroglial protein S100B and visually evoked event-related potentials before and after antidepressant treatment. *Psychopharm.,* **178**, 161–166.

Hjorth, S. and Auerbach, S.B. (1994). Further evidence for the importance of 5-HT_{1A} autoreceptors in the action of selective serotonin reuptake inhibitors. *Eur J Pharmacol.,* **260**, 251–255.

Holmes, A.J. and Pizzagalli, D.A. (2008). Spatiotemporal dynamics of error processing dysfunctions in major depressive disorder. *Arch Gen Psychiatry,* **65**, 179–188.

Hsu, F.C., Garside, M.J. Massey, A.E., and McAllister-Williams, R.H. (2003). Effects of a single dose of cortisol on the neural correlates of episodic memory and error processing in healthy volunteers. *Psychopharm.,* **167**, 431–442.

Hunter, A.M., Leuchter, A.F., Morgan, M.L. et al. (2005). Neurophysiologic correlates of side effects in normal subjects randomized to venlafaxine or placebo. *Neuropsychopharm,* **30**, 792–799.

Hunter, A.M., Leuchter, A.F., Morgan, M.L., and Cook, I.A. (2006). Changes in brain function (quantitative EEG cordance). during placebo lead-in and treatment outcomes in clinical trials for major depression. *Am J Psychiatry,* **163**, 1426–1432.

Ising, M., Horstmann, S., Kloiber, S. et al. (2007). Combined dexamethasone/corticotropin releasing hormone test predicts treatment response in major depression – a potential biomarker? *Biol Psychiatry,* **62**, 47–54.

John, E.R., Prichep, L.S., Fridman, J., and Easton, P. (1988). Neurometrics: computer-assisted differential diagnosis of brain dysfunctions. *Science,* **239**, 162–169.

Juckel, G., Molnar, M., Hegerl, U., Csepe, V., and Karmos, G. (1997). Auditory-evoked potentials as indicator of brain serotonergic activity--first evidence in behaving cats. *Biol Psychiatry,* **41**, 1181–1195.

Juckel, G., Hegerl, U., Molnar, M., Csepe, V., and Karmos, G. (1999). Auditory evoked potentials reflect serotonergic neuronal activity—a study in behaving cats administered drugs acting on 5-HT1A autoreceptors in the dorsal raphe nucleus. *Neuropsychopharm,* **21**, 710–716.

Juckel, G., Pogarell, O., Augustin, H. et al. (2007). Differential prediction of first clinical response to serotonergic and noradrenergic antidepressants using the loudness dependence of auditory evoked potentials in patients with major depressive disorder. *J Clin Psychiatry,* **68**, 1206–1212.

Kawasaki, T., Tanaka, S., Wang, J., Hokama, H., and Hiramatsu, K. (2004). Abnormalities of P300 cortical current density in unmedicated depressed patients revealed by LORETA analysis of event-related potentials. *Psychiatry & Clinical Neurosciences,* **58**, 68–75.

Klimesch, W. (1999). EEG alpha and theta oscillations reflect cognitive and memory performance: a review and analysis. *Brain Res Brain Res Rev.,* **29**, 169–195.

Knott, V.J., Telner, J.I., Lapierre, Y.D., Browne. M., and Horn. E.R. (1996). Quantitative EEG in the prediction of antidepressant response to imipramine. *J Affect Disord.,* **39**, 175–184.

Knott, V., Mahoney, C., Kennedy, S., and Evans, K. (2002). EEG correlates of acute and chronic paroxetine treatment in depression. *J Affect Disord.,* **69**, 241–249.

Knyazev, G.G. (2007). Motivation, emotion, and their inhibitory control mirrored in brain oscillations. *Neurosci Biobehav Rev.,* **31**, 377–395.

Kupfer, D.J., Foster, F.G., Reich, L., Thompson, S.K., and Weiss, B. (1976). EEG sleep changes as predictors in depression. *Am J Psychiatry,* **133**, 622–626.

Lee, T.W., Yu, Y.W., Chen, T.J., and Tsai, S.J. (2005). Loudness dependence of the auditory evoked potential and response to antidepressants in Chinese patients with major depression. *J Psychiatry Neurosci.,* **30**, 202–205.

Leuchter, A.F., Cook, I.A., Lufkin, R.B. et al. (1994). Cordance: a new method for assessment of cerebral perfusion and metabolism using quantitative electroencephalography. *Neuroimage,* **1**, 208–219.

Leuchter, A.F., Uijtdehaage, S.H., Cook, .IA., O'Hara, R., and Mandelkern, M. (1999). Relationship between brain electrical activity and cortical perfusion in normal subjects. *Psychiatry Res.,* **90**, 125–140.

Leuchter, A.F., Cook, I.A., Witte, E.A., Morgan, M., and Abrams, M. (2002). Changes in brain function of depressed subjects during treatment with placebo. *Am J Psychiatry,* **159**, 122–129.

Linka, T., Muller, B.W., Bender, S., and Sartory, G. (2004). The intensity dependence of the auditory evoked N1 component as a predictor of response to Citalopram treatment in patients with major depression. *Neurosci Lett.,* **367**, 375–378.

Linka, T., Muller, B.W., Bender, S., Sartory, G., and Gastpar, M. (2005). The intensity dependence of auditory evoked ERP components predicts responsiveness to reboxetine treatment in major depression. *Pharmacopsychiat.,* **38**, 139–143.

Linka, T., Sartory, G., Bender, S., Gastpar, M., and Muller, B.W. (2007). The intensity dependence of auditory ERP components in unmedicated patients with major depression and healthy controls. An analysis of group differences. *J Affect Disord.,* **103**, 139–145.

Massey, A.E., Marsh, V.R., and McAllister-Williams, R.H. (2004). Lack of effect of tryptophan depletion on the loudness dependency of auditory event related potentials in healthy volunteers. *Biol Psychology,* **65**, 137–145.

Mayberg, H.S. (1997). Limbic-cortical dysregulation: a proposed model of depression. *Journal of Neuropsychiatry & Clinical Neurosciences,* **9**, 471–481.

Mayberg, H.S., Lozano, A.M., Voon, V. et al. (2005). Deep brain stimulation for treatment-resistant depression. *Neuron,* **45**, 651–660.

McAllister-Williams, R.H. and Massey, A.E. (2003). EEG effects of buspirone and pindolol: a method of examining 5-HT(1A) receptor function in humans. *Psychopharm*, **166**, 284–293.

Miller, J.M., Oquendo, M.A., Ogden, R.T., Mann, J.J., and Parsey, R.V. (2008). Serotonin transporter binding as a possible predictor of one-year remission in major depressive disorder. *J Psychiatr Res.,*

Moore, P., Landolt, H.P., Seifritz, E. et al. (2000). Clinical and physiological consequences of rapid tryptophan depletion. *Neuropsychopharm.*, **23**, 601–622.

Morgan, M.L., Witte, E.A., Cook, I.A., Leuchter, A.F., Abrams, M., and Siegman, B. (2005). Influence of age, gender, health status, and depression on quantitative EEG. *Neuropsychobiol.*, **52**, 71–76.

Mulert, C., Jager, L., Schmitt, R. et al. (2004a). Integration of fMRI and simultaneous EEG: towards a comprehensive understanding of localization and time-course of brain activity in target detection. *Neuroimage*, **22**, 83–94.

Mulert, C., Pogarell, O., Juckel, G. et al. (2004b). The neural basis of the P300 potential. Focus on the time-course of the underlying cortical generators. *European Archives of Psychiatry & Clinical Neuroscience*, **254**, 190–198.

Mulert, C., Juckel, G., Brunnmeier, M. et al. (2007a). Prediction of treatment response in major depression: integration of concepts. *J Affect Disord.*, **98**, 215–225.

Mulert, C., Juckel, G., Brunnmeier, M. et al. (2007b). Rostral anterior cingulate cortex activity in the theta band predicts response to antidepressive medication. Clinical EEG & Neuroscience: Official *Journal of the EEG & Clinical Neuroscience Society*, (ENCS) **38**, 78–81.

O'Donnell, B.F., Vohs, J.L., Hetrick, W.P., Carroll, C.A., and Shekhar, A. (2004). Auditory event-related potential abnormalities in bipolar disorder and schizophrenia. *Int J Psychophysiol.*, **53**, 45–55.

O'Neill, B.V., Croft, R.J., and Nathan, P.J. (2008). The loudness dependence of the auditory evoked potential (LDAEP) as an in vivo biomarker of central serotonergic function in humans: rationale, evaluation and review of findings. *Hum Psychopharmacol.*, **23**, 355–370.

Paige, S.R., Fitzpatrick, D.F., Kline, J.P., Balogh, S.E., and Hendricks, S.E. (1994). Event-related potential amplitude/intensity slopes predict response to antidepressants. *Neuropsychobiol.*, **30**, 197–201.

Paige, S.R., Hendricks, S.E., Fitzpatrick, D.F., Balogh, S., Burke, W.J. (1995). Amplitude/intensity functions of auditory event-related potentials predict responsiveness to bupropion in major depressive disorder. *Psychopharm Bull.*, **31**, 243–248.

Pascual-Marqui, R.D., Michel, C.M., and Lehmann, D. (1994). Low resolution electromagnetic tomography: a new method for localizing electrical activity in the brain. *Int J Psychophysiol.*, **18**, 49–65.

Pascual-Marqui, R.D., Lehmann, D., Koenig, T. et al. (1999). Low resolution brain electromagnetic tomography (LORETA) functional imaging in acute, neuroleptic-naive, first-episode, productive schizophrenia. *Psychiatry Res.*, **90**, 169–179.

Perlis, R.H. (2007). Pharmacogenetic studies of antidepressant response: how far from the clinic? *Psychiatr Clin North Am.*, **30**, 125–138.

Phillips, M.A., Oxtoby, E.K., Langley, R.W., Bradshaw, C.M., and Szabadi, E. (2000). Effects of acute tryptophan depletion on prepulse inhibition of the acoustic startle (eyeblink) response and the N1/P2 auditory evoked response in man. *J Psychopharm.*, **14**, 258–265.

Pizzagalli, D., Pascual-Marqui, R.D., Nitschke, J.B. et al. (2001). Anterior cingulate activity as a predictor of degree of treatment response in major depression: evidence from brain electrical tomography analysis. *Am J Psychiatry*, **158**, 405–415.

Pizzagalli, D.A., Oakes, T.R. and Davidson, R.J. (2003). Coupling of theta activity and glucose metabolism in the human rostral anterior cingulate cortex: an EEG/PET study of normal and depressed subjects. *Psychophys.*, **40**, 939–949.

Prichep, L.S., Mas, F., Hollander, E. et al. (1993). Quantitative electroencephalographic subtyping of obsessive-compulsive disorder. *Psychiatry Res.*, **50**, 25–32.

Putnam, K.M. and McSweeney, L.B. (2008). Depressive symptoms and baseline prefrontal EEG alpha activity: a study utilizing Ecological Momentary Assessment. *Biol Psychology*, **77**, 237–240.

Reid, S.A., Duke, L.M., and Allen, J.J. (1998). Resting frontal electroencephalographic asymmetry in depression: inconsistencies suggest the need to identify mediating factors. *Psychophys.*, **35**, 389–404.

Reilly, J.G., McTavish, S.F., Young, A.H. (1997). Rapid depletion of plasma tryptophan: a review of studies and experimental methodology. J *Psychopharm.*, **11**, 381–392.

Ruchsow, M., Grothe, J., Spitzer, M., and Kiefer, M. (2002). Human anterior cingulate cortex is activated by negative feedback: Evidence from event-related potentials in a guessing task. *Neurosci Lett.*, **325**, 203–206.

Saxena, S., Brody, A.L., Ho, M.L., Zohrabi, N., Maidment, K.M., and Baxter, L.R., Jr. (2003). Differential brain metabolic predictors of response to paroxetine in obsessive-compulsive disorder versus major depression. *Am J Psychiatry*, **160**, 522–532.

Seminowicz, D.A., Mayberg, H.S., McIntosh, A.R. et al. (2004). Limbic-frontal circuitry in major depression: a path modeling metanalysis. *Neuroimage*, **22**, 409–418.

Serretti, A., Artioli, P., and Quartesan, R. (2005). Pharmacogenetics in the treatment of depression: pharmacodynamic studies. *Pharmacogenetics & Genomics*, **15**, 61–67.

Smith, G.S., Reynolds, C.F., III, Pollock, B. et al. (1999). Cerebral glucose metabolic response to combined total sleep deprivation and antidepressant treatment in geriatric depression. *Am J Psychiatry*, **156**, 683–689.

Souza, V.B., Muir, W.J., Walker, M.T. et al. (1995). Auditory P300 event-related potentials and neuropsychological performance in schizophrenia and bipolar affective disorder. *Biol Psychiatry*, **37**, 300–310.

Stubbeman, W.F., Leuchter, A.F., Cook, I.A. et al. (2004). Pretreatment neurophysiologic function and ECT response in depression. *Journal of ECT.*, **20**, 142–144.

Suffin, S.C. and Emory, W.H. (1995). Neurometric subgroups in attentional and affective disorders and their association with pharmacotherapeutic outcome. *Clin Electroencephalogr.*, **26**, 76–83.

Trivedi, M.H., Rush, A.J., Wisniewski, S.R. et al. (2006). Evaluation of outcomes with citalopram for depression using measurement-based care in STAR*D: implications for clinical practice. *Am J Psychiatry*, **163**, 28–40.

Ulrich, G., Renfordt, E., Zeller, G., and Frick, K. (1984). Interrelation between changes in the EEG and psychopathology under pharmacotherapy for endogenous depression. A contribution to the predictor question. *Pharmacopsychiat.*, **17**, 178–183.

Ulrich, G. and Frick, K. (1986). A new quantitative approach to the assessment of stages of vigilance as defined by spatiotemporal EEG patterning. *Percept Mot Skills*, **62**, 567–576.

Ulrich, G., Haug, H.J., Stieglitz, R.D., and Fahndrich, E. (1988). Are there distinct biochemical subtypes of depression? EEG characteristics of clinically defined on-drug responders and non-responders. J *Affect Disord.*, **15**, 181–185.

Vidal, F., Hasbroucq, T., Grapperon, J., and Bonnet, M. (2000). Is the 'error negativity' specific to errors? *Biol Psychology*, **51**, 109–128.

Volpe, U., Mucci, A., Bucci, P., Merlotti, E., Galderisi, S., and Maj, M. (2007). The cortical generators of P3a and P3b: a LORETA study. *Brain Res Bull.*, **73**, 220–230.

Wu, J., Buchsbaum, M.S., Gillin, J.C. et al. (1999). Prediction of antidepressant effects of sleep deprivation by metabolic rates in the ventral anterior cingulate and medial prefrontal cortex. *Am J Psychiatry*, **156**, 1149–1158.

Chapter 25

Can we use magnetic/electric fields to help in treatment-resistant depression?

Thomas E. Schlaepfer and Bettina Bewernick

Antidepressant drugs – which are associated with modulation of monoaminergic neurotransmission and/or regulation of the hypothalamic-pituitary-adrenal axis (Mason and Pariante, 2006) – are effective in improving depressive symptoms in major depression (Mann, 2005). Traditionally, antidepressant drugs were mainly found by serendipitous observations of antidepressant effects of substances such as iproniazid (originally developed as a treatment for tuberculosis) or imipramine (originally developed as a treatment for schizophrenia). In particular, increasing levels of monoamine neurotransmitters in the synaptic cleft are associated with improvements of depressive symptoms. This insight led to a more targeted drug discovery process, resulting in drugs with fewer side effects, such as SSRIs . These medications, in conjunction with certain methods of psychotherapy and electroconvulsive therapy, are effective at alleviating depressive symptomatology in most patients (Andrews and Nemeroff, 1994; Mann, 2005). However, these treatments do not work for all patients. Indeed, 8–13% of patients suffering from major depression have a poor outcome after five years of treatment (Keller et al. 1992). A more recent study found that 63.2% of patients included in the STAR-D study were not treated to remission the acute study phase (Rush et al. 2006). Patients who do not respond to known treatment combination including electroconvulsive therapy are thus referred to as suffering from treatment-resistant depression (TRD). A need for the development of alternative treatments for resistant depression which are effective, have fewer side effects or have longer lasting antidepressant effects has been identified (Nestler, 1998; Schlaepfer and Kosel, 2004).

Psychotropic drugs work by altering neurochemistry to a large extent in widespread regions of the brain, many of which may be unrelated to depression. It might well be that more focused, targeted treatment approaches that modulate specific networks in the brain will prove a more effective approach to help treatment-resistant patients. Indeed, this novel approach might lead to the discovery of novel antidepressant treatments that are not or not only based on effects on monoaminergic neurotransmission. Whereas existing depression treatments approach this disease as a general brain dysfunction, a more complete and appropriate treatment will arise from thinking of depression as a dysfunction of specific brain networks that mediate mood and reward signals, in particular, the cortical–limbic–thalamic–striatal network (Mayberg, 2002). This conceptualization leads to novel ideas about targeted neuromodulatory treatments which might be able to positively influence or reset dysfunctional parts of a network processing affective stimuli. Some of the experimental and clinical evidence relevant to the ideas presented here are also discussed in Chapters 12 and 13 of this book. Moreover, this and the last chapters in this book (Chapter 23, 24, 26, and 27) specifically discuss the more recent developments in the treatment of affective disorders.

Repetitive transcranial magnetic stimulation and magnetic seizure therapy

Transcranial Magnetic Stimulation (TMS) refers to a technique delivering magnetic pulses to the cortex using a handheld stimulating coil, which is applied directly to the head. The equipment necessary to deliver TMS consists of two parts: a stimulator, which generates brief pulses of strong electrical currents whose frequency and intensity can be varied and a stimulation coil connected to the stimulator. The magnetic field generated at the coil passes unimpeded through scalp and skull and induces an electrical current in the underlying tissue, which in turn depolarizes neurons. The main advantage of this method of stimulation is its non-invasiveness and the possibility to stimulate very small brain volumes. With recent technology, single-, paired-, or repetitive magnetic pulses can be generated and delivered. Cortical excitability may be increased or decreased depending on stimulation frequency (Hallett, 2000), and TMS has been shown to modify regional cerebral blood flow (Bohning et al. 2000; Catafau et al. 2001).

With the possibility of stimulating the motor cortex non-invasively, TMS replaced high-voltage transcutaneous electrical stimulation previously used in clinical studies to measure variables such as central motor conduction time. Altered conduction time can be associated with a variety of neurological disorders such as multiple sclerosis, amyotrophic lateral sclerosis, cervical myelopathy, and degenerative ataxic disorders. TMS has great potential in the intraoperative monitoring of the integrity of motor tracts during surgery of the brain and spinal tract (Murray, 1991). TMS has found widespread diagnostic use in neurology for demyelinating disorders involving the excitability and the connections of the motor cortex with other parts of the nervous system involved in motor function (Ziemann and Hallett, 2000).

In 1987 Bickford extended the field of TMS research into neuropsychiatry: He was the first to describe transient mood elevation in several normal volunteers receiving single-pulse stimulations to the motor cortex (Bickford et al. 1987). This was the starting point of the scientific investigation of effects of depolarizing magnetic fields in a variety of neuropsychiatric disorders. Soon after, open studies of the effects of TMS on patients with major depression were conducted using single-pulse stimulations at frequencies less than 0.3 Hz (Grisaru et al. 1994; Höflich et al. 1993; Kolbinger et al. 1995). In these studies relatively large areas under the vertex were stimulated bilaterally and involved only very few subjects. More recent work has suggested that both slow and fast rTMS may have some value in depression.

Because of its ability to focally interfere with cortical circuits, rTMS has been proposed and subsequently researched as a putative therapeutic approach in refractory major depression (Nemeroff, 1996; Nestler, 1998). As in the studies of mood modulation by rTMS, the dorsolateral prefrontal cortex (DLPFC) has been the most important target for stimulation in major depression studies. George et al. reported the first open study of the effects of rTMS in six patients with refractory depression treated with five daily rTMS sessions to the left DLPFC (George et al. 1995). They demonstrated that two patients in this study experienced improvement as assessed by a reduction of 26% in the Hamilton Rating Scale for Depression (HRSD) scores. Open and blinded studies of rTMS to the left DLPFC followed with varying results. A relatively large open study demonstrated that 42% of 56 patients responded to 5 daily rTMS sessions; the elderly exhibited a considerably lower response rate (Figiel et al. 1998). A two-week treatment study resulted in a 41% decrease in HRSD scores in another open trial (Triggs et al. 1999).

In the sham-controlled, single-blinded studies of rTMS in treatment-resistant depression, effect sizes have varied considerably. In a within-subject crossover, sham-controlled study of 12 depressed patients treated for two weeks with stimulation to the left DLPFC only somewhat modest antidepressant efficacy of rTMS was found (George et al. 1997). In a more recent study, an antidepressant effect in 20 subjects that was statistically different from sham stimulation using similar stimulation parameters in a parallel design, but still only of modest clinical impact, was demonstrated (Berman et al. 2000). In some studies a low stimulation intensity of 80% of motor threshold was used. Generally, it seems that higher intensity may be more effective, though Loo et al. found no differences between active and sham rTMS using a much higher stimulation intensity (110% of motor threshold) (Loo et al. 1999), an observation which was confirmed in a relatively older outpatient patient group (Schlaepfer et al. 2001). In a large sham-controlled trial with 71 patients that utilized low frequency rTMS, it was demonstrated that 1 Hz stimulation to the right DLPFC was significantly more effective than sham stimulation (Klein et al. 1999). It is unclear whether stimulation of the left dorsolateral prefrontal cortex at these parameters would have had the same effect. The effect of frequency was compared in a study in which 18 patients were randomized to single-pulse TMS, 10 Hz rTMS, and sham rTMS delivered to the left DLPFC. A sham-controlled trial in which 20 patients were randomly assigned to receive an equivalent number of pulses at 5 Hz or 20 Hz over two weeks was reported in which both active groups experienced a 45% reduction in depression severity ratings and none of the patients responded to the sham stimulation (George et al. 2000a). This suggests that lower frequencies may have therapeutic efficacy as well, which is important because slow rTMS is associated with a lower seizure risk.

There are indications that TMS stimulation at higher amplitudes might be more efficacious (Padberg et al. 2002). A negative correlation between the distance from the coil to the cortex and antidepressant response expressed as the percentage of HAMD rating decrease before and after treatment in a relatively older patient group with treatment refractory major depression was reported (Mosimann et al. 2002). This study demonstrated that there might be a process of prefrontal atrophy that outpaces motor cortex atrophy in chronically depressed middle-aged subjects.

These observations together with the established fact that therapeutic seizures have a strong and reliable effect in depression lead to the development of another method, which uses rTMS at convulsive levels as a more targeted form of convulsive therapy (see Lisanby, this volume). Efficacy and side effects of electroconvulsive therapy (ECT) seem to be dependent upon the path of the current passed through the brain (Sackeim et al. 1993). Therefore targeting seizures to focal cortical areas, such as regions of the prefrontal cortex, may reduce some of the side effects of convulsive treatment. Magnetic seizure therapy (MST) has now been tested in proof of concept studies both in nonhuman primates and patients (Lisanby et al. 2001b) and preliminary results on cognitive side effects of the treatment compared to those of ECT have been obtained (Lisanby et al. 2001a). Additional research is obviously needed to evaluate the putative clinical efficacy of this approach and to determine if it has significant advantages over ECT in terms of similar effects and a better side effect profile.

A recent large and well-designed study in 301 patients with major depression who had not benefited from prior drug treatment, transcranial magnetic stimulation was effective in treating major depression with minimal side effects (O'Reardon et al. 2007). This is certainly an important step forward in developing TMS for depression; data from this trial are currently being used to seek FDA approval.

The method of meta-analysis has been applied to the body of literature in the field of rTMS in depression (Burt et al. 2002; Holtzheimer et al. 2001; Martin et al. 2002, 2003; McNamara et al. 2001). While all of those analyses selected slightly different studies and different metaanalytic methods were appl, including different studies and applying different methods of analysis, they find that the antidepressant effect of rTMS is higher than the one of sham treatment. Overall this antidepressant effect is mild to moderate and the reviews do not agree in terms of clinical signifi-cance of the method (Schlaepfer et al. 2003).

Vagus nerve stimulation

Vagus nerve stimulation (VNS) therapy is a type of treatment where a small electrical pulse is administered through an implanted neurostimulator to a bipolar lead attached to the left vagus nerve (George et al. 2000b, c; Kosel and Schlaepfer, 2002; Schlaepfer and Kosel, 2004). This procedure has been studied in patients with treatment-resistant epilepsy and has been demonstrated to be effective in reducing seizure frequency (Ben-Menachem et al. 1994; The Vagus Nerve Stimulation Study Group, 1995; Handforth et al. 1998; Morris and Mueller, 1999). Interestingly, significant and clinically meaningful antidepressant effects of VNS in epilepsy patients have been described, independent of reduction of seizure frequency (Elger et al. 2000; Harden et al. 2000; Helmstaedter et al. 2001).

The precise mechanism by which VNS might influence depressive symptoms is not known, but VNS clearly has effects on brain function (Groves and Brown, 2005; Kosel and Schlaepfer, 2002). Preliminary evidence for the mode of action of putative antidepressant effect was obtained from brain-imaging studies indicating that VNS affects the metabolism of limbic structures relevant to mood regulation (Henry et al. 1999). VNS has been shown to induce c-fos immunolabeling in several forebrain structures, including the posterior cortical amygdaloid nucleus, cingulate and retrosplenial cortex, ventromedial and arcuate hypothalamic nuclei (Naritoku et al. 1995). Another potential mechanism of action, supported by both animal and human studies might be that VNS influences monoaminergic neurotransmission. Unlike other antidepressants, VNS seems not to be associated with an initial reduction in the firing rates of serotonergic neurons; in an animal study raphe neuron firing rates progressively increased over two weeks which could be an explanation for the slow and progressive increase of antidepressant response in clinical VNS studies (Dorr and Debonnel, 2006). Reviews on the emerging body on functional neuroimaging effects (PET, SPECT, fMRI) of VNS found the data difficult to reconcile, mainly because of the small sample sizes, different diagnoses, different types of concomitant antidepressant therapies and different time point of scans obtained (Chae et al. 2003).

Several studies assessing antidepressant properties of VNS in treatment-resistant depression have been conducted so far. The first open, unblinded four-centre pilot study (D01) of 60 patients showed efficacy in very treatment-resistant patients, of whom 30.5% met criteria for response after three months of VNS (Rush et al. 2000). The authors found, that the number of unsuccessful adequate antidepressant treatment trials (rated by the Antidepressant Treatment History Form [ATHF], Prudic et al. 1990) during the current episode was inversely correlated with VNS response. The response rate was 50% in patients with 2–3 failed trials in the current episode, 29.1% after 4–7 failed trials, and 0% after more than 7 failed trials (Sackeim, 2001). The authors concluded that VNS is most effective in patients with moderate but not extreme levels of resistance to conventional antidepressant treatments.

A subsequent sham-controlled, multisite, double-blind trial (D02) in a larger sample did not demonstrate superiority of active VNS treatment over sham treatment after three months. In the active VNS group ($n = 112$) 15.2% of the patients met criteria for response versus 10.0% in the sham group (Rush et al. 2005a, b), despite excluding patients with more than six adequate antidepressant medication trials (as measured by the ATHF, Prudic et al. 1990). The authors suggested that the lack of superiority of active versus sham treatment could have been due to lower stimulation current. While in the first three months of VNS Therapy output current in the D01 study ranged from 0.25 mA to 3.00 mA (median of 0.75 mA; mean 0.96 mA ± 0.54) (Sackeim et al. 2001), in the D02 study output current ranged from 0.25 mA to 3.00 mA, (median 0.75 mA; mean 0.67 ± 0.33) (Rush et al. 2005b). Longer term outcomes following the first three months of VNS in the D02 study revealed that at one year of VNS Therapy 29.8% had responded and 17.1% had remitted (mean output current 1.0 mA) (range 0–2 mA).

The results of one year of VNS in the D02 study were significantly superior to outcomes at one year in a cluster matched but more randomized comparison sample of patients receiving treatment as usual (TAU) (George et al. 2005). Response rates as measured by the HRSD24 were 29.8% (D02) and 12.5% (TAU, $n = 104$) at one year. This TAU sample was acquired initially to define prospectively the outcome of TAU on such patients. In both the long-term TAU and VNS samples, medications and psychotherapy could be added or dropped and doses could be changed, and other non-pharmacological treatments (ECT, TMS, light therapy) could be used. A careful examination of the potential contributions to the differential outcomes in these two samples failed to reveal that any baseline covariate, intercurrent treatment, or medication management differences could account for the difference in outcome. In summary, results of open label, uncontrolled trials examining efficacy of VNS in treatment-resistant major depression seem to point to both acute and longer term effectiveness.

A European study of VNS for treatment-resistant depression (D03) was able to point to antidepressant properties of VNS in a very treatment-resistant patient population, even if due to the protocol limitation the putative contribution of the placebo effect cannot be assessed (Schlaepfer et al. 2008).

Deep brain stimulation

Recent advances in stereotaxic neurosurgical methods have provided a novel and promising technique for alleviating depression in treatment-resistant patients. This technique is deep brain stimulation (DBS), and refers to the stereotaxic placement of unilateral or bilateral electrodes in target brain regions connected to a permanently implanted neurostimulator, which electrically stimulates that brain region (Schlaepfer and Lieb, 2005). Today, DBS is widely used as a treatment for symptoms of Parkinson's disease (Ghika et al. 1998; Greenberg and Rezai, 2003). In these patients, electrodes are placed in the subthalamic nucleus or the globus pallidus internus, and provide immediate recovery to otherwise debilitating motor symptoms. In psychiatric disorders, DBS is used in patients with refractory obsessive compulsive and Tourette's disorders, and preliminary results suggest that DBS is an effective treatment (Abelson et al. 2005; Flaherty et al. 2005; Gross, 2004) and stimulation of the nucleus accumbens for this indication has been proposed by one of the authors (Sturm et al. 2003). One group has recently reported the use of DBS in patients with major depression (Mayberg et al. 2005a).

The exact neurobiological mechanisms by which DBS exerts effects on brain tissue are not yet fully understood (Hardesty and Sackeim, 2007). On the neuronal level, excitatory and inhibitory processes might play a role (McIntyre et al. 2004). Most probably, DBS leads to a functional lesion of the surrounding tissue. Further mechanisms are depolarization blockade of current dependent ion channels (Beurrier et al. 2001), exhaustion of the neurotransmitter pool (Zucker and Regehr, 2002), or synaptic inhibition (Dostrovsky et al. 2000). Today, it is unknown which part of the neuron (e.g. cell body, axon) is primarily modulated by DBS. Certainly, the stimulation volume is not a fixed area around the electrode and the effect on neuronal tissue is variable. The effect of DBS on neurons depends on different factors: the physiological properties of the surrounding brain tissue, the geometric configuration of the electrode and the distance and orientation of the neuronal elements towards the electrode (Kringelbach et al. 2007). Stimulation parameters (frequency, amplitude, pulse width, duration) clearly have an impact on the effect (Ranck, 1975). With commonly used methods a relatively large volume of neural tissue is influenced (Kringelbach et al. 2007).

Neurophysiologic recordings during stimulation have demonstrated that the oscillatory activity between brain structures is modulated by DBS in patients with movement disorders (Kringelbach et al. 2007). Changes in neurotransmitter release (glutamate, dopamine) and brain-derived neurotrophic factor (BDNF) in response to stimulation have been reported (Hilker et al. 2002; Stefani et al. 2006). Functional neuroimaging data have demonstrated that DBS changes the activity of brain areas far beyond the targeted region, and so complex neural networks are modulated (Kringelbach et al. 2007; Mayberg et al. 2005b; Schnitzler and Gross, 2005; Stefurak et al. 2003). These results appear to match the long-term changes described in psychiatric patients. The reversibility of DBS effects is presumed but not proven; it is conceivable that network alterations made by DBS could eventually persist after stimulation is stopped. In summary, short-term changes can explain the acute effects of DBS in movement disorders. In psychiatric disorders, long-term changes in symptoms have been described. These can only result from long-lasting, complex modulation of neural networks (McIntyre et al. 2004).

The anterior limb of the internal capsule is a prominent target for DBS in depression. Historic lesion studies contributed to the hypothesis that the inactivation of larger brain areas inhibits dysfunctional connections through this region. The role of the internal capsule in depression is unclear; interest in this brain region for depression is an outgrowth of its use as a target in OCD. After one month of DBS there was a substantial reduction in depression in a majority of patients, by Montgomery-Asberg Depression Rating scores. This outcome remained stable with some fluctuation over half a year (Greenberg and Malone, 2007).

The subgenual cingulate cortex (Brodman Area cg25) has been stimulated with DBS (Mayberg, 1997). This region modulates negative mood states, is involved in the onset of sadness, and seems to be involved in the effect of some antidepressant drugs. The rostral part of the cingulate cortex plays a role in modulating the network associated with depression. Mayberg and colleagues demonstrated that two months after surgery five of six patients met the criterion for clinical response

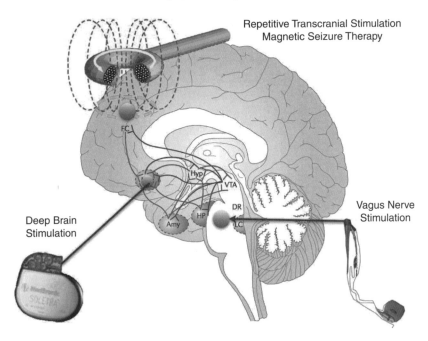

Fig. 25.1 The figure shows schematically that the described targeted neuromodulatory interventions might act on a network that processes affective stimuli at different sites. This network has been identified and described using functional neuroimaging methods in depressed patients. See colour plate section for colour version.

(fall in baseline HDRS score by 50%). After six months, four patients showed sustained response. Several neuropsychological functions that were impaired at baseline were significantly improved. A reduction in the pathological hyperactivity in this region has also been demonstrated using oxygen1-water Positron Emission Tomography (PET) in this study. During the blinded sham stimulation phase in one patient the condition worsened considerably showing that continued stimulation was required in this patient to prevent depression. No adverse events from stimulation were observed (Mayberg, 1997).

Our group selected the nucleus accumbens as a target for DBS because of its prominent role in the reward system. The nucleus accumbens regulates motivation for motor activity associated with the processing of emotions in the limbic system. Modulation of this structure was associated with changes in the symptoms of anhedonia and mood in three depressed patients (Schlaepfer et al. 2007). The stimulation current correlated negatively with anhedonia ratings. Normalization of brain metabolism in fronto-striatal networks as a result of stimulation was also observed. No side effects were observed from DBS. Results of those intial three and further eight patients in this study show acute as well as long-term antidepressant effects of DBS at this target.

In summary, DBS is a unique and promising method for the treatment of therapy-resistant psychiatric patients. The method consists of manipulating pathological neuronal networks in a localized and precise manner. Initial studies showed promising effects in psychiatric disorders, but the number of patients involved is too small for generalization. Still, the logic and specificity of the DBS approach gives new hope to the many therapy-resistant psychiatric patients. To date, no fundamental ethical objections to its use in psychiatric disorders have appeared, but until substantial clinical data is available, mandatory standards are needed.

References

Abelson, J.L., Curtis, G.C., Sagher, O. et al. (2005). Deep brain stimulation for refractory obsessive-compulsive disorder. *Biol Psychiatry,* **57,** 510–516.

Andrews, J.M. and Nemeroff, C.B. (1994). Contemporary management of depression. *Am J Med.,* **97,** 24S–32S.

Ben-Menachem, E., Manon-Espaillat, R., Ristanovic, R. et al. (1994). Vagus nerve stimulation for treatment of partial seizures: 1. A controlled study of effect on seizures. First international vagus nerve stimulation study group. *Epilepsia,* **35,** 616–626.

Berman, R.M., Narasimhan, M., Sanacora, G. et al. (2000). A randomized clinical trial of repetitive transcranial magnetic stimulation in the treatment of major depression. *Biol Psychiatry,* **47,** 332–337.

Beurrier, C., Bioulac, B., Audin, J., and Hammond, C. (2001). High-frequency stimulation produces a transient blockade of voltage-gated currents in subthalamic neurons. *J Neurophysiol.,* **85,** 1351–1356.

Bickford, R.G., Guidi, M., Fortesque, P., and Swenson, M. (1987). Magnetic stimulation of human peripheral nerve and brain: response enhancement by combined magnetoelectrical technique. *Neurosurgery,* **20,** 110–116.

Bohning, D.E., Shastri, A., Wasserman, E.M. et al. (2000). BOLD-fMRI response to single-pulse transcranial magnetic stimulation (TMS). *Journal of Magnetic Resonance Imaging,* **11,** 569–574.

Burt, T., Lisanby, S.H., and Sackeim, H.A. (2002). Neuropsychiatric applications of transcranial magnetic stimulation: a meta analysis. *Int J Neuropsychopharmacol,* **5,** 73–103.

Catafau, A., Perez, V., Gironell, A. et al. (2001). SPECT mapping of cerebral activity changes induced by repetitive transcranial magnetic stimulation in depressed patients. A pilot study. *Psychiat Res.,* **106,** 151–160.

Chae, J.H., Nahas, Z., Lomarev, M. et al. (2003). A review of functional neuroimaging studies of vagus nerve stimulation (VNS). *J Psychiatr Res.,* **37,** 443–455.

Dorr, A.E. and Debonnel, G. (2006). Effect of vagus nerve stimulation on serotonergic and noradrenergic transmission. *J Pharmacol Exp Ther.,* **318,** 890–898.

Dostrovsky, J.O., Levy, R., Wu, J.P., Hutchison, W.D., Tasker, R.R., and Lozano, A.M. (2000). Microstimulation-induced inhibition of neuronal firing in human globus pallidus. *J Neurophysiol.,* **84,** 570–574.

Elger, G., Hoppe, C., Falkai, P., Rush, A., and Elger, C. (2000). Vagus nerve stimulation is associated with mood improvements in epilepsy patients. *Epilepsy Res,* **42,** 203–210.

Figiel, G.S., Epstein, C., Mcdonald, W.M. et al. (1998). The use of rapid-rate transcranial magnetic stimulation (rTMS). in refractory depressed patients. *J Neuropsychiatry Clin Neurosci.,* **10,** 20–25.

Flaherty, A.W., Williams, Z.M., Amirnovin, R. et al. (2005). Deep brain stimulation of the anterior internal capsule for the treatment of Tourette syndrome: technical case report. *Neurosurgery,* **57,** E403; discussion E403.

George, M.S., Wasserman, E.M., Williams, W.A. et al. (1995). Daily repetitive transcranial magnetic stimulation (rTMS) improves mood in depression. *Neuroreport,* **6,** 1853–1856.

George, M.S., Wassermann, E.M., Kimbrell, T.A. et al. (1997). Mood improvement following daily left prefrontal repetitive transcranial magnetic stimulation in patients with depression: a placebo-controlled crossover trial. *Am J Psychiatry,* **154,** 1752–1756.

George, M., Nahas, Z., Molloy, M. et al. (2000a). A controlled trial of daily left prefrontal cortex TMS for treating depression. *Biol Psychiatry,* **48,** 962–970.

George, M., Sackeim, H., Marangell, L. et al. (2000b). Vagus nerve stimulation. A potential therapy for resistant depression? *Psychiatr Clin North Am.,* **23,** 757–783.

George, M., Sackeim, H., Rush, A. et al. (2000c). Vagus nerve stimulation: a new tool for brain research and therapy. *Biol Psychiatry,* **47,** 287–295.

George, M.S., Rush, A.J., Marangell, L.B. et al. (2005). A one-year comparison of vagus nerve stimulation with treatment as usual for treatment-resistant depression. *Biol Psychiatry,* **58,** 364–373.

Ghika, J., Villemure, J.G., Fankhauser, H., Favre, J., Assal, G., and Ghika-Schmid, F. (1998). Efficiency and safety of bilateral contemporaneous pallidal stimulation (deep brain stimulation) in levodopa-responsive patients with Parkinson's disease with severe motor fluctuations: a 2-year follow-up review. *J Neurosurg.,* **89,** 713–718.

Greenberg, B. and Malone, D. (2007). Preliminary results from DBS multicenter study in depression. *Providence,* Rhode Island, Personal Communication.

Greenberg, B.D. and Rezai, A.R. (2003). Mechanisms and the current state of deep brain stimulation in neuropsychiatry. *CNS Spectr.,* **8,** 522–526.

Grisaru, N., Yaroslavsky, Y., Abarbanel, J.M., Lamberg, T., and Belmaker, R. (1994). Transcranial magnetic stimultation in depression and schizophrenia. *European Neuropsychopharmacology,* **4,** 287–288.

Gross, R.E. (2004). Deep brain stimulation in the treatment of neurological and psychiatric disease. *Expert Rev Neurother.,* **4,** 465–478.

Groves, D.A. and Brown, V.J. (2005). Vagal nerve stimulation: a review of its applications and potential mechanisms that mediate its clinical effects. *Neurosci Biobehav Rev.,* **29,** 493–500.

Hallett, M. (2000). Transcranial magnetic stimulation and the brain. *Nature,* **406,** 147–150.

Handforth, A., Degiorgio, C., Schachter, S., Uthman, B., Naritoku, D., and Tecoma, E. (1998). Vagus nerve stimulation therapy for partial-onset seizures: a randomized activecontrol trial. *Neurology,* **51,** 48–55.

Harden, C.L., Pulver, M.C., Ravdin, L.D., Nikolov, B., Halper, J.P., and Labar, D.R. (2000). A pilot study of mood in epilepsy patients treated with vagus nerve stimulation. *Epilepsy Behav.,* **1,** 93–99.

Hardesty, D.E. and Sackeim, H.A. (2007). Deep brain stimulation in movement and psychiatric disorders. *Biol Psychiatry,* **61,** 831–835.

Helmstaedter, C., Hoppe, C., and Elger, C.E. (2001). Memory alterations during acute high-intensity vagus nerve stimulation. *Epilepsy Research,* **47,** 37–42.

Henry, T.R., Votaw, J.R., Pennell, P.B. et al. (1999). Acute blood flow changes and efficacy of vagus nerve stimulation in partial epilepsy. *Neurology*, **52**, 1166–1173.

Hilker, R., Voges, J., Thiel, A. et al. (2002). Deep brain stimulation of the subthalamic nucleus versus levodopa challenge in Parkinson's disease: measuring the on- and off-conditions with FDG-PET. *J Neural Transm.*, **109**, 1257–1264.

Höflich, G., Kasper, S., Hufnagel, A., Ruhrmann, S., and Möller, H.J. (1993). Application of transcranial magnetic stimulation in the treatment of drug-resistant major depression: a report of two cases. *Human Psychopharmacology*, **8**, 361–365.

Holtzheimer, P.E., 3rd, Russo, J., and Avery, D.H. (2001). A meta-analysis of repetitive transcranial magnetic stimulation in the treatment of depression. *Psychopharmacol Bull.*, **35**, 149–169.

Keller, M.B., Lavori, P.W., Mueller, T.I. et al. (1992). Time to recovery, chronicity, and levels of psychopathology in major depression. A 5-year prospective follow-up of 431 subjects. *Arch Gen Psychiatry*, **49**, 809–816.

Klein, E., Kreinin, I., Chistyakov, A. et al. (1999). Therapeutic efficacy of right prefrontal slow repetitive transcranial magnetic stimulation in major depression: a double-blind controlled study. *Arch Gen Psychiatry*, **56**, 315–320.

Kolbinger, H.M., Höflich, G., Hufnagel, A., Möller, H.J., and Kasper, S. (1995). Transcranial magnetic stimulation (TMS). in the treatment of major depression. *Human Psychopharmacology*, **10**, 305–310.

Kosel, M. and Schlaepfer, T.E. (2002). Mechanisms and state of the art of vagus nerve stimulation. *The Journal of ECT*, **18**, 189–192.

Kringelbach, M.L., Jenkinson, N., Owen, S.L., and Aziz, T.Z. (2007). Translational principles of deep brain stimulation. *Nat Rev Neurosci.*, **8**, 623–635.

Lisanby, S.H., Luber, B., Finck, A.D., Schroeder, C., and Sackeim, H.A. (2001a). Deliberate seizure induction with repetitive transcranial magnetic stimulation in nonhuman primates. *Arch Gen Psychiatry*, **58**, 199–200.

Lisanby, S.H., Schlaepfer, T.E., Fisch, H.U., and Sackeim, H.A. (2001b). Magnetic seizure therapy of major depression. *Arch Gen Psychiatry*, **58**, 303–305.

Loo, C., Mitchell, P., Sachdev, P., Mcdarmont, B., Parker, G., and Gandevia, S. (1999). Double-blind controlled investigation of transcranial magnetic stimulation for the treatment of resistant major depression. *Am J Psychiatry*, **156**, 946–948.

Mann, J.J. (2005). The medical management of depression. *N Engl J Med.*, **353**, 1819–1834.

Martin, J., Barbanoj, M., Schlaepfer, T. et al (2002). *Transcranial magnetic stimulation for treating depression*. (*Cochrane Review*). Oxford: The Cochrane Library.

Martin, J.L., Barbanoj, M.J., Schlaepfer, T.E., Thompson, E., Perez, V., and Kulisevsky, J. (2003). Effectiveness of repetitive transcranial magnetic stimulation for the treatment of depression: systematic review and meta-analysis. *British Journal of Psychiatry*, **182**, 480–491.

Mason, B.L. and Pariante, C.M. (2006). The effects of antidepressants on the hypothalamic-pituitary-adrenal axis. *Drug News Perspect.*, **19**, 603–608.

Mayberg, H.S. (1997). Limbic-cortical dysregulation: a proposed model of depression. *Journal of Neuropsychiatry*, **9**, 471–481.

Mayberg, H.S. (2002). Modulating limbic-cortical circuits in depression: targets of antidepressant treatments. *Semin Clin Neuropsychiatry*, **7**, 255–268.

Mayberg, H.S., Lozano, A.M., Voon, V. et al. (2005a). Deep brain stimulation for treatment-resistant depression. *Neuron*, **45**, 651–660.

Mayberg, H.S., Lozano, A.M., Voon, V. et al. (2005b). Deep brain stimulation for treatment-resistant depression. *Neuron*, **45**, 651–660.

Mcintyre, C.C., Savasta, M., Kerkerian-le Goff, L., and Vitek, J.L. (2004). Uncovering the mechanism(s) of action of deep brain stimulation: activation, inhibition, or both. *Clin Neurophysiol.*, **115**, 1239–1248.

Mcnamara, B., Ray, J.L., Arthurs, O.J., and Boniface, S. (2001). Transcranial magnetic stimulation for depression and other psychiatric disorders. *Psychol Med.*, **31**, 1141–1146.

Morris, G.L.3rd and Mueller, W.M. (1999). Long-term treatment with vagus nerve stimulation in patients with refractory epilepsy. The vagus nerve stimulation study group E01-E05. *Neurology*, **53**, 1731–1735.

Mosimann, U., Marré, S.C., Werlen, S. et al. (2002). Antidepressant effects of repetitive transcranial magnetic stimulation in the elderly correlation between effect size and coil-cortex distance. *Archives of General Psychiatry*, **59**, 560–561.

Murray, N.M.F. (1991). Magnetic stimulation of cortex: clinical applications. *Journal of Clinical Neurophysiology*, **8**, 66–76.

Naritoku, D.K., Terry, W.J., and Helfert, R.H. (1995). Regional induction of fos immunoreactivity in the brain by anticonvulsant stimulation of the vagus nerve. *Epilepsy Res.*, **22**, 53–62.

Nemeroff, C. (1996). Augmentation strategies in patients with refractory depression. *Depress Anxiety*, **4**, 169–181.

Nestler, E. (1998). Antidepressant treatments in the 21st century. *Biol Psychiatriy*, **44**, 526–533.

O'Reardon, J.P., Solvason, H.B., Janicak, P.G. et al, (2007). Efficacy and safety of transcranial magnetic stimulation in the acute treatment of major depression: a multisite randomized controlled trial. *Biol Psychiatry*, **62**, 1208–1216.

Padberg, F., Zwanzger, P., Keck, M. et al. (2002). Repetitive transcranial magnetic stimulation (rTMS) in major depression. relation between efficacy and stimulation intensity. *Neuropsychopharmacology*, **27**, 638.

Prudic, J., Sackeim, H.A., and Devanand, D. P. (1990). Medication resistance and clinical response to electroconvulsive therapy. *Psychiatry Res.*, **31**, 287–296.

Ranck, J.B., Jr. (1975). Which elements are excited in electrical stimulation of mammalian central nervous system: a review. *Brain Res*, **98**, 417–440.

Rush, A.J., George, M.S., Sackeim, H.A. et al. (2000). Vagus nerve stimulation (VNS) for treatment-resistant depression: a multicenter study. *Biol Psychiatry*, **47**, 276–286.

Rush, A.J., Marangell, L.B., Sackeim, H.A. et al. (2005a). Vagus nerve stimulation for treatment-resistant depression: a randomized, controlled acute phase trial. *Biol Psychiatry*, **58**, 347–354.

Rush, A.J., Sackeim, H.A. et al. (2005b). Effects of 12 months of vagus nerve stimulation in treatment-resistant depression: a naturalistic study. *Biol Psychiatry*, **58**, 355–363.

Rush, A.J., Trivedi, M.H., Wisniewski, S.R. et al. (2006). Acute and longer-term outcomes in depressed outpatients requiring one or several treatment steps: a STAR*D report. *Am J Psychiatry*, **163**, 1905–1917.

Sackeim, H.A. (2001). The definition and meaning of treatment-resistant depression. *J Clin Psychiatry*, **62** Supplement **16**, 10–17.

Sackeim, H.A., Keilp, J.G., Rush, A.J. et al. (2001). The effects of vagus nerve stimulation on cognitive performance in patients with treatment-resistant depression. *Neuropsychiatry Neuropsychol Behav Neurol.*, **14**, 53–62.

Sackeim, H.A., Prudic, J., Devanand, D.P. et al. (1993). Effects of stimulus intensity and electrode placement on the efficacy and cognitive effects of electroconvulsive therapy. *N Engl J Med.*, **328**, 839–846.

Schlaepfer, T.E., Mosimann, U.P., Schmitt, W.J., Fisch, H.U., and Pearlson, G. D. (2001). Repetitive transcranial magnetic stimulation (rTMS) in elderly patients with major depression. *Biol Psychiatry*, **8S**, 160.

Schlaepfer, T.E., Kosel, M., and Nemeroff, C.B. (2003). Efficacy of repetitive transcranial magnetic stimulation (rTMS) in the treatment of affective disorders. *Neuropsychopharmacology*, **28**, 201–205.

Schlaepfer, T.E. and Kosel, M. (2004). Novel physical treatments for major depression: vagus nerve stimulation, transcranial magnetic stimulation and magnetic seizure therapy. *Current Opinion in Psychiatry*, **17**, 15–20.

Schlaepfer, T. and Lieb, K. (2005). Deep brain stimulation for treatment refractory depression. *Lancet,* **366,** 1420–1422.

Schlaepfer, T.E., Cohen, M.X., Frick, C. et al. (2007). Deep brain stimulation to reward circuitry alleviates anhedonia in refractory major depression. *Neuropsychopharmacology,* **33,** 368–377.

Schlaepfer, T., Frick, C., Zobel, A. et al. (2008). Vagus nerve stimulation for depression: efficacy and safety in a European study *Psychological Medicine,* **38,** 651–662.

Schnitzler, A. and Gross, J. (2005). Normal and pathological oscillatory communication in the brain. *Nat Rev Neurosci.,* **6,** 285–296.

Stefani, A., Fedele, E., Galati, S. et al. (2006). Deep brain stimulation in Parkinson's disease patients: biochemical evidence. *J Neural Transm.,* Supplement 401–408.

Stefurak, T., Mikulis, D., Mayberg, H. et al. (2003). Deep brain stimulation for Parkinson's disease dissociates mood and motor circuits: a functional MRI case study. *Mov Disord.,* **18,** 1508–1516.

Sturm, V., Lenartz, D., Koulousakis, A. et al. (2003). The nucleus accumbens: a target for deep brain stimulation in obsessive-compulsive- and anxiety-disorders. *J Chem Neuroanat.,* **26,** 293–299.

The Vagus Nerve Stimulation Study Group. (1995). A randomized controlled trial of chronic vagus nerve stimulation for treatment of medically intractable seizures: the vagus nerve stimulation study group. *Neurology,* **45,** 224–230.

Triggs, W.J., Mccoy, K.J.M., Greer, R. et al. (1999). Effects of left frontal transcranial magnetic simulation on depressed mood, cognition, and corticomotor threshold. *Biol Psychiatry,* **45,** 1440–1445.

Ziemann, U. and Hallett, M. (2000). Basic neurophysiological studies with TMS. In George, M.S. and Belmaker, R. H. (eds.) *Transcranial Magnetic Stimulation in Neuropsychiatry.* Washington DC, American Psychiatric Press.

Zucker, R.S. and Regehr, W.G. (2002). Short-term synaptic plasticity. *Annu Rev Physiol.,* **64,** 355–405.

Chapter 26

Antiglucocorticoids in the treatment of affective disorders: from preclinical to clinical studies

Sarah E. Gartside, Keith S. Reid, and I. Nicol Ferrier

Introduction

It has been known for over half a century that there is an association between major depression and hypercortisolaemia. This change is found in many patients, especially in those who are psychotic or have the so-called melancholic form of the disorder, but is less commonly found in less severe depressions in community samples. The hypercortisolaemia is characterized by a change in the diurnal rhythm of cortisol secretion with higher levels in the morning and a reduction of the normal nadir. In major depression the phenomenon is generally state related, that is, it improves as patients' mood improves. The mechanism underlying the cortisol disturbance is not clear. It does not simply relate to stress or anxiety since the phenomenon is found much more markedly in patients with depression rather than those with anxiety and/or stress. However it may well link to persistent effects of stress of a variety of kinds in childhood with a re-setting of the hypothalamic-pituitary-adrenal (HPA) axis – an issue which is dealt with in greater detail in several other Chapters of this book (Chapters 5, 7–9, 11, 15, 16, 19, and 21). Several studies investigating the pathophysiology of major depression have highlighted dysregulation of the glucocorticoid receptor (GR) as underpinning the hypercortisolaemia phenomenon.

Several pieces of research have suggested that raised cortisol is a marker of prognosis and that persistent hypercortisolaemia is likely to identify those patients who are either not improving or are likely to be vulnerable to relapse. There is evidence that HPA dysregulation in depression is associated with a number of negative outcomes. Thus, a meta-analysis of the dexamethasone suppression test (DST) as a predictor of treatment outcome concluded that although DST status at baseline was not predictive of response to antidepressant treatment, persistent non-suppression DST after treatment was associated with high risk of early relapse and poor outcome after discharge from hospital (Ribeiro et al. 1993). For example, in a study of depressed patients treated with the SSRI fluoxetine (Young et al. 2004b), non-responders showed abnormal HPA axis reactivity, while responders did not differ from healthy controls. More recently, a research group at the Max Planck Institute in Munich has shown that treatment response in 50 depressed patients was predicted by the cortisol response to the combined dexamethasone/corticotrophin-releasing hormone (CRH) challenge test – in that treatment responders showed 'a more pronounced normalization of an initially dysregulated HPA-axis' (Hennings et al. 2008). The mechanism whereby hypercortisolaemia mitigates against treatment response is currently under investigation (see later). There is also evidence that manipulation of the HPA axis can alter cognitive function in normal human subjects, particularly related to working and episodic memory. This raises the question of whether cognitive outcomes in affective disorder are associated with the presence or absence and/or degree of hypercortisolaemia.

As discussed above, hypercortisolaemia may be associated with a number of the symptoms or signs of major depression and impact on the cognitive changes associated with the disorder. The data suggest that hypercortisolaemia is associated with poor prognosis and poor treatment response. These observations have given rise to a series of studies investigating the role of drugs which might reduce the impact of cortisol on the patient. These treatments go under the general name of 'antiglucocorticoids'.

This chapter primarily outlines the current understanding of glucocorticoid receptors in the brain. We also examine the synthesis of glucocorticoids and how antiglucocorticoids interfere with normal steroid synthesis and activity. We then give an account of preclinical studies on the effects of antiglucocorticoids, particularly focusing on hippocampal neurogenesis, dendritic organization, hippocampal and prefrontal functional plasticity, and 5-HT neurotransmission. The chapter concludes with a review of the clinical evidence for the efficacy of antiglucocorticoids in terms of affective and neuropsychological outcomes. Finally we provide an overview of the subject and highlight future directions for research. This is also the last chapter to discuss the differences and similarities between depression and bipolar disorder, together with Chapter 6, 21, and 22. Moreover, this and the last chapters in this book (Chapter 23, 24, 25, and 27) specifically discuss the more recent developments in the treatment of affective disorders.

Physiology and pharmacology of glucocorticoids

Glucocorticoid receptors in the brain

The actions of glucocorticoids (cortisol in man and corticosterone in rodents) in the brain are mediated by two receptors, the glucocorticoid receptor (GR) and the mineralocorticoid receptor (MR). GR and MR are members of the superfamily of steroid receptors. They are soluble intracellular proteins that act as ligand-inducible transcription factors, binding to DNA to alter gene expression. GR and MR are products of distinct genes but they have similar protein structures. Their homology in the DNA-binding domain is particularly high and they bind to the same so-called glucocorticoid response element (GRE) consisting of the 15 nucleotide sequence AGAACAnnnTGTTCT (Funder, 1997). While there is high homology in the DNA-binding domain, the two receptors differ markedly in the steroid-binding domain, meaning that MR and GR differ in their ligand-binding properties. Some evidence suggests that MR binds cortisol and corticosterone with much higher affinity ($K_d \sim 0.5$–2 nM) than does GR ($K_d \sim 10$–20 nM) meaning that while MRs are close to saturated even at low concentrations of cortisol or corticosterone, GR are only significantly occupied by relatively high circulating cortisol/corticosterone concentrations (Reul and de Kloet, 1985; De Kloet et al. 1998). Thus GRs may be seen as having particular importance in mediating the effects of elevated levels of glucocorticoids. However this conclusion has more recently been questioned (Pace and Spencer, 2005) and remains a moot point.

In the absence of ligand, GR and MR exist in the cytoplasm in a complex with heat shock proteins (Pratt and Toft, 1997; Schoneveld et al. 2004). In the presence of endogenous or exogenous agonist, dimers of liganded receptors form and translocate to the nucleus. These dimers can bind to GREs in the promoter regions of certain genes and induce or repress their transcription. For some genes, binding of the liganded receptor alone to the GRE is sufficient to regulate transcription. Other genes however require a glucocorticoid response unit (GRU) comprising the bound receptor in a complex with other co-factors. This dependence on the presence of other co-factors allows for potential tissue and cellular specificity in the response of a given gene to corticosteroids. Additionally, liganded receptors may repress transcription by competitive blockade of the binding of transcriptional promoters at sites adjacent to the GRE. Glucocorticoid receptors may even regulate transcription in genes which do not have a GRE, by binding to and inactivating other transcriptional factors. These multiple mechanisms allow for both positive and negative regulation of a wide variety of genes with cellular selectivity (for reviews see Buckingham, 2006; Schoneveld et al. 2004).

Glucocorticoid receptors have been shown to be widely expressed in the central nervous system (CNS) with highest densities in cortical regions including prefrontal cortex, in limbic areas including hippocampus and amygdala, and in the thalamus and hypothalamus (Ahima and Harlan, 1990; Cintra et al. 1994; Fuxe et al. 1985a, b; Fuxe et al. 1987; Morimoto et al. 1996). In the cortex expression is concentrated in pyramidal cells, while in the hippocampus both pyramidal and granule cells express GR (see Fig. 26.1a and b).

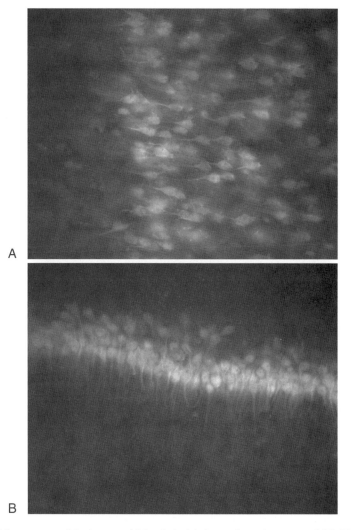

Fig. 26.1 GR immunoreactivity in pyramidal cells in (a) the prefrontal cortex and (b) CA1 region of the hippocampus of an adult male Lister-hooded rat. GR antibody from Santa Cruz Biotechnology, CA, visualized with FITC goat anti-rabbit secondary. In (a) medial surface is at the right hand side of the image.

In the paraventricular nucleus of the hypothalamus GRs are concentrated in parvocellular corticotrophs. GRs have also been shown to be present in the cell bodies of ascending 5-HT neurones (Harfstrand et al. 1986). Indeed in a recent study we have observed that all 5-HT neurones in both the dorsal and median raphe nuclei express GR (Gartside et al. unpublished). Some evidence also indicates GR localization in noradrenergic and dopaminergic neurones, although there is inconsistency in the literature particularly with respect to DA neurones of the VTA (Czyrak and Chocyk, 2001; Harfstrand et al. 1986; own unpublished).

Mapping of MR in the CNS has been less comprehensive and data are less consistent. However, a widespread distribution has been noted (Ahima et al. 1991) with particularly high MR density in hippocampal, thalamic, and hypothalamic regions (Ahima et al. 1991; Agarwal et al. 1993; Ito et al. 2000; Han et al. 2005). Our recent studies confirm the presence of MR in the hippocampus where it is located in both pyramidal and granule cells and we have also observed MR immunoreactivity in the prefrontal cortex where it is concentrated in pyramidal cells (Gartside et al. unpublished). Few studies have examined the presence of MR in monoaminergic neurones, however we have found extensive co-localization of MR immunoreactivity with the 5-HT cellular marker tryptophan hydroxylase (TPH) in the midbrain raphe nuclei (Gartside et al. unpublished).

An important issue in the distribution of MR is to comment on the apparent mismatch in the reported distributions of MR mRNA and protein. This may be explained by the existence of several variants in the 5' untranslated region of the MR gene (Kwak et al. 1993) which may affect the translational efficiency of the gene (Kozak, 1991).

A final point on the distribution of GR and MR is to note that GR and MR are frequently found in the same brain regions and indeed in the same cell types. Thus, for example, a very high proportion of (if not all) cortical and hippocampal pyramidal cells and 5-HT neurones of the DRN express GR and MR, indicating that in all likelihood these receptors are co-localized within individual cells.

Synthesis of glucocorticoids

Glucocorticoids are synthesized from cholesterol in the adrenal cortex under the regulation of adrenocorticotropic hormone (ACTH) in a pathway involving multiple enzymatic steps. Initially the side chain is cleaved from cholesterol by the action of a cytochrome P450 enzyme known as P450 side chain cleavage (P450scc, CYP11A1, or 20,22 desmolase). The resulting pregnenolone is the precursor for both glucocorticoid hormones (in the zona fasciculata) and mineralocorticoid hormones in the (zona glomerulosa); see Fig. 26.2. In man the superior activity of 17α-hydroxylase (CYP17A1) in the zona fasciculata ensures that cortisol rather than corticosterone is the major glucocorticoid hormone.

Antiglucocorticoid treatments

Inhibitors of glucocorticoid synthesis

Ketoconazole

Ketoconazole (an antifungal agent) inhibits 17α-hydroxylase (CYP17 17,20-lyase) which converts pregnenolone to 17α-hydroxypregnenolone, and 11β-hydroxylase (CYP11B1) which converts 11-deoxycortisol to cortisol and 11-deoxycorticosterone to corticosterone. Ketoconazole inhibits the synthesis not only of cortisol and corticosterone, but also of dehydroepiandrosterone (DHEA) and the sex steroids oestrogen and testosterone. In the rat, the effect of ketoconazole on trough levels of corticosterone has not been investigated. However, administration of ketoconazole has been shown to block rises in plasma corticosterone induced by a number of stimuli including

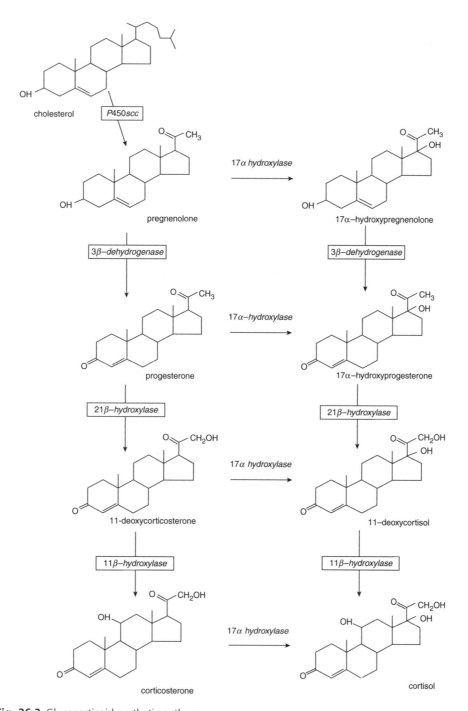

Fig. 26.2 Glucocorticoid synthetic pathways.

cocaine (Goeders et al. 1998) and exposure to cat scent (Cohen et al. 2000). Ketoconazole also tends to increase plasma ACTH (Burrin et al. 1986; Smagin and Goeders, 2004); an effect which is probably the result of decreased glucocorticoid mediated negative feedback on ACTH secretion.

Clinically, ketoconazole is used in the treatment of systemic mycoses and in Cushing's syndrome. Ketoconazole has been demonstrated to decrease serum concentrations of cortisol in man. This has been shown by both serum assay and in vitro assay of tumour-secreted cortisol (Farwell et al. 1988), and has been shown in normal subjects, at treatment doses for infection (Pont et al. 1984). However, Deuschle and colleagues found that administration of a pharmacological dose of ketoconazole did not greatly affect cortisol levels at 8.30 am in 10 healthy young men (Deuschle et al. 2003). The same data included a demonstrable decrease in CSF cortisol in elderly subjects (Deuschle et al. 2003). It would seem that the basal properties of the HPA axis of the subject are important in determining the effect of ketoconazole, that is, lower levels = less effect and age and sex differences may also be important. This theme is worth considering in the later parts of this chapter where we consider experimental attempts to manipulate the HPA axis in various cohorts.

Metyrapone

Metyrapone (Metopirone) is more selective than ketoconazole in its mechanisms of action with respect to steroid synthesis as it blocks only the final step in the production of cortisol or corticosterone. Thus metyrapone is without direct effects on sex steroids or DHEA. It is unclear whether metyrapone reduces levels of corticosterone during the diurnal cycle in rats, but evidence consistently indicates that single or repeated injections of metyrapone can block increases in plasma corticosterone induced by physical and psychological stressors (Herman et al. 1992; Krugers et al. 2000; Smith-Swintosky et al. 1996). In man the suppression of cortisol levels by metyrapone has been confirmed in Cushing's disease and in depression (Nussey et al. 1988; Young et al. 1994).

Aminoglutethimide

Aminoglutethimide inhibits the initial side chain cleavage reaction catalysed by P450scc which converts cholesterol to pregnenolone. As this is the first step in the synthesis of all steroids (including aldosterone, cortisol/corticosterone, and sex steroids), the actions of aminoglutethimide are non-selective.

Glucocorticoid receptor antagonists

A major hurdle in the development of selective GR antagonists has been the fact that GRs show close structural similarities with other members of the steroid receptor superfamily. In particular

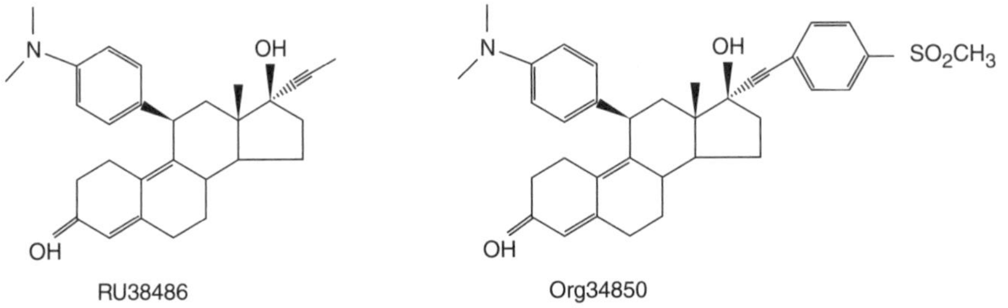

RU38486   Org34850

Fig. 26.3 Chemical structure of two steroidal GR antagonists drugs RU486 and Org 34850.

there is high amino acid homology between the GR and progesterone receptor (PR) and even closer structural similarity if the three-dimensional conformation of hydrophobic residues of the receptors is considered. Thus far, the majority of compounds shown to have appreciable affinity for the GR are analogues of the endogenous ligands cortisol or corticosterone. The most frequently used 'GR antagonist' is RU38486, now known as RU486, developed by Roussel-Uclaf and marketed as mifepristone (Fig. 26.3). This drug crosses the blood–brain barrier and is a potent antagonist of GRs. However, it is even more potent as an antagonist of PRs; a feature which limits its use in the treatment of psychiatric disorders particularly in women, and which explains its use as a means of termination of pregnancy. Although generally referred to as an antagonist, it should be noted that some evidence indicates that RU486 is partial agonist at both the PR and GR (Laue et al. 1988). Org 34850 is one of a series of GR antagonists developed by Organon Laboratories (Fig. 26.3). It freely crosses the blood–brain barrier and has greater GR/PR selectivity than does RU486 but it is less potent (Peeters et al. 2004). Org 34850 has been used in some preclinical studies.

Dehydroepiandrosterone

Dehydroepiandrosterone is a steroid hormone produced from 17-α-hydroxypregnenolone by the action of 17,20 lyase (or 17,20 desmolase), in the zona reticularis of the adrenal gland. DHEA (like its sulphated metabolite DHEA-S) has been shown to be a negative modulator of $GABA_A$ receptor function. However, in addition to this action, DHEA has recognized 'antiglucocorticoid effects' opposing the physiological actions of GR agonists (Aoki et al. 2004; Kalimi et al. 1994). The mechanism of this effect is not entirely clear: evidence indicates that DHEA does not bind to the GR-binding site and so is not a classical competitive antagonist (Muller et al. 2004). However DHEA has been demonstrated in some studies to block the activation-induced nuclear translocation of GRs (Cardounel et al. 1999; Saponaro et al. 2007; but see Muller et al. 2004).

Preclinical studies on the effects of antiglucocorticoids

Over the past 20 or more years, a huge body of data from preclinical studies on the effects of glucocorticoids and/or stress on brain structure and function has accumulated. Much evidence indicates that stress and glucocorticoid hormones have important effects on brain function many of which are mediated by GRs. Given the wealth of data on the effects of antiglucocorticoids on various indices of brain structure and function, this review must necessarily be limited. Here we focus on the effects of antiglucocorticoids on (i) neurogenesis and dendritic organization, (ii) functional plasticity in the hippocampus and prefrontal cortex, and (iii) 5-HT function, as potentially important processes mediating the clinical mood and cognitive effects of antiglucocorticoid therapies in depressed patients. The effects of the antiglucocorticoids metyrapone and ketoconazole (as inhibitors of glucocorticoid synthesis), DHEA (inhibitor of GR activation), and RU486 and Org 34850 as direct GR antagonists will be reviewed.

Endogenous glucocorticoid tone

Determining the effects of antiglucocorticoid strategies on outcome measures of relevance to the mood and cognitive symptoms of depression is complicated by the activation of GRs by endogenous glucocorticoids. The magnitude of this GR activation will inevitably determine the magnitude of effect of the antiglucocorticoids. However, it is worthy of note that the response to underlying GR activation may present either as a threshold effect or as a continuous dose-response curve. In some cases an elevated level of glucocorticoid is explicit in the experimental design. Indeed, it may be argued that most relevant to the use of antiglucocorticoids in the treatment of depression, are studies in which the antiglucocorticoid is given against a background of elevated endogenous glucocorticoids or flattened glucocorticoid rhythm engendered by administration of exogenous glucocorticoids, or acute stress. However, it should also be noted that many drugs which may be part of an experimental design (including antidepressants, psychostimulants, and anaesthetics) can also elevate glucocorticoid levels, as can prior chronic stress. Finally, even where elevated corticosterone is not a factor in the experimental design there is nevertheless a degree of endogenous activation of GRs which, it should be remembered, varies markedly through the diurnal cycle. Thus when examining the effects of antiglucocorticoid treatments, it is important that the level of endogenous glucocorticoid stimulation against which the antiglucocorticoid strategy mitigates is considered in the interpretation of the results.

Hippocampal neurogenesis

The dentate gyrus of the hippocampus is unusual in being one of the few sites of neurogenesis in the adult brain (see also Chapter 11 in this book). Given the negative impact of stress (see below), and the positive modulation by antidepressant drugs (Duman et al. 2001; Huang and Herbert, 2006), changes in hippocampal neurogenesis have been suggested as a potentially important process in the development and the resolution of affective disorders (Duman, 2004; Herbert, 2008). Both corticosterone (Cameron and Gould, 1994; Pinnock et al. 2007; Wong and Herbert, 2006) and stress (Falconer and Galea, 2003; Heine et al. 2005; Malberg and Duman, 2003) have been shown to have a negative impact on the numbers of new neurones arising in the dentate gyrus of the hippocampus. Interestingly, it has recently been shown that flattening the diurnal rhythm of corticosterone has a negative impact on neurogenesis as well as on the stimulation of neurogenesis by antidepressants and other factors (Huang and Herbert, 2006; Pinnock and Herbert, 2008).

Although few dividing cells appear to express GRs (Garcia et al. 2004), several pieces of evidence suggest that the effects of stress and corticosterone on neurogenesis are mediated by GRs (rather than MRs). Thus, the effects of corticosterone and stress on neurogenesis are mimicked by the selective GR agonist dexamethasone (Kanagawa et al. 2006; Kim et al. 2004; Yu et al. 2004). Importantly the inhibitory effect of exogenous corticosterone on neurogenesis has been reported to be blocked by both DHEA (Karishma and Herbert, 2002) and RU486 (Oomen et al. 2007). RU486 administration also blocked the effect of stress on hippocampal neurogenesis (Mayer et al. 2006).

Few studies have directly examined neurogenesis in otherwise naïve animals treated with antiglucocorticoids. However, chronic DHEA administration was shown to increase neurogenesis in the hippocampus (Karishma and Herbert, 2002) while repeated RU486 treatment reportedly fails to alter neurogenesis in unstressed control animals (Mayer et al. 2006; Oomen et al. 2007). The failure of RU486 to alter neurogenesis in unstressed or normocortisolaemic animals may be explained by its partial agonist action, which means that an agonist effect predominates at low corticosterone levels. Alternatively, it may reflect low constitutive repression of neurogenesis by endogenous corticosterone through GRs. This latter explanation would be consistent with the finding that neurogenesis is unaltered in adult mice with a brain-specific disruption of GR (Gass et al. 2000). However, it should be noted that an important role for corticosterone (probably through MRs) is suggested by the stimulatory effect of adrenalectomy on neurogenesis (Cameron and Gould, 1994; Krugers et al. 2007). Studies on the effects of full GR antagonists (i.e. without partial agonist activity) on neurogenesis may help to resolve this issue.

Dendritic organization

In addition to influencing the number of new neurones, glucocorticoids have long been known to play a role in determining the structural plasticity of existing mature neurons. Thus both chronic corticosterone and chronic restraint stress have been shown to induce atrophy of the apical dendrites of pyramidal neurons in the CA3 region of the hippocampus (Magarinos and McEwen, 1995; Watanabe et al. 1992a, b; Woolley et al. 1990). Importantly this effect of corticosterone is also observed when a chronically high but flattened profile is achieved (Bisagno et al. 2000). Similar effects of corticosterone or stress have been observed in prefrontal cortex pyramidal cells (Cook and Wellman, 2004; Wellman, 2001).

Surprisingly, the relative roles of GR and MRs in these effects of stress and corticosterone have not been thoroughly characterized. While the 3β-hydroxysteroid dehydrogenase inhibitor cyanoketone, blocked the 'pruning' effect of stress on the apical dendrites of CA3 pyramidal neurones (Magarinos and McEwen, 1995), this drug inhibits the synthesis of both glucocorticoids and mineralocorticoids. In a recent study, Cerqueira and co-workers (Cerqueira et al. 2007b) showed that dexamethasone mimicked the effect of corticosterone on dendritic structure in the prefrontal cortex suggesting that this effect is mediated by GRs. In vitro, the BDNF-induced increase in hippocampal spine formation has been shown to be mitigated by dexamethasone administration (an effect which was blocked by RU486) (Kumamaru et al. 2008). However, it was recently reported that four days of RU486 administration failed to alter the changes in dendritic structure in CA1 neurones which occurred in response to the stress of handling and vehicle administration (Alfarez et al. 2008). These latter data argue against the importance of GR activation in the dendritic reorganizational response to stress.

As is the case for neurogenesis, relatively few studies have probed the effects of antiglucocorticoid drug treatments of naïve animals on dendritic structure. Margarinos and McEwen (Magarinos and McEwen, 1995) observed that cyanoketone treatment had no effect on either basal or apical dendrites of CA3 pyramidal cells in unstressed rats. Interestingly, the same group had previously reported that treatment of female rats with RU486 inhibits the decrease in spine density which normally occurs between proestrus and oestrus (Woolley and McEwen, 1993). This was interpreted as involving antiprogesterone effect of RU486 but might in part be mediated by GR blockade.

Hippocampal and prefrontal functional plasticity

Hippocampus

The phenomena of long-term potentiation (LTP) and long-term depression (LTD) in the Ammon's horn and the dentate gyrus of the hippocampus are well described. These functional plasticity responses to differing electrophysiological stimulus parameters are thought to underlie some of the cognitive functions of the hippocampus. The modulation of this synaptic plasticity by stress and glucocorticoids has been extensively studied. LTP in the hippocampus is reduced by both corticosterone (Pavlides et al. 1993) and stress (Foy et al. 1987; Shors et al. 1989; 1990a). LTD has been shown to be increased by stress (Xu et al. 1997; Yang et al. 2008). A role for GR in the effects of corticosterone and stress is indicated by the reports that a selective GR agonist depressed LTP and enhanced LTD in the dentate gyrus in vivo (Pavlides et al. 1995). Similarly a GR agonist has been shown to reduce LTP in CA1 in vitro (Pavlides et al. 1996). Finally, the suppressant effects of stressors on LTP in dentate gyrus and CA1 have been shown to be blocked by prior administration of RU486, or another GR antagonist RU40555 (Avital et al. 2006; Kohda et al. 2007; Yang et al. 2008).

Some studies have also examined the effects of antiglucocorticoids in otherwise naïve animals on functional plasticity in the hippocampus. It is consistently reported that acute administration of RU486, or RU40555, fails to alter the induction of LTP in CA1 and dentate gyrus in adult unstressed animals (Avital et al. 2006; Kohda et al. 2007; Yang et al. 2008). LTD was also unaffected by GR antagonist administration (Avital et al. 2006; Yang et al. 2008). However, it is of note that in an earlier study it was reported that chronic treatment with RU486 did block age-related changes in LTP in CA1 (Talmi et al. 1996).

Prefrontal cortex

Neurons of the prefrontal cortex also display plasticity of function exemplified by the LTP and LTD responses of the medial prefrontal pyramidal cells to stimulation of CA1/subiculum afferents (Burette et al. 1997; Jay et al. 1995; Takita et al. 1999). The hippocampal-prefrontal LTP response has been shown to be impaired by stress (Cerqueira et al. 2007a; Rocher et al. 2004): an effect which is reportedly reversed by administration of RU486 (Mailliet et al. 2008). Interestingly restraint stress has also been shown to decrease 5-HT-induced EPSCs in pyramidal cells in layer V of prefrontal cortex. This effect of restraint stress was mimicked by chronic corticosterone treatment and blocked by RU486 (Liu and Aghajanian, 2008). The effects of GR antagonists on prefrontal plasticity in normocortisolaemic animals has not widely investigated however, acute RU486 was shown to be without effect on LTP in the prefrontal cortex (Mailliet et al. 2008).

5-HT neurotransmission

A huge body of evidence implicates 5-HT neurotransmission in the regulation of mood and in cognitive function. Hence dysfunction of 5-HT neurotransmission is a candidate mechanism to explain alterations in mood and cognition in affective disorders. The effects of glucocorticoids on aspects of 5-HT neurotransmission have been the subject of many studies. One of the most consistent findings is that chronic elevation of glucocorticoid levels, by corticosterone administration or stress, causes functional desensitization of the 5-HT$_{1A}$ autoreceptor (Fairchild et al. 2003; Lanfumey et al. 1999). We have also seen functional 5-HT$_{1A}$ autoreceptor desensitization when the corticosterone rhythm is flattened at a level around the mid-diurnal level (Gartside et al. 2003; Leitch et al. 2003). To our knowledge the relative roles of GR and MR in the corticosterone-induced desensitization of the 5-HT$_{1A}$ autoreceptor have not been systematically investigated. One study in mice with a genetically engineered GR impairment indicated that the effects of stress on 5-HT$_{1A}$ autoreceptor sensitivity are mediated through the GR (Froger et al. 2004). However, in an electrophysiological study we found that in unstressed animals chronic blockade of GRs by administration of RU486 in the diet had no effect on 5-HT$_{1A}$ autoreceptor function (Gartside and Judge, unpublished). We have also found that, chronic administration of GR antagonists (Org 34850 and Org 34517) fails to alter 5-HT$_{1A}$ autoreceptor sensitivity measured using microdialysis (Johnson et al. 2007). Taken together these data suggest that GRs mediate regulation of 5-HT$_{1A}$ autoreceptor sensitivity but only when GR activation is elevated. Extrapolating this to human clinical data, the monoaminergic and HPA systems interact in ways that may be relevant to pharmacotherapy.

As noted above, not only do depressed patients frequently exhibit elevation of cortisol and flattening of the diurnal rhythm, but also many of the antidepressant drugs with which patients are treated tend to increase glucocorticoid release (Fuller et al. 1996; Golden et al. 1989; Lotrich et al. 2005). In a series of recent studies we have examined the impact of GR antagonists, on neurochemical responses to a 5-HT reuptake inhibitor antidepressant, fluoxetine. We found that GR antagonists in combination with fluoxetine both hastened the development of autoreceptor desensitization and augmented the effect of the SSRI on extracellular 5-HT levels (Johnson et al. 2007). However, it is of note that the GR antagonists alone had no effect on basal extracellular 5-HT. Further studies have indicated that the mechanism by which GR antagonists augment the fluoxetine-induced increase in extracellular 5-HT is by enhancing the downregulation of the 5-HT transporter protein which follows chronic blockade by the SSRI (Johnson et al. 2008).

Preclinical summary

The data discussed above indicate that glucocorticoids have an important impact on several processes which may be key mediators of mood and cognitive function. For the majority of these processes the evidence suggests the involvement of GRs, although in some cases MRs may also play a role. A key point is that GR antagonists as well as antiglucocorticoids have been shown to have most effect in the context of raised corticosterone or flattened diurnal rhythm.

Clinical evidence for efficacy of the antiglucocorticoids in mood and cognitive disorders

We have carried out a literature search for studies which examine the clinical effects of antigluco-corticoid treatments focusing on those which have ratings of depression or cognitive perform-ance as their main outcome measure. Neither the conceptual nor the evidential fields are simple. To begin with, the life course of normal healthy adults can include affective symptoms not amounting to affective disorder and forgetfulness not amounting to a dementing disorder, and hypercortisolaemia is only part of a very complex functional response to stress. Then, there are phenomenological overlaps between cognitive symptoms of affective disorders and affective symptoms of those disorders which affect cognition. This presents measurement problems. Furthermore, some apparently healthy individuals and unaffected relatives of affective probands carry disturbances of the HPA axis without manifesting clinical problems outside of the labora-tory. Finally there are those disorders outside our affective-cognitive remit, such as schizophre-nia, HIV, and dementia which present both affective and neuropsychiatric signs and symptoms, and which have attracted a lot of interest among investigators. The complex interactions of these different syndromes and the various disturbances of the HPA axis and monoaminergic systems make experimental design a significant challenge, and it is with humility that we discuss the experimental data from our own and others' attempts.

The search terms used included drug names and known synonyms and wildcard searches for psychol*, psychia*, cognit*, and other relevant clinical terms. We also hand-searched bibliogra-phies of major review articles, including the recent Cochrane meta-analysis of 'antiglucocorticoid treatments for affective disorders' by Gallagher and colleagues (Gallagher et al. 2008). Where randomized control trials (RCTs) are available these have been presented. Open label studies and case reports are included in the absence of controlled data, to provide context. Below we present our synthesis of this data. We would like to signpost the interesting data concerning related interventions for organic and schizophreniform disorders; we have not felt able to deal with those topics comprehensively here.

Affective outcomes: glucocorticoid synthesis inhibitors

Glucocorticoid synthesis inhibitors as monotherapy

The original open label trials of glucocorticoid synthesis inhibitors in the treatment of depression have been followed by some, albeit heterogeneous and small, blinded-placebo-controlled trials.

In an open uncontrolled cohort of ten hypercortisolaemic depressed patients treated with ketoconazole over six weeks, five subjects remitted, two partially remitted, and three dropped out because of incidental illness or side effects. Serum cortisol concentrations reduced in the cohort, and the association can be interpreted as supporting the hypothesis that hypercortisolaemia is associated with psychopathology (Wolkowitz et al. 1993). A second open cohort comprising eight depressed patients administered ketoconazole over four weeks showed reduction in depression symptoms with five remissions and three partial responses, as well as an increase in sensitivity of their prolactin response to d-fenfluramine (indicative of normalization of 5-HT function) (Thakore and Dinan, 1995). Once again association with change in the endocrine biochemical marker was proposed as evidence of the importance of cortisol in determining the course of the affective disorder.

Thirteen of a cohort of 20 psychotic and non-psychotic depressed patients showed a response to combinations of the glucocorticoid synthesis inhibitors ketoconazole, aminoglutethimide, and metyrapone. The analysis in this open and uncontrolled trial did not include cortisol assays, but was noted that psychotic patients had more of a trend to improvement than non-psychotic patients (Ghadirian et al. 1995). This may reflect an 'antipsychotic' effect, greater regression to the mean in the more disturbed group of patients, or even may be stretched by the ambitious to a significant clinical anticortisolaemic effect given the association of severity with cortisolaemia.

There are further data, including an interesting case report and an uncontrolled trial, to support the efficacy of combinations of glucocorticoid synthesis inhibitors in the treatment of affective disorders. Thus, a hypercortisolaemic lady with treatment-resistant depression and suicidality achieved a rapid and sustained remission on a combination of aminoglutethimide and metyrapone. Remission persisted for at least two years following cessation of treatment (Murphy, 1991). These findings led to an uncontrolled study in 20 patients with treatment-resistant depression of combined aminoglutethimide, metyrapone, and/or ketoconazole, along with a small dose of cortisol for eight weeks. Patients were free of antidepressant medication though some were taking chloral hydrate and/or benzodiazepines. The authors found a reduction in Hamilton Depression Rating Scales (HRDS), which correlated with reduction in DHEA-S levels. However, the previous associations between depressive remission and cortisol reduction were not replicated (Murphy et al. 1998).

These open trials must be seen as inferior to higher forms of evidence, but the interesting observations concerning cortisol provide a conceptual framework for consideration of any further positive results.

A six-week double-blind placebo-controlled trial involving 16 patients with treatment refractory major depressive disorder was conducted. Of the eight patients in each arm, two responded in the ketoconazole arm as opposed to none in the placebo arm: a result seen as a demonstration of 'limited efficacy' by the authors (Malison et al. 1999). We remain unsure whether cortisol data are available on these patients. In a four-week double-blind randomized controlled trial, 20 depressed participants with or without hypercortisolaemia were randomized to ketoconazole or placebo. An interaction between hypercortisolaemia and ketoconazole treatment was observed. When compared to placebo, ketoconazole was associated with some improvement in depression ratings although interestingly, this effect was only observed in patients with pre-existing hypercortisolemia (Wolkowitz et al. 1999a). We would be keen to see replication of these data, perhaps combining cortisol response over time including serial cortisol data over remission periods following the intervention. Even more useful would be a randomized controlled trial of a selected cohort of hypercortisolaemic depressed patients, or further well-powered a priori attempts to use cortisol levels as a predictive factor with regard to ketoconazole treatment under randomized blinded conditions.

The small total number of participants in experimental mental health treatment series reduces sensitivity for rare psychiatric adverse events. However, we note a case report of a 'mentally healthy man' who experienced ego-dystonic obsessional suicidal ideation and imagery following administration and re-administration of ketoconazole for fungal infection (Fisch and Lahad, 1991). If ketoconazole were to become a widely used psychiatric treatment, it would be important to be vigilant for adverse effects of this type, given that the patients involved may be already at increased risk of these phenomena.

In summary, cortisol synthesis inhibitors had initially promising results beginning with uncontrolled trials, which hinted at the importance of changes in cortisol and known serotonergic but cortisol-sensitive processes to the success of the intervention. This relationship between hypercortisolaemia and treatment efficacy is compatible with the results of the best randomized control data, but larger trials are necessary.

Glucocorticoid synthesis inhibitors as adjuncts to antidepressant drugs

In addition to studies examining the efficacy of glucocorticoid synthesis inhibitors as sole treatments for major depression, several studies have examined the potential of these inhibitors as an adjunct to established antidepressant treatments. An open uncontrolled cohort of nine depressed patients showed improvement in depression rating scales following augmentation with metyrapone of the strongly serotonergic tricyclic antidepressant imipramine (Rogoz et al. 2004). The design involved washout, treatment for six weeks with imipramine, and then treatment for six weeks with imipramine and metyrapone together. The authors reported that an improvement in depressive outcomes occurred mainly during the metyrapone augmentation phase of the study. This did not appear to be the result of a pharmacokinetic interaction as serum concentrations of imipramine and desipramine were not increased by metyrapone (Rogoz et al. 2004). This trial hints towards the interactions between the HPA-axis and serotonergic systems which were described above in the preclinical section. The authors are to be praised for their inclusion of the relevant data to exclude possible pharmacokinetic confounds.

In a double-blind cross-over trial O'Dwyer and colleagues demonstrated a significant average reduction in HDRS in eight participants (O'Dwyer et al. 1995). They compared metyrapone together with physiological hydrocortisone replacement against placebo in patients some of whom were on continued stable antidepressant medication although others were drug free (O'Dwyer et al. 1995). The team explicitly stated that they were investigating a 'block and replace' protocol with their use of hydrocortisone. The response in clinical depression scores and serum cortisol diverged after treatment ceased. The clinical improvement was maintained although their plasma cortisol returned to pre-treatment levels.

In a randomized controlled trial by Jahn and colleagues, first-episode and recurrently depressed patients were randomized to receive a serotonergic antidepressant (fluvoxamine or nefazodone) with placebo or metyrapone for five weeks (Jahn et al. 2004). Serotonergic antidepressant choice was clinical and related to inhibited or agitated subtype. A priori remission outcomes for the whole depressed group were significantly greater for adjunct metyrapone (23/33, 70%) versus placebo adjunct (13/30, 43%). Although there was no significant association with between higher basal cortisol levels and successful metyrapone treatment, those treated with metyrapone did have characteristic alterations in the HPA axis (Jahn et al. 2004). We note once again the successful use of serotonergics in combination with manipulation of the HPA axis – how crucial is the proposed synergy? Would efficacy in non-adjunctively treated patients rely on endogenous monoaminergic drive?

Affective outcomes: glucocorticoid receptor antagonists

There are substantial data and commentaries referring to the use of the PR and GR antagonist mifepristone, (RU486), alone and as an adjuncts in the treatment of psychiatric and behavioural syndromes.

Glucocorticoid receptor antagonists as monotherapy

The original eight-week uncontrolled trial in antidepressant-free patients with major depression by Murphy and colleagues showed some response in three out of four participants during and after mifepristone treatment (Murphy et al. 1993). ACTH, DHEA, and cortisol rose during treatment indicative of effective blockade of GR-mediated negative feedback. In a subsequent study, 20 patients with psychotic depression participated in an uncontrolled open trial of six days of mifepristone followed by eight weeks of inpatient observation (Simpson et al. 2005). It is hard to separate the effect of this mifepristone from other therapeutic events that were occurring in the inpatient setting. Nonetheless some clinical improvement was noted, particularly at the start of the observation, coincident with mifepristone (Simpson et al. 2005).

Of five participants with psychotic major depressive disorder in an eight-day cross-over double-blind trial, all showed some improvement in HDRS and four showed some improvement on the Brief Psychiatric Rating Scale (BPRS) in their treatment phase (Belanoff et al. 2001). The largest trial of mifepristone as monotherapy in the treatment of psychosis in depression involved 221 patients (DeBattista et al. 2006). The BPRS was employed in this double-blind randomized controlled trial in which placebo was compared with mifepristone given for seven days followed by an extended observation period. Antidepressant and antipsychotic use in the preceding week was an exclusion criterion, but some treatments were allowed after day seven of treatment. The data indicated that patients in the mifepristone group were more likely to have met the a priori 30% reduction in BPRS than those in the placebo group (DeBattista et al. 2006). Once again the statistical and clinical inferences made from this drew debate, for example, that the number needed to treat was relatively high at NNT = 17 suggesting only a minimal clinical benefit (Rubin and Carroll, 2006).

Glucocorticoid receptor antagonists as adjuncts to antidepressant drugs

In a double-blind design lasting eight days, 30 participants with psychotic major depression the majority of whom were on stable antidepressant medication, were randomized to mifepristone or placebo in addition to continued psychotropic treatment (Flores et al. 2006). There were no significant differences between the two groups in their receipt of concomitant medications, but as these were standard outpatient regimens, a degree of serotonergic drive will likely have been present. Significant reductions in the positive subscale of the BPRS, but non-significant reductions in the HDRS and the full BPRS, were demonstrated. Neuroendocrine responses were also recorded, and included an increase of serum cortisol indicative of GR blockade (Flores et al. 2006). The statistical and clinical interpretation were criticized in the same journal (Carroll and Rubin, 2006).

Our group has conducted a double-blind cross-over trial of mifepristone as adjunctive treatment in 20 depressed adults with bipolar disorder (Young et al. 2004a). The study design involved two three-week blocks in which treatment (mifepristone or placebo) was given for only the first week of the block and established mood stabilizers, antidepressant, and/or antipsychotic medication was continued throughout. Mood outcomes (HDRS and MADRS) were improved in the mifepristone phase at day 21 while there was no change in ratings in the placebo treatment block, but effects were not statistically significant. It is of note that in this cohort mifepristone was well tolerated and there were no adverse-event related drop-outs (Young et al. 2004a). Cognitive data are re-presented in the section on cognitive outcomes below.

Mifepristone treatment of mood outcomes in major depressive disorder and bipolar disorder is therefore supported by at least some large-scale randomized controlled data meeting a priori criteria. The large-scale data do not throw much direct light on the HPA interactions, and have been questioned, but suggest efficacy.

Affective outcomes: DHEA

The effects of the antiglucocorticoid DHEA on mood have also been examined in several trials in mood disorders.

DHEA as monotherapy

Bloch and colleagues investigated the responses of 17 drug-free men and women with midlife dysthymia in a double-blind cross-over treatment paradigm with three phases, free of other medications (Bloch et al. 1999). These were 6 weeks of placebo, 3 weeks of 90 mg of DHEA and 3 weeks of 450 mg DHEA. Mood symptoms improved most on the treatment arms. Cortisol levels were not recorded. Mood symptoms or changes broadly did not correlate with other hormonal assays including DHEA or sex hormones, except for an association between change in plasma DHEA-S and change in Beck Depression Inventory (BDI) scores (Bloch et al. 1999). This trial was extended to include more patients with major depression and showed similar clinical results (Schmidt et al. 2005).

An open label study in six drug-free depressed patients aged 51–72 who had low DHEA and/ or DHEA sulphate (DHEA-S), suggested that 30–90 mg DHEA improved some mood symptoms (Wolkowitz et al. 1997). DHEA concentrations and DHEA/cortisol ratios increased, and cortisol levels non-significantly decreased.

DHEA as adjunct to antidepressants

The findings of the open label study described above (Wolkowitz et al. 1997) were followed up by a double-blind randomized placebo-controlled trial in a larger cohort by the same team (Wolkowitz et al. 1999b). This cohort of 22 clinically depressed patients was different from the first and included two bipolar (but non-rapid cycling) patients. Unlike the original study, the majority of patients in this trial were stabilized on antidepressant medication while only a minority were drug-free. Neuroendocrine data were not presented. The intervention arm had a 5/11 response rate in HDRS, as opposed to 0/11 in the placebo arm (Wolkowitz et al. 1999b).

Cognitive outcomes

Our literature search revealed no data for the effects of glucocorticoid synthesis inhibitors on cognitive measures relevant to the cognitive dysfunction characteristic of affective disorders. However, several studies have examined the effects of the GR antagonist RU486 and the inhibitor of GR activation DHEA on neurocognitive outcomes in healthy and patient populations. These data are presented and commented on below.

Cognitive outcomes: RU486

The preclinical summary showed evidence that hypercortisolaemia can be damaging to the cortex and its function. Noting evidence of links between cognition and the HPA axis, and the observation that Alzheimer's disease is associated with HPA dysregulation, Pomara et al. hypothesized that mifepristone might be useful in the treatment of Alzheimer's disease (Pomara et al. 2002). They investigated this hypothesis using a pilot, single-site, randomized, placebo-controlled, double-blind six-week trial. Recruitment was truncated by unexpected withdrawal of the agent from the trial by the pharmaceutical provider. Despite the unexpectedly small sample, and an attrition rate of a third, leaving six patients, some subtests of cognition were improved on an intention to treat analysis (Pomara et al. 2002). The authors suggested further work with better-tolerated antiglucocorticoids.

In our double-blind cross-over trial of mifepristone as adjunctive treatment in bipolar disorder described above, spatial working memory outcomes were improved in the mifepristone phase at day 21 (see Fig. 26.4). A post hoc analysis revealed that area under the curve for baseline cortisol correlated significantly with percentage improvement in spatial working memory, consistent with the neurocognitive effect being most pronounced in those with hypercortisolaemia (Young et al. 2004a). Interestingly these effects were not seen in a second, comparable, cohort with stable symptomatic schizophrenia (Gallagher et al. 2005), perhaps suggesting that the effect is not generic across functional illnesses. Other literature has been published on various outcomes in schizophrenia and is well worth reading. The other trails of RU486 in affective illness (reviewed above) have not reported on cognitive outcomes however, this is clearly an area which warrants further investigation.

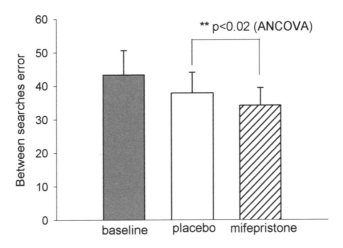

Fig. 26.4 Mifepristone significantly improved performance in a spatial working memory paradigm in bipolar depressed patients. Graph shows between searches errors at baseline and on day 21 of the cross-over placebo and mifepristone treatment arms (Young et al. 2004a). The experimental paradigm involved searching for items with increasing numbers of boxes in a virtual scenario. According to the game rules, the item will not repeat its position. Errors are instances where the participant searches the same position twice despite awareness of the rules. A significant main effect of treatment phase (Mifepristone versus Placebo) was found by ANCOVA (F1,16 = 7.87, *p* = 0.013) Further analysis showed significantly better relative improvements against baseline for mifepristone as compared to placebo. Order of cross-over did not demonstrate a significant effect. Data are mean + standard error of the mean (*n* = 19).

Cognitive outcomes: DHEA

In view of the observations that DHEA levels fall with age and that cognitive performance also declines with age, several investigators have examined the effects of DHEA administration on cognition in healthy elderly subjects on cognition. In one study the administration of 50 mg daily for two weeks improved attention, while recall following stress was reduced, and spatial memory showed no change (Wolf et al. 1997). However after Bonferroni correction for multiple tests, no significant outcomes were achieved (Wolf et al. 1997). Other studies and a meta-analysis also show heterogeneity, across and within gender in the elderly, with regard to correlations between cognition and endocrine status, before and after DHEA supplementation, and invited further study (Grimley Evans et al. 2006). However, a recent large ($n = 225$) year long double-blinded randomized controlled trial of the use of physiological replacement DHEA doses in older healthy men and women (aged 55–85 years) was comprehensively negative with regard to 'cognitive, emotional, sexual or other benefits' (Kritz-Silverstein et al. 2008).

In a trial from our group, a placebo-controlled double-blind randomized cross-over study in healthy young men found that despite their relatively high basal DHEA levels, these individuals had some improvement in memory (and mood) following DHEA administration (Alhaj et al. 2006). Improvements included subjective memory and mood as measured by visual analogue scale, and objective recall accuracy in an episodic memory task (see Fig. 26.5). The paradigm of the working memory test was active recall (rather than recognition) of the gender of voice in which a word was spoken on previous presentation. The difference in the findings of our own study and that of Kritz-Silverstein and colleagues (Kritz-Silverstein et al. 2008) may be due either to the high dose of DHEA used (450 mg), increased neural plasticity in a young university

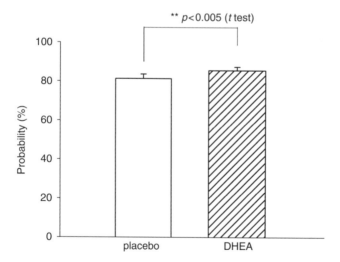

Fig. 26.5 DHEA significantly increased performance in an episodic memory recall paradigm in healthy male volunteers. Graph shows probability of accurate recall in a source memory paradigm following placebo or DHEA treatment in a cross-over study (Alhaj and colleagues, reproduced by kind permission). The task involved a study phase in which subjects were aurally presented words spoken in either a male or female voice. The test phase involved the visual presentation of a mixture of 'old' (i.e. from the study phase) and 'new' words. Accurate recall was defined as the probability of a word being correctly identified as old and assigned the correct gender of the voice that spoke it in the study phase. Data are mean + standard error of the mean ($n=24$). $P < 0.005$ paired t test.

population, or specific improvements in memory which were more sensitively brought out by this particular paradigm (Alhaj et al. 2006).

Studies examining cognitive outcomes in affective disorders following DHEA treatment are few. However, in the open label study by Wolkowitz and colleagues described above (Wolkowitz et al. 1997), DHEA reportedly improved some cognitive aspects of depression, including memory. Unfortunately cognitive outcomes were not measured in the expanded cohort (Wolkowitz et al. 1999b). However, in the trial by Bloch and colleagues which showed positive outcomes for affective symptoms, DHEA failed to influence cognitive outcomes despite being administered at relatively high doses (90 mg and 450 mg) (Bloch et al. 1999).

Discussion

As can be seen there is suggestive but not conclusive evidence that various ways of interfering with the impact of cortisol on the brain can improve outcomes in patients with affective disturbances. The mechanism of any efficacy remains uncertain, although the themes of pre-existing hypercortisaemia and serotonergic modulation appear to us to be exciting. Other studies on this topic are required, as discussed in a recent Cochrane review of 'antiglucocorticoid treatments for mood disorders' (Gallagher et al. 2008). The Cochrane review however, could not provide a sensitivity analysis of baseline hypercortisolaemia within a priori boundaries.

While monotherapy studies with antiglucocorticoid agents are required particularly for licensing purposes it seems likely that the main benefit of this approach will be as an adjunctive treatment of other known antidepressants. However, this remains to be tested in pragmatic clinical trials. It is not clear what the best outcome measure to look at the effect of antiglucocorticoid is. Nor is it clear whether these drugs are only effective in patients who are substantially hypercortisolaemic and further clarification, particularly in large naturalistic studies at this point, would be welcomed. Such studies need to be informed by a greater wealth of preclinical data with development of more selective agents. The best outcome measures for antiglucocorticoid therapies in animal studies is also uncertain. There is the prospect that a greater breadth and depth of understanding in this field will inform the design of treatments for depression which should in turn improve outcome in a number of domains.

References

Agarwal, M.K., Mirshahi, F., Mirshahi, M., and Rostene, W. (1993). Immunochemical detection of the mineralocorticoid receptor in rat brain. *Neuroendocrinology, 58*, 575–580.

Ahima, R.S. and Harlan, R.E. (1990). Charting of type II glucocorticoid receptor-like immunoreactivity in the rat central nervous system. *Neuroscience, 39*, 579–604.

Ahima, R., Krozowski, Z., and Harlan, R. (1991). Type I corticosteroid receptor-like immunoreactivity in the rat CNS: distribution and regulation by corticosteroids. *J Comp Neurol., 313*, 522–538.

Alfarez, D.N., Karst, H., Velzing, E.H., Joels, M., and Krugers, H.J. (2008). Opposite effects of glucocorticoid receptor activation on hippocampal CA1 dendritic complexity in chronically stressed and handled animals. *Hippocampus, 18*, 20–28.

Alhaj, H.A., Massey, A.E., and McAllister-Williams, R.H. (2006). Effects of DHEA administration on episodic memory, cortisol and mood in healthy young men: a double-blind, placebo-controlled study. *Psychopharmacology (Berl)., 188*, 541–551.

Aoki, K., Taniguchi, H., Ito, Y. et al. (2004). Dehydroepiandrosterone decreases elevated hepatic glucose production in C57BL/KsJ-db/db mice. *Life Sci., 74*, 3075–3084.

Avital, A., Segal, M. and Richter-Levin, G. (2006). Contrasting roles of corticosteroid receptors in hippocampal plasticity. *J Neurosci., 26*, 9130–9134.

Belanoff, J.K., Flores, B.H., Kalezhan, M., Sund, B., and Schatzberg, A.F. (2001). Rapid reversal of psychotic depression using mifepristone. *J Clin Psychopharmacol., 21*, 516–521.

Bisagno, V., Ferrini, M., Rios, H., Zieher, L.M., and Wikinski, S.I. (2000). Chronic corticosterone impairs inhibitory avoidance in rats: possible link with atrophy of hippocampal CA3 neurons. *Pharmacol Biochem Behav., 66*, 235–240.

Bloch, M., Schmidt, P.J., Danaceau, M.A., Adams, L.F., and Rubinow, D.R. (1999). Dehydroepiandrosterone treatment of midlife dysthymia. *Biol Psychiatry, 45*, 1533–1541.

Buckingham, J.C. (2006). Glucocorticoids: exemplars of multi-tasking. *Br J Pharmacol., 147* Suppl 1, S258–268.

Burette, F., Jay, T.M., and Laroche, S. (1997). Reversal of LTP in the hippocampal afferent fiber system to the prefrontal cortex in vivo with low-frequency patterns of stimulation that do not produce LTD. *J Neurophysiol., 78*, 1155–1160.

Burrin, J.M., Yeo, T.H., Ashby, M.J., and Bloom, S.R. (1986). Effect of ketoconazole on adrenocorticotrophic hormone secretion in vitro and in vivo. *J Endocrinol., 108*, 37–41.

Cameron, H.A. and Gould, E. (1994). Adult neurogenesis is regulated by adrenal steroids in the dentate gyrus. *Neuroscience, 61*, 203–209.

Cardounel, A., Regelson, W., and Kalimi, M. (1999). Dehydroepiandrosterone protects hippocampal neurons against neurotoxin-induced cell death: mechanism of action. *Proc Soc Exp Biol Med., 222*, 145–149.

Carroll, B.J. and Rubin, R.T. (2006). Is mifepristone useful in psychotic depression? *Neuropsychopharmacology, 31*, 2793–2794; author reply 95–7.

Cerqueira, J.J., Mailliet, F., Almeida, O.F., Jay, T.M., and Sousa, N. (2007a). The prefrontal cortex as a key target of the maladaptive response to stress. *J Neurosci., 27*, 2781–2787.

Cerqueira, J.J., Taipa, R., Uylings, H.B., Almeida, O.F., and Sousa, N. (2007b). Specific configuration of dendritic degeneration in pyramidal neurons of the medial prefrontal cortex induced by differing corticosteroid regimens. *Cereb Cortex, 17*, 1998–2006.

Cintra, A., Zoli, M., Rosen, L. et al. (1994). Mapping and computer assisted morphometry and microdensitometry of glucocorticoid receptor immunoreactive neurons and glial cells in the rat central nervous system. *Neuroscience, 62*, 843–897.

Cohen, H., Benjamin, J., Kaplan, Z., and Kotler, M. (2000). Administration of high-dose ketoconazole, an inhibitor of steroid synthesis, prevents posttraumatic anxiety in an animal model. *Eur Neuropsychopharmacol., 10*, 429–435.

Cook, S.C. and Wellman, C.L. (2004). Chronic stress alters dendritic morphology in rat medial prefrontal cortex. *J Neurobiol., 60*, 236–248.

Czyrak, A. and Chocyk, A. (2001). Search for the presence of glucocorticoid receptors in dopaminergic neurons of rat ventral tegmental area and substantia nigra. *Pol J Pharmacol., 53*, 681–684.

De Kloet, E.R., Vreugdenhil, E., Oitzl, M.S., and Joels, M. (1998). Brain corticosteroid receptor balance in health and disease. *Endocr Rev., 19*, 269–301.

DeBattista, C., Belanoff, J., Glass, S. et al. (2006). Mifepristone versus placebo in the treatment of psychosis in patients with psychotic major depression. *Biol Psychiatry, 60*, 1343–1349.

Deuschle, M., Lecei, O., Stalla, G.K. et al. (2003). Steroid synthesis inhibition with ketoconazole and its effect upon the regulation of the hypothalamus-pituitary-adrenal system in healthy humans. *Neuropsychopharmacology, 28*, 379–383.

Duman, R.S., Nakagawa, S., and Malberg, J. (2001). Regulation of adult neurogenesis by antidepressant treatment. *Neuropsychopharmacology, 25*, 836–844.

Duman, R.S. (2004). Depression: a case of neuronal life and death? *Biol Psychiatry, 56*, 140–145.

Fairchild, G., Leitch, M.M., and Ingram, C.D. (2003). Acute and chronic effects of corticosterone on 5-HT$_{1A}$ receptor-mediated autoinhibition in the rat dorsal raphe nucleus. *Neuropharmacology, 45*, 925–934.

Falconer, E.M. and Galea, L.A. (2003). Sex differences in cell proliferation, cell death and defensive behavior following acute predator odor stress in adult rats. *Brain Res.*, **975**, 22–36.

Farwell, A.P., Devlin, J.T., and Stewart, J.A. (1988). Total suppression of cortisol excretion by ketoconazole in the therapy of the ectopic adrenocorticotropic hormone syndrome. *Am J Med.*, **84**, 1063–1066.

Fisch, R.Z. and Lahad, A. (1991). Drug induced suicidal ideation. *Isr J Psychiatry Relat Sci.*, **28**, 41–43.

Flores, B.H., Kenna, H., Keller, J., Solvason, H.B., and Schatzberg, A.F. (2006). Clinical and biological effects of mifepristone treatment for psychotic depression. *Neuropsychopharmacology*, **31**, 628–636.

Froger, N., Palazzo, E., Boni, C. et al. (2004). Neurochemical and behavioral alterations in glucocorticoid receptor-impaired transgenic mice after chronic mild stress. *J Neurosci.*, **24**, 2787–2796.

Fuller, R.W., Perry, K.W., Hemrick-Luecke, S.K., and Engleman, E. (1996). Serum corticosterone increases reflect enhanced uptake inhibitor-induced elevation of extracellular 5-hydroxytryptamine in rat hypothalamus. *J Pharm Pharmacol.*, **48**, 68–70.

Funder, J.W. (1997). Glucocorticoid and mineralocorticoid receptors: biology and clinical relevance. *Annu Rev Med.*, **48**, 231–240.

Fuxe, K., Harfstrand, A., Agnati, L.F. et al. (1985a). Immunocytochemical studies on the localization of glucocorticoid receptor immunoreactive nerve cells in the lower brain stem and spinal cord of the male rat using a monoclonal antibody against rat liver glucocorticoid receptor. *Neurosci Lett.*, **60**, 1–6.

Fuxe, K., Wikstrom, A.C., Okret, S. et al. (1985b). Mapping of glucocorticoid receptor immunoreactive neurons in the rat tel- and diencephalon using a monoclonal antibody against rat liver glucocorticoid receptor. *Endocrinology*, **117**, 1803–1812.

Fuxe, K., Cintra, A., Agnati, L.F. et al. (1987). Studies on the cellular localization and distribution of glucocorticoid receptor and estrogen receptor immunoreactivity in the central nervous system of the rat and their relationship to the monoaminergic and peptidergic neurons of the brain. *J Steroid Biochem.*, **27**, 159–170.

Gallagher, P., Watson, S., Smith, M.S., Ferrier, I.N., and Young, A.H. (2005). Effects of adjunctive mifepristone (RU-486) administration on neurocognitive function and symptoms in schizophrenia. *Biol Psychiatry*, **57**, 155–161.

Gallagher, P., Malik, N., Newham, J., Young, A.H., Ferrier, I.N., and Mackin, P. (2008). Antiglucocorticoid treatments for mood disorders. *Cochrane Database Syst Rev.*, CD005168.

Garcia, A., Steiner, B., Kronenberg, G., Bick-Sander, A., and Kempermann, G. (2004). Age-dependent expression of glucocorticoid- and mineralocorticoid receptors on neural precursor cell populations in the adult murine hippocampus. *Aging Cell*, **3**, 363–371.

Gartside, S.E., Leitch, M.M., and Young, A.H. (2003). Altered glucocorticoid rhythm attenuates the ability of a chronic SSRI to elevate forebrain 5-HT: implications for the treatment of depression. *Neuropsychopharmacology*, **28**, 1572–1578.

Gass, P., Kretz, O., Wolfer, D.P. et al. (2000). Genetic disruption of mineralocorticoid receptor leads to impaired neurogenesis and granule cell degeneration in the hippocampus of adult mice. *EMBO Rep.*, **1**, 447–451.

Ghadirian, A.M., Engelsmann, F., Dhar, V. et al. (1995). The psychotropic effects of inhibitors of steroid biosynthesis in depressed patients refractory to treatment. *Biol Psychiatry*, **37**, 369–375.

Goeders, N.E., Peltier, R.L., and Guerin, G.F. (1998). Ketoconazole reduces low dose cocaine self-administration in rats. *Drug Alcohol Depend.*, **53**, 67–77.

Golden, R.N., Hsiao, J., Lane, E., Hicks, R., Rogers, S., and Potter, W.Z. (1989). The effects of intravenous clomipramine on neurohormones in normal subjects. *J Clin Endocrinol Metab.*, **68**, 632–637.

Grimley Evans, J., Malouf, R., Huppert, F., and van Niekerk, J.K. (2006). Dehydroepiandrosterone (DHEA) supplementation for cognitive function in healthy elderly people. *Cochrane Database Syst Rev.*, CD006221.

Han, F., Ozawa, H., Matsuda, K., Nishi, M., and Kawata, M. (2005). Colocalization of mineralocorticoid receptor and glucocorticoid receptor in the hippocampus and hypothalamus. *Neurosci Res.*, **51**, 371–381.

Harfstrand, A., Fuxe, K., Cintra, A. et al. (1986). Glucocorticoid receptor immunoreactivity in monoaminergic neurons of rat brain. *Proc Natl Acad Sci USA*, **83**, 9779–9783.

Heine, V.M., Zareno, J., Maslam, S., Joels, M., and Lucassen, P.J. (2005). Chronic stress in the adult dentate gyrus reduces cell proliferation near the vasculature and VEGF and Flk-1 protein expression. *Eur J Neurosci.*, **21**, 1304–1314.

Hennings, J.M., Owashi, T., Binder, E.B. et al. (2008). Clinical characteristics and treatment outcome in a representative sample of depressed inpatients – Findings from the Munich Antidepressant Response Signature (MARS) project. *J Psychiatr Res.*

Herbert, J. (2008). Neurogenesis and depression: breakthrough or blind alley? *J Neuroendocrinol.*, **20**, 413–414.

Herman, J.P., Schafer, M.K., Thompson, R.C., and Watson, S.J. (1992). Rapid regulation of corticotropin-releasing hormone gene transcription in vivo. *Mol Endocrinol.*, **6**, 1061–1069.

Huang, G.J. and Herbert, J. (2006). Stimulation of neurogenesis in the hippocampus of the adult rat by fluoxetine requires rhythmic change in corticosterone. *Biol Psychiatry*, **59**, 619–624.

Ito, T., Morita, N., Nishi, M., and Kawata, M. (2000). In vitro and in vivo immunocytochemistry for the distribution of mineralocorticoid receptor with the use of specific antibody. *Neurosci Res.*, **37**, 173–182.

Jahn, H., Schick, M., Kiefer, F., Kellner, M., Yassouridis, A. and Wiedemann, K. (2004). Metyrapone as additive treatment in major depression: a double-blind and placebo-controlled trial. *Arch Gen Psychiatry*, **61**, 1235–1244.

Jay, T.M., Burette, F., and Laroche, S. (1995). NMDA receptor-dependent long-term potentiation in the hippocampal afferent fibre system to the prefrontal cortex in the rat. *Eur J Neurosci.*, **7**, 247–250.

Johnson, D.A., Grant, E.J., Ingram, C.D., and Gartside, S.E. (2007). Glucocorticoid receptor antagonists hasten and augment neurochemical responses to a selective serotonin reuptake inhibitor antidepressant. *Biol Psychiatry*,

Johnson, D.A., Ingram, C.D., Grant, E.J., Craighead, M. and Gartside, S.E. (2008). Glucocorticoid receptor antagonism augments fluoxetine-induced downregulation of the 5-HT transporter. *Neuropsychopharmacology*,

Kalimi, M., Shafagoj, Y., Loria, R., Padgett, D., and Regelson, W. (1994). Anti-glucocorticoid effects of dehydroepiandrosterone (DHEA). *Mol Cell Biochem.*, **131**, 99–104.

Kanagawa, T., Tomimatsu, T., Hayashi, S. et al. (2006). The effects of repeated corticosteroid administration on the neurogenesis in the neonatal rat. *Am J Obstet Gynecol.*, **194**, 231–238.

Karishma, K.K. and Herbert, J. (2002). Dehydroepiandrosterone (DHEA) stimulates neurogenesis in the hippocampus of the rat, promotes survival of newly formed neurons and prevents corticosterone-induced suppression. *Eur J Neurosci.*, **16**, 445–453.

Kim, J.B., Ju, J.Y., Kim, J.H. et al. (2004). Dexamethasone inhibits proliferation of adult hippocampal neurogenesis in vivo and in vitro. *Brain Res.*, **1027**, 1–10.

Kohda, K., Harada, K., Kato, K. et al. (2007). Glucocorticoid receptor activation is involved in producing abnormal phenotypes of single-prolonged stress rats: a putative post-traumatic stress disorder model. *Neuroscience*, **148**, 22–33.

Kozak, M. (1991). An analysis of vertebrate mRNA sequences: intimations of translational control. *J Cell Biol.*, **115**, 887–903.

Kritz-Silverstein, D., von Muhlen, D., Laughlin, G.A. and Bettencourt, R. (2008). Effects of dehydroepiandrosterone supplementation on cognitive function and quality of life: the DHEA and well-ness (DAWN) trial. *J Am Geriatr Soc.*

Krugers, H.J., Maslam, S., Korf, J., Joels, M. and Holsboer, F. (2000). The corticosterone synthesis inhibitor metyrapone prevents hypoxia/ischemia-induced loss of synaptic function in the rat hippocampus. *Stroke*, **31**, 1162–1172.

Krugers, H.J., van der Linden, S., van Olst, E. et al. (2007). Dissociation between apoptosis, neurogenesis, and synaptic potentiation in the dentate gyrus of adrenalectomized rats. *Synapse*, **61**, 221–230.

Kumamaru, E., Numakawa, T., Adachi, N. et al. (2008). Glucocorticoid prevents brain-derived neurotrophic factor-mediated maturation of synaptic function in developing hippocampal neurons through reduction in the activity of mitogen-activated protein kinase. *Mol Endocrinol.*, **22**, 546–558.

Kwak, S.P., Patel, P.D., Thompson, R.C., Akil, H., and Watson, S.J. (1993). 5'-Heterogeneity of the mineralocorticoid receptor messenger ribonucleic acid: differential expression and regulation of splice variants within the rat hippocampus. *Endocrinology*, **133**, 2344–2350.

Lanfumey, L., Pardon, M.C., Laaris, N. et al. (1999). 5-HT$_{1A}$ autoreceptor desensitization by chronic ultramild stress in mice. *Neuroreport*, **10**, 3369–3374.

Laue, L., Gallucci, W., Loriaux, D.L., Udelsman, R., and Chrousos, G.P. (1988). The antiglucocorticoid and antiprogestin steroid RU 486: its glucocorticoid agonist effect is inadequate to prevent adrenal insufficiency in primates. *J Clin Endocrinol Metab.*, **67**, 602–606.

Leitch, M.M., Ingram, C.D., Young, A.H., McQuade, R., and Gartside, S.E. (2003). Flattening the corticosterone rhythm attenuates 5-HT1A autoreceptor function in the rat: relevance for depression. *Neuropsychopharmacology*, **28**, 119–125.

Liu, R.J. and Aghajanian, G.K. (2008). Stress blunts serotonin- and hypocretin-evoked EPSCs in prefrontal cortex: role of corticosterone-mediated apical dendritic atrophy. *Proc Natl Acad Sci USA*, **105**, 359–364.

Lotrich, F.E., Bies, R., Muldoon, M.F., Manuck, S.B., Smith, G.S., and Pollock, B.G. (2005). Neuroendocrine response to intravenous citalopram in healthy control subjects: pharmacokinetic influences. *Psychopharmacology (Berl).*, **178**, 268–275.

Magarinos, A.M. and McEwen, B.S. (1995). Stress-induced atrophy of apical dendrites of hippocampal CA3c neurons: comparison of stressors. *Neuroscience*, **69**, 83–88.

Mailliet, F., Qi, H., Rocher, C., Spedding, M., Svenningsson, P., and Jay, T.M. (2008). Protection of stress-induced impairment of hippocampal/prefrontal LTP through blockade of glucocorticoid receptors Implication of MEK signaling. *Exp Neurol.*, **211**, 593–6.

Malberg, J.E. and Duman, R.S. (2003). Cell proliferation in adult hippocampus is decreased by inescapable stress: reversal by fluoxetine treatment. *Neuropsychopharmacology*, **28**, 1562–71.

Malison, R.T., Anand, A., Pelton, G.H. et al. (1999). Limited efficacy of ketoconazole in treatment-refractory major depression. *J Clin Psychopharmacol.*, **19**, 466–470.

Mayer, J.L., Klumpers, L., Maslam, S., de Kloet, E.R., Joels, M., and Lucassen, P.J. (2006). Brief treatment with the glucocorticoid receptor antagonist mifepristone normalises the corticosterone-induced reduction of adult hippocampal neurogenesis. *J Neuroendocrinol.*, **18**, 629–631.

Morimoto, M., Morita, N., Ozawa, H., Yokoyama, K., and Kawata, M. (1996). Distribution of glucocorticoid receptor immunoreactivity and mRNA in the rat brain: an immunohistochemical and in situ hybridization study. *Neurosci Res.*, **26**, 235–269.

Muller, C., Cluzeaud, F., Pinon, G.M., Rafestin-Oblin, M.E. and Morfin, R. (2004). Dehydroepiandrosterone and its 7-hydroxylated metabolites do not interfere with the transactivation and cellular trafficking of the glucocorticoid receptor. *J Steroid Biochem Mol Biol.*, **92**, 469–476.

Murphy, B.E. (1991). Treatment of major depression with steroid suppressive drugs. *J Steroid Biochem Mol Biol.*, **39**, 239–244.

Murphy, B.E., Filipini, D., and Ghadirian, A.M. (1993). Possible use of glucocorticoid receptor antagonists in the treatment of major depression: preliminary results using RU 486. *J Psychiatry Neurosci.*, **18**, 209–213.

Murphy, B.E., Ghadirian, A.M., and Dhar, V. (1998). Neuroendocrine responses to inhibitors of steroid biosynthesis in patients with major depression resistant to antidepressant therapy. *Can J Psychiatry,* **43**, 279–286.

Nussey, S.S., Price, P., Jenkins, J.S., Altaher, A.R., Gillham, B., and Jones, M.T. (1988). The combined use of sodium valproate and metyrapone in the treatment of Cushing's syndrome. *Clin Endocrinol (Oxf).*, **28**, 373–380.

O'Dwyer, A.M., Lightman, S.L., Marks, M.N., and Checkley, S.A. (1995). Treatment of major depression with metyrapone and hydrocortisone. *J Affect Disord.*, **33**, 123–128.

Oomen, C.A., Mayer, J.L., de Kloet, E.R., Joels, M., and Lucassen, P.J. (2007). Brief treatment with the glucocorticoid receptor antagonist mifepristone normalizes the reduction in neurogenesis after chronic stress. *Eur J Neurosci.*, **26**, 3395–3401.

Pace, T.W. and Spencer, R.L. (2005). Disruption of mineralocorticoid receptor function increases corticosterone responding to a mild, but not moderate, psychological stressor. *Am J Physiol Endocrinol Metab.*, **288**, E1082–8.

Pavlides, C., Ogawa, S., Kimura, A., and McEwen, B.S. (1996). Role of adrenal steroid mineralocorticoid and glucocorticoid receptors in long-term potentiation in the CA1 field of hippocampal slices. *Brain Res.*, **738**, 229–235.

Pavlides, C., Watanabe, Y., and McEwen, B.S. (1993). Effects of glucocorticoids on hippocampal long-term potentiation. *Hippocampus,* **3**, 183–192.

Pavlides, C., Watanabe, Y., Magarinos, A.M., and McEwen, B.S. (1995). Opposing roles of type I and type II adrenal steroid receptors in hippocampal long-term potentiation. *Neuroscience,* **68**, 387–394.

Peeters, B.W., Tonnaer, J.A., Groen, M.B. et al. (2004). Glucocorticoid receptor antagonists: new tools to investigate disorders characterized by cortisol hypersecretion. *Stress,* **7**, 233–241.

Pinnock, S.B., Balendra, R., Chan, M., Hunt, L.T., Turner-Stokes, T., and Herbert, J. (2007). Interactions between nitric oxide and corticosterone in the regulation of progenitor cell proliferation in the dentate gyrus of the adult rat. *Neuropsychopharmacology,* **32**, 493–504.

Pomara, N., Doraiswamy, P.M., Tun, H., and Ferris, S. (2002). Mifepristone (RU 486) for Alzheimer's disease. *Neurology,* **58**, 1436.

Pont, A., Graybill, J.R., Craven, P.C. *et al.* (1984). High-dose ketoconazole therapy and adrenal and testicular function in humans. *Arch Intern Med.*, **144**, 2150–2153.

Pratt, W.B. and Toft, D.O. (1997). Steroid receptor interactions with heat shock protein and immunophilin chaperones. *Endocr Rev.*, **18**, 306–360.

Reul, J.M. and de Kloet, E.R. (1985). Two receptor systems for corticosterone in rat brain: microdistribution and differential occupation. *Endocrinology,* **117**, 2505–2511.

Ribeiro, S.C., Tandon, R., Grunhaus, L., and Greden, J.F. (1993). The DST as a predictor of outcome in depression: a meta-analysis. *Am J Psychiatry,* **150**, 1618–1629.

Rocher, C., Spedding, M., Munoz, C., and Jay, T.M. (2004). Acute stress-induced changes in hippocampal/prefrontal circuits in rats: effects of antidepressants. *Cereb Cortex,* **14**, 224–229.

Rogoz, Z., Skuza, G., Wojcikowski, J. et al. (2004). Effect of metyrapone supplementation on imipramine therapy in patients with treatment-resistant unipolar depression. *Pol J Pharmacol.*, **56**, 849–855.

Rubin, R.T. and Carroll, B.J. (2006). Claims for mifepristone in neuropsychiatric disorders: commentary on DeBattista and Belanoff, and Neigh and Nemeroff. *Trends Endocrinol Metab.*, **17**, 384–5; author reply 87–9.

Saponaro, S., Guarnieri, V., Pescarmona, G.P., and Silvagno, F. (2007). Long-term exposure to dehydroepiandrosterone affects the transcriptional activity of the glucocorticoid receptor. *J Steroid Biochem Mol Biol.*, **103**, 129–136.

Schmidt, P.J., Daly, R.C., Bloch, M. et al. (2005). Dehydroepiandrosterone monotherapy in midlife-onset major and minor depression. *Arch Gen Psychiatry*, **62**, 154–162.

Schoneveld, O.J., Gaemers, I.C., and Lamers, W.H. (2004). Mechanisms of glucocorticoid signalling. *Biochim Biophys Acta.*, **1680**, 114–128.

Simpson, G.M., El Sheshai, A., Loza, N. et al. (2005). An 8-week open-label trial of a 6-day course of mifepristone for the treatment of psychotic depression. *J Clin Psychiatry*, **66**, 598–602.

Smagin, G.N. and Goeders, N.E. (2004). Effects of acute and chronic ketoconazole administration on hypothalamo – pituitary – adrenal axis activity and brain corticotropin-releasing hormone. *Psychoneuroendocrinology*, **29**, 1223–1228.

Smith-Swintosky, V.L., Pettigrew, L.C., Sapolsky, R.M. et al. (1996). Metyrapone, an inhibitor of glucocorticoid production, reduces brain injury induced by focal and global ischemia and seizures. *J Cereb Blood Flow Metab.*, **16**, 585–598.

Takita, M., Izaki, Y., Jay, T.M., Kaneko, H., and Suzuki, S.S. (1999). Induction of stable long-term depression in vivo in the hippocampal-prefrontal cortex pathway. *Eur J Neurosci.*, **11**, 4145–4148.

Talmi, M., Carlier, E., Bengelloun, W., and Soumireu-Mourat, B. (1996). Chronic RU486 treatment reduces age-related alterations of mouse hippocampal function. *Neurobiol Aging*, **17**, 9–14.

Thakore, J.H. and Dinan, T.G. (1995). Cortisol synthesis inhibition: a new treatment strategy for the clinical and endocrine manifestations of depression. *Biol Psychiatry*, **37**, 364–368.

Watanabe, Y., Gould, E., Cameron, H.A., Daniels, D.C., and McEwen, B.S. (1992a). Phenytoin prevents stress- and corticosterone-induced atrophy of CA3 pyramidal neurons. *Hippocampus*, **2**, 431–435.

Watanabe, Y., Gould, E. and McEwen, B.S. (1992b). Stress induces atrophy of apical dendrites of hippocampal CA3 pyramidal neurons. *Brain Res.*, **588**, 341–345.

Wellman, C.L. (2001). Dendritic reorganization in pyramidal neurons in medial prefrontal cortex after chronic corticosterone administration. *J Neurobiol.*, **49**, 245–253.

Wolf, O.T., Neumann, O., Hellhammer, D.H. et al. (1997). Effects of a two-week physiological dehydroepiandrosterone substitution on cognitive performance and well-being in healthy elderly women and men. *J Clin Endocrinol Metab.*, **82**, 2363–2367.

Wolkowitz, O.M., Reus, V.I., Manfredi, F., Ingbar, J., Brizendine, L. and Weingartner, H. (1993). Ketoconazole administration in hypercortisolemic depression. *Am J Psychiatry*, **150**, 810–812.

Wolkowitz, O.M., Reus, V.I., Roberts, E. et al. (1997). Dehydroepiandrosterone (DHEA) treatment of depression. *Biol Psychiatry*, **41**, 311–318.

Wolkowitz, O.M., Reus, V.I., Chan, T. et al. (1999a). Antiglucocorticoid treatment of depression: double-blind ketoconazole. *Biol Psychiatry*, **45**, 1070–1074.

Wolkowitz, O.M., Reus, V.I., Keebler, A. et al. (1999b). Double-blind treatment of major depression with dehydroepiandrosterone. *Am J Psychiatry*, **156**, 646–649.

Wong, E.Y. and Herbert, J. (2006). Raised circulating corticosterone inhibits neuronal differentiation of progenitor cells in the adult hippocampus. *Neuroscience*, **137**, 83–92.

Woolley, C.S., Gould, E., and McEwen, B.S. (1990). Exposure to excess glucocorticoids alters dendritic morphology of adult hippocampal pyramidal neurons. *Brain Res.*, **531**, 225–231.

Woolley, C.S. and McEwen, B.S. (1993). Roles of estradiol and progesterone in regulation of hippocampal dendritic spine density during the estrous cycle in the rat. *J Comp Neurol.*, **336**, 293–306.

Yang, P.C., Yang, C.H., Huang, C.C., and Hsu, K.S. (2008). Phosphatidylinositol 3–kinase activation is required for stress protocol-induced modification of hippocampal synaptic plasticity. *J Biol Chem.*, **283**, 2631–2643.

Young, E.A., Haskett, R.F., Grunhaus, L. et al. (1994). Increased evening activation of the hypothalamic-pituitary-adrenal axis in depressed patients. *Arch Gen Psychiatry,* **51**, 701–707.

Young, A.H., Gallagher, P., Watson, S., Del-Estal, D., Owen, B.M. and Ferrier, I.N. (2004a). Improvements in neurocognitive function and mood following adjunctive treatment with mifepristone (RU-486) in bipolar disorder. *Neuropsychopharmacology,* **29,** 1538–1545.

Young, E.A., Altemus, M., Lopez, J.F. et al. (2004b). HPA axis activation in major depression and response to fluoxetine: a pilot study. *Psychoneuroendocrinology,* **29**, 1198–1204.

Yu, I.T., Lee, S.H., Lee, Y.S., and Son, H. (2004). Differential effects of corticosterone and dexamethasone on hippocampal neurogenesis in vitro. *Biochem Biophys Res Commun.,* **317**, 484–490.

Chapter 27

How can we use current knowledge to improve antidepressant treatments?

David Nutt and Christopher A. Lowry

Introduction

The theme of this book is depression and especially the relationship of depression to stress – both physical and psychological. So how can the information we have gained in this excellent series of discussions help us in the development of new treatment approaches to depression? In this chapter we review some aspects of knowledge relating to depression antidepressants and stress which give potential new directions for new antidepressants and suggest lines of research investigation that may prove fruitful in future.

Where are we now?

The first antidepressants – the monoamine oxidase inhibitors (MAOIs) and the tricyclic antidepressants (TCAs) were discovered by serendipity over 50 years ago. Within a decade their mode of action had been identified as relating to increasing the action of the amine neurotransmitters 5-hydroxytryptamine (5-HT) and/or noradrenaline and possibly dopamine (for review see Slattery et al. 2004). Intriguingly other antidepressant treatments, in particular electroconvulsive therapy (ECT), were also found to work on the same neurotransmitters (Nutt and Glue 1992). Since then one can argue that there have been no significant new insights or developments of truly new antidepressant mechanisms as all currently available drugs increase amine function either through re-uptake blockade, enzyme inhibition, or by blocking inhibitory auto receptors (Slattery et al. 2004). Of course, the process of evolution of antidepressant drugs has lead to major advances in terms of safety – for example, the newer antidepressants especially the selective serotonin re-uptake inhibitors (SSRIs) are better tolerated and much less dangerous in overdose than the original TCAs (Nutt, 2005) and this has significantly improved their utility in clinical practice with more patients who need them being prescribed and able to tolerate them. However, a significant proportion of patients do not make a full response and so there is still a great need for new interventions.

At least one potential novel treatment has come and gone with the demise of the tachykinin receptor NK1 [substance P] antagonists being a particular disappointment especially after the initial promising clinical trial of the Merck lead compound (Kramer et al. 1998). This target was something of a serendipitous one also as the original target indications were pain and nausea. So how can we develop new antidepressants based on scientific hypotheses?

Stress: the good and the bad

Bad stress and new drug targets

Much of the research detailed in this book relates to the negative effects that stress has on mood and the molecular mechanisms that may explain this association. Clearly one of the few things that all psychiatrists agree on is that stress is a risk factor for relapse in depression and so drugs that interfere with elements of the stress response are clear targets for new treatments. Some of the most obvious of these are listed in Table 27.1 and are discussed in other chapters in this volume. Some target the hypothalamic-pituitary-adrenal (HPA) axis systems that regulate the stress response (see Chapters 5, 7–9, 11, 15, 16, 19, 21, and 26), while others the peripheral immune regulatory pathways that seem important in depression and medical illness or during treatment with immune modulators such as interferon (see Chapters 10, 11, 16, and 17).

Good stress: vaccination against depression?

Although the concept of good stress seems paradoxical, it has been around for many decades in the concept of 'toughening up'. Simply put this concept suggests that exposure to a stressor that can be overcome or successfully resisted leads the organism to develop greater stress-resistance – or resilience – in future. Gaining control over a stressor leads to the ability to combat future stressors more readily, and this can be seen in both the psychological and medical fields. For instance, prolonged maternal separation of young rat pups leads to a supersensitive HPA axis system that is believed to lead to vulnerability to stress-induced depression later in life. However, shorter periods of separation as a neonate have the opposite effect, making the rat more resilient to other stressors when adult, perhaps because they lead to greater input from the mother after the separation (so called neonatal handling effect). It is thought that similar processes apply to humans and

Table 27.1 Possible targets to prevent/reverse stress-induced depression based on research discussed in other chapters in this volume

Brain systems
• CRF1 receptor antagonists
• V3a receptor antagonists
• GR receptors antagonists
• Block excessive cortisol synthesis e.g. metyrapone/ketaconazole
• *Stop excessive awakening rise of cortisol in depressed people*
Peripheral immune systems
• TNFα and IL-6 receptor antagonists
• *IFNα receptor antagonists or uptake blockers*
• *P38 blockers*
(Those in italics are still theoretical)

Abbreviations: CRF1 receptor, corticotropin-releasing factor type I receptor; IFNa, interferon alpha receptor; P38, P38 mitogen-activated protein kinase (MAPK); TNFα receptor, tumour necrosis factor alpha receptor; V3a, vasopressin type 3a receptor that a degree of stress in childhood such that the child and parent can successfully deal with and overcome it, will produce a more resilient adult.

For centuries vaccination approaches have been used to give immune resilience to humans and other animals, and more recently they have been used to augment anti-cancer treatment. In a trial of Mycobacterium vaccae augmentation of chemotherapy O'Brien et al. (2004) noted that 'M. vaccae treatment improved scores for global health status, physical functioning, role limited to emotional health, cognitive functioning, bodily pain, vitality'. This statement is very reminiscent of the original observations on the antidepressant effects of the MAOI isoniazid in treatment of tuberculosis (TB) during the 1950s when patients were found to feel better even though their lung disease did not improve! So how might M. vaccae be having this beneficial action on mood?

One exciting possibility is that there is a positive link between immune activation in certain organs and mood-regulating neuronal populations. Recent work from Lowry et al. (2007) gives strong evidence for this assertion. They found that in a model where M. vaccae was being given subcutaneously to mice to promote immune activation, the rats showed an antidepressant response as indicated by reduced immobility in the forced swim test (Fig. 27.1). Moreover this inoculation procedure was found to increase 5-HT metabolism in medial prefrontal cortex (mPFC), a brain region intimately involved in stress resilience (see Chapter 12). The link between peripheral immune activation and the mPFC was shown to be via M. vaccae activation of a specific subset of 5-HT-containing neurons in the interfascicular part of the dorsal raphe nucleus (DRI). These neurones project specifically to a distributed system implicated in the pathophysiology of depression, including the mPFC, frontal, cingulate, and entorhinal cortices, hippocampus and midline thalamus (Drevets et al. 2008; Lowry et al. 2008).

The exact circuit from the periphery to the raphe is still being worked out but these data raise two important new approaches to antidepressant treatments. The first is that it might be possible to use a similar inoculation to augment antidepressant treatments in humans, just as it is being used to augment anti-cancer drugs. It also raises the possibility that inoculation alone might have

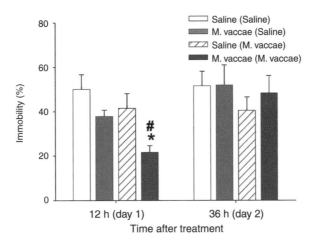

Fig. 27.1 M. vaccae inoculation in preimmunized mice produces an antidepressant-like effect in the forced swim test. Treatments consisted of preimmunization (in parentheses) with either s.c. saline or M. vaccae followed by challenge with s.c. saline or M. vaccae. # P < 0.05 compared with M. vaccae-preimmunized, saline-challenged control group. * P < 0.01 compared with saline-preimmunized, M. vaccae-challenged control group. (adapted from Lowry et al. 2007, with permission)

antidepressant – or at least – some resilience-inducing actions on mood. Secondly, if the inter-fascicular part of the dorsal raphe nucleus is central to 5-HT-mediated antidepressant responses then targeting treatments that just activate this subset of 5-HT neurones might be a novel way to find antidepressant drugs that would be free of unwanted 5-HT actions, so would not lead to adverse effects such as sexual dysfunction, headache, nausea, and so on.

Interestingly, the long-term benefits of *M. vaccae*, for example, the emotional and cognitive effects observed in cancer patients, might be due to the regulatory effects of *M. vaccae* to prevent the chronic inflammation that is commonly observed in depressed patients (Rook and Lowry, 2008).

Optimizing current pharmacological approaches

5-HT

The SSRIs are the current first-line treatment of depression for reasons of safety tolerability and cost. However in terms of efficacy they are no better than the earlier TCAs and indeed may be less effective in older male patients (Joyce and Paykel, 2006). They also have some adverse effects, especially jitteriness (which can lead to anxiety and panic attacks and thence to non-compliance) at the start of treatment in patients so predisposed and they take several weeks for their full thera-peutic benefit to become manifest. As the pharmacology of the 5-HT system becomes better understood and receptor-selective antagonists become available for rodent studies there is evi-dence that the initial jitteriness is due to stimulation of post-synaptic 5-HT2C receptors (Bagdy et al. 2001), whereas the delay in response is due to the progressive time it takes for the 5HT1A autoreceptor to desensitize (Artigas et al. 2001).

The advent of 5HT2C receptor antagonist drugs with human safety data, for example, ago-melatine (Millan et al. 2005) means that the jitteriness theory can now be tested in humans, and if verified then combinations of SSRIs and 5HT2C receptor antagonists might have real clinical benefits. Attempts to mimic 5HT1A receptor desensitization by the use of antagonists has proved effective in rodent models but no selective antagonists appear to have been tested in human augmentation studies yet. Currently the only human efficacy evidence we have for this approach consists of studies where beta-adrenoceptor blockers which also have 5HT1A antagonist proper-ties have been used. Most data are with pindolol where some promising early data have not been consistently replicated – perhaps due to the difficulty in achieving high 5HT1A receptor blockade without using doses that are not well tolerated (Martinez et al. 2001).

Are there other ways to rapidly promote 5-HT function in the brain? One that was being utilized for therapeutic purposes until the rave culture of the 1980s lead to its being made illegal is 3,4-methylenedioxymethamfetamine (MDMA), otherwise given the popular misnomer of ecstasy. This drug is chemically related to stimulants such as amfetamine but has relative selec-tivity for 5-HT rather than for noradrenaline or dopamine release (Green et al. 2003). In low to medium doses and in therapeutic settings MDMA seems quite safe and works quickly to promote a sense of well-being and psychic warmth with empathy. Although the banning of ecstasy use effectively stopped research for nearly twenty years this situation is gradually being reversed with trials in post-traumatic stress disorder (PTSD) and depression now underway (see Sessa and Nutt, 2007). If these trials prove the value of this approach then medicinal chemistry approaches might possibly improve on the 5-HT-releasing properties of MDMA-like compounds and so produce a new generation of 5-HT-promoting agents as potential new antidepressants.

Of course the issue of their legal status will concern many main-stream pharma companies as ecstasy and related drugs are currently class A. However, recent assessments of their harms relative to other controlled drugs do not appear to justify this level of control (Nutt et al 2007a).

Moreover, in other branches of medicine, especially pain, drug regulatory class does not seem to be a barrier to effective treatments, so why should it limit treatments for depression, a disorder that causes more global suffering than pain syndromes?

Noradrenaline and dopamine

Agents, especially re-uptake blockers, that target noradrenaline are well established as effective antidepressant treatments – they include the TCAs desipramine and lofepramine as well as the α2-adrenoceptor antagonist mirtazapine. These often provide more energy and motivation than SSRIs though they are less effective against anxiety and obsessive symptoms of depression. Of course mixed 5-HT and noradrenaline re-uptake blockers (misleadingly called SNRIs which does not mean selective noradrenaline re-uptake inhibitors but serotonin noradrenaline re-uptake inhibitors) now exist, for example, venlafaxine and duloxetine. The theory behind these is that they can give the best of both worlds and there is some evidence of increased efficacy especially in severe depression when high doses are used (Anderson et al. 2008).

Use of dopamine-selective agents in treatment of depression are quite rare – indeed the only one that has been studied is nomifensine which was withdrawn due to some cases of haemolytic anaemia, and tianeptine which was too stimulant-like so was withdrawn. Bupropion however is a weak dopamine and noradrenaline re-uptake blocker and/or releasing agent which has particular value in retarded apathetic depression probably by enhancing dopamine-mediated drive (Nutt et al. 2007b). The idea of combining all three properties in a single molecule – the so-called triple uptake blocker – is appealing especially as it seems that ECT and the MAOIs might have this broad an action (Nutt and Glue, 1992). However, the ideal ratio of re-uptake blockade of each neurotransmitter is not known and early experience with compounds that were potent at all three re-uptake sites was an unacceptable level of adverse effects. Also there is always a risk with drugs that markedly stimulate dopamine release that they might be subject to abuse.

Can we target cognitions in depression?

Just as the brain mechanisms of antidepressant actions are becoming more understood there is a parallel growing knowledge of the brain mechanisms underlying the cognitive problems that are so characteristic of depression. These include negative cognitive schemas and pessimistic views that underpin and explain many of the features of depressive mood and which are the target of interventions such a cognitive behavioural therapy (CBT). It now seems from the work of Harmer and colleagues (see Chapter 13) that these cognitive processes are associated with detectable alterations in brain function as revealed by excessive amygdala activation in functional Magnetic Resonance Imaging (fMRI) studies. Cognitive set can also be tested in normal volunteers and in this population cognitive set is also affected by antidepressant drugs, so offering a novel paradigm for screening potential new antidepressants before moving to patient studies (Harmer et al. 2004).

Moreover, 5-HT appears to play a significant role in cognitive attitude; reducing brain 5-HT function by the technique of rapid tryptophan depletion leads to more negative cognitive processes, in the direction of those found in depression (Hayward et al. 2005), and conversely increasing 5-HT has the opposite effect (Murphy et al. 2006). This observation parallels the findings in depressed patients recovered on SSRIs that tryptophan depletion can lead to relapse (Delgado et al. 1990) and that recovered drug-free depressives are also made vulnerable to relapse if exposed to tryptophan depletion (Smith et al. 1997). Similar findings also apply in anxiety disorders (Argyropolous et al. 2004; Bell et al. 2002).

Cognitive set therefore seems to be quite 5-HT sensitive and one way of conceptualizing this and the effects of antidepressant drugs on it is given in Fig. 27.2. Here we see that the position

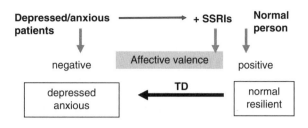

Fig. 27.2 5-HT levels and cognitive set: TD = tryptophan depletion

of an individual on the negative affect axis of Clark and Watson (1991) is under 5-HT control. Low levels of 5-HT produce a state of high negative affect whereas this reduces to normal under the influence of the SSRIs, which also provide a greater degree of resilience to stress. The benefits of the antidepressants are undone when 5-HT levels fall under tryptophan depletion, and in normal volunteers 5-HT depletion reduces resilience (Richell et al. 2005).

Unlearning depression?

There may be other ways to tackle cognitive dysfunction other than by giving drugs to directly affect them. Clearly CBT is a powerful psychotherapeutic approach that over time alters cognitive set through a process of learning new positive attitudes and cognitions. One exciting new area of research is that of enhancing psychotherapy by using pro-learning drugs. It is well established that glutamate processes especially those acting through the N-methyl-D-aspartate (NMDA) receptor are involved in many learning processes and this has been utilized in animal models of extinction learning to accelerate the learning of adaptive responses that effectively 'overwrite' aversive memories (Davis et al. 2006). In humans it is possible to use the anti-TB drug – D-cycloserine – as an indirect NMDA receptor glutamate modifier and studies where this has been used to amplify the effects of psychotherapy in certain phobias have shown clinically relevant benefits (Ressler et al. 2004). Could D-cycloserine be used to augment or accelerate the psychotherapeutic process with CBT? Only controlled trials will let us know but there is certainly a good reason for doing them.

Conclusions

There are many potential new approaches to the development of new antidepressant treatments. Some are based on current knowledge and involve evolution of current proven drug treatment strategies especially those relating to the potentiation of 5-HT function. Anti-stress agents are more blue-sky but nevertheless well founded in contemporary understanding of the factors leading to and perpetuating depression. Completely novel approaches such as inoculation and drug-assisted cognitive remodelling are testable and may prove to be the next real advance.

References

Anderson, I.M., Ferrier, I.N., Baldwin, R.D.C. et al. (2008). Evidence-based guidelines for treating depressive disorders with antidepressants: a revision of the 2000 British Association for Psychopharmacology guidelines. *J Psychopharmacol.*, **22**, 343–396.

Argyropoulos, S., Hood, S.D., Adrover, M. et al. (2004). Tryptophan depletion reverses the therapeutic effect of selective serotonin reuptake inhibitors in social anxiety disorder. *Biol Psychiatr.*, **56**, 503–509.

Artigas, F., Celada, P., Laruelle, M., and Adell, A. (2001). How does pindolol improve antidepressant action? *Trends Pharmacol Sci.*, **22**, 224–228.

Bagdy, G., Graf, M., Anheuer, Z.E., Modos, E.A., and Kantor, S. (2001). Anxiety-like effects induced by acute fluoxetine, sertraline or m-CPP treatment are reversed by pretreatment with the 5-HT2C receptor antagonist SB-242084 but not the 5-HT1A receptor antagonist WAY-100635. *Int J Neuropsychopharmacol.*, **4(4)**, 399–408.

Bell, C., Forshall, S., Adrover, M. et al. (2002). Does 5-HT restrain panic? A tryptophan depletion study in panic disorder patients recovered on paroxetine. *J Psychopharmacol.*, **16**, 5–14.

Clark, L.A. and Watson, D. (1991). Tripartite model of anxiety and depression: psychometric evidence and taxonomic implications. *J Abnorm Psychol.*, **100**, 316–336.

Davis, M., Myers, K.M., Chhatwal, J., and Ressler, K.J. (2006). Pharmacological treatments that facilitate extinction of fear: relevance to psychotherapy. *NeuroRx.*, **3**, 82–96.

Delgado, P.L., Charney, D.S., Price, L.H., Aghajanian, G.K, Landis, H., and Heninger, G.R. (1990). Serotonin function and the mechanism of antidepressant action. Reversal of antidepressant-induced remission by rapid depletion of plasma tryptophan. *Arch Gen Psychiatry.*, **47**, 411–418.

Drevets, W.C., Price, J.L., and Furey, M.L. (2008). Brain structural and functional abnormalities in mood disorders: implications for neurocircuitry models of depression. *Brain Struct Funct.*, 2008 Aug 13. (Epub ahead of print).

Green, A.R., Mechan, A.O., Elliott, J.M., O'Shea, E., and Colado, M.I. (2003). The pharmacology and clinical pharmacology of 3,4-methylenedioxymethamphetamine (MDMA, "ecstasy"). *Pharmacol Rev.*, **55**, 463–508.

Harmer, C.J., Shelley, N.C., Cowen, P.J., Goodwin, and G.M. (2004). Increased positive versus negative affective perception and memory in healthy volunteers following selective serotonin and norepinephrine reuptake inhibition. *Am J Psychiatry.*, **161**, 1256–1263.

Hayward, G., Goodwin, G.M., Cowen, P.J., and Harmer, C.J. (2005). Low-dose tryptophan depletion in recovered depressed patients induces changes in cognitive processing without depressive symptoms. *Biol Psychiatry.*, **57**, 517–524.

Joyce, P.R. and Paykel, E.S. (2006). Advances in the treatment of affective disorders. *Aust N Z J Psychiatry.*, **40**, 379–380.

Kramer, M.S., Cutler, N., Feighner, J. et al. (1998). Distinct mechanism for antidepressant activity by blockade of central substance P receptors. *Science*, **281**, 1640–1645.

Lowry, C.A., Hollis, J.H., de Vries, A. et al. (2007). Identification of an immune-responsive mesolimbocortical serotonergic system: potential role in regulation of emotional behavior. *Neuroscience*, **146**, 756–772.

Lowry, C.A., Evans, A.K., Gasser, P.J., Hale, M.W., Staub, D.R., and Shekhar, A. (2008). Topographic organization and chemoarchitecture of the dorsal raphe nucleus and the median raphe nucleus. In Monti, J.M., Pandi-Perumal, S.R., Jacobs, B.L., and Nutt, D.J. (eds.) *Serotonin and Sleep: Molecular, Functional and Clinical Aspects*, pp. 25–67. Basel, Switzerland, Birkhauser Verlag AG.

Martinez, D., Hwang, D.R., Mawlawi,O. et al. (2001). Differential occupancy of somatodendritic and postsynaptic 5HT1A receptors by pindolol: a dose-occupancy study with (^{11}C)WAY100635 and Positron Emission Tomography in humans. *Neuropsychopharmacology*, **24**, 209–229.

Millan, M.J., Mauricette, B., Gobert, A., and Dekeyne, A. (2005). Anxiolytic properties of agomelatine, an antidepressant with melatonergic and serotonergic properties: role of 5HT2C receptor blockade. *Psychopharmacology*, **177**, 448–459.

Murphy, S.E., Longhitano, C., Ayres, R.E., Cowen, P.J., and Harmer, C.J. (2006). Tryptophan supplementation induces a positive bias in the processing of emotional material in healthy female volunteers. *Psychopharmacology (Berlin)*, **187**, 121–130.

Nutt, D.J, and Glue, P. (1992). The neurobiology of ECT: animal studies. In Coffey, C.E. (ed.) *ECT: From Research to Clinical Practice.* pp. 241–265.

Nutt, D.J (2005). Death by tricyclic: the real antidepressant scandal? *J Psychopharmacol.*, **19**, 123.

Nutt, D.J., King, L.A., Saulsbury, W., and Blakemore, C. (2007a). Developing a rational scale for assessing the risks of drugs of potential misuse. *Lancet*, **369**, 1047–1053.

Nutt, D., Demyttenaere, K., Janka, Z. et al. (2007b). The other face of depression, reduced positive affect: the role of catecholamines in causation and cure. *J Psychopharmacol.*, **21**, 461–471.

O'Brien, M.E.R., Anderson, H., Kaukel, E. et al. (2004). SRL172 (killed *Mycobacterium vaccae*) in addition to standard chemotherapy improves quality of life without affecting survival in patients with advanced small-cell lung cancer: phase III results. *Ann Oncol.*, **15**, 906–914.

Ressler, K.J, Rothbaum, B.O., Tannenbaum, L. et al. (2004). Cognitive enhancers as adjuncts to psychoptherapy: use of D-Cycloserine in phobic individuals to facilitate extinction of fear. *Arch Gen Psychiatry.*, **61**, 1136–1144.

Richell, R.A., Deakin, J.F., and Anderson, I.M. (2005). Effect of acute tryptophan depletion on the response to controllable and uncontrollable noise stress. *Biol Psychiatry.*, **57**, 295–300.

Rook, G.A.W., and Lowry, C.A. (2008). The hygiene hypothesis and psychiatric disorders, *Trends Immunol.*, **29**, 150–158.

Sessa, B. and Nutt, D.J. (2007). MDMA, politics and medical research: have we thrown the baby out with the bathwater? *J Psychopharmacol.*, **21**, 787–791.

Slattery, D.A., Hudson, A.L, and Nutt, D.J. (2004). Invited review: the evolution of antidepressant mechanisms. *Fundamental and Clinical Pharmacology*, **18**, 1–21.

Smith, K.A., Fairburn, C.G., and Cowen, P.J. (1997). Relapse of depression after rapid depletion of tryptophan. *Lancet*, **349**, 915–919.

Index